# THE CALORIEKING®
## Calorie, Fat & Carbohydrate Counter

## EXTRA DIET GUIDES & COUNTERS

# Weight Control Tips

## ✅ Eat & Drink Sensibly

- Avoid fad diets. Eat 3 sensible portion-controlled meals daily.
- Limit fats, high-fat foods/snacks and sugar. Eat adequate fresh fruit & vegetables.
- Limit soft drinks, energy drinks, fruit juice and alcohol. Quench your thirst on water. (See Sample Meal Plan ~ Page 11)

## ✅ Exercise Daily

- Aim for at least 30 minutes daily – even in 5-10 minute lots. For motivation, find an exercise buddy, personal trainer or join a gym. *(Extra Notes ~ Page 12)*

## ✅ Reshape Eating Behaviors

- Be aware of eating and shopping behaviors that lead to overeating.
- Also focus on social and emotional situations that may trigger compulsive eating. *(Extra Notes ~ Page 14)*

## ✅ Keep a Food & Exercise Journal

- A journal helps you see exactly what you eat and drink, and how much you exercise. *(Extra Notes ~ Page 15)*
- An excellent motivator and proven weight loss aid. Keeps you honest!

## ✅ Arrange Moral Support

- Gain the support of family and friends.
- Get extra professional help if required, from your doctor, dietitian, psychologist, exercise trainer, or slimming group.
- Beware of family saboteurs who discourage you from adopting a healthier lifestyle!

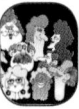

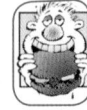

---

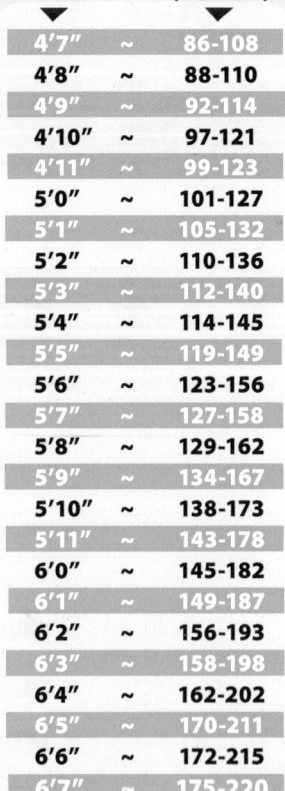

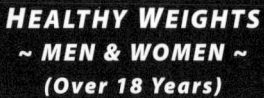

### HEALTHY WEIGHTS
### ~ MEN & WOMEN ~
### (Over 18 Years)

Based on weights with least risk of disease or death from heart disease, diabetes, stroke and cancer.

Based on Body Mass Index of 20-25

BMI calculated as: $\dfrac{\text{Weight (kg)}}{\text{Height (m)}^2}$

| Height (No Shoes) Ft Ins | | Healthy Weight Range (Pounds) |
|---|---|---|
| 4'7" | ~ | 86-108 |
| 4'8" | ~ | 88-110 |
| 4'9" | ~ | 92-114 |
| 4'10" | ~ | 97-121 |
| 4'11" | ~ | 99-123 |
| 5'0" | ~ | 101-127 |
| 5'1" | ~ | 105-132 |
| 5'2" | ~ | 110-136 |
| 5'3" | ~ | 112-140 |
| 5'4" | ~ | 114-145 |
| 5'5" | ~ | 119-149 |
| 5'6" | ~ | 123-156 |
| 5'7" | ~ | 127-158 |
| 5'8" | ~ | 129-162 |
| 5'9" | ~ | 134-167 |
| 5'10" | ~ | 138-173 |
| 5'11" | ~ | 143-178 |
| 6'0" | ~ | 145-182 |
| 6'1" | ~ | 149-187 |
| 6'2" | ~ | 156-193 |
| 6'3" | ~ | 158-198 |
| 6'4" | ~ | 162-202 |
| 6'5" | ~ | 170-211 |
| 6'6" | ~ | 172-215 |
| 6'7" | ~ | 175-220 |

---

### DOCTOR CHECK-UP

*Ask your doctor to check your blood pressure, blood sugar and blood cholesterol levels.*

## Body Fat Distribution & Health

Moderate amounts of body fat do not compromise health. However, excess fat above the hips carries a far greater health risk than fat on or below the hips - better to be a 'pear-shape' than an 'apple-shape'.

**Abdominal obesity** greatly increases the risk of developing diabetes, heart disease, high blood fats, hypertension, stroke, sleep apnea, arthritis and some cancers. So-called 'cellulite' carries no extra health risk.

**Waist Circumference** directly reflects the increased health risk of abdominal obesity. Waist size associated with a high health risk:

**Men** ~ Over 40 inches   **Women** ~ Over 35 inches

## Body Mass Index (BMI)

BMI is a general (but not specific) indicator of body fatness. Although BMI alone is not diagnostic, the higher the BMI, the greater the health risk of developing diabetes, high blood pressure and heart disease. BMI does not apply to heavily muscled persons. BMI is used in a different way for children.

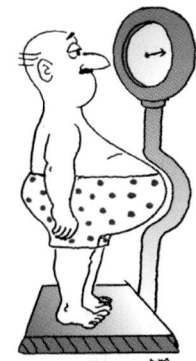

*Abdominal obesity greatly increases the risk of ill-health and earlier death.*

**Check Your BMI:** Find your height (no shoes) - look across the row to the weight nearest your own. Then track down to BMI.

| Ht | WEIGHT (LBS) ~ ADULTS | | | | | | | | | | | | | |
|------|-----|-----|-----|-----|-----|-----|-----|-----|-----|-----|-----|-----|-----|-----|
| 5'1" | 100 | 106 | 111 | 116 | 122 | 127 | 132 | 137 | 143 | 148 | 153 | 158 | 185 | 211 |
| 5'2" | 104 | 109 | 115 | 120 | 126 | 131 | 136 | 142 | 147 | 153 | 158 | 164 | 191 | 218 |
| 5'3" | 107 | 113 | 118 | 124 | 130 | 135 | 141 | 146 | 152 | 158 | 163 | 169 | 197 | 225 |
| 5'4" | 110 | 116 | 122 | 128 | 134 | 140 | 145 | 151 | 157 | 163 | 169 | 174 | 204 | 232 |
| 5'5" | 114 | 120 | 126 | 132 | 138 | 144 | 150 | 156 | 162 | 168 | 174 | 180 | 210 | 240 |
| 5'6" | 118 | 124 | 130 | 136 | 142 | 148 | 155 | 161 | 167 | 173 | 179 | 186 | 216 | 247 |
| 5'7" | 121 | 127 | 134 | 140 | 146 | 153 | 159 | 166 | 172 | 178 | 185 | 191 | 223 | 255 |
| 5'8" | 125 | 131 | 138 | 144 | 151 | 158 | 164 | 171 | 177 | 184 | 190 | 197 | 230 | 262 |
| 5'9" | 128 | 135 | 142 | 149 | 155 | 162 | 169 | 176 | 182 | 189 | 196 | 206 | 236 | 270 |
| 5'10" | 132 | 139 | 146 | 153 | 160 | 167 | 174 | 181 | 188 | 195 | 202 | 207 | 243 | 278 |
| 5'11" | 136 | 143 | 150 | 157 | 165 | 172 | 179 | 186 | 193 | 200 | 208 | 215 | 250 | 286 |
| 6'0" | 140 | 147 | 154 | 162 | 169 | 177 | 184 | 191 | 199 | 206 | 213 | 221 | 258 | 294 |
| 6'1" | 144 | 151 | 159 | 166 | 174 | 182 | 189 | 197 | 204 | 212 | 219 | 227 | 265 | 302 |
| 6'2" | 148 | 155 | 163 | 171 | 179 | 186 | 194 | 202 | 210 | 218 | 225 | 233 | 272 | 311 |
| 6'3" | 152 | 160 | 168 | 176 | 184 | 192 | 200 | 208 | 216 | 224 | 232 | 240 | 279 | 319 |
| 6'4" | 156 | 164 | 172 | 180 | 189 | 197 | 205 | 213 | 221 | 230 | 238 | 246 | 287 | 328 |

**BMI** 19 20 21 22 23 24 25 26 27 28 29 30 35 40

**BMI Classification:**

**BMI Below 19**
Underweight

**BMI 19-24.9**
Healthy Weight
(Low Health Risk)

**BMI 25-29.9**
Overweight
(Moderate Health Risk)

**BMI 30-40**
Obese (High Health Risk)

**BMI Over 40**
Morbid Obesity
(Very High Risk)

Interactive BMI Calculator
www.calorieking.com

## Calories in Food

Calories in food are derived from protein, fat and carbohydrate. Alcohol also provides calories. Vitamins, minerals and water provide no calories.

### Calorie Values Per Gram

| | |
|---|---|
| Fat/Oil | ~ 9 Calories |
| Carbohydrate | ~ 4 Calories |
| Protein | ~ 4 Calories |
| Alcohol | ~ 7 Calories |

Note that fats have over double the calories of protein and carbohydrate. The higher the fat content of food, the higher the calories.

### Sample Calculation

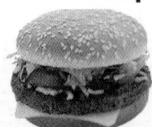

**QUARTER POUNDER®
WITH CHEESE
has 510 calories
derived from:**

| | |
|---|---|
| 26g Fat (x 9 cals/gram) | = 234 |
| 40g Carbohyd.(x 4 cals/gram) | = 160 |
| 29g Protein (x 4 cals/gram) | = 116 |
| Total Calories | = 510 |

## Calorie Levels for Weight Loss

Start with a calorie-controlled diet that allows a moderate weight loss of ½ - 1 pound per week. Weight loss is usually much greater in the first few weeks due to extra fluid losses.

Note: It is better to increase exercise rather than lessen food calories too drastically.

### Suggested Calories for Weight Loss

| | | |
|---|---|---|
| **Women:** | **Non-active** | **1000 - 1200** |
| | Active | 1200 - 1500 |
| **Men:** | **Non-active** | **1200 - 1500** |
| | Active | 1500 - 1800 |
| **Teenagers:** | | **1200 - 1800** |

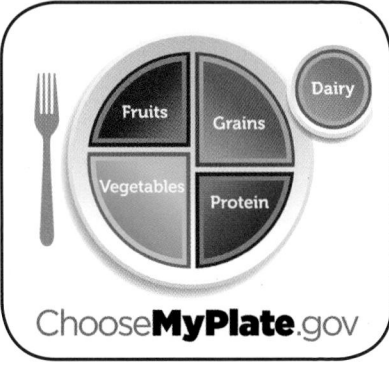

## ChooseMyPlate.gov

The MyPlate symbol represents the recommended proportion of foods from each food group. It focuses on the importance of making smart food choices in every food group, every day. Daily physical activity is also important. *(More info: www.ChooseMyPlate.gov)*

## Examples of Single Serving Sizes

**Grains (Eat 6 servings per day):**
- 1 slice wholegrain bread (1 oz)
- ½ bun, small bagel or English muffin
- 4 small crackers or 1 tortilla
- 1 oz ready-to-eat wholegrain cereal
- ½ cup cooked cereal, rice or pasta

**Vegetables (Eat 3-5 servings per day):**
- 1 cup raw leafy vegetables
- 1½ cups raw chopped vegetables
- ½ cup cooked vegetables
- ½ - ¾ cup vegetable juice

**Fruit (Eat 3-5 servings per day):**
- 1 medium apple, orange, banana
- ½ cup canned fruit (in own juice)
- ¼ cup dried fruit
- ½ cup fruit juice (unsweetened)
- ¼ medium avocado

**Protein (2-3 servings per day):**
- 2-3 oz (cooked) lean meat/poultry/fish
- 2 eggs or 6 oz tofu or ¼ cup nuts
- 1 cup (cooked) dried beans or chickpeas

**Dairy (2-3 servings per day):**
- 1 cup (8 fl.oz) milk/soy (enriched)/yogurt
- 1½ oz cheese or ½ cup cottage cheese

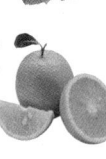

## Portion Size Counts!

Food portion size is critical to controlling calorie intake for weight control.

Super-sized food servings have become more common when eating out and in the home. This can mean a day's worth of calories being consumed in one meal; or a snack being equivalent to a full meal.

It is easy to underestimate portion size of foods and drinks, and unwittingly consume excess calories – even if the fat content is low or even zero!

To more accurately estimate portion size of different foods, weigh and measure your food with food scales, measuring spoons and cups. Better control of calories will result.

**For a visual idea of portion sizes, visit www.CalorieKing.com** See examples (fries and cola) on this page.

## Allow for Extra Calories in Packaged Food

The actual weight of packaged foods is usually 5-10% more than the label net weight (the minimum legal weight) – and in some cases up to 50% more. However, manufacturers calculate the calories based on the net weight. For actual calories, weigh the product and calculate the extra calories.

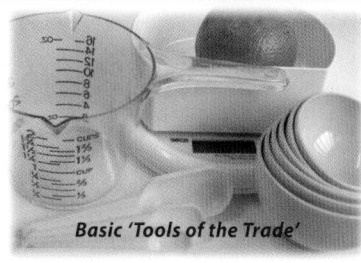

*Basic 'Tools of the Trade'*

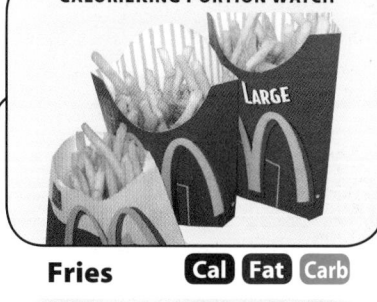

**CALORIEKING PORTION WATCH**

| Fries | Cal | Fat | Carb |
|-------|-----|-----|------|
| Small | 230 | 11 | 29 |
| Medium | 380 | 19 | 48 |
| Large | 500 | 25 | 63 |

**CALORIEKING PORTION WATCH**

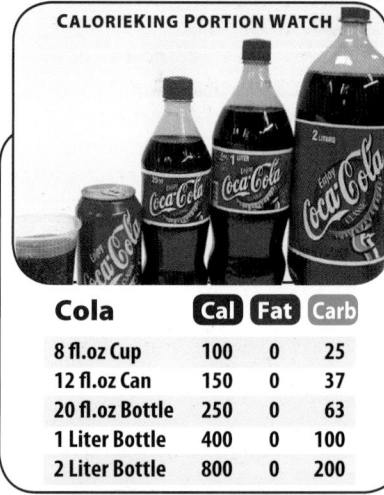

| Cola | Cal | Fat | Carb |
|------|-----|-----|------|
| 8 fl.oz Cup | 100 | 0 | 25 |
| 12 fl.oz Can | 150 | 0 | 37 |
| 20 fl.oz Bottle | 250 | 0 | 63 |
| 1 Liter Bottle | 400 | 0 | 100 |
| 2 Liter Bottle | 800 | 0 | 200 |

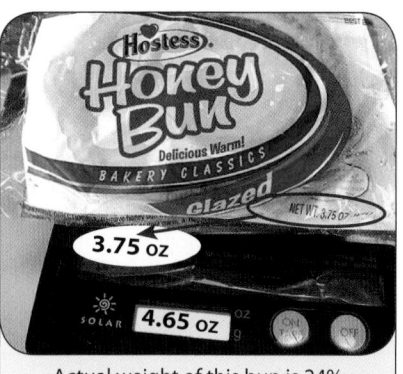

NET WT. 3.75 OZ

3.75 OZ

4.65 OZ

Actual weight of this bun is 24% more than the stated net weight.

# Recommended Fat Intake

## ▶ Fat in the Diet

Fats in the diet are essential for good health. However, too much fat can contribute to obesity and a higher risk of heart disease, high blood pressure, diabetes, gallstone and certain cancers.

Dietary fat and oils have over double the calories of carbohydrates and protein. (Example: Changing from whole-milk to non-fat milk halves the calories.)

## ▶ Beware low-fat foods

It is a mistake to think that eating low-fat or fat-free foods allows you to eat double the quantity. You can end up with even more calories than eating smaller amounts of regular-fat products.

Food products which are fat-free but high in calories include soda drinks, fruit juices, beer, alcoholic spirits, sugar and candy. Bread, rice and pasta also have negligible fat but need to be eaten in controlled amounts.

Ultimately, **it is food portion size as well as total calories that count** whether from fat, carbohydrate or protein. Remember, cows get fat on grass!

### MAXIMUM DESIRABLE FAT INTAKE (DAILY)

| Calories | Fat |
|---|---|
| 1200 cals | 30g fat |
| 1500 cals | 40g fat |
| 1800 cals | 50g fat |
| 2000 cals | 60g fat |
| 2200 cals | 70g fat |
| 2500 cals | 80g fat |
| 3000 cals | 110g fat |

### ZERO GRAMS TRANS FAT

*Don't be fooled by **Zero Grams Trans Fat** boldly displayed on some high-fat snacks. They are still high in fat and calories.*

*Examples: Cheetos 99c pkg ~ 24g fat, 380 cals*
*Lay's Chips (2¾ oz pkg) ~ 27g fat, 430 calories*

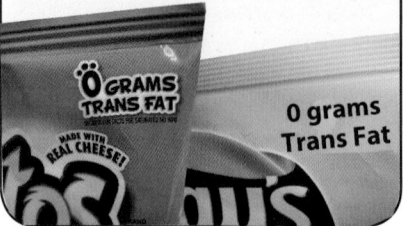

0 grams
Trans Fat

*Reduced fat and fat-free foods are not necessarily low calorie. Portion size is still important.*

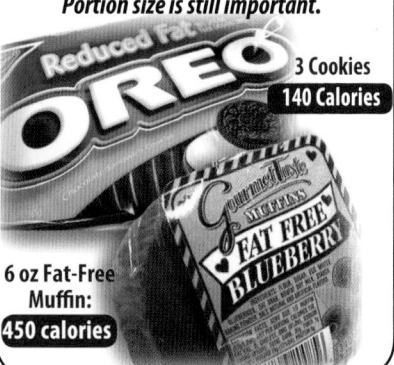

3 Cookies
140 Calories

6 oz Fat-Free Muffin:
450 calories

### FOOD LABEL MEANINGS

**FDA Nutrition Claim Definitions**
(All are on a Per Serving Basis)

*Low Calorie:* 40 Calories or less

*Light or Lite:* One third fewer calories or, 50% or less fat than regular product

*Fat-Free:* Less than half a gram of fat

*Low-Fat:* 3 grams or less of fat

*Reduced Fat:* 25% less fat than regular product

*Fewer or Less Calories:* At least 25% fewer calories than regular product

## ▶ Meats, Poultry, Fish

- **Choose lean cuts** of meat with little marbling. **Trim all visible fat** from meat and remove the skin from poultry. Removal of fat after cooking, is okay (to prevent dryness). Choose 'extra lean' ground beef.
- **Avoid high-fat meat products** such as salami, bacon, sausage and franks.
- **Broil or bake. Avoid frying in oil.** Allow casseroles to cool and skim off surface fat.
- **Avoid fried fish,** frozen fish in batter and canned fish in oil.

## ▶ Fats & Oils

- **Use minimal amounts** of all types of fat and oil. All are high in calories.
- **Choose** 'light' and 'reduced fat' spreads but still use sparingly.
- Use minimal amounts of oil when stir-frying. Use no-stick sprays like Pam.

## ▶ Salad Dressings & Sauces

- **Avoid regular mayonnaise and oil dressings.** Choose 'light', 'reduced fat' or 'fat-free' brands.
- **Choose low-fat or fat-free sauces** (mainly tomato-based). Avoid 'pesto', 'alfredo', 'cheese' and 'creamy' sauces.

## ▶ Milk, Cheese

- **Choose low-fat or nonfat milks and yogurts.** Avoid full-cream milk, cream, Half & Half.
- **Cheese:** Choose fat-free, and low-fat cheese. Part-skim ricotta is still high in fat. Low-fat cottage cheese is a good choice. Cheese substitutes can still be high in fat.

## ▶ Snacks, Cookies, Candy

- **Avoid** high-fat snacks such as potato chips, corn/tortilla chips, cheese puffs, buttered popcorn, chocolate and carob bars.

## ▶ Desserts/Sweets

- **Avoid high-fat desserts,** such as cake, pie, pastries, cheesecake, full-fat puddings.
- **Choose** fresh fruits, fresh fruit salad, canned fruit in water pack, low-fat ice cream. Use low-fat yogurt in place of cream.

## ▶ Fast-Foods & Take-Out

*Check the Fast-Foods Section of this book for actual fat and calorie counts.*

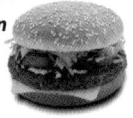

- **Avoid deep-fried foods such as** chicken, french fries and onion rings.
- **Pizzas:** Avoid sausage/pepperoni. Choose vegetarian topping and modest quantity of cheese. Eat a moderate serving. Eat extra salad and fresh fruit.
- **Hamburgers:** Choose medium size, lower fat burgers. Avoid bacon. Have a side salad (with fat-free dressing).
- **Delis:** Choose sandwiches/bread rolls, pitas with low-fat fillings and plain salad. Limit meat/cheese to small portions.
- **Coffees:** Avoid large sizes of latte and frappuccino. Request nonfat milk and no whipped cream. Avoid cookies and pastries.

*Extra Information: www.CalorieKing.com*

### FRYING ADDS FAT!

*The greater the surface area of potato exposed to fat or oil, the higher the fat content and calories.*

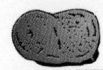 **Whole Potato (3 oz)**
**0g Fat** 65 Cals

 **Roasted Potato (3 oz)**
**5g Fat** 155 Cals

 **Fries (Large cut, 3 oz)**
**12g Fat** 220 Cals

 **Fries (Small, 3 oz)**
**15g Fat** 265 Cals

 **Potato Chips (3 oz)**
**30g Fat** 450 Cals

# Carbohydrates ~ Friend or Foe?

## Naturally-Friendly Carbs

- **Carbohydrate foods in their more natural forms** (not overly processed) are essential to good health. They are the main source of fuel for the body, and also provide important vitamins, minerals, antioxidants and fiber – all of which help protect against heart disease, diabetes, hypertension, constipation-related ailments and many other diseases.

- Carbohydrates even help the body produce serotonin, the 'feel good' brain chemical that helps control appetite and overeating. Too little serotonin can lead to mood swings and depression.

## Carbohydrates are found
in different forms in food as:

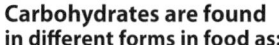

- Sugars in fruit, sugar cane, milk
- Starches in whole grains, legumes, nuts, seeds and vegetables
- Dietary fiber (See Fiber Guide ~ Page 264)

*Glycemic Index & Diabetes ~ Page 21*

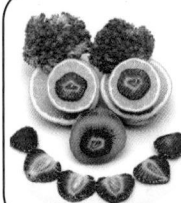

*Carbohydrate foods (minimally processed) are essential to good health.*

*Be sure to eat adequate fruit and vegetables (5 - 7 servings) every day.*

| Calories (Daily) | Carbohydrate (Grams) | Percent Carbohydrate Calories |
|---|---|---|
| **RECOMMENDED CARBOHYDRATE INTAKE** | | |
| 1200 cals | 100-120g | 35-40% |
| 1500 cals | 140-170g | 40-45% |
| 1800 cals | 180-200g | 40-45% |
| 2000 cals | 200-250g | 40-50% |
| 2500 cals | 310-350g | 50-55% |
| 3000 cals | 410-450g | 55-65% |

## How Much Do We Need?

- As shown in the chart, well-balanced diets above 2000 calories contain 50-60% of total calories from carbohydrates.
- At lower calorie levels used for weight control (1200-1500 calories), carbohydrates account for as little as 40% of total calories. This is because protein calories have nutritional priority.
- Carbohydrates & Diabetes ~ *See Page 21*

## Low-Carbohydrate Diets

- Popular low-carbohydrate diets are extreme in their recommendations to initially cut carb intake to as little as 20 grams per day – the amount in 1 thick slice of bread, or 1 medium apple, or 1 small potato.

  This greatly increases the risk of nutritional deficiencies and compromises health, particularly if fat intake is excessive through fatty meats, high-fat dairy products, and fried foods.

- While overweight Americans do need to reduce carbohydrate intake, it should be done **sensibly as part of reducing portion size and total calories.**

- Simply eating 'low-carb' food products without regard to portion size, calories or fats, will do little to promote weight loss or good health.

- **Low-carb diets (and indeed any diet) only work if total calories are reduced.**

- Refined sugars should be one of the first targets in reducing carb intake.

*Extra Info ~ www.CalorieKing.com*

**FAT MATTERS
CARBS COUNT
BUT
CALORIES ARE
KING!**

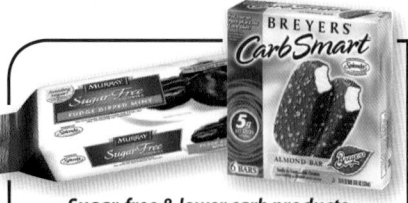

*Sugar-free & lower carb products may still be high in calories and fat.*

- **Excess Sugar:** Many overweight, inactive people consume over 500 calories of refined sugars per day, either self-added or as part of food products. This is equivalent to over 30 level teaspoons – a significant amount in weight control terms. Halving this amount would be reasonable and worthwhile.

  **Note: Naturally occurring sugars** in fruits, vegetables and milk are fine when consumed in normal recommended amounts. These foods are also rich in other nutrients.

  Refined sugar is referred to as having **'empty calories'**. Sugar supplies calories but negligible nutrients and no fiber.

- **Most sugar in our diet is 'hidden'** in processed foods such as soft drinks, fruit drinks, candy, cookies, cake, jam, sauces, ice cream, desserts, canned foods, and processed breakfast cereals.

  For serious weight control, severely limit these foods and substitute healthier higher fiber wholefoods.

  **Note:** Be careful not to substitute sugar-rich foods with high-fat foods which might boost calories even more!

- **Be aware that sugar comes in different forms** such as sucrose, glucose, fructose, malt, high-fructose corn syrup, molasses, honey and maple syrup. Check the label.

- **Sugar alcohols** such as sorbitol, mannitol and maltitol are carb-based and have ½ - ¾ the calories of regular sugar. While not counted as sugar on food labels, they do add to the carb count. Excess amounts can cause bloating, gas and diarrhea.

- **Sugar-free sweeteners** make it easy to reduce sugar in drinks and recipes. However, use minimally since research suggests possible ill-effects of some artificial sweeteners on gut microbes. This may increase the risk of glucose intolerance and an increase in appetite.

  **Note:** Most recipes can be adapted to contain less sugar with little effect on taste.

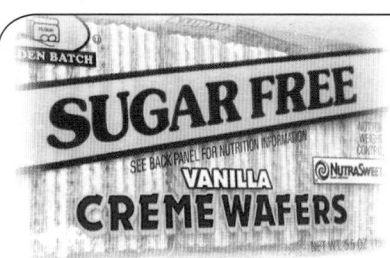

*Sugar-free snacks and foods may be higher in fat and calories than the regular product.*

| Example | ~ Creme Wafers (3): |
|---------|---------------------|
| Regular | ~ 115 cals, 6g fat |
| Sugar-Free | ~ 160 cals, 10g fat |

## SUGAR CONTENT OF SOME COMMON FOODS

**Teaspoons of Sugar**

| | |
|---|---|
| *Coca Cola* or *Pepsi*, 12 fl.oz | 10 |
| 20 fl.oz size | 17 |
| Iced Tea, sweetened, 12 fl.oz | 8 |
| Chocolate Milk, 12 fl.oz | 6 |
| *Honey Smacks* Cereal, ¾ cup, 1 oz | 4 |
| Popcorn, caramel, 1 cup | 3.5 |
| Chocolate Bar, 1.5 oz | 6 |
| *M&M's* 1.7 oz pkg | 7 |
| Muffin, large, 4 oz | 6 |
| Choc Chip Cookie, 1 oz | 2 |
| Donut, iced | 6 |
| Apple Pie, 1 piece | 7 |
| *Jell-O*, ½ cup | 4.5 |
| Jam, 1 Tbsp, ¾ oz | 2.5 |
| Syrup, maple, 1 Tbsp | 3 |

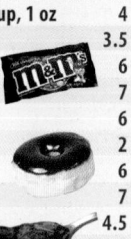

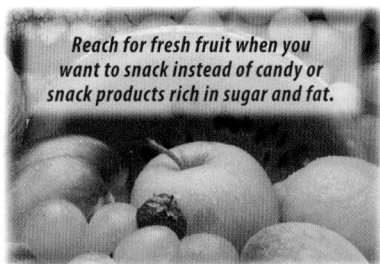

*Reach for fresh fruit when you want to snack instead of candy or snack products rich in sugar and fat.*

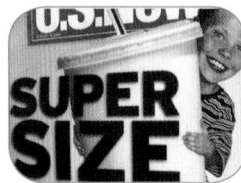

### The XL Generation

Some 15% of American kids and adolescents are overweight; and childhood obesity has doubled over the last 20 years. Diabetes, high blood pressure and high cholesterol are major problem areas for overweight children and adolescents, as are depression, low self-esteem, sleep apnea and bone joint problems.

To address this problem, cooperation is required between kids, parents, schools and government. Weight control is a family and community affair.

## Five Simple Tips To Get Started:

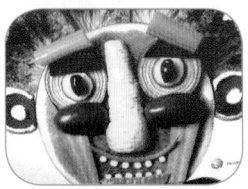

### ❶ Watch Soda Intake

Limit soda and sugary drinks to one serving on the weekends. Soda should not be an everyday beverage – water should be. When at restaurants or using a soda fountain, choose small servings with ice or choose diet soda instead. Schools should provide water and restrict access to soda as should parents when eating out or in the home!

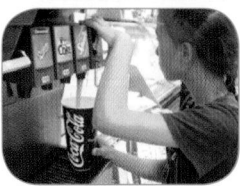

### ❷ Cut back on Fast-Foods and Eating Out

Many more calories are consumed when you eat out. Healthy meals prepared at home are best for the whole family.

### ❸ Say "No" to Super-Sizing

When meals are upsized, loads more calories are consumed. Choose sensible portion sizes when eating out and at home. Use smaller plates and choose smaller packages.

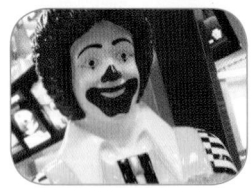

### ❹ Limit Between-Meal Snacking

Watch out for high-fat and high-calorie snacks – they can have more calories than a meal! Keep your eye on portion sizes and limit salty snack foods and candy to parties and special occasions. Choose fresh fruit, vegetables, nuts and low-fat milk instead.

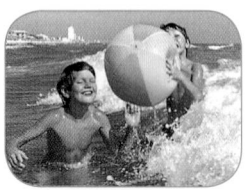

### ❺ Get Moving ~ Watch Less TV

Kids need at least 60 minutes of physical activity every day. It's critical for their fitness, and greatly lessens the risk of obesity.

Encourage kids to be active out of school hours. Wearing a pedometer can be highly motivational for kids to move more – as can playing dance video games such as *Dance Dance Revolution. Dance Central* (XBox360) and *Wii Fit (Nintendo)* are also excellent fitness motivators.

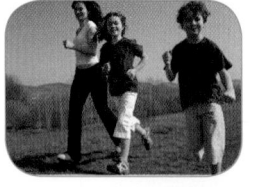

**Limit TV and non-active computer games** to just one hour per day. Also limit the accompanying snacks! Include exercise in family activities.

*Extra information and tips ~ www.CalorieKing.com*

**For Healthy, Overweight Persons ~ Not for Persons With Any Medical Condition**
**~ Please Check With Your Doctor & Dietitian ~**

## Breakfast (approx. 300 cal)

| | |
|---|---|
| | 1 Small Fruit or ½ oz Dried Fruit |
| Plus | Cereal: 1½ oz Dry (high fiber) |
| | or 1 cup cooked Oatmeal |
| Plus | ½ oz Almonds/Seeds |
| Plus | Milk (from daily allowance) or Yogurt (low-fat) |

### Daily Milk Allowance (approx.160 calories)
2 cups Non-Fat Milk or 1½ cups Low-fat (1%) Milk
or equivalent Soy Drink, Yogurt, Cheese, Tofu

### Fat Allowance (140 calories; 15g Fat)
4 tsp Fat or 6-8 tsp Diet Margarine or 3 tsp Oil
or 1½ Tbsp Mayonnaise or ½ medium Avocado
or 1½ Tbsp Peanut Butter or 30g Nuts/Seeds

## Breakfast ~ Choice 2

| | |
|---|---|
| | 1 Small Fruit |
| Plus | 2 Eggs (no added fat) |
| | or 2 oz Cheese (low-fat) |
| | or 4 oz Cottage Cheese (low-fat) |
| | or 2 oz Lean/Canadian Bacon |
| Plus | 1 Tomato |
| Plus | 1 Slice Wholegrain Toast |

## Between Meals

Water, Coffee, Tea, Diet drinks,
Fruit from main meals; Raw vegetable
pieces, Milk from Daily Allowance

## Lunch (approx. 440 calories)

| | |
|---|---|
| | 2 slices Wholegrain Bread (2 oz) |
| | or 4 Crispbreads/Crackers or 6" Pita |
| Plus | 2 oz lean Meat, Chicken or Turkey |
| | or 3½oz Tuna (in water) or 2½ oz Salmon |
| | or 1 oz Cheese or ½ cup (4 oz) Cottage Cheese |
| | or ½ cup (4 oz) Ricotta Cheese (low-fat) |
| | or ½ cup (4 oz) Fruit Yogurt (low-fat) |
| | or ½ cup (4 oz) Bean Salad |
| Plus | Large Salad (Oil-free dressing) |
| Plus | 1 small Fruit or ½ oz Dried Fruit |

## Dinner (approx. 360 calories)

| | |
|---|---|
| | Soup (fat-free) |
| Plus | 3 oz lean Meat (cooked weight) |
| | or 4 oz Chicken Breast (no skin) |
| | or 3 oz Chicken Thigh/Leg (no skin) |
| | or 5 oz Fish (grilled, no fat) |
| | or ¾ cup (6 oz) Beans (Soy, Kidney, Pinto etc)/Lentils |
| | or Low-fat Entree (e.g. Lean Cuisine) |
| Plus | 1 small Potato |
| | or ½ cup Rice/Pasta/Sweet Corn |
| | or 1 slice Wholegrain Bread |
| Plus | 2-3 servings Vegetables/Salad |
| Plus | 1 small Fruit + Diet Gelatin Dessert |

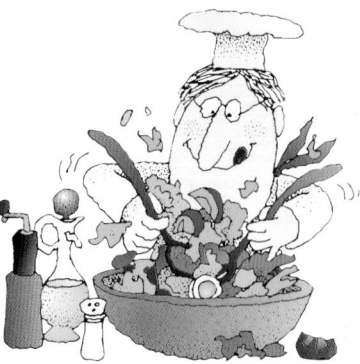

# Exercise & Weight Control

- **Persons who exercise regularly lose more weight** and keep it off longer than non-exercisers. Blood glucose control also improves.
- **Exercise also improves general health and well-being.** Mood, confidence and self-esteem are enhanced by a sense of control and accomplishment.
- **Exercise is a good way to 'wake up' a sluggish metabolism** and burn excess body fat.
- **Aerobic (huff and puff) exercise most days** is great for burning calories and for cardiovascular fitness. But, it is strength training that mainly builds the muscles that burn calories.
- **Strength training is the key to retaining or rebuilding muscles.** As we age, we lose some 6 pounds of muscle per decade. This results in a lower metabolism and fewer calories burnt.

  Muscles are the furnaces that burn calories. The more muscle you have, the more calories burnt – and as a bonus, the more food you can eat.

- **Regular strength training (2-3 times weekly)** can increase our metabolic rate for several days following exercise – with up to an extra 100 calories per day being burnt.

  While 2-3 pounds of muscle may be gained in the first 8-10 weeks, weight from exercised muscles is ok. It is excess fat (particularly abdominal fat) that is a potential health hazard.

  Gaining muscle and losing fat also helps body reshaping - even if the scales don't show it.

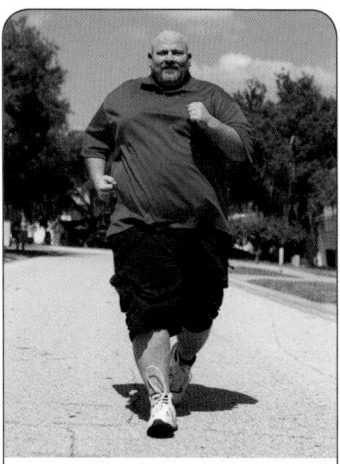

*Brisk walking each day is a safe and effective way to burn calories and keep fit.*
*Try it – you'll like it!*
Be sure to wear sun-protective clothing.

- **Avoid injury** by beginning with walking, low impact aerobics, or weight-supported exercise (e.g. swimming, cycling). Avoid competitive sports. Allow 2-3 days of recovery between strength training sessions. Get professional advice.
- **How Much?** Start with 10-20 minutes per day and progress to 30-60 minutes per day. Also walk up stairs instead of using elevators. Take a brisk walk at lunch. Use an exercise bike, treadmill or stair machine while watching TV. Walk the dog.
- **How Often?** While aerobic fitness may require only 3-4 sessions weekly, **weight control is a daily event which requires daily exercise to burn calories.** Also add in strength training 2-3 times weekly.

**Note:** Persons on cholesterol-lowering statin drugs may experience muscle pains and weakness (as well as damage to muscle ultrastructure). Supplementing with coenzyme Q10, magnesium, selenium, vitamins D and K2, may be beneficial. Check with you Healthcare provider.

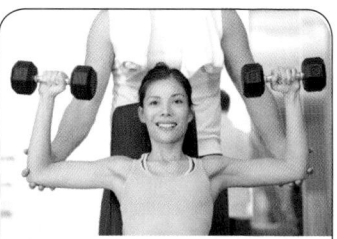

*Strength training is the key to retain or rebuild muscles.*
*Exercized muscles burn extra calories even while you sleep.*
*For extra guidance and motivation, seek a qualified trainer or join a gym.*

# Calories Used in Exercise

| LIGHT | MODERATE | HEAVY |
|---|---|---|
| 130 lbs ~ 3 Cals/Min | 130 lbs ~ 5 Cals/Min | 130 lbs ~ 8 Cals/Min |
| 170 lbs ~ 4 Cals/Min | 170 lbs ~ 6 Cals/Min | 170 lbs ~ 10 Cals/Min |
| 220 lbs ~ 5 Cals/Min | 220 lbs ~ 7 Cals/Min | 220 lbs ~ 12 Cals/Min |

**LIGHT**
- Walking, slow
- Cycling, light
- Frisbee playing
- Gardening, light
- Golf, social
- Tennis, doubles
- Housework, cleaning
- Calisthenics, light
- Bowling
- Ping-pong, social
- Ice Skating, light
- Aquarobics, light
- Skate Boarding
- Line/Square Dancing
- Tai Chi, Yoga
- Volleyball

**MODERATE**
- Walking, brisk
- Cycling, moderate
- Swimming, crawl
- Weight-training, light
- Tennis, moderate
- Racquetball, beginners
- Aerobics, light
- Football, touch
- Basketball, Baseball
- Walking Downstairs
- Snow Skiing (downhill)
- Shovelling snow
- Dancing (ballroom)
- Rowing, moderate
- Volleyball, competitive

**HEAVY**
- Walking (power), Jogging
- Cycling (vigorous)
- Swimming, strenuous
- Weight-training, heavy
- Wrestling/Judo, advanced
- Racquetball, advanced
- Tae Bo, Kick Boxing
- Football, training
- Basketball (Pro)
- Climbing Stairs
- Skipping Rope
- Skiing (cross country)
- Aquarobics, advanced
- Dancing (strenuous), Zumba
- Rowing, vigorous
- Martial Arts

Note: Only those sports or activities that are sustained over a period of time (e.g running)
qualify for heavy exercise. Stop-start sports such as tennis are considered 'moderate'.

## WALKING PROGRAM

### USE DISTANCE, STEPS OR TIME

| Weeks | Distance | Steps Pedometer | Time |
|---|---|---|---|
| 1-2 | 1 mile | 2000 | 20 mins |
| 3-5 | 1.5 miles | 3000 | 28 mins |
| 6-8 | 2 miles | 3500 | 35 mins |
| 9-10 | 2.5 miles | 4500 | 45 mins |
| 11+ | 3.5 miles | 6000 | 60 mins |

## 10,000 STEPS PER DAY

A pedometer can motivate you to be more active. It clips to your belt or waist band and registers each step.

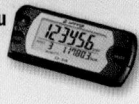

Alternatively, use a *Fitbit*, *Garmin* or *Striiv* activity tracker, or your smartphone inbuilt accelerometer.

Aim for 8,000 - 10,000 steps per day, inead of an average of only 3,000 - 4,000 steps.

# Reshaping Eating Behaviors

- Eating is a behavior that is largely controlled by people with whom we live or socialize, places in which we carry out our lives, and our emotions. Become aware of those situations that commonly lead to extra food being eaten.

- We may also be unaware of 'bad' eating habits that can lead to excess calorie intake; e.g. eating quickly, large mouthfuls, eating when tense or bored, finishing a large serving of food when not hungry.

**Tips to help uncover and correct those 'bad' or problem eating habits:**

- **Don't eat while engaged in other activities;** for example, watching TV, reading. Eat only at the table, not at the fridge or while standing.

- **Don't eat quickly.** Chewing slowly allows time to register a feeling of fullness. Don't use fingers, only utensils. Cut food into smaller pieces. Don't load your fork until the previous mouthful is finished.

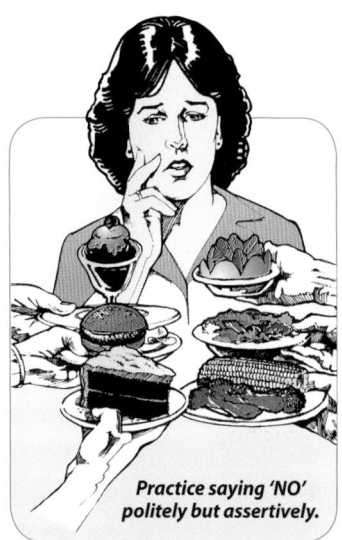

*Practice saying 'NO' politely but assertively.*

- **Don't purchase problem high calorie foods.** Shop from a set list to prevent impulse buying. Avoid shopping with children.

- **Buy snack foods** in the smallest package. The larger the serving size or package, the more you are likely to eat or drink.

- **Plan meals in advance. Stick to a set menu.**

- **Plan a strategy to avoid uncontrolled eating** and drinking at social events, or when your emotions urge you to binge.

  Rehearse repeatedly in your mind exactly what you will do in such situations. Remind yourself several times each day that you are in charge of your actions and that you can be strong-willed. Seek counseling or coaching on various strategies.

- **Distract yourself** when you feel the urge to snack impulsively. Engage in some activity that will distract you from thinking about food. Examples: go for a walk, brush your teeth, phone a friend.

  If you eat out of boredom, find some new hobby or interest that gets you out of the house. Even enrol in an adult education class.

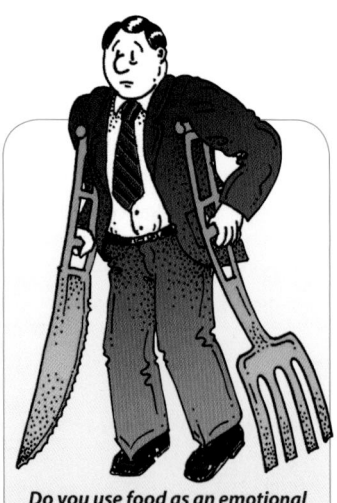

*Do you use food as an emotional crutch? If so, professional counseling may be helpful.*

**The food journal is the most powerful proven aid for dieters.** Persons who keep a food and exercise journal not only lose more weight, they also keep it off. Here are some of the reasons:

- **Recording your eating and exercise habits** jolts you into realizing just what you do eat and drink each day; and also whether you exercise sufficiently.

- **Helps you identify problem foods** and drinks with excessive calories and fat.

- **Helps identify moods,** situations and events that lead to excessive eating of unwanted calories. You can then plan to overcome or avoid them.

- **Prevents 'calorie amnesia',** the forgetfulness that leads to rebound weight gain after successful weight loss. Recording puts you back on the right track.

- **Helps you develop greater self-discipline.** You will think twice about overindulging if you have to record it - especially if someone checks your journal regularly. It certainly keeps you honest!

- **Motivates you** to carefully plan your meals and to exercise each day.

- **Serves as a check system** for your doctor, dietitian or counselor to assess your progress and make recommendations.

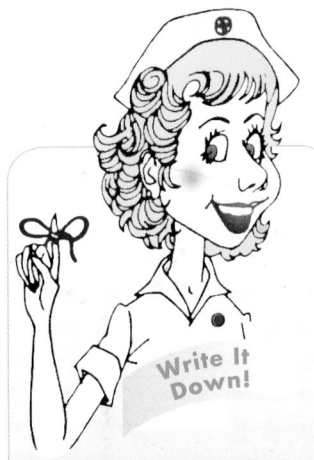

Write It Down!

*"Keeping a journal gives me feedback on exactly what I eat and drink each day.*

*It helps prevent 'calorie amnesia' and reminds me to exercise each day.*

*It's a 'must' for successful weight control!"*

## 3 Easy Ways to Track Your Food & Exercise Calories!

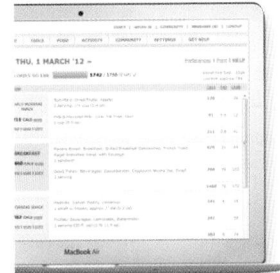

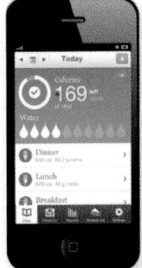

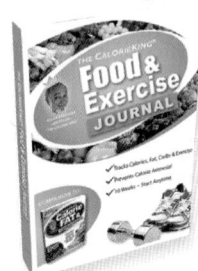

### CalorieKing Online
Part of a comprehensive personalized program that includes tools, reports and a supportive community.

### iPhone
Make smart food choices wherever you are! ControlMyWeight is easy to use & always with you.

### Book
A 10-week journal that fits in your pocket. Includes Weekly Summary page and Progress Checklist

*Extra Information ~ CalorieKing.com*

# Diabetes Guide
## (In Association with Joslin Diabetes Center)

## What is Diabetes?

**Diabetes occurs when the body has difficulty processing glucose sugar in the blood.**

- **After digestion,** sugar and starches are changed into **glucose** – the simplest form of sugar vital for body energy and growth.

- Insulin is the hormone which acts like a key that opens the door to body cells and allows glucose to enter.

- **Without enough insulin,** glucose builds up in the blood and passes into the urine. High blood glucose levels lead to frequent urination, extreme thirst, and tiredness.

- **Untreated diabetes increases the risk of damage to nerves and blood vessels.** This, in turn, increases the risk of heart disease, stroke, blindness, kidney damage, foot ulcers and gangrene (with amputation), impotence and other complications.

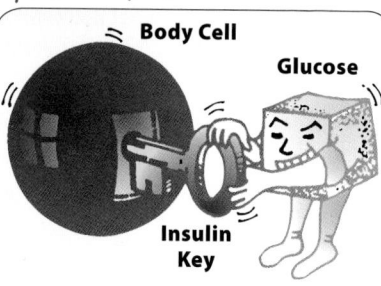

*Insulin acts like a key. It opens the door to body cells and allows glucose to enter.*

*People with type 1 diabetes and some with type 2 have too few or no keys and require insulin injections.*

*Others (primarily type 2) make enough insulin but the body doesn't use it as well as it should – particularly if obese and inactive.*

## SYMPTOMS OF DIABETES

- Frequent urination
- Extreme thirst
- Unusual hunger
- Rapid weight loss
- Extreme fatigue
- Blurred vision
- Skin infections that are slow to heal
- Tingling/numbness in feet

**DON'T IGNORE DIABETES**
**IT'S A SERIOUS DISEASE!**

*Note: Diabetes can be present even with no symptoms.*

## TYPE 2 DIABETES

- Occurs in 90% of diabetes cases
- Occurs mainly in adults - particularly in overweight and inactive persons
- Insulin is produced but body cells resist its action and glucose cannot enter cells
- Usually treated with meal planning and physical activity. Sometimes requires medication (pills or insulin)

## TYPE 1 DIABETES

- Occurs in 10% of diabetes cases
- Usually in children and young adults
- Pancreas produces little or no insulin. Daily insulin injections (or use of an insulin pump) are necessary, as well as:
  - matching pre-meal insulin to the amount of carbohydrate eaten
  - weight control and regular physical activity

## GESTATIONAL DIABETES

- Occurs in some women during pregnancy. It usually disappears after the baby's birth.
- Women who have had gestational diabetes still have a high risk of developing type 2 diabetes within 5 to 10 years. One in 3 do.
- Requires weight control, a healthy lifestyle and regular medical checks during and after pregnancy.

## Are You At Risk for Diabetes?

### *Pre-Diabetes ~ An Early Warning!*

Pre-diabetes means your blood glucose levels are higher than normal, but not high enough to be called diabetes.

**If you have pre-diabetes, you have a higher risk for getting diabetes later on.**

The good news is that you can start taking steps to prevent diabetes by making healthy lifestyle changes – such as losing weight if overweight, and being more physically active.

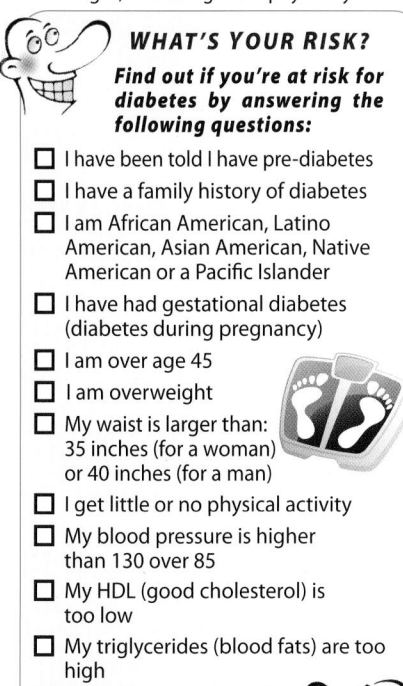

### *WHAT'S YOUR RISK?*

*Find out if you're at risk for diabetes by answering the following questions:*

☐ I have been told I have pre-diabetes

☐ I have a family history of diabetes

☐ I am African American, Latino American, Asian American, Native American or a Pacific Islander

☐ I have had gestational diabetes (diabetes during pregnancy)

☐ I am over age 45

☐ I am overweight

☐ My waist is larger than: 35 inches (for a woman) or 40 inches (for a man)

☐ I get little or no physical activity

☐ My blood pressure is higher than 130 over 85

☐ My HDL (good cholesterol) is too low

☐ My triglycerides (blood fats) are too high

#### ✔ CHECK YOUR RESULT

• If you've put a check mark in two or more of the boxes, you may be more likely to develop type 2 diabetes.

• Talk with your healthcare provider to see if you should have a blood test for diabetes.

### BLOOD GLUCOSE CLASSIFICATION OF DIABETES

| | |
|---|---|
| **Normal:** | **Below 100 mg/dl*** |
| **Pre-Diabetes:** | **100-125 mg/dl*** |
| **Diabetes:** | **Over 125 mg/dl*** |

**(*Fasting Blood Glucose)**

#### *KNOW YOUR BGL*

*(Blood Glucose Level)*
*Everyone over the age of 45 should have a blood glucose test every three years.*

## Importance of Weight Control

• **Type 2 diabetes** is more common in people who are overweight.

• **Being overweight** means that your insulin doesn't work as well to control blood glucose levels.

• **Losing just 10 to 20 pounds** can help you better manage your diabetes and lower your risk for heart disease.

### Keys to weight control include:

• Follow a healthy eating plan

• Control food portions.

• Be physically active every day. Track your daily activity.

• Keep food records ~ *See Page 15*

• Get the support of family and friends.

• **Work with a registered dietitian** who can help you reach a weight that's ideal for you.

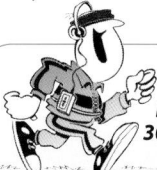

#### *KEEP MOVING!*

*Every day, do at least 30 minutes of moderate intensity exercise.*
*(even in 5-minute sets)*

*It's the key to improving insulin action.*
*Add muscle strength training 3-4 times a week to double the benefits.*

## Managing Diabetes

Don't battle diabetes alone. Establish a partnership with your doctor, dietitian, certified diabetes educator, and pharmacist.

### Extra Support:
- American Association of Diabetes Educators
- American Diabetes Association
- Joslin Diabetes Center
- Juvenile Diabetes Research Foundation
- National Diabetes Education Program

### Hints to keep blood glucose within safe limits:

- **Control your food intake.** Know what and when you will eat. Seek referral to a dietitian for expert advice.

- **Exercise regularly.** It assists weight control and can improve sensitivity of body cells to insulin. Plan physical activity into your daily routine.

- **Monitor your blood glucose** at home and work with a blood glucose meter. It will help you become familiar with your blood glucose patterns, and the effects of food, activity and medication.

- **Take insulin or oral medication as prescribed.** If on insulin, know what action to take if hypoglycemia (low blood glucose) occurs. Also educate your family and friends. More Info: www.joslin.org

## Be Heart Smart ~ Know Your ABCs

If you have diabetes, you are at a higher risk for heart attack and stroke than someone without diabetes. But you can fight back!

### Be smart about your heart!

Take control of the ABCs of diabetes and live a long and healthy life. Talk to your healthcare provider about your ABC targets.

### Ⓐ is for A1C
The A1C (A-one-C) test – short for hemoglobin A1C. It reflects your average blood glucose (sugar) over the last 3 months.
**Suggested Target: Below 7%**

### Ⓑ is for Blood Pressure
High blood pressure makes your heart work too hard.
**Suggested Target: Below 130/80**

### Ⓒ is for Cholesterol
Bad cholesterol, or LDL, can build up and clog your arteries. **Suggested Target: Below 100**

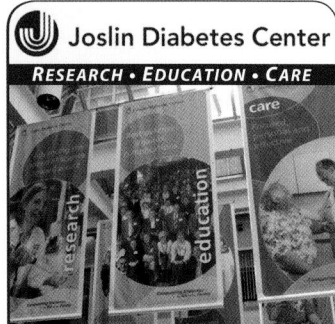

**Joslin Diabetes Center**
*RESEARCH • EDUCATION • CARE*

Joslin Diabetes Center, an affiliate of Harvard Medical School, is the world's largest diabetes research center, diabetes clinic and provider of diabetes education.

*MORE INFORMATION*
www.joslin.org or call 800-344-4501

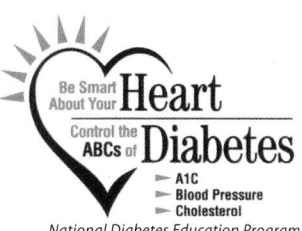

Be Smart About Your **Heart**
Control the **Diabetes**
ABCs of
➤ A1C
➤ Blood Pressure
➤ Cholesterol

*National Diabetes Education Program*

**Be smart about your heart!**

**Take control of the ABC's of diabetes and live a long and healthy life.**

**Talk to your healthcare provider about your ABC targets.**

**Take action now to lower your risk for heart attack, stroke and other diabetes problems.**

◄ *Note: These targets are suggested by the National Institutes for Health and the American Diabetes Association*

**Guidelines for choosing a healthy diet apply equally to people with or without diabetes.** Eating a wide variety of foods that are mainly low in fat, low in refined sugars, and high in fiber, is recommended.

However, actual food quantities, as well as when you eat, will also influence control of blood glucose. Your dietitian will individualize a meal plan to suit your food preferences, lifestyle and medical status.

## Here are a few tips:

- **Maintain a healthy weight.** If overweight, even a modest weight loss plus daily physical activity can help manage blood glucose in type 2 diabetes.

- **Don't skip meals.** If you take insulin or an oral hypoglycemic agent, regular meals are important.

  **If on insulin,** eat meals at the same time each day. Eat a similar amount of food at each meal. Eating about the same amount of carbohydrate over the day will make best use of insulin and prevent wide variations in blood glucose levels.

- **Know which foods contain carbohydrate;** and learn how to check the *Nutrition Facts Label* on foods. Check the serving size, total fat and total carbohydrate – not just the sugar content. All carbohydrate breaks down to sugars after digestion.

- **Choose wholegrain breads, cereals and pasta.** Eat fresh fruits, vegetables and legumes. These foods contain more fiber and slow the release of glucose into your blood after a meal.

- **Limit foods high in saturated fat, trans fat and cholesterol.** Enjoy fish, soy foods, and other foods rich in omega-3 fats. *(Extra Notes: Page 259)*

- **Limit sugars and foods high in added sugar** particularly if overweight. Small amounts of sugar as part of a meal may occasionally be okay. Check with your dietitian. *(Extra Notes: Page 9)*

*Eat a well-balanced with foods high in fiber and low in saturated fat.*

*A fiber-rich diet assists the growth of friendly gut microbes that can benefit our metabolism, weight and blood glucose levels – as well as hunger, mood and our immune system.*
*(Also see Fiber Guide ~ Page 264)*

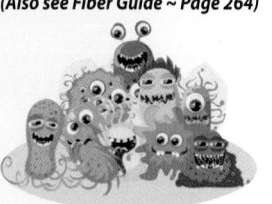

### ALCOHOL TIPS

- **If you drink alcohol, have only moderate amounts:**
  **Men ~ 1-2 drinks/day**
  **Women ~ 1 drink/day**
  For some people, safe drinking will mean no alcoholic drinks at all.
  *(Also see Alcohol Guide ~ Page 23)*

- **Drink along with your food** – especially if you use insulin or diabetes pills.

- **Do not omit any carb food** in exchange for an alcoholic drink. However, non-alcoholic beers (12 fl oz) count as one carb exchange.

- **Alcohol increases the risk of hypoglycemia** (low blood sugar) and drug interactions if you take insulin and certain types of diabetes pills.

- **Check with your doctor and dietitian.**
  *Extra Info: www.joslin.org*

## ...ate Method – An Easy Way ...o Eat Healthfully

The plate method is a helpful tool to guide your food choices until you see a dietitian for your own meal plan.

**For a healthy meal:**

- Fill half of your plate with non-starchy vegetables (broccoli, green beans, carrots).
- Fill a quarter of your plate with carbohydrate (wholegrain bread, pasta, potato, brown rice).
- Fill the other quarter of your plate with 3-4 ounces of lean meat, poultry, or fish.
- Use 1-2 teaspoons of tub margarine or a heart-healthy vegetable oil.
- Add a small piece of fruit or 8 ounces of skim/low-fat milk or yogurt.

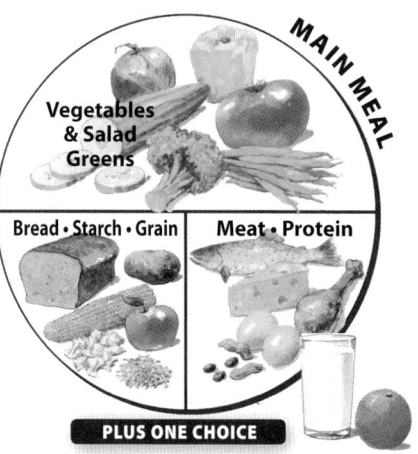

Milk, Fruit, Dessert or other Carb Food

## How Much Carbohydrate Should You Eat?

A dietitian can best determine how much carbohydrate you need at each of your meals, based on your lifestyle, food preferences, and overall diabetes control.

Until you see a dietitian, aim to keep the amount of carbohydrate you eat the same at each of your meals.

### CARB CHOICES MEAL PLAN
**One Carb Choice = 15 Grams of Carb**

**The amount in:** 1 slice Bread **or** ¾ cup Cereal (unsweetened) **or** 1 small Potato **or** 1 small Fruit

**Breakfast**
- Eat 2-3 carb choices (30-45 grams)
- Include a low-fat protein source such as egg whites or skim milk.

**Lunch and Dinner**
- Eat 3-4 carb choices (45-60 grams carb)
- Include fruit and non-starchy vegetables. Choose small portions of low-fat protein foods.

**Snacks:** If needed, eat 1-2 carb choices (15-30 grams carb).

*Note: Above plan is for adults. Carbohydrate amounts will vary with physical activity level.*

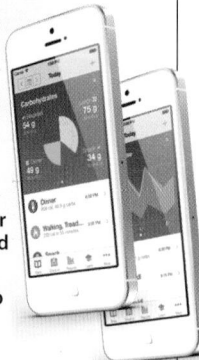
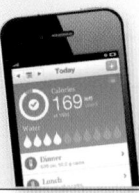
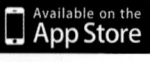

## Carb Type Affects Blood Glucose

The various forms of carbohydrate affect blood glucose levels in different ways. It is difficult to predict the effect of particular foods, sugars, or meals, simply by their carbohydrate content.

Thus the same amount of carbohydrate from different foods may affect blood sugar levels very differently. **Many factors affect the rate of digestion and absorption such as:**

- the type of sugar, starch, and fiber
- the degree of processing and cooking (which increases digestion rate)
- the amount of protein and fat (which slow stomach emptying and digestion).

## Glycemic Index (GI)

**The GI is a method of ranking carbo-hydrate foods on a scale (0-100)** according to how they affect blood glucose levels. (See next column).

**The higher the GI value,** the greater the food's ability to rapidly raise blood glucose levels; and the more insulin that is needed by the body (not desirable).

**Eating low-GI foods may lead to better control of blood glucose and insulin levels** (which in turn lowers the risk of damage to blood vessels and nerves). The slower digestion of low-GI foods may also help to delay hunger pangs and benefit weight control.

## Cautionary Notes on GI

**Choosing low-GI foods is not a license to eat unlimited amounts.** Calorie restriction and portion control for weight control is of prime importance.

**Also remember, low-GI foods are carbo-hydrate foods** and must still be counted as part of any dietetic carbohydrate plan.

**GI is not meant to be used by itself** without regard to portion size, and other dietary recommendations for healthy eating. Foods are not good or bad on the basis of their GI.

While GI may be a helpful tool for some people with diabetes, what is most important is to control the total amount of carbohydrate that you eat.

### LOWER-GLYCEMIC FOODS

*Slower-Acting Carbohydrates*
These foods are more slowly digested and absorbed. They help maintain more even blood glucose levels, as long as excessive amounts are not eaten. Use these foods regularly but still limit portion size for weight control.
*Examples:*
- Dried beans, peas, lentils
- Nuts and seeds
- Wholegrain breads
- Bran cereals, oats
- Sweet corn, barley, quinoa buckwheat
- Wholegrain pasta, basmati rice
- Fresh fruit: apples, avocados, bananas (firm), berries, cherries, grapefruit, grapes, olives, oranges, pears, plums. Fresh juices.
- Vegetables: broccoli, yam, nopales, salad greens
- Milk, yogurt, soy drinks
- Dark chocolate, cacao
- Sugar alcohols (sorbitol, maltitol)

### HIGHER-GLYCEMIC FOODS

*Quicker-Acting Carbohydrates*
These foods more rapidly raise blood glucose levels. Eat only in moderation.
- White bread, rice cakes, bagels, croissants, doughnuts
- Low-fiber cereals: Cornflakes, *Rice Krispies, Froot Loops*
- White potatoes, white rice
- Watermelon, ripe bananas, cantaloupe, pineapple
- Soda, sugar-sweetened sports and energy drinks
- Sugar, candy, popcorn (plain)
- Ice cream (low-fat), frozen yogurt

*High-GI fruits and potatoes are still healthy choices when eaten in moderate amounts.*

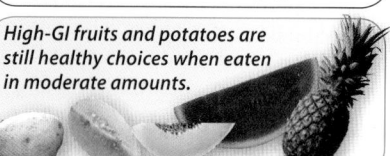

» **Calorie and fat values have been rounded off.**
**Calories** ~ to the nearest 5 or 10 calories.
**Fat** ~ to nearest half gram. **Note:** Trace amounts of fat (less than 0.3 grams) have been treated as zero.

» **Carbohydrate figures** in this book are for total carbohydrate, and not **Net Carbs** (which deducts fiber, polydextrose and sugar alcohols from total carbs).

» Because manufacturers' figures on labels are rounded off, figures in this book may differ slightly from the label. Serving sizes may also vary.

## IMPORTANT DISCLAIMER

* The authors and publishers of this book are not physicians and are not licensed to give medical advice. This book is not a substitute for professional advice. Users should consult their medical professional before making any health, medical or other decisions based on the material contained herein.

* This book is a compilation of original material from other sources intended for educational purposes only. Because food manufacturers constantly change their products, only they are the authoritative source for food's most current nutritional information.

* Persons using the information herein for any medical purposes, such as matching insulin dosage to carbohydrate intake, should not rely solely on the accuracy of figures herein and should independently check food labels or contact the food manufacturer for the latest data.

### Canadian Readers:

Please note that figures in this book are based on U.S. food products and restaurants. Equivalent Canadian foods may vary and should be checked independently.

### * WARRANTY DISCLAIMER:

THE AUTHOR AND PUBLISHER DISCLAIM ANY LIABILITY ARISING DIRECTLY OR INDIRECTLY FROM THE USE OF THIS BOOK. THE INFORMATION HEREIN IS PROVIDED "AS IS" AND WITHOUT ANY WARRANTY EXPRESSED OR IMPLIED. ALL DIRECT, INDIRECT, SPECIAL, INCIDENTAL, CONSEQUENTIAL OR PUNITIVE DAMAGES ARISING FROM ANY USE OF THIS INFORMATION IS DISCLAIMED AND EXCLUDED.

This information is also provided subject to Family Health Publications' Terms and Conditions found at the website, www.calorieking.com/terms and incorporated herein.

**C** ~ Calories
**F** ~ Fat (grams)
**Cb** ~ Carbohydrate (grams)

### Abbreviations

tsp = teaspoon
Tbsp or T = Tablespoon
oz = ounce(s)
c = cup
fl.oz = fluid ounce(s)
g = gram(s)
avg = average
pkg = package

### Volume Measures

(All measures are level)
3 tsp = 1 Tbsp
2 Tbsp = 1 fl.oz
½ cup = 4 fl.oz
1 cup = 8 fl.oz
2 cups = 1 Pint
2 Pints = 1 Quart

Note: 8 oz weight is not the same as 8 fl oz volume (space occupied). Dense foods weigh more per set volume. Examples:
1 cup popcorn weighs ½ oz
1 cup milk weighs 8½ oz
1 cup pudding weighs 10 oz

### Metric Conversion

½ oz = 14 grams
1 oz = 28.4 grams
2 oz = 57 grams
3½ oz = 100 grams
1 fl.oz = 30 mls
1 cup (8 fl.oz) = 240 mls
33 fl.oz = 1 liter (volume)

## INFORMATION SOURCES

• U.S. Dept. of Agriculture
• U.S. Food Manufacturers
• Food Industry Boards & Councils
• Author extrapolations

## FEEDBACK WELCOME!

Please contact the author with your queries and suggestions.
feedback@calorieking.com

- **Health Hazards: Excessive alcohol intake** contributes to obesity, high blood pressure, stroke, heart and liver disease, some cancers, and even impotence. **Concentration and short-term memory** are reduced as well as athletic performance.

  **Other alcohol hazards include:** Fetal Alcohol Syndrome, stomach upsets, gut dysbiosis, menstrual problems, depression, snoring, sleep problems, work absenteeism, impaired judgement, risky behaviors and social/family problems.

- **Alcohol contributes to obesity** through its high calories and by lessening the body's ability to burn fat. Fat storage is promoted, particularly in the belly – a health danger zone. Alcohol can also stimulate the appetite; and weaken the dieter's resolve!

- **Alcohol is potentially more harmful while dieting:** Blood sugar levels may drop with resultant fatigue and further impairment of concentration, reflexes and driving skills.

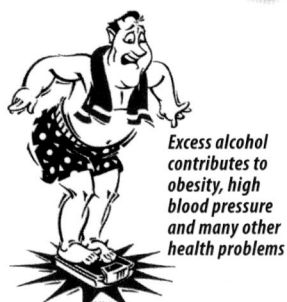

*Excess alcohol contributes to obesity, high blood pressure and many other health problems*

### LOWER RISK ALCOHOL LIMITS

**WOMEN:**
No more than
**1 drink** per day

**MEN:**
No more than
**2 drinks** per day
(Over 65 y.o. ~ 1 drink)

(At least 2 days a week should be alcohol-free)

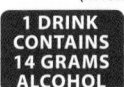
**1 DRINK CONTAINS 14 GRAMS ALCOHOL**
→ 12 fl.oz Regular Beer (5% Alc.)
→ OR 14 fl.oz Light Beer (4.2% Alc.)
→ OR 5 fl.oz Wine (12% Alc.)
→ OR 1½ fl.oz Spirits (80 Proof)

**Note: You cannot save daily drinks for one occasion.**
**Binge drinking is particularly harmful:**
**4 drinks for males or 3 drinks for females (within 2 hours).**

### HOW TO CALCULATE ALCOHOL CONTENT

Percent alcohol on label refers to alcohol volume (ml alcohol/100ml).
Note: 100ml = 3½ fl.oz

To convert to grams (weight) of alcohol, multiply the alcohol volume by 0.8 – since 1 ml of alcohol weighs only 0.8 grams.

*EXAMPLE:*
*12 fl.oz Can Beer*
*(5% alcohol)*
5% alc. volume
= 5% of 12 fl.oz = 0.6 fl.oz
= 18ml alcohol (Note: 1 fl.oz = 30ml)
Weight (18ml x 0.8) = 14.4g alcohol

For some people, safe drinking means no alcohol at all. Even one drink may impair driving skills, particularly if tired. For women who drink frequently, breast cancer risk is increased by 9% for each drink after the first drink. In men, just 2 drinks a day doubles the risk of cancers of the mouth and throat.

**It is advisable not to drink at all if you are:**

- pregnant, trying to conceive or breastfeeding
- taking medication or have liver or heart disease (unless approved by your doctor or pharmacist)
- planning to drive, use machinery or play sports
- studying or needing to concentrate
- a child or adolescent

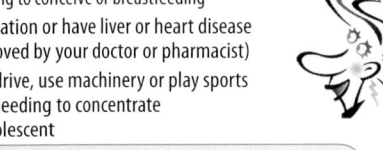
Women and adolescents are more prone to alcohol's ill-effects due to their lower body weight, smaller livers and lesser capacity to metabolize alcohol. As we age, our ability to handle alcohol decreases.

### GOVERNMENT WARNINGS!

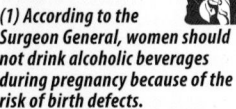

*(1) According to the Surgeon General, women should not drink alcoholic beverages during pregnancy because of the risk of birth defects.*

*(2) Consumption of alcoholic beverages impairs your ability to drive a car or operate machinery, and may cause health problems.*

### EXTRA INFORMATION
*Alcohol & Diabetes ~ See Page 19*
*Alcohol & The Heart ~ See Page 18*
*Tips to Avoid Harmful Drinking ~ Page 19*

## Quick Guide    Alc ~ Alcohol (Grams)

### Beer:
Cb ~ Carbohydrate

**Beer Contains Zero Fat:**

| Regular Beer (5% Alc. Vol.): | C | Alc | Cb |
|---|---|---|---|
| 7 fl.oz Glass | 80 | 8.5 | 4 |
| 12 fl.oz Bottle/Can/Glass | 140 | 14 | 10 |
| 16 fl.oz Bottle/Can | 185 | 19 | 13 |
| 22 fl.oz Bottle | 260 | 26 | 18 |
| 24 fl.oz Can | 280 | 28 | 20 |
| 32 fl.oz Bottle | 370 | 38 | 28 |
| 40 fl.oz Bottle | 470 | 47 | 35 |
| 50 fl.oz Football | 590 | 59 | 50 |
| **Light Beer (4.2% Alc. Vol.):** | | | |
| 7 fl.oz Glass | 65 | 7 | 4 |
| 12 fl.oz Bottle/Can/Glass | 110 | 12 | 7 |
| 16 fl.oz Bottle/Can | 145 | 16 | 9 |
| 22 fl.oz Bottle | 200 | 22 | 13 |
| 24 fl.oz Can | 220 | 24 | 14 |

**Non-Alcoholic Brews:**
(Less than 0.5% alcohol by volume)

| | C | Alc | Cb |
|---|---|---|---|
| Average all Brands, 12 fl.oz | 70 | 1 | 14 |

## Beer ~ Brands

Note: Figure shown are the United States except for the states of Utah, Colorado, Kansas and Oklahoma who have certain restrictions limiting the alcohol content to not more than 4% by volume (3.2% by weight).
*Percentage alcohol listed is by volume - not by weight.*
*Per 12 fl.oz Serving*

| | C | Alc | Cb |
|---|---|---|---|
| **Amstel,** Light (3.5%) | 95 | 10 | 5 |
| **Anchor:** Porter (5.6%) | 210 | 15 | 23 |
| Steam (4.9%) | 160 | 14 | 14 |
| **Asahi:** Kuronama (5.3%) | 165 | 14 | 14 |
| Select (4.7%) | 140 | 13 | 11 |
| Super Dry (4.9%) | 150 | 14 | 11 |
| **Bass,** Pale Ale (5.1%) | 155 | 14 | 12 |
| **Beck's:** Original (5%) | 145 | 14 | 10 |
| Premier Light (2.3%) | 65 | 7 | 4 |
| Sapphire (6%) | 160 | 17 | 9 |
| **Big Sky:** Original IPA (6.2%) | 195 | 18 | 17 |
| Moose Drool (5.3%) | 175 | 15 | 16 |
| Scape Goat (4.7%) | 155 | 14 | 14 |
| Trout Slayer Ale ( 4.7%) | 145 | 14 | 12 |
| **Blatz:** Original (4.6%) | 145 | 13 | 13 |
| Light (3.9%) | 110 | 11 | 8 |
| **Blue Moon:** Belgian White (5.4%) | 165 | 15 | 13 |
| Grand Cru Ale (8.2%) | 230 | 21 | 14 |
| Harvest Pumpkin Ale (5.7%) | 185 | 16 | 16 |
| Spring Ale (5.4%) | 155 | 16 | 12 |
| Winter Abbey Ale (5.6%) | 180 | 16 | 15 |
| **Bohemia** (4.73%) | 140 | 14 | 12 |

## Brands (Cont)    Alc ~ Alcohol (Grams)

*Per 12 fl.oz Serving*

| | C | Alc | Cb |
|---|---|---|---|
| **Bud,** Ice (5.5%) | 120 | 16 | 4 |
| **Bud Light:** Regular (4.2%) | 110 | 12 | 7 |
| & Clamato Chelada (4.2%) | 150 | 12 | 16 |
| Extra Lime (4.2%) | 160 | 12 | 17 |
| Lime (4.2%) | 115 | 12 | 8 |
| Lime-A-Rita (8%), 8 oz | 220 | 15 | 29 |
| Lime Straw-Ber-Rita (8%), 8 oz | 200 | 15 | 24 |
| **Budweiser:** Lager (5%) | 145 | 14 | 11 |
| & Clamato Picante Chelada (5%) | 200 | 14 | 23 |
| Black Crown (6%) | 165 | 17 | 10 |
| Select (4.3%) | 100 | 12 | 3 |
| Select 55 (2.4%) | 55 | 7 | 2 |
| **Busch:** Original (4.3%) | 115 | 12 | 7 |
| Ice (5.9%) | 135 | 17 | 4 |
| Light (4.1%) | 95 | 12 | 3 |
| NA (0.4%) | 60 | 1 | 13 |
| **Carlsberg,** Pilsner (5%) | 135 | 14 | 10 |
| **Carta Blanca** (4.6%) | 145 | 13 | 11 |
| **Castlemaine XXXX,** | | | |
| Bitter (4.6%) | 140 | 14 | 10 |
| **Cerveza,** Aguila (4%) | 125 | 11 | 11 |
| **Colt 45,** Malt Liquor (5.6%) | 155 | 16 | 11 |
| **Coors:** Banquet (5%) | 145 | 14 | 11 |
| Extra Gold (5%) | 150 | 14 | 12 |
| Light (4.2%) | 100 | 12 | 5 |
| **Corona:** Extra (4.6%) | 150 | 13 | 14 |
| Light (4.1%) | 100 | 12 | 5 |
| **Dos Equis XX:** Ambar (4.7%) | 145 | 14 | 12 |
| Lager (4.5%) | 140 | 13 | 11 |
| **Fosters:** Lager (5%) | 145 | 14 | 11 |
| Premium Ale (5.5%) | 160 | 16 | 13 |
| **Genesee:** Lager (4.5%) | 150 | 13 | 14 |
| Genny Light Lager (4%) | 100 | 10 | 4 |
| **George Killian's,** Irish Red (5.4%) | 170 | 16 | 15 |
| **Grolsch:** Blonde (2.8%) | 120 | 8 | 16 |
| Light (3.6%) | 95 | 11 | 6 |
| Premium (5%) | 145 | 14 | 10 |
| **Guinness:** Draught (4%) | 125 | 12 | 10 |
| Extra Stout (6%) | 175 | 17 | 14 |
| Blonde American (5%) | 150 | 14 | 11 |
| Nitro IPA (5.8%), 11.2oz | 155 | 19 | 5 |
| **Hamm's:** Original (4.7%) | 145 | 13 | 12 |
| Special Light (3.9%) | 110 | 12 | 8 |
| **Heineken:** Lager (5%) | 140 | 14 | 10 |
| Special Dark (5%) | 165 | 14 | 15 |
| Premium Light (3.5%) | 100 | 10 | 7 |
| **Hurricane:** Malt Liquor (6%) | 140 | 17 | 4 |
| High Gravity (8.1%) | 185 | 23 | 6 |
| **Icehouse:** Original (5.5%) | 150 | 16 | 10 |
| Light (5%) | 125 | 14 | 7 |
| **Keystone:** Ice (5.9%) | 145 | 17 | 6 |
| Light (4.1%) | 105 | 12 | 5 |

## Brands (Cont)   Alc ~ Alcohol (Grams)      Cb ~ Carbohydrate

**Beer Contains Zero Fat:**
*Per 12 fl.oz Serving*

| | C | Alc | Cb |
|---|---|---|---|
| **King Cobra** (6%) | 135 | 17 | 4 |
| **Kirin:** Ichiban (5%) | 145 | 14 | 11 |
| Light (3.2%) | 95 | 9 | 8 |
| **Kokanee Glacier** (5%) | 145 | 14 | 11 |
| **Labatt:** Blue (5%) | 135 | 14 | 10 |
| Blue Light (4%) | 110 | 11 | 8 |
| Ultra Light, 52 Calories (2.2%) | 52 | 6 | 2 |
| **Landshark,** Lager (4.6%) | 150 | 13 | 13 |
| **Leinenkugel's:** Original (4.6%) | 150 | 13 | 14 |
| Summer Shandy (4.2%) | 135 | 12 | 12 |
| **Lone Star:** Pale Lager (4.65%) | 135 | 13 | 11 |
| Light (3.85%) | 110 | 11 | 8 |
| **Lowenbrau,** Original (5%) | 140 | 14 | 12 |
| **Magic Hat,** #9 (5.1% alc) | 165 | 15 | 15 |
| **Magnum,** Malt Liquor (5.6%) | 155 | 16 | 11 |
| **Michelob:** Amber Bock (5.1%) | 150 | 14 | 12 |
| Lager (4.8%) | 160 | 14 | 14 |
| Light (4.1%) | 120 | 12 | 9 |
| Golden Draft Light (4.1%) | 110 | 12 | 7 |
| Ultra (4.2%) | 95 | 12 | 2.5 |
| Ultra Fruit Flavors (4%) | 95 | 11 | 5.5 |
| **Mickey's,** Malt Liquor (5.6%) | 155 | 16 | 11 |
| **Miller:** Chill, 100 Calorie (4.2%) | 100 | 12 | 4 |
| Genuine Draft /High Life (4.6%) | 145 | 13 | 13 |
| High Life Light (4.1%) | 110 | 12 | 7 |
| Lite (4.2%) | 95 | 12 | 3 |
| MGD 64 (2.8%) | 65 | 8 | 2.5 |
| **Milwaukee's Best:** | | | |
| Ice (5.9%) | 145 | 17 | 7 |
| Light (4.1%) | 100 | 12 | 3.5 |
| Premium (4.3%) | 130 | 12 | 11 |
| **Minnesota's Best,** Original (4.9%) | 140 | 14 | 10 |
| **Modelo,** Especial (4.4%) | 145 | 13 | 14 |
| **Molson Canadian:** Ice (5.6%) | 170 | 16 | 14 |
| Lager (5%) | 150 | 14 | 11 |
| Light (3.9%) | 120 | 11 | 10 |
| **Moosehead,** Lager (5%) | 150 | 14 | 11 |
| **Natural:** Ice (5.9%) | 130 | 17 | 4 |
| Light (4.2%) | 95 | 12 | 3 |
| **Negra Modelo** (5.4%) | 175 | 15 | 16 |
| **Newcastle,** Brown Ale (4.7%) | 130 | 13 | 10 |
| **O'Douls:** Amber (0.4%) | 90 | 1 | 18 |
| Original (0.4%) | 65 | 1 | 13 |
| **Old Milwaukee:** | | | |
| Ice (5.5%) | 150 | 16 | 10 |
| Lager (4.5%) | 150 | 13 | 15 |
| Light (4.3%) | 125 | 12 | 10 |
| **Old Style:** Lager (4.7%) | 145 | 13 | 12 |
| Light (4.2%) | 115 | 12 | 7 |
| **Pabst:** Blue Ribbon (4.7%) | 145 | 13 | 12 |
| Light (3.9%) | 110 | 11 | 8 |

*Per 12 fl.oz Serving Unless Indicated*

| | C | Alc | Cb |
|---|---|---|---|
| **Pacifico,** Clara (4.4%) | 145 | 13 | 13 |
| **Piels,** Lager (4.3%) | 125 | 12 | 9 |
| **Pilsner Urquell,** Lager (4.4%) | 155 | 13 | 16 |
| **Point:** Amber Classic (4.7%) | 160 | 14 | 14 |
| Special Lager (4.7%) | 150 | 14 | 12 |
| **Redbridge,** Lager (4%) | 135 | 10 | 14 |
| **Red Dog,** Lager (5%) | 145 | 14 | 12 |
| **Red Hook:** ESB (5.8%) | 185 | 16 | 16 |
| India Pale Ale (4.7%) | 190 | 13 | 19 |
| **Red Stripe,** Jamaican Ale (5%) | 155 | 14 | 14 |
| **Redd's,** Apple Ale (5%) | 165 | 14 | 17 |
| **Samuel Adams:** | | | |
| Boston Lager (4.9%) | 175 | 14 | 17 |
| **Sam Adams,** Light Lager (4%) | 120 | 13 | 8 |
| **Sapporo,** Prem. Lager (4.9%) | 135 | 14 | 9 |
| **Schaefer:** Lager (4.6%) | 145 | 13 | 12 |
| Light (3.9%) | 110 | 11 | 8 |
| **Schell's:** Deer (4.7%) | 145 | 14 | 13 |
| Light (3.5%) | 100 | 10 | 7 |
| **Schlitz:** Pale Lager (4.6%) | 145 | 13 | 12 |
| Light (3.8%) | 110 | 11 | 8 |
| **Schmidt's:** Pale Lager (4.6%) | 145 | 13 | 13 |
| Light (3.8%) | 110 | 11 | 8 |
| **Sheaf,** Stout (5.7%) | 190 | 16 | 19 |
| **Shock Top:** Belgian White (5.2%) | 165 | 15 | 15 |
| Lemon Shandy (4.2%) | 145 | 12 | 15 |
| **Sierra Nevada:** Bigfoot (9.6%) | 330 | 28 | 32 |
| Draft Pale Ale (5%) | 155 | 14 | 13 |
| Pale Ale (5.6%) | 175 | 16 | 14 |
| Porter (5.6%) | 195 | 16 | 18 |
| **Sol** (4.2%) | 130 | 12 | 11 |
| **Southpaw,** Light (5%) | 125 | 14 | 7 |
| **Sparks,** Lager (6%) | 250 | 17 | 34 |
| **Steel Reserve:** | | | |
| High Gravity Malt Liquor (8.1%) | 220 | 23 | 15 |
| Steel 6 (6%) | 160 | 17 | 11 |
| **Stella Artois,** Pale Lager (5%) | 155 | 14 | 13 |
| **Stroh's:** Pale Lager (4.6%) | 145 | 13 | 12 |
| Light (3.9%) | 115 | 11 | 7 |
| **Tecate:** Pale Lager (4.6%) | 140 | 13 | 11 |
| Light (4%) | 110 | 10 | 8 |
| **Third Shift,** Amber Lager (5.3%) | 185 | 15 | 18 |
| **Trader Jose:** | | | |
| Premium Lager (5%), 11.2 fl.oz | 145 | 14 | 14 |
| Light (3.8%), 11.2 fl.oz | 105 | 14 | 8 |
| **Widmer,** Hefewéizen (4.9%) | 155 | 14 | 13 |
| **Wild Blue,** Lager (8%) | 240 | 23 | 20 |
| **ZeigenBock,** Amber (4.9%) | 145 | 14 | 11 |

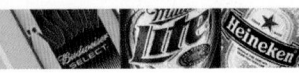
**Alc** ~ Alcohol (Grams)    **Cb** ~ Carbohydrate

## Cider ~ Alcoholic/Hard

*Per 12 fl.oz Unless Indicated*

| | C | Alc | Cb |
|---|---|---|---|
| **Ace:** Cider (5%), average all flavors | 155 | 14 | 12 |
| Joker (6.9%) | 120 | 20 | 12 |
| **Angry Orchard:** Apple Ginger (5%) | 200 | 14 | 26 |
| Crisp Apple (5%) | 220 | 14 | 31 |
| Traditional Dry (5.5%) | 180 | 16 | 20 |
| **Crispin:** Original (5%) | 150 | 14 | 15 |
| Blackberry (5%) | 160 | 14 | 16 |
| Brut (5.5%) | 165 | 16 | 14 |
| Pacific Pear (4.5%) | 160 | 13 | 17 |
| **Hornsby's:** | | | |
| Amber (5.5%), 12 fl.oz | 180 | 16 | 19 |
| Crisp (5.5%), 12 fl.oz | 190 | 16 | 26 |
| **Johnny Appleseed,** (5.5%) | 210 | 16 | 26 |
| **Magners,** (4.5%) | 125 | 13 | 9 |
| **Michelob,** Ultra Light Cider (4%) | 120 | 10 | 10 |
| **Smith & Forge,** (6%) | 220 | 17 | 26 |
| **Stella Artois Cidre,** (4.5%) | 170 | 13 | 21 |
| **Strongbow:** | | | |
| Gold Apple (5%), 11.2 fl.oz | 170 | 13 | 20 |
| Honey & Apple (5%), 11.2 fl.oz | 195 | 13 | 26 |
| **Woodchuck:** Amber (5%) | 200 | 14 | 21 |
| 802 (5%) | 180 | 14 | 16 |
| Granny Smith (5%) | 160 | 14 | 11 |
| Pear (4%) | 150 | 12 | 18 |
| Raspberry (4%) | 170 | 12 | 22 |
| **Wyder's:** Pear (4%) | 140 | 12 | 22 |
| Raspberry (4%) | 120 | 12 | 17 |
| Reposado (6.9%) | 250 | 19 | 30 |

## Quick Guide

### Table Wines:
*Average all Varieties (11.5% Alc.)*
*(Wine Contains Zero Fat)*

| | C | Alc | Cb |
|---|---|---|---|
| **4 fl.oz,** 1 small wine glass OR ½ large wine glass | 100 | 12 | 3 |
| **6 fl.oz,** (¾ large wine glass) | 145 | 18 | 5 |
| **8 fl.oz,** (1 large wine glass) | 195 | 25 | 7 |
| **½ Carafe/Bottle,** 12 fl.oz | 295 | 37 | 10 |
| **1 Bottle,** 750ml, 25.4 fl.oz | 620 | 78 | 21 |

## Table Wines

**Red:** *Per 4 fl.oz*

| | C | Alc | Cb |
|---|---|---|---|
| Burgundy/Cabernet/Merlot, av. | 100 | 11 | 4 |

**White:** *Per 4 fl.oz*

| | C | Alc | Cb |
|---|---|---|---|
| Dry (Chenin; Fume Blanc; Chardonnay) | 95 | 11 | 4 |
| Sparkling, 4 fl.oz | 95 | 11 | 4 |
| Zinfandel Sweet, (Moselle/Sauterne), 4 fl.oz | 85 | 11 | 2 |

## Table Wines (Cont)

| | C | Alc | Cb |
|---|---|---|---|
| **Champagne:** *Per 4 fl.oz* | | | |
| Average all types, 1 glass | 85 | 11 | 2 |
| with Orange Jce (3:1 orange) | 75 | 8 | 4 |
| with Orange Jce (1:1 orange) | 65 | 5 | 7 |
| **Mulled Wine** *(Gluhwein),* 4 fl.oz | 180 | 14 | 20 |
| **Non-Alcoholic Wine:** *Less than 0.5% Alcohol* | | | |
| *Ariel:* White varieties, average, 4 fl.oz | 35 | 0.5 | 8 |
| Red varieties, average, 4 fl.oz | 25 | 0.5 | 5 |
| **Reduced Alcohol Wine:** | | | |
| Average all types, (6%), 4 fl.oz | 80 | 6 | 10 |
| *Skinnygirl,* Red/White, (8.5%), 5 fl.oz | 100 | 10 | 5 |
| **Sake** *(Gekkeikan),* (16%), 4 fl.oz | 120 | 15 | 5 |
| **Sangria** *(Skinnygirl),* (4%), 5 fl.oz | 130 | 5 | 23 |

## Flavored Wines

***Average All Brands (6% alcohol)***
*(Arbor Mist, Wild Vines, Boone's Farm):*

| | C | Alc | Cb |
|---|---|---|---|
| 1 small wine glass, 4 fl.oz | 80 | 6 | 10 |
| 1 large wine glass, 8 fl.oz | 160 | 11 | 20 |
| 1 bottle, 750 ml (25.4 fl.oz) | 510 | 35 | 64 |

## Dessert Wines

| | C | Alc | Cb |
|---|---|---|---|
| **Madeira** (18%), 2 oz | 85 | 9 | 5 |
| **Marsala** (18%), 2 oz | 110 | 9 | 11 |
| **Port,** Muscatel (18%), 2 oz | 85 | 9 | 5 |
| **Sherry** (15%), 2 oz: | | | |
| Dry, 1 Sherry glass | 90 | 7 | 7 |
| Sweet/Cream, average | 90 | 7 | 8 |
| **Vermouth** *(Martini & Rossi):* | | | |
| Extra Dry (18%), 2 oz | 65 | 9 | 2 |
| Martini Rosso (16%), 2 oz | 90 | 8 | 8 |

## Cooking Wines

**Holland House:**

| | C | Alc | Cb |
|---|---|---|---|
| **Marsala,** (14%), 2 T., 1 fl.oz | 45 | 4 | 4 |
| **Red/White,** (10%): 2 T., 1 fl.oz | 20 | 2 | 1 |
| 1 cup, 8 fl.oz | 160 | 24 | 8 |
| **Sherry,** (17%), 2 Tbsp, 1 fl.oz | 45 | 5 | 2 |

### Cooking with Wine:
For alcohol to evaporate, sufficient heat and cooking time (at least 30 minutes) is required.
**Red and white table wines** would then contain negligible residual calories.
**Sweetened wines** (marsala/sherry) would contain 10 calories per 1 fl.oz.
**Flambé Desserts:** Only surface alcohol is burned off, so negligible reduction in alcohol or calories.

## Quick Guide
### Alc ~ Alcohol (Grams)

**Spirits/Liquors:**
*Includss Bourbon, Brandy, Gin, Rum, Scotch, Tequila, Vodka, Whiskey.*
Note: All spirits with same alcohol proof have similar calories and zero fat.

| Average All Brands | C | Alc | Cb |
|---|---|---|---|
| **80 Proof (40% Alcohol by Volume):** | | | |
| 1 fl.oz | 65 | 9.5 | 0 |
| 1.5 fl.oz (1 shot) | 100 | 14 | 0 |
| 3 fl.oz (Double shot) | 195 | 28 | 0 |
| ½ Bottle, 350 ml (12 fl.oz) | 770 | 113 | 0 |
| 1 Bottle, 700 ml (24 fl.oz) | 1540 | 227 | 0 |
| **86 Proof (43% Alc):** | | | |
| 1 fl.oz | 70 | 10 | 0 |
| 1.5 fl.oz (1 shot) | 105 | 15 | 0 |
| 1 Bottle (24 fl.oz) | 1670 | 247 | 0 |
| **100 Proof (50% Alc),** | | | |
| 1.5 fl.oz | 125 | 18 | 0 |
| **Shochu (Soju),** | | | |
| average all types (25% alc) 2 fl.oz | 65 | 12 | 0 |

## Flavored Spirits

| | C | Alc | Cb |
|---|---|---|---|
| **Captain Morgan:** *Per 1.5 fl.oz* | | | |
| **Original** (35%) | 85 | 12 | 0.5 |
| **Black Spiced** (47.3%) | 115 | 14 | 1 |
| **Parrot Bay** (21%), average | 90 | 7.5 | 10 |
| **Silver Spiced** (35%) | 95 | 12 | 2 |
| **Malibu Rum,** | | | |
| Original/Fruit Flavors (21%), 1.5 fl.oz | 80 | 8 | 8 |
| **Southern Comfort** (35%), 1.5 fl.oz | 100 | 13 | 3 |

## Hard Lemonade, Sodas & Tea

| | C | Alc | Cb |
|---|---|---|---|
| **Margaritaville:** *Per 12 fl.oz* | | | |
| **Lime Margarita** (8%) | 310 | 23 | 30 |
| **Paradise Punch** (8%) | 340 | 23 | 46 |
| **Mike's:** | | | |
| **Lemonade:** | | | |
| Hard (5%), 11.2 fl.oz | 220 | 13 | 33 |
| Harder (8%) average, 16 fl.oz | 395 | 31 | 44 |
| **Margarita,** 11.2 fl.oz | 220 | 14 | 34 |
| **Punch :** | | | |
| Hard Mango (5.5%), 11.2 fl.oz | 230 | 15 | 33 |
| Harder (8%), 12 fl.oz | 300 | 23 | 36 |
| **Sparks:** *Per 16 fl.oz Can* | | | |
| **Blackberry** (8%) | 385 | 31 | 44 |
| **Iced Tea** (8%) | 375 | 31 | 41 |
| **Lemonade** (8%) | 345 | 31 | 36 |
| **Original** (6%) | 335 | 23 | 45 |
| **Twisted Tea:** Original (5%) | 220 | 14 | 31 |
| Half & Half (5%) | 260 | 14 | 34 |

## Coolers & Premix Cocktails

**Ready-To-Drink:**
*Zero Fat Unless Indicated*

| | C | Alc | Cb |
|---|---|---|---|
| **Bacardi:** *Per 4 fl.oz* | | | |
| **Party Drinks (Ready To Pour):** | | | |
| Bahama Mama; Mai Tai (10%) | 130 | 9 | 16 |
| Mojito (15%) | 160 | 14 | 16 |
| Rum Island Ice Tea (12.5%) | 150 | 12 | 16 |
| **Bacardi Silver:** *Per 12 fl.oz* | | | |
| Lemonade/Sangria (6%), av. | 270 | 17 | 41 |
| Raz/Strawberry (5%) | 240 | 14 | 36 |
| Mojito (5%) | 240 | 14 | 36 |
| **Bartles & Jaymes:** *Per 11.2 fl.oz* | | | |
| **Malt Based Coolers** (3.2%): | | | |
| Exotic Berry | 195 | 9 | 31 |
| Margarita | 245 | 9 | 43 |
| Pina Colada | 250 | 9 | 45 |
| Sangria | 240 | 9 | 40 |
| Strawberry Daiquiri | 205 | 9 | 34 |
| **Captain Morgan's,** | | | |
| Parrot Bay (4.1%), all var. av., 11.2 fl.oz | 210 | 10 | 35 |
| **Chi Chi's:** Long Is. Iced Tea, 4 fl.oz | 145 | 12 | 17 |
| Mexican Mudslide, 4 fl.oz (8g fat) | 240 | 1.5 | 42 |
| Mojito, 4 fl.oz | 160 | 11 | 21 |
| Pina Colada, 4 fl.oz (6g fat) | 240 | 4 | 42 |
| White Russian, 4 fl.oz (7g fat) | 245 | 1.5 | 43 |
| **Daily's,** Frozen Pouches (5%), | | | |
| average all flavors, 10 fl.oz | 285 | 12 | 47 |
| **Jack Daniels,** Country Cocktails (4.8%), | | | |
| average all varieties, 10 fl.oz | 200 | 9 | 30 |
| **Jose Cuervo:** | | | |
| **Margaritas:** | | | |
| Classic Lime (10%), 6 fl.oz | 210 | 14 | 29 |
| Golden (12.7%), 4.7 fl.oz | 170 | 14 | 19 |
| **Seagram's:** | | | |
| **Escapes Coolers** (3.2%): | | | |
| Bahama Mama, 11.2 fl.oz | 200 | 9 | 36 |
| Strawb. Daiquiri, 11.2 fl.oz | 225 | 9 | 41 |
| **Skinnygirl:** | | | |
| Vodka with flavors (30%), 1.5 fl.oz | 75 | 11 | 0 |
| Cocktails (10%), av., 3 fl.oz | 70 | 8 | 4 |
| **Smirnoff:** | | | |
| **Frozen Lemonades (5%),** av,, 10 oz | 285 | 12 | 53 |
| **Ice,** 4.5%: | | | |
| Cherry Lime, 12 oz | 250 | 13 | 30 |
| Mango/Pineapple, 12 oz | 220 | 13 | 35 |
| Raspberry/Tropical Fruit, 12 oz | 230 | 13 | 38 |
| **TGI Friday's:** | | | |
| **On The Rocks:** *Per 6 fl.oz* | | | |
| Long Island Ice Tea (15%) | 250 | 21 | 28 |
| Margarita (7.5%) | 185 | 11 | 29 |
| Mudslide (10%) | 365 | 14 | 31 |
| **Blenders** (12.5%), | | | |
| Mudslide, 6 fl.oz | 365 | 18 | 31 |

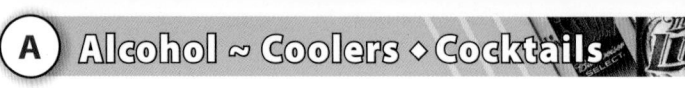
## Coolers & Premix Cocktails (Cont)

**Ready-To-Drink:**

| | **C** | **Alc** | **Cb** |
|---|---|---|---|
| **The Club Premix Cocktails:** *Per 3.4 oz Serving (½ can)* | | | |
| Censored on Beach; Margarita (7.5%) | 105 | 6 | 17 |
| Gin/Vodka Martini (21%), average | 155 | 17 | 0.2 |
| Long Island Ice Tea (15%) | 145 | 12 | 17 |
| Manhattan (17%) | 115 | 13 | 5 |
| Mudslide/Pina Colada (10%), average | 200 | 8 | 16 |
| Screwdriver (7.5%) | 95 | 6 | 14 |
| Whiskey Sour (10%) | 95 | 8 | 11 |

## Shooters

*Alc ~ Alcohol (Grams)*

| | **C** | | |
|---|---|---|---|
| Alabama Slammer | 110 | 14 | 2 |
| Amaretto Sour | 120 | 6 | 19 |
| B52 | 145 | 14 | 11 |
| Beam Me Up Scotty | 145 | 13 | 13 |
| Blue Tequila | 160 | 18 | 6 |
| Jager Bomb | 205 | 8 | 30 |
| Jager Bomb, w/ Sugar-Free Red Bull | 155 | 8 | 18 |
| Jell-O Shot: 3 oz, with 1.5 oz Vodka | 180 | 14 | 19 |
| with Diet Jell-O | 110 | 14 | 0 |
| Kamikaze | 75 | 8 | 3 |
| Kool-Aid | 160 | 15 | 14 |
| Orgasm | 100 | 12 | 6 |
| Peppermint Patty | 195 | 8 | 11 |
| Stinger | 170 | 18 | 12 |
| Surfer on Acid | 90 | 7 | 11 |

## Cocktail Mixers ~ Non-Alcoholic

| | **C** | | |
|---|---|---|---|
| **Bacardi:** *Per 8 fl.oz, Prepared from 2 fl.oz Concentrate* | | | |
| Daiquiris; Rum Runner | 120 | 0 | 32 |
| Margarita | 90 | 0 | 25 |
| Mojito | 110 | 0 | 30 |
| Pina Colada | 170 | 0 | 36 |
| **Baja Bob's:** *Per 4 fl.oz* | | | |
| Cranberry Cosmo Martini | 10 | 0 | 2 |
| Pina Colada | 30 | 0 | 4 |
| **Jose Cuervo:** | | | |
| Margaritas: Av. all flav., 4 fl.oz | 85 | 0 | 21 |
| Light (Sugar Free), Lime, 4 fl.oz | 5 | 0 | 1 |
| **Mr & Mrs T:** | | | |
| Bloody Mary: Original, 5 oz | 30 | 0 | 7 |
| Bold & Spicy, 4 oz | 35 | 0 | 7 |
| Mai Tai | 130 | 0 | 32 |
| Margarita | 100 | 0 | 26 |
| Pina Colada | 170 | 0 | 44 |
| Strawberry Daiquiri | 180 | 0 | 46 |
| **TGI Friday's:** | | | |
| Mudslide, 2.3 fl.oz | 110 | 0 | 23 |
| Cosmo; Berrytini, 2 fl.oz | 80 | 0 | 20 |
| Strawb. Daiquiri; Marg., 4 fl.oz | 190 | 0 | 46 |

## Cocktails

*Alc ~ Alcohol (Grams)*

**Made to Standard Recipes (Standard Size):**
*(Main Reference: The New American Bartender's Guide)*
*Zero Fat Unless Indicated*

| | **C** | **Alc** | **Cb** |
|---|---|---|---|
| Adios Mother F. | 260 | 23 | 23 |
| Bacardi & Coke (with 1.5 oz Bacardi) | 160 | 14 | 17 |
| Bellini, 4.5 fl.oz | 95 | 11 | 7 |
| Bloody Mary (with 1.5 oz Vodka) | 125 | 10 | 7 |
| Blushin' Russian (20g fat) | 405 | 14 | 23 |
| Bourbon & Soda (with 2 oz Bourbon) | 130 | 19 | 0 |
| Brandy Alexander (10g fat) | 300 | 20 | 15 |
| Chupa Naranjas (with 1.5 oz Tequila) | 150 | 16 | 8 |
| Cosmopolitan | 215 | 24 | 12 |
| Daiquiri (w/ 2 oz Rum), av. all types | 140 | 19 | 4 |
| Frozen Daiquiri (with 2 oz Rum): | | | |
| without fruit | 155 | 19 | 6 |
| with fruit (with 1.5 oz Rum) | 145 | 14 | 11 |
| Grasshopper | 260 | 17 | 28 |
| Greyhound (with 1.5 oz Vodka) | 170 | 14 | 17 |
| Harvey Wallbanger (2 oz) | 200 | 19 | 17 |
| Highball (1.5 oz Whiskey) | 100 | 14 | 0 |
| Irish Coffee (10g fat) | 205 | 14 | 2 |
| Kahlua Mudslide: with milk (3g fat) | 145 | 11 | 12 |
| with cream (12g fat) | 230 | 11 | 10 |
| Lemon Drop, 4 fl.oz | 130 | 14 | 10 |
| Long Island Iced Tea (with 3 oz Cola) | 270 | 19 | 32 |
| with 3 oz Diet Cola | 235 | 19 | 22 |
| Mai Tai (with 2 oz Rum) | 290 | 24 | 33 |
| Manhattan | 130 | 17 | 5 |
| Margarita | 160 | 18 | 7 |
| Martini: Dry, with 1.5 oz gin | 100 | 14 | 0 |
| Sour Apple, w/ 2 oz Vodka/1 oz Schnapps | 250 | 31 | 10 |
| Mint Julep (with 2½ oz Bourbon) | 180 | 24 | 4 |
| Mojito (with 2 oz rum) | 170 | 19 | 9 |
| Moscow Mule | 185 | 14 | 24 |
| Pina Colada (10g fat), 6 oz | 250 | 15 | 18 |
| Red Bull & Vodka (with 1.5 oz vodka) | 210 | 14 | 28 |
| with Sugar Free Red Bull | 105 | 14 | 3 |
| Rum & Coke (with 1.5 oz Rum) | 160 | 14 | 17 |
| Sangria: with 1 oz Fruit Juice, 5 oz | 120 | 12 | 9 |
| with 0.5 oz Brandy, 5.5 oz | 150 | 17 | 9 |
| Screwdriver | 160 | 14 | 15 |
| Sex On The Beach | 235 | 19 | 25 |
| Spritzer (with 3 oz Wine) | 65 | 8 | 2 |
| Tequila Sunrise | 200 | 14 | 25 |
| Tom Collins (with 2 oz Gin) | 210 | 19 | 18 |
| Vodka Soda (with 1.5 oz Vodka) | 100 | 14 | 0 |
| Vodka Tonic (with 1.5 oz Vodka) | 165 | 14 | 18 |
| Whiskey Sour (w/ 2 oz Whiskey) | 155 | 19 | 7 |
| White Russian (10g fat) | 240 | 19 | 7 |
| **Non-Alcoholic:** | | | |
| Cinderella | 45 | 0 | 11 |
| Shirley Temple (with 6 oz Ginger Ale) | 140 | 0 | 34 |

# Alcohol ~ Liqueurs  A

## Liqueurs/Cordials     C  Alc  Cb

*Per 1 fl.oz*

| | C | Alc | Cb |
|---|---|---|---|
| Advocaat (36 Proof; 2g fat) | 85 | 4 | 9 |
| Alizé: Cognac (80 Proof) | 70 | 9 | 2 |
| Gold/Red Passion (32 Proof) | 105 | 4 | 11 |
| Amaretto (56 Proof) | 110 | 7 | 17 |
| Baileys Irish Cream (34 Proof; 4g fat) | 100 | 4 | 8 |
| Benedictine (80 Proof) | 90 | 9 | 5 |
| Chambord (33 Proof) | 105 | 4 | 11 |
| Chartreuse (80 Proof) | 100 | 9 | 9 |
| Cherry Brandy (48 Proof) | 80 | 6 | 9 |
| Coffee Liqueur (53 Proof) | 115 | 7 | 16 |
| Cointreau (80 Proof) | 95 | 9 | 7 |
| Creme de Cacao (54 Proof) | 100 | 6 | 15 |
| Creme de Menthe (72 Proof) | 125 | 9 | 14 |
| Curacao (70 Proof) | 95 | 8 | 6 |
| Drambuie (80 Proof) | 105 | 9 | 9 |
| Frangelico (40 Proof) | 65 | 5 | 12 |
| Galliano (86 Proof) | 100 | 10 | 8 |
| Grand Marnier (80 Proof) | 100 | 9 | 7 |
| Kahlua (40 Proof) | 85 | 5 | 14 |
| Kirsch (68 Proof) | 80 | 8 | 6 |
| Midori (42 Proof) | 80 | 5 | 11 |
| Ouzo (80 Proof) | 105 | 9 | 11 |
| Pernod (80 Proof) | 75 | 9 | 11 |
| Sambuca (84 Proof) | 100 | 10 | 11 |
| Schnapps (100 Proof) | 115 | 12 | 9 |
| Southern Comfort (70 Proof) | 65 | 8 | 3 |

## Liqueur Coffee & Hot Drinks

*Per Standard Drink*

| | C | Alc | Cb |
|---|---|---|---|
| **Liqueur Coffee:** Av. all types | 200 | 10 | 10 |
| Irish, 1.5 oz Whiskey & 1 oz whip | 205 | 9 | 4 |
| **Hot Toddy,** with 1½ oz liquor, av. all | 170 | 9 | 19 |
| **Mulled Wine** *(Glühwein)*, 4 fl.oz, av | 195 | 14 | 25 |

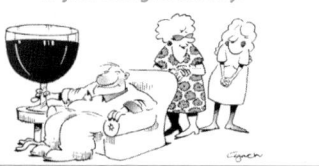

*"The doctor told him to cut down to just one glass a day."*

## TEN TIPS TO AVOID HARMFUL DRINKING

1. **Add up the alcohol** you typically drink each day and on social occasions. How does this compare with 'low risk' amounts? *(See page 23)*

2. **Compare the alcohol content** of different drinks and select the lowest. Request half shots of alcohol in cocktails and mixed drinks. Dilute them and keep topping off with non-alcoholic drinks.

3. **Go easy on 'Light' beers.** At 4% alcohol, on average, they are still high in alcohol compared to regular beer (5% alcohol).

4. **Try low alcohol or non-alcohol** alternatives such as fruit juices and mineral water. Take your own to parties.

5. **Before drinking alcohol,** quench your thirst with water and non-alcoholic drinks – particularly after vigorous exercise or sports.

6. **Slow the rate of drinking.** Chugging or drinking fast is the major cause of illness and death from alcohol poisoning.

7. **Avoid drinking in 'rounds'.**

8. **Have a non-alcoholic 'spacer'** between drinks (e.g. mineral water, orange juice).

9. **Don't drink on an empty stomach.** Food slows the rate of alcohol absorption.

10. **Keep track of the number of drinks** and know when to stop. Stick to a set limit.

*Note: Alcohol can be very dangerous when taken with prescription or street drugs, or when you are very tired.*

**Extra Info: www.CalorieKing.com**

## Cocktail Mixers & Extracts

| | C | Alc | Cb |
|---|---|---|---|
| Angostura Bitters, ¼ tsp | 2 | 0 | 0.5 |
| Grenadine, ½ tsp | 6 | 0 | 2 |
| Lime/Lemon Juice, 2 Tbsp, 1 oz | 10 | 0 | 2 |
| Maraschino Cherry, 1 small | 8 | 0 | 2 |
| Simple Syrup, 1 Tbsp, av. | 50 | 0 | 14 |
| Sweet & Sour Mix, 2 Tbsp, 1 oz | 30 | 0 | 7 |
| Tonic Water, 8 fl.oz | 80 | 0 | 22 |
| **Flavor Extracts** *(McCormick)*: | | | |
| Pure Lemon (83%), 1 tsp | 0 | 3.5 | 0 |
| Pure Vanilla (35%), 1tsp | 0 | 1.5 | 0 |

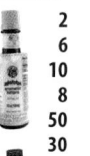

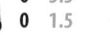

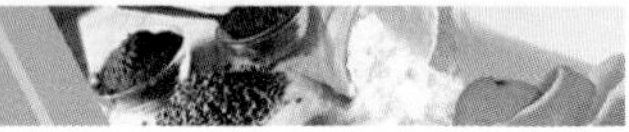

## Baking Ingredients

| Baking Ingredients | C | F | Cb |
|---|---|---|---|
| **Almond Paste**, (Marzipan), 2 Tbsp | 170 | 7 | 24 |
| **Apple Pie Filling**, Sweetened, 9.4 oz | 290 | 0 | 69 |
| **Aquafaba** (Bean Water), ¼ c., 2 oz | 10 | 0 | 2 |
| **Baking Powder:** Regular, 1 tsp | 5 | 0 | 1 |
| Cream of Tartar, 1 tsp | 10 | 0 | 2 |
| Baking Mix (*Bisquick*): Original, ⅓ cup, 1.5 oz | 160 | 5 | 26 |
| **Batter Mix** (*Golden Dipt*), All Purpose, ¼ cup | 100 | 0 | 20 |
| **Butter/Margarine**, ½ cup, 4 oz | 800 | 88 | 1 |
| Stick (*Land O' Lakes*), 0.5 oz | 100 | 11 | 0 |
| **Cacao Butter**, 2 Tbsp, 1 oz | 240 | 28 | 0 |
| **Cacao Nibs**, raw, 3 Tbsp, 1 oz | 180 | 14 | 8 |
| **Cacao Powder,** raw: 1 Tbsp, 0.3 oz | 35 | 2 | 3 |
| ¼ cup, 1 oz | 150 | 9 | 11 |
| **Carob Flour**, ½ cup | 115 | 0.5 | 46 |
| **Chocolate Baking Bars:** *Average all Brands* | | | |
| Sweet (*Baker's*): | | | |
| 1 oz portion | 120 | 7 | 16 |
| 4 oz bar | 470 | 28 | 64 |
| Semi-sweet, 1 oz | 140 | 9 | 16 |
| White Baking, 1 oz | 160 | 9 | 16 |
| Unsweetened: 1 oz | 140 | 14 | 8 |
| Grated, 1 cup, 4.5 oz | 660 | 69 | 39 |
| **Chocolate Baking Chips:** *Average all Brands* | | | |
| Milk Choc./Semi Sweet, 1 oz | 140 | 8 | 18 |
| ½ cup, 3 oz | 420 | 24 | 54 |
| 1 cup, 6 oz | 840 | 48 | 108 |
| Dark, 1 Tbsp, 0.5 oz | 70 | 5 | 3 |
| Mini Kisses (*Hershey*), 1 piece | 5 | 0.5 | 1 |
| **Cocoa Powder**, unsweetened: | | | |
| 1 Tbsp, 0.2 oz | 15 | 0.5 | 3 |
| ⅓ cup, 1 oz | 60 | 4 | 17 |
| **Coconut**, dried: | | | |
| Sweetened/Flaked: | | | |
| 1 oz | 130 | 8 | 15 |
| ½ cup, 1.3 oz | 195 | 12 | 22 |
| Toasted (*Baker's*), 1 oz | 170 | 13 | 13 |
| Unsweetened, 1 oz | 190 | 18 | 7 |
| **Coconut Cream/Milk** ~ *See Page 89* | | | |
| **Coconut Manna** (*Nutiva*), 1 Tbsp | 100 | 9 | 3 |
| **Cornstarch**, 1 Tbsp | 30 | 0 | 7 |
| **Eggs:** Large (1) | 75 | 5 | 0 |
| Jumbo (1) | 90 | 6 | 0.5 |
| **Egg White:** 1 Egg White | 15 | 0 | 0 |
| ½ cup (4 egg whites), 4 oz | 60 | 0 | 1 |
| **Flour:** Whole Wheat, 1 cup, 4.2 oz | 400 | 2 | 84 |
| White: 1 Tbsp, 0.3 oz | 25 | 0 | 5.5 |
| 1 cup, 4.2 oz | 400 | 1 | 88 |

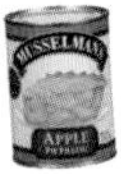

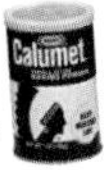

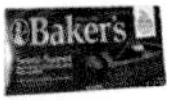

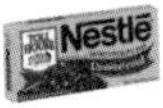

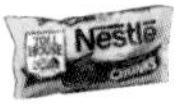

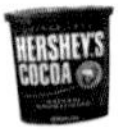

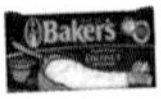

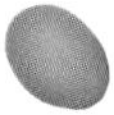

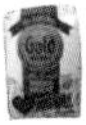

| | C | F | Cb |
|---|---|---|---|
| **Flavor Extracts:** *Av. all Brands* | | | |
| Imitation, 1 tsp | 10 | 0 | 2 |
| Pure Extract, 1 tsp | 10 | 0 | 0.5 |
| Almond; Vanilla, 1 tsp | 10 | 0 | 0.5 |
| **Fruit Pectin:** Swtnd, ¼ tsp | 5 | 0 | 1 |
| Unsweetened, ¼ tsp | 0 | 0 | 0 |
| **Gelatin**, dry, unsweetened, 0.3 oz | 20 | 0 | 0 |
| **Glaze** (*Duncan Hines*): Choc., 2 T. | 150 | 7 | 21 |
| Vanilla, 2 Tbsp | 140 | 6 | 22 |
| *Golden Dipt*, Batter Mix ¼ cup, 1 oz | 100 | 0 | 23 |
| **Honey**, ½ cup, 6 oz | 515 | 0 | 140 |
| **Lemon/Orange Peel**, ¼ cup | 25 | 0 | 6 |
| **Lighter Bake** (*Sunsweet*): (Butter & Oil replacement) | | | |
| 1 Tbsp, ½ oz | 35 | 0 | 9 |
| ¼ Cup, 2.7 oz | 140 | 0 | 36 |
| **Milk:** Whole, 1 cup, 8 fl.oz | 150 | 8 | 12 |
| 2%, 1 cup, 8 fl.oz | 120 | 5 | 12 |
| 1%, 1 cup, 8 fl.oz | 100 | 2.5 | 12 |
| Fat-Free, 1 cup, 8 fl.oz | 90 | 0.5 | 13 |
| **Pastry** ~ *See Page 134* | | | |
| **Pie Crusts** ~ *See Page 134* | | | |
| **Pie Fillings, Fruits** ~ *See Page 134* | | | |
| Lemon Creme, ⅓ cup | 130 | 1.5 | 28 |
| Mincemeat, 3.5 oz | 190 | 5 | 45 |
| Pumpkin, 1 cup, 9.3 oz | 270 | 1.5 | 60 |
| **Prune Puree**, ¼ cup, 3 oz | 220 | 0 | 55 |
| **Raisins**, ½ cup, 2.8 oz | 240 | 0.5 | 63 |
| **Rennin**, 0.4 oz pkt | 10 | 0 | 2 |
| **Soy Milk** ~ *See Pages 49-50* | | | |
| **Sprinkles**, all types, 1 tsp | 20 | 1 | 3 |
| **Sugar:** 1 Tbsp, 0.5 oz | 55 | 0 | 14 |
| 1 oz | 110 | 0 | 28 |
| 1 cup, 7 oz | 775 | 0 | 195 |
| 16 oz (1 lb) | 1760 | 0 | 454 |
| **Sweeteners & Sugar Substitutes** ~ *See Page 156* | | | |
| **Vinegar**, average all types, 1 oz | 5 | 0 | 1 |
| **Whey**, sweet, dry, 1 oz | 100 | 0.5 | 21 |
| **Yeast:** | | | |
| Active, dry, 0.3 oz pkg | 25 | 0.5 | 3 |
| Bakers, compressed, 1 oz | 30 | 0 | 5 |
| *Fleischmann's*, 0.6 oz pkg | 0 | 0 | 0 |

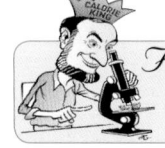

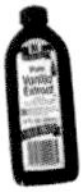

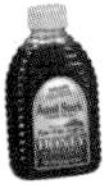

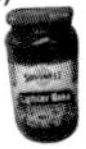

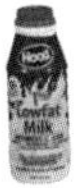

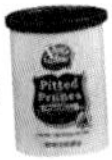

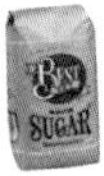

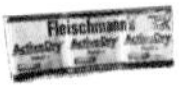

*ℱor* Full Nutritional Data & Product Updates
~ *See Author's Website*
www.CalorieKing.com

Note: Actual weight of bars is usually 5-10% more than label Net Weight. Weigh bar and allow extra calories.

| Bars ~ Brands | C | F | Cb |
|---|---|---|---|

*Per Bar*

**AdvantEdge** ~ *See EAS*

**Annie's Homegrown:**

**Organic Granola Bars:** *Per 1 oz Bar*

| | C | F | Cb |
|---|---|---|---|
| Berry Berry | 120 | 3.5 | 20 |
| Chocolate Chip | 120 | 4 | 19 |
| PB & J; Peanut Butter | 120 | 4.5 | 18 |

**Atkins:**

**Meal Bars:**

| | C | F | Cb |
|---|---|---|---|
| Blueberry Greek Yogurt Bar, 1.7 oz | 200 | 8 | 22 |
| Chocolate Chip Cookie Dough, 2 oz | 220 | 10 | 32 |
| Chocolate Chip Granola, 1.7 oz | 200 | 9 | 19 |
| Choc. Peanut Butter, 2 oz | 250 | 14 | 23 |
| Choc. Peanut Butter Pretzel, 1.7 oz | 210 | 10 | 19 |
| Cinnamon Bun; Mudslide, 1.7 oz | 210 | 10 | 19 |
| Cookies 'n Crème, 1.7 oz | 200 | 11 | 19 |
| Strawb. Almond, 1.7 oz | 200 | 9 | 20 |

**Snack Bars:** *Per 1.6 oz bar*

| | C | F | Cb |
|---|---|---|---|
| Caramel Chocolate Nut Roll | 190 | 13 | 19 |
| Caramel Chocolate Peanut Nougat | 170 | 11 | 20 |
| Caramel Double Chocolate Crunch | 160 | 9 | 22 |
| Cashew Trail Mix Bar | 170 | 11 | 19 |
| Chocolate Chip Crisp | 140 | 6 | 17 |
| Chocolate Hazelnut | 180 | 14 | 18 |
| Chocolate Oatmeal Fiber | 130 | 5 | 24 |
| Classic Trail Mix | 190 | 15 | 13 |
| Cranberry Almond Bar | 150 | 6 | 16 |
| Coconut Almond Delight | 200 | 15 | 18 |
| Dark Choc. Almond Coconut Crunch | 190 | 15 | 17 |
| Dark Chocolate Decadence Bar | 160 | 9 | 22 |
| Sweet & Salty Trail Mix | 190 | 14 | 15 |
| Triple Chocolate | 160 | 9 | 17 |

*Note: Snack Bars Carb figure includes 4-15g sugar alcohol*

**Attune Bars:**

**Probiotic Bars:** *Per 0.7 oz Bar*

| | C | F | Cb |
|---|---|---|---|
| Dark Chocolate | 80 | 6 | 11 |
| Milk Choc. Crisp | 90 | 6 | 12 |
| Mint Chocolate | 90 | 6 | 12 |

**Balance:**

**Original Bars:**

| | C | F | Cb |
|---|---|---|---|
| Average, 1.8 oz | 200 | 7 | 21 |
| Dark Chocolate varieties, 1.6 oz | 180 | 6 | 20 |
| Bare, av., 1.2 oz | 160 | 9 | 17 |
| Bites, 1 pouch, 1.5 oz | 190 | 7 | 20 |

**Cascadian Farms** *(General Mills):*

| | C | F | Cb |
|---|---|---|---|
| Chewy Granola, av. all var., 1.2 oz | 135 | 3 | 26 |
| Crunchy Granola, all var., 2 bars, 1.4 oz | 185 | 8 | 27 |
| Granola Bark, average, 1 oz piece | 140 | 8 | 16 |
| Protein Granola Bars, av. all var., 1.8 oz | 250 | 15 | 21 |

*Per Bar*

**Clif:**

| | C | F | Cb |
|---|---|---|---|
| **Original:** Av. all varieties., 2.4 oz | 240 | 5 | 45 |
| Mini size, average, 1.2 oz | 100 | 2.5 | 17 |
| **Builder's:** Av. all varieties, 2.4 oz | 270 | 8 | 30 |
| Max, average all varieties, 3.4 oz | 385 | 13 | 40 |
| **Dark Choc.:** Cherry Almond, 1.4 oz | 180 | 9 | 23 |
| Average other varieties, 1.4 oz | 195 | 11 | 20 |
| **Kid,** ZBar, av. all varieties, 1.3 oz | 125 | 3.5 | 23 |
| **Mojo,** average, 1.6 oz | 190 | 11 | 21 |

**Corazonas:**

**Heartbar Oatmeal Squares:** *Per 1.8 oz Bar*

| | C | F | Cb |
|---|---|---|---|
| PB Oatmeal; White Choc. Macad. | 200 | 7 | 29 |
| Average other varieties | 185 | 7 | 28 |

**Curate:**

| | C | F | Cb |
|---|---|---|---|
| Balsamic Fig & Hazelnut, 1.6 oz | 190 | 9 | 23 |
| Av. other varieties, 1.6 oz | 195 | 10 | 21 |
| Kid's, av. all flavors, 1.2 oz | 160 | 7 | 20 |

**Detour:**

| | C | F | Cb |
|---|---|---|---|
| **Original,** Caramel Peanut, 3 oz | 350 | 11 | 32 |

**Lean Muscle:**

| | C | F | Cb |
|---|---|---|---|
| Cookie Dough Caramel Crisp, 3.2 oz | 370 | 12 | 33 |
| P'nut Butter Choc. Crunch, 3.2 oz | 420 | 18 | 33 |

**Lower Sugar,** average all varieties,

| | C | F | Cb |
|---|---|---|---|
| 1.4 oz | 170 | 5.5 | 16 |
| 2.8 oz Bar | 340 | 11 | 33 |

*Note: Low Sugar Bars Carb figures include 12-28g sugar alcohol*

**Simple:**

| | C | F | Cb |
|---|---|---|---|
| Full size, 20g Protein, av., 2.1 oz | 230 | 8 | 24 |
| Snack size, 10g Protein, av., 1 oz | 110 | 4 | 11 |

**Smart:** Coconut Almond, 1.3 oz | 150 | 5 | 16

| | C | F | Cb |
|---|---|---|---|
| Fruit varieties, 1.3 oz | 135 | 2.5 | 18 |
| Peanut Butter Chocolate, 1.3 oz | 160 | 6 | 16 |

**dotFIT:**

**dotBAR:**

| | C | F | Cb |
|---|---|---|---|
| Double Choc. Brownie, 3.3 oz | 370 | 13 | 38 |
| Peanut Butter Cup, 3.3 oz | 370 | 13 | 38 |

*Note: dotBARS Carb figure includes 21g sugar alcohol*

**dotSTICK,** Iced, av. all var., 2 oz | 190 | 6 | 26

*Note: dotSTICK Bars Carb figure includes 8g sugar alcohol*

**EAS:**

**AdvantEDGE:**

| | C | F | Cb |
|---|---|---|---|
| Carb Control, average all varieties, 2 oz | 235 | 8 | 27 |

*Note: Carbohydrate figures includs 17-19g sugar alcohol*

| | C | F | Cb |
|---|---|---|---|
| **Lean**, average all varieties, 1.8 oz | 210 | 7 | 22 |
| **Myoplex 30,** av. all varieties, 3 oz | 355 | 11 | 35 |
| **Extend Bar:** Crunch, av., 1.4 oz | 150 | 2.5 | 30 |
| Anytime, av. all varieties, 1.4 oz | 145 | 4 | 22 |

*Note: Carbohydrate figures include 4-9g sugar alcohol*

## Bars ~ Brands (Cont) | C | F | Cb

*Per Bar*

| | C | F | Cb |
|---|---|---|---|
| **Fiber One:** 90-Calorie Bar, | | | |
| av. all varieties, 0.8 oz | 90 | 2 | 17 |
| **Cheesecake Bar,** all flavors, 1.4 oz | 150 | 6 | 24 |
| **Chewy:** Protein Caramel Nut, 1.2 oz | 130 | 6 | 16 |
| Other Protein Nut Varieties, 1.2 oz | 140 | 6 | 17 |
| Oat Varieties, average, 1.4 oz | 140 | 4 | 29 |
| **General Mills:** *Per 1.6 oz Bar* | | | |
| Milk 'n Cereal Bar, | | | |
| Honey Nut Cheerios | 160 | 4 | 28 |
| **Glenny's:** *Per 1 oz Bar* | | | |
| **Cashew/Cranberry & Almond,** av. | 145 | 7 | 17 |
| **Cherry & Almond** | 130 | 6 | 18 |
| **Classic Fruit & Nut** | 140 | 6 | 18 |
| **Peanuts & Peanut Butter** | 170 | 13 | 10 |
| **Glucerna:** | | | |
| **Crispy Delights,** | | | |
| Peanut/Choc. Chip, av., 1.4 oz | 150 | 5 | 20 |
| *Note: Carbohydrate figure includes 7g sugar alcohol* | | | |
| **Mini Snack Bar,** average, 0.7 oz | 80 | 3.5 | 10 |
| *Note: Carbohydrate figure includes 2-5 g sugar alcohol* | | | |
| **Great Value** *(Walmart):* | | | |
| **Chewy Granola:** 90 calorie, 0.8 oz | 90 | 1.5 | 18 |
| Peanut Butter Choc Chip, 0.8 oz | 100 | 2.5 | 19 |
| **Chewy Fiber,** av., 1.4 oz | 140 | 4 | 29 |
| **Crunchy Granola,** 2-bar pkg, 1.4 oz | 200 | 7 | 29 |
| **Fruit & Grains,** av., 1.3 oz | 140 | 2.5 | 25 |
| **Sweet & Salty,** Almond, 1.2 oz | 160 | 8 | 20 |
| **Trail Mix,** Fruit & Nut, 1.2 oz | 140 | 4 | 24 |
| **Health Valley:** | | | |
| **Cobbler Cereal Bars,** 1.3 oz | 130 | 2.5 | 27 |
| **HMR,** Benefit Bars, av. all, 1.4 oz | 160 | 5 | 22 |
| **Init:** | | | |
| **Dark Choc.,** av., 1.4 oz | 180 | 10 | 23 |
| **Mixed Nut & Sweet Berries,** 1.4 oz | 180 | 9 | 24 |
| **Rstd Nuts & Honey Chipotle,** 1.4 oz | 190 | 13 | 18 |
| **Jenny Craig:** S'mores, 1.3 oz | 140 | 4 | 22 |
| Yogurt Dream Bar, 1.2 oz | 130 | 4.5 | 20 |
| **Kashi:** Cereal Bars, 1.3 oz | 130 | 3 | 24 |
| **Granola & Seed Bars:** | | | |
| 1 Bar, av. all varieties, 1.2 oz | 145 | 4 | 24 |
| 2 Bars, av. all varieties, 1.4 oz | 180 | 7 | 27 |
| **Granola Bars:** | | | |
| Chewy, average all varieties, 1.3 oz | 135 | 3 | 21 |
| Crunchy, all varieties, | | | |
| 2 bars, 1.4 oz | 170 | 6 | 26 |
| Layered, av. all, 1 oz | 125 | 4 | 21 |
| **Savory Bars,** av., 1 oz | 140 | 5 | 20 |
| **Kellogg's:** | | | |
| **Cinnabon Bar,** Original, 1.3 oz | 150 | 4.5 | 26 |
| **Fiber Plus,** Protein, av., 1.4 oz | 170 | 8 | 18 |
| **Nutrigrain** ~ *See page 33* | | | |
| **Special K** ~ *See page 34* | | | |

*Per Bar*

| | C | F | Cb |
|---|---|---|---|
| **Kind:** *Per 1.4 oz Bar* | | | |
| **Fruit & Nut:** | | | |
| Almond & Apricot | 180 | 10 | 23 |
| Apple Cinnamon & Pecan | 190 | 12 | 20 |
| Nut Delight | 210 | 16 | 20 |
| **Healthy Grains,** av. all varieties, 1.2 oz | 145 | 5 | 24 |
| **Nuts & Spices:** | | | |
| Cashew & Ginger Spices | 200 | 14 | 16 |
| Madagascar Vanilla Almond | 210 | 16 | 14 |
| Average other varieties | 200 | 14 | 16 |
| **Plus:** | | | |
| PB with. Dark Choc. | 200 | 13 | 17 |
| Average other varieties | 185 | 12 | 20 |
| **Strong & Kind,** all varieties, 1.6 oz | 230 | 16 | 15 |
| **Kudos,** av. all varieties, 0.9 oz | 100 | 3 | 17 |
| **Labrada:** | | | |
| **Cookie Roll,** Cinnamon Bun, 2.8 oz | 300 | 8 | 35 |
| **Lean Body Protein Bar:** | | | |
| Caramel Peanut; S'mores | 360 | 14 | 33 |
| P'nut Butter & Jelly | 350 | 12 | 36 |
| **Larabar:** | | | |
| **Apple Pie,** 1.6 oz | 190 | 10 | 24 |
| **Cherry Pie,** 1.7 oz | 200 | 8 | 30 |
| **Chocolate Chip Brownie,** 1.6 oz | 200 | 9 | 31 |
| **Peanut Butter & Jelly,** 1.7 oz | 210 | 10 | 27 |
| **Strawberry Shortcake,** 1.6 oz | 200 | 11 | 24 |
| **Lindora,** av. all varieties, 1.6 oz | 155 | 5 | 15 |
| **Luna:** | | | |
| **Regular,** av., 1.69 oz | 190 | 6 | 26 |
| **Dark Chocolate,** (5g Sugar), | | | |
| av. all varieties, 1.5 oz | 180 | 8 | 20 |
| **Protein,** av. all varieties, 1.6 oz | 180 | 7 | 21 |
| **Marathon** *(Snickers):* | | | |
| **Energy:** Chewy, av. all var., 2 oz | 210 | 8 | 26 |
| Crunchy, Dark Chocolate, 1.6 oz | 150 | 4.5 | 22 |
| **Protein,** average all, 2.8 oz | 285 | 9 | 40 |
| **Market Pantry** *(Target):* | | | |
| **Granola Bars:** | | | |
| Chewy: Choc Chip, 0.8 oz | 100 | 3 | 17 |
| Choc. Chunk; S'Mores, 0.8 oz | 90 | 1.5 | 18 |
| Crunchy, Oats & Honey, 1.5 oz | 180 | 6 | 28 |
| **Mariani:** *Per 1.4 oz Bar* | | | |
| **Honey Bars:** Cranb.; Granola, av. | 170 | 8 | 23 |
| Sesame | 200 | 14 | 16 |
| **Medifast:** Chewy, all var., 1.3 oz | 110 | 3 | 15 |
| Crunch, av. all varieties, 1.2 oz | 110 | 3 | 13 |
| *Note: Crunch Bars Carb figure includes 2-3g sugar alcohol* | | | |
| Maintenance, Cararmel Nut, 1.5 oz | 170 | 5 | 22 |
| **Meta,** average all varieties, 1.41 oz | 150 | 3 | 31 |

| **Bars ~ Brands (Cont)** | **C** | **F** | **Cb** |
|---|---|---|---|

*Per Bar*

**Met-Rx:**

**Big 100,** av. all varieties, 3.5 oz — 375 — 6 — 49

**Big 100 Colossal:**

Av. all var., 3.5 oz — 410 — 13 — 45

Minis, av. all varieties, 1.2 oz — 130 — 4 — 15

**Prime,** average all varieties, 2.3 oz — 210 — 5 — 29

**Protein Plus,**

Chocolate Chocolate Chunk, 3.2 oz — 310 — 10 — 29

**Mojo Bars** ~ *See List*

**Muscle Milk** *(Cytosport):*

**Collegiate,** av. all varieties, 1.4 oz — 170 — 6 — 18

**High Protein,** av. all varieties, 2.6 oz — 315 — 11 — 30

**Protein Crunch,**

Chocolate PB, 2.9 oz — 360 — 13 — 31

**Protein Snack,** all varieties, 1.6 oz — 190 — 6 — 19

**Naure's Path:**

**Chewy,** average all varieties, 1.2 oz — 140 — 4 — 25

**Crunchy,** average all varieties, 1.4 oz — 190 — 7 — 28

**Qi'a Superfood Snack Bar,** av. 1.3 oz — 185 — 9 — 19

**Nature Valley:**

**Crunchy Granola Bars:**

Apple Crisp (2), 1.5 oz — 170 — 7 — 26

Average other var. (2), 1.5 oz — 185 — 7 — 28

**Granola Thins,** av. all var., 0.6 oz — 85 — 4.5 — 11

**Protein,** all varieties, 1.4 oz — 190 — 12 — 14

**Sweet & Salty,** 1.3 oz — 165 — 8 — 21

**Trail Mix,** Chewy, av. all, 1.3 oz — 135 — 4 — 25

**Yogurt,** Chewy, all varieties, 1.2 oz — 140 — 4 — 26

**NuGo:**

**Dark,** average all varieties — 200 — 5 — 29

**Family:** Choc. Banana — 190 — 2.5 — 25

Av. other varieties — 170 — 3 — 26

**Fiber:** Orange Cranberry — 130 — 3 — 32

Coconut Macaroon; P'nut Choc Chip — 160 — 6 — 28

Average other varieties — 140 — 4 — 30

**Gluten Free,** average all varieties — 180 — 4 — 28

**Organic,** all varieties — 190 — 5 — 26

**Slim:** Espresso — 170 — 5 — 20

Average other varieties — 185 — 5 — 19

**Smarte Carb:** Choc. Black Berry — 150 — 3 — 22

Peanut Butter Crunch — 190 — 4 — 19

*Note: Smarte Carb Bars Carb figure includes 12-16 g sugar alcohol*

**Stronger:**

Cookies 'N Crm; Caramel Pretzel, av. — 290 — 7 — 36

Average other varieties — 315 — 12 — 35

**Nutri-Grain** *(Kellogg's):*

Fruit Crunch (2), 1.5 oz — 185 — 7 — 29

Harvest, 1.5 oz — 180 — 5 — 34

Soft Baked B'fast Cereal Bars,

average all varieteies, 1.3 oz — 125 — 3.5 — 24

*Per Bar*

| | **C** | **F** | **Cb** |
|---|---|---|---|

**Nutrilite** *(Amway Global):*

**Energy Bars:** Choc. Nut Roll, 1.6 oz — 180 — 6 — 16

Mixed Berry Smoothie, 1.6 oz — 180 — 4 — 28

**Whey Protein,** av. all varieties, 2.5 oz — 300 — 25 — 28

**NutriSystem:**

**Granola Breakfast Bars:**

Chewy Chocolate Chip — 150 — 2 — 27

Peanut Butter — 160 — 5 — 25

**Odwalla:**

**Chewy**

Choc. Alm. Coconut, 1.6 oz — 200 — 8 — 29

White Chocolate Macadamia — 210 — 10 — 27

**Nourishing:** *Per 2 oz Bar*

Choco-walla — 210 — 5 — 39

Dark Chocolate Chip Walnut — 220 — 7 — 36

**Protein,** Choc. Chip Peanut, 2 oz — 230 — 8 — 33

**Superfood:** *Per 2 oz Bar*

Original — 210 — 4.5 — 39

Berries GoMega — 210 — 6 — 36

Blueberry Swirl — 200 — 3 — 41

Strawberry Pomegranate — 200 — 2 — 42

**Oh Yeah!** *(ISS):*

**Original,** 3 oz — 380 — 19 — 31

**Good Grab,** P'nut Butter Crunch, 1.6 oz — 190 — 10 — 19

**One Bar,** 2.1 oz — 220 — 7 — 23

*Note: One Bar Carb figure includes 10g sugar alcohol*

**Victory Bars,** av. all varieties, 2.3 oz — 200 — 6 — 26

**Optifast,** 800 Bars, average, 1.6 oz — 165 — 4 — 20

**PowerBar:**

**Harvest Energy:** Cranb. Oatmeal — 130 — 2.5 — 23

Peanut Butter Choc Chip — 220 — 10 — 22

Rstd Peanut Butter — 140 — 4.5 — 21

Toffee Chocolate Chip — 210 — 9 — 23

**Performance Energy: Bars:**

Nutty Berry; PB & Jelly, average — 220 — 4 — 39

Wafers, average all varieties, 1 pkt — 175 — 4.5 — 31

**Protein & Recovery:**

12g Protein, Triple Threat, av. all — 190 — 8 — 24

20g Protein Plus, Choc. Mint Cookie — 270 — 8 — 30

30g Protein Plus, av. all varieties — 335 — 10 — 40

**Power Crunch** *(BNRG),*

Orig. Protein Bar, av. all var., 1.4 oz — 205 — 12 — 10

**PR Bar:** Chocolate Peanut. 1.8 oz — 200 — 7 — 22

Yogurt Berry, 1.8 oz — 210 — 7 — 22

Granola, Oatmeal Raisin, 1.8 oz — 210 — 7 — 22

**Premier Nutrition:**

**Premier Protein:**

Fiber Bars, average all var., 1.8 oz — 195 — 7 — 26

*Note: Fiber Bars Carb figure includes 3-8g sugar alcohol*

Protein Bars, average all var., 2.5 oz — 280 — 7 — 24

Note: Actual weight of bars is usually 5-10% more than label Net Weight. Weigh bar and allow extra calories.

### Bars ~ Brands (Cont)

| Per Bar | C | F | Cb |
|---|---|---|---|
| **Promax:** | | | |
| **Gluten-Free,** av. all varieties, 2.6 oz | 285 | 8 | 37 |
| **Lower Sugar,** av. all varieties, 2.4 oz | 230 | 7 | 33 |
| **Pro Series,** av. all varieties, 3.17 oz | 340 | 12 | 39 |
| **Proti Bars** (Bariatrix), av. all var. | 160 | 5.5 | 16 |
| **PureFit,** av. all varieties, 2 oz | 220 | 7 | 25 |
| **Pure Protein:** | | | |
| **Hi Protein,** average all varieties: | | | |
| 1.8 oz bar | 190 | 5 | 18 |
| 1.9 oz | 200 | 5 | 22 |
| 2.8 oz bar | 300 | 10 | 28 |
| Note: Hi Protein Bars Carb figure includes 5-8g Sugar Alcohol | | | |
| **Quaker:** | | | |
| **Baked Bars:** | | | |
| Protein, average all varieties, 1.7 oz | 190 | 6 | 25 |
| Soft Baked, av. all, 1.5 oz | 140 | 3.5 | 26 |
| **Granola Bars:** | | | |
| Chewy: 25% Less Sugar, Choc. Chip, 08 oz | 100 | 3.5 | 17 |
| 90 Calories, av. all var., 1 oz | 90 | 2 | 19 |
| Big, average all varieties, 1.5 oz | 170 | 6 | 29 |
| Dipps, Caramel Nut | 140 | 6 | 21 |
| Yogurt, all varieties, 1.2 oz | 150 | 4.5 | 25 |
| Quinoa, average all varieties, 1.3 oz | 150 | 6 | 24 |
| **Oatmeal To Go,** | | | |
| Regular, average all varieties, 2 oz | 220 | 4 | 43 |
| **Real Medleys,** av. all varieties, 1.3 oz | 170 | 7 | 25 |
| **Quest Bar:** | | | |
| **Protein Bar,** | | | |
| average all varieties | 185 | 8 | 22 |
| Note: Protein Bars Carb figure includes 1-6g Sugar Alccohol | | | |
| **Revival Soy** (Direct): | | | |
| Chocolate Temptation | 270 | 7 | 32 |
| Marshmallow Crunch | 220 | 2.5 | 30 |
| Peanut Pal | 240 | 6 | 28 |
| **Low Carb**, average all varieties | 235 | 8 | 31 |
| Note: Low Carb Bars Carb figure includes 20-22g Sugar Alcohol | | | |
| **Slim-Fast:** | | | |
| **Meal Bars:** | | | |
| Chewy Chocolate Crisp, 1.7 oz | 200 | 6 | 25 |
| Chocolate P'nut Caramel, 1.6 oz | 200 | 7 | 21 |
| Sweet & Salty Choc. Almond, 1.6 oz | 200 | 8 | 21 |
| **Snack Bars,** average all flavors | 100 | 3 | 16 |
| **SoyJoy Bars,** av. all var., 1 oz | 135 | 6 | 16 |
| **Solo,** GI, av. all, 1.8 oz | 200 | 7 | 26 |

| Per Bar | C | F | Cb |
|---|---|---|---|
| **Special K:** | | | |
| **Cereal Bars,** av. all varieties, 0.8 oz | 90 | 1.5 | 17 |
| **Chewy Nut Bars,** Cranb Almond, 1.2oz | 150 | 6 | 21 |
| **Chewy Snack Bars,** | | | |
| av. all varieties, 0.9 oz | 100 | 2 | 19 |
| **Protein Granola Bars,** | | | |
| all varieties, 1 bar, 0.9 oz | 110 | 3 | 17 |
| **Protein Meal,** av. all varieties, 1.6 oz | 175 | 5 | 25 |
| **Supreme Protein:** | | | |
| **High Protein:** | | | |
| PB Crunch | 400 | 18 | 26 |
| Cookies & Cream | 370 | 14 | 30 |
| Rocky Road Brownie | 410 | 18 | 32 |
| Note: High Protein Bars Carb figure includes 14-15g sugar alcohol | | | |
| **thinkThin:** | | | |
| **High Protein,** Choc. Strawb., 2oz | 250 | 9 | 24 |
| Note: Carb figure includes 12g sugar alcohol | | | |
| **Protein Nut,** average all var., 1.4 oz | 190 | 12 | 16 |
| **Tiger's Milk:** | | | |
| Protein Rich, 1.2 oz | 140 | 5 | 19 |
| Peanut Butter Crunch, 1.2 oz | 150 | 6 | 18 |
| King Size, average all varieties, 2 oz | 225 | 9 | 28 |
| **Toaster Strudel** ~ see page 64 | | | |
| **Trader Joe's:** | | | |
| **Chewy Coated Granola Bars, 6-Packs:** | | | |
| Chocolate Chip, 1.3 oz | 150 | 4 | 26 |
| Peanut Butter, 1.3 oz | 170 | 8 | 19 |
| Vanilla Almond, 1.3 oz | 150 | 6 | 22 |
| **Fruit Bars:** Fig 1.5 oz | 120 | 2 | 24 |
| Average other varieties, 1.5 oz | 140 | 2.5 | 27 |
| **Granola Bars, 6-packs:** | | | |
| Fiberful, 1.3 oz | 120 | 3.5 | 22 |
| Trail Mix, 1.3 oz | 150 | 5 | 23 |
| **Tri-O-Plex** (Chef Jay's): | | | |
| **High Protein,** | | | |
| Ban. Walnut, 4.2 oz | 405 | 14 | 40 |
| **Duo,** Bursting Peanut Butter | 395 | 17 | 35 |
| **Usana:** | | | |
| Berry Nutty, 1.4 oz | 160 | 8 | 22 |
| Choco Chip, 1.4 oz | 160 | 5 | 17 |
| Peanutt Bliss, 1.2 oz | 160 | 6 | 18 |
| **Zone Perfect:** | | | |
| Choc, Chip Cookie Dough, 1.5 oz | 180 | 5 | 24 |
| Chocolate Peanut Butter, 1.8 oz | 210 | 7 | 24 |
| Dark Choc., av. all, 1.5 oz | 190 | 6 | 22 |
| Fudge Graham, 1.8 oz | 210 | 7 | 23 |
| Strawberry Yogurt, 1.8 oz | 200 | 6 | 25 |
| Sweet & Salty, Cashew Pretzel, 1.6 oz | 200 | 7 | 23 |

## Cocoa & Hot Chocolate  **C**  **F**  **Cb**

**Cocoa:**

| | C | F | Cb |
|---|---|---|---|
| Small (8 fl.oz): | | | |
| with Whole Milk | 205 | 8.5 | 22 |
| with Nonfat Milk | 145 | 1 | 23 |
| Tall (12 fl.oz): with Whole Milk | 280 | 12 | 26 |
| with Nonfat Milk | 185 | 1 | 28 |

**Hot Chocolate:**

| | C | F | Cb |
|---|---|---|---|
| Small (8 fl.oz): with Whole Milk | 180 | 7 | 26 |
| with Nonfat Milk | 140 | 2 | 27 |
| Tall (12 fl.oz): with Whole Milk | 260 | 10 | 36 |
| with Nonfat Milk | 190 | 2 | 37 |
| **Cinnabon,** Mochalatta Chill, 16 oz | 420 | 17 | 63 |
| **Swiss Miss,** Mixes, av., 1 packet | 120 | 2.5 | 22 |

## Cocoa - Chocolate Mixes

***Add extra cals/fat/carbohydrate for milk***
**Carnation Breakfast Drinks** ~ *See Page 38*
**Carnation:** *Per 3 Tbsp*

| | C | F | Cb |
|---|---|---|---|
| Malted Milk: Original | 90 | 2 | 15 |
| Chocolate | 90 | 1 | 18 |

**Ghirardelli:**

| | C | F | Cb |
|---|---|---|---|
| Chocolate Mocha, 3 Tbsp, 1.2 oz | 120 | 1.5 | 29 |
| Double Chocolate, 3 Tbsp, 1.3 oz | 120 | 1.5 | 30 |

**Hershey's,** Cocoa,

| | C | F | Cb |
|---|---|---|---|
| Natural, unsweetened, 1 Tbsp, 0.2 oz | 10 | 0.5 | 3 |

**Land O Lakes:**

| | C | F | Cb |
|---|---|---|---|
| Arctic White Coccoa, 1.3 oz | 160 | 6 | 26 |
| Other varieties, 1.3 oz | 140 | 3.5 | 26 |

**Nestle:** *Per Per Single Serve Envelope*

| | C | F | Cb |
|---|---|---|---|
| Chocolate Caramel | 100 | 3 | 19 |
| Dark Chocolate | 100 | 3 | 19 |
| Rich Milk Chocolate: | | | |
| Regular | 80 | 3 | 14 |
| Fat Free | 25 | 0 | 5 |
| No Sugar Added | 50 | 0 | 9 |

**Nesquik Powder:** *Per 2 Tbsp*

| | C | F | Cb |
|---|---|---|---|
| Chocolate; Strawberry | 60 | 0.5 | 15 |
| Chocolate; Strawb., No Added Sugar | 35 | 1 | 7 |

**Ovaltine,** All Natural Cocoa Mixes,

| | C | F | Cb |
|---|---|---|---|
| average all varieties, 2 Tbsp | 40 | 0 | 10 |

**Swiss Miss:** *Per Single Serve Envelope*

| | C | F | Cb |
|---|---|---|---|
| **Breakfast Blends:** Great Start | 60 | 1 | 11 |
| Pick Me Up | 110 | 2 | 23 |

**Classics, Milk Chocolate:**

| | C | F | Cb |
|---|---|---|---|
| Hot Cocoa Mix | 90 | 2 | 16 |
| No Added Sugar | 60 | 1 | 10 |
| with Marshmallow | 90 | 2 | 16 |
| Rich Chocolate | 120 | 2 | 23 |

## Instant Coffee  **C**  **F**  **Cb**

**Powder/Granules:** *Regular or Decaffeinated,*

| | C | F | Cb |
|---|---|---|---|
| 1 level tsp | 2 | 0 | 0.5 |
| 1 rounded tsp | 4 | 0 | 1 |
| **Ground,** 3 tsp | 7 | 0 | 2 |
| **Brewed/Percolated,** 1 cup, 8 fl.oz | 4 | 0 | 1 |

**Coffee with Milk/Cream/Creamers:** *Per 8 oz Cup*

| | C | F | Cb |
|---|---|---|---|
| **Black:** | 4 | 0 | 1 |
| with Whole Milk: Dash, 1 Tbsp | 15 | 0.5 | 2 |
| 2 Tbsp, 1 fl.oz | 25 | 1 | 2.5 |
| with 2% Milk, 2 Tbsp | 20 | 0.5 | 2.5 |
| with 1% Milk, 2 Tbsp | 20 | 0.5 | 2.5 |
| with Fat Free Milk, 2 Tbsp | 15 | 0 | 2.5 |
| with Soy Milk: 1 Tbsp | 10 | 0 | 1.5 |
| 2 Tbsp, 1 oz | 15 | 0.5 | 2 |
| with Half & Half: 2 Tbsp | 50 | 3 | 3 |
| ¼ cup, 2 fl.oz | 90 | 6 | 4 |
| with Cream (light coffee), 2 Tbsp | 65 | 6 | 2 |
| with Coffee Mate: Liquid, reg., 1 T. | 20 | 1 | 3 |
| Liquid Fat Free, 1 Tbsp | 25 | 0 | 2 |
| Powder, 1 heaping tsp | 15 | 1 | 2 |
| **Sugar ~ Add Extra:** 1 heaping tsp | 25 | 0 | 6 |
| Single portion, 1 package | 25 | 0 | 6 |
| **Sweeteners,** *(Equal/Splenda/Sweet N Low),* Powder, 1 package | 0 | 0 | 0 |

## Flavored Coffee Mixes

**Chicory:**

| | C | F | Cb |
|---|---|---|---|
| Instant Coffee, 1 tsp | 5 | 0 | 1 |
| Coffee Essence, 1 tsp | 15 | 0 | 4 |

**Caffé D'Vita:**

| | C | F | Cb |
|---|---|---|---|
| Mixes, average all varieties, 3 tsp, | 60 | 1.5 | 11 |
| Sugar Free Mixes, 2 tsp | 35 | 2 | 3 |

**General Foods International:**

| | C | F | Cb |
|---|---|---|---|
| Average all varieties, 0.5 oz | 60 | 3 | 10 |
| Sugar-free, av. all varieties, 1 tsp | 30 | 2.5 | 2 |
| Cappuccino Coolers, all varieties, 0.5 oz | 60 | 0 | 15 |

**Hills Bros:** *Per 3 Tbsp, 1 oz*

| | C | F | Cb |
|---|---|---|---|
| Cappuccino: French Vanilla | 120 | 4.5 | 19 |
| Chocolate Hazelnut | 110 | 3.5 | 19 |
| Classic Cappuccino | 120 | 5 | 17 |
| Dark Chocolate | 110 | 4 | 19 |
| Mocha Mint | 120 | 4 | 20 |

| | C | F | Cb |
|---|---|---|---|
| **Nescafe,** Memento, 1 stick, average all varieties | 100 | 2.5 | 19 |
| **Starbucks,** VIA, Iced Coffee, all varieties, 1 stick/packet | 100 | 0 | 24 |

## Coffee Shops/Restaurants

*Per 8 fl.oz Cup (Unless Indicated)*

| | C | F | Cb |
|---|---|---|---|
| **Coffee,** Regular/Percolated/Filtered | 5 | 0 | 0 |
| **Americano Drip Coffee,** 1 cup | 7.5 | 0 | 1 |
| **Cafe Au Lait:** 1 cup, 8 fl.oz | 60 | 3.5 | 5 |
| Nonfat Milk, 1 cup, 8 fl.oz | 35 | 0 | 5 |
| **Caffe Latté:** | | | |
| 8 fl.oz cup: with Whole Milk | 110 | 6 | 9 |
| with 2% Milk | 100 | 3.5 | 9 |
| with Nonfat Milk | 70 | 0 | 10 |
| 12 fl.oz: with Whole Milk | 180 | 9 | 14 |
| with Nonfat Milk | 100 | 0 | 15 |
| 16 fl.oz: with Whole Milk | 220 | 11 | 18 |
| with Nonfat Milk | 130 | 0 | 19 |
| **Cafe Mocha (Mochaccino):** 8 fl.oz | 150 | 6 | 20 |
| 12 fl.oz | 230 | 9 | 31 |
| 16 fl.oz | 290 | 12 | 41 |
| **Cappuccino:** | | | |
| 8 fl.oz cup: with Whole Milk | 90 | 3.5 | 7 |
| with 2% Milk | 80 | 3 | 8 |
| with Nonfat Milk | 50 | 0 | 8 |
| 12 fl.oz: with Whole Milk | 110 | 6 | 9 |
| with 2% Milk | 90 | 3.5 | 9 |
| with Nonfat Milk | 60 | 0 | 9 |
| 16 fl.oz: with Whole Milk | 140 | 7 | 11 |
| with 2% Milk | 120 | 3.5 | 11 |
| with Nonfat Milk | 80 | 0 | 12 |
| **Mocha:** *With Cream* | | | |
| 8 fl.oz: with Whole Milk | 200 | 11 | 22 |
| with Nonfat Milk | 160 | 6 | 22 |
| 12 fl.oz: Whole Milk | 290 | 15 | 33 |
| with Nonfat Milk | 230 | 8 | 34 |
| **Iced Mocha:** *Without Cream* | | | |
| 12 fl.oz: with Whole Milk | 170 | 6 | 26 |
| with Nonfat Milk | 130 | 2 | 27 |
| **Espresso:** Single (Solo), 1 fl.oz | 5 | 0 | 1 |
| Double (Doppio), 2 fl.oz | 10 | 0 | 2 |
| **Espresso con Panna,** | | | |
| (w/ dollop wh. cream), solo, 1 fl.oz | 30 | 2.5 | 2 |
| **Espresso Macchiato,** solo, 1 fl.oz | 5 | 0 | 1 |
| **Frappuccino:** Tall, 12 fl.oz | 180 | 2.5 | 37 |
| Grande, 16 fl.oz | 240 | 3 | 48 |
| **Frappuccino Mocha:** | | | |
| (with Cream): Tall, 12 fl.oz | 280 | 11 | 43 |
| Grande, 16 fl.oz | 380 | 15 | 57 |
| **Iced Latte,** Similar to Caffe Latte | | | |

**McCafe (McDonald's)** ~ *See Fast Food, Page 216*
**Starbucks** ~ *See Fast-Foods Section , Page 243*

## Coffee Substitute Mixes    C   F   Cb

**Roasted Cereal Beverages ~** *(No Caffeine)*

| | C | F | Cb |
|---|---|---|---|
| **Cafix,** Instant Beverage, 1 tsp | 5 | 0 | 1 |
| **Kaffree Roma,** Instant Beverage, 1 tsp | 10 | 0 | 2 |
| **Teeccino,** Herbal Coffees, 1 tsp | 10 | 0 | 2 |

## Irish & Liqueur Coffees

| | C | F | Cb |
|---|---|---|---|
| **Irish Coffee,** without sugar | 175 | 10 | 0 |
| **Liqueur Coffee,** with cream, all varieties, av., 1 fl.oz | 100 | 5 | 7 |

## Coffee Extras

| | C | F | Cb |
|---|---|---|---|
| Chocolate (Cocoa) Topping, ½ tsp | 5 | 0 | 1 |
| Flavored Syrups: Regular, 2 Tbsp | 80 | 0 | 20 |
| Sugar-free, 2 Tbsp | 0 | 0 | 0 |
| Half & Half Cream: 2 Tbsp | 40 | 3.5 | 1 |
| Single serve pkg, ⅜ fl.oz | 15 | 1.5 | 0.5 |
| Light whipped cream, 2 Tbsp | 15 | 1.5 | 1 |
| Marshmallows, miniature (2) | 5 | 0 | 1 |
| **Sugar:** | | | |
| 1 single portion package | 20 | 0 | 5 |
| 1 level tsp | 15 | 0 | 4 |
| 1 heaping tsp | 25 | 0 | 6 |
| *Equal/Splenda/Sweet 'N Low* | 0 | 0 | 0 |

## Coffee Shop ~ Cakes, Cookies

| | C | F | Cb |
|---|---|---|---|
| **Cookies:** | | | |
| Biscotti, 1 oz | 140 | 6.5 | 18 |
| Chocolate Chip, 3 oz | 350 | 15 | 54 |
| Oatmeal Raisin, 3 oz | 350 | 12 | 56 |
| Peanut Butter, 3 oz | 410 | 25 | 39 |
| White Choc. Macadamia, 3.33 oz | 420 | 20 | 55 |
| **Cakes/Pastries:** | | | |
| Almond Croissant, 5 oz | 620 | 35 | 67 |
| Apple Danish, 5 oz | 450 | 18 | 67 |
| Banana Walnut, 4.5 oz | 410 | 17 | 60 |
| Brownie, 3 oz | 390 | 24 | 42 |
| Bundt, Chocolate, 4 oz | 440 | 21 | 61 |
| Carrot Cake, 4 oz | 400 | 22 | 45 |
| Chocolate Cake, 5 oz | 530 | 28 | 65 |
| Crumble Coffee Cake, 4.5 oz | 500 | 25 | 65 |
| Cupcake, 3 oz | 330 | 16 | 43 |
| Pound Cake, av., 3 oz | 330 | 17 | 40 |
| **Cinnamon Roll,** 6 oz | 500 | 15 | 83 |
| **Donuts:** | | | |
| Sugared, 1.8 oz | 220 | 11 | 27 |
| Glazed, 2 oz | 250 | 12 | 34 |
| **Pretzel,** large, 4 oz | 290 | 5 | 52 |

**Starbucks Bakery Items** ~ *See Page 244*

## READY TO DRINK COFFEE  C  F  Cb

### Bottled & Chilled:

| | | | |
|---|---|---|---|
| **Full Throttle Coffee & Energy** ~ *See Page 38* | | | |
| **International Delight,** | | | |
| Iced, all flavors, 8 fl.oz | **150** | 2.5 | 29 |
| **Java Monster Energy** ~ *See Page 39* | | | |
| **Kahlua,** Cappuccino Shake, 10.5 fl.oz | **130** | 2 | 24 |
| **Starbucks:** | | | |
| **Doubleshot Coffee & Protein (20g):** *Per 11 fl.oz Can* | | | |
| Dark Chocolate | **210** | 2.5 | 33 |
| Vanilla Bean | **200** | 2.5 | 34 |
| **Doubleshot Energy:** *Per 15 fl.oz Can* | | | |
| Coffee Drink | **210** | 2.5 | 36 |
| Hazelnut Drink | **210** | 3 | 31 |
| Mocha Drink | **200** | 2.5 | 33 |
| Vanilla Drink | **210** | 2.5 | 34 |
| Light | **130** | 2.5 | 20 |
| White Chocolate Drink | **210** | 3 | 31 |
| **Doubleshot Espresso:** *Per 6.5 fl.oz Can* | | | |
| Espresso & Cream | **140** | 6 | 18 |
| Espresso & Cream Light | **70** | 4 | 5 |
| **Frappuccino Coffee Drink:** *Per 9.5 fl.oz Bottle* | | | |
| Mocha | **180** | 3 | 33 |
| Light Mocha | **100** | 3 | 12 |
| Vanilla | **200** | 3 | 37 |
| **Iced Coffee:** *Per 11 fl.oz Bottle* | | | |
| Coffee: with Milk | **110** | 0.5 | 23 |
| Light | **50** | 1 | 11 |
| Caramel | **110** | 0.5 | |
| Vanilla | **120** | 0.5 | 22 |
| **Iced Espresso Classics (Chilled):** *Per 8 fl.oz Bottle* | | | |
| Caffe Mocha | **140** | 2.5 | 23 |
| Caramel Macchiato | **130** | 2.5 | 21 |
| Vanilla Latte | **130** | 2.5 | 21 |
| **Skinny:** Caramel Macchiato | **70** | 0 | 10 |
| Vanilla Latte | **70** | 0 | 10 |
| **Starbucks Refreshers** ~ *See Page 40* | | | |
| **TruMoo:** | | | |
| **Coffee Milk:** | | | |
| Low-Fat (1%), 1 cup, 8 fl.oz | **130** | 2.5 | 20 |
| Fat-Free, 1 cup, 8 fl.oz | **110** | 0 | 20 |

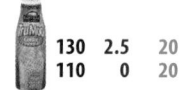

### Tips to Reduce the Calories in Your Coffee Drinks:

- Request non-fat milk in place of whole or 2% milk
- Downsize to 8 fl.oz or 12 fl.oz
- Avoid cream on frappuccinos
- Replace sugar with *Equal, Splenda, Stevia* or *Sweet 'N Low*
- Avoid syrup add-ons

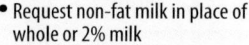

## CAFFEINE COUNTER

Moderate caffeine intake is not harmful to healthy adults. However, frequent large amounts (over 350mg/day) may cause dependency ('caffeinism') and adversely affect health. **To be safe, limit caffeine to 200mg/day.** Avoid if pregnant, breast feeding, a child under 8, have sleep problems, an overactive bladder or heart arrhythmia.

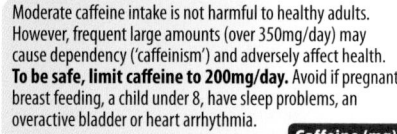

**Caffeine (mg)**

| | |
|---|---|
| **Coffee: Instant:** Weak, 1 level teaspoon | 30 |
| Medium, 1 rounded teaspoon | 60 |
| Strong, 1 heaping teaspoon | 100 |
| **Decaffeinated**, 1 rounded teaspoon | 2 |
| **Bags (Folgers)**, 1 bag (6-8 fl.oz) | 115 |
| **Ground**, 1 Tbsp, 0.2 oz | 60 |
| **Bottled (Ready-To-Drink)**, 9.5 fl.oz | 70 |
| **Coffee Shop:** Brewed, 8 fl.oz | 110 -150 |
| **Cappuccino/Latte:** 1 cup, 8 fl.oz | 75 |
| Tall, 12 fl.oz | 110 |
| Large, 16 fl.oz | 150 |
| **Decappuccino**, decaffeinated | 5 |
| **Espresso:** Regular/Single/Solo | 75 |
| Double/Doppio | 150 |
| Iced Coffee w/o Milk, 12 fl.oz | 140 |
| Latte, 1 cup, 8 fl.oz | 75 |
| Mocha, 1 cup, 8 fl.oz | 90 |
| Hot Chocolate, 8 fl.oz | 15 |
| **Black Tea:** Weak, 1 cup | 20 |
| Medium Strength, 1 cup | 40 |
| Strong, 1 cup | 70 |
| Decaffeinated Tea, 1 cup | 0-5 |
| Herbal Tea, 1 cup | 0 |
| **Green Tea**, 1 cup | 20 |
| **Iced Tea**, tall glass/can, 12 fl.oz | 20-30 |
| **Soft Drinks:** *Per 12 fl.oz Can* | |
| Coca-Cola; Pepsi (Regular/Diet) | 35 |
| Diet Coke; TAB; RC Cola (Regular) | 45 |
| Dr. Pepper; Sunkist Orange | 40 |
| Pepsi One; Mountain Dew; Mellow Yellow; Surge | 55 |
| Pepsi Max (Regular/Diet) Sun Drop (Reg/Diet) | 70 |
| 7-Up, Fanta, Sprite, Fresca, Diet Rite Cola | 0 |
| **Energy Drinks (with added caffeine):** | |
| *(AMP, Adrenaline Rush, Full Throttle Monster, No Fear, Red Bull, Rockstar)* | |
| **Average all brands:** 8 fl.oz | 80 |
| 16 fl.oz | 160 |
| **NOS Energy**, 16 fl.oz | 260 |
| **Chocolate Bars:** Milk Chocolate, 2 oz | 20 |
| Dark Chocolate, 2 oz | 30 |
| **Choc Chip Cookies**, 2 medium, 2 oz | 6 |
| **Chocolate Syrup**, 2 Tbsp, 1.4 oz | 5 |
| **Guarana**, *GNC*, 1 tablet | 90 |
| **Medicinals:** *Excedrin Extra*/Migraine, 1 tab. | 65 |
| *Jet Alert/NoDoz*, 1 tablet | 200 |
| *Stay Awake (Walgreens), Vivarin*, 1 tab. | 200 |

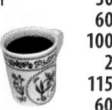
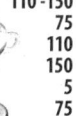
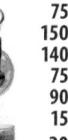
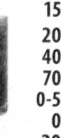
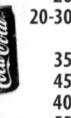
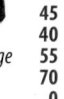
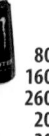
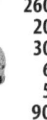
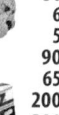

## Energy/Protein Drinks

| | C | F | Cb |
|---|---|---|---|
| 5-hour Energy, 2 fl.oz | 4 | 0 | 1 |
| **A.B.B:** | | | |
| **Energy:** Speed Shot, 8.5 fl.oz | 0 | 0 | 0 |
| Ripped Force, 18 fl.oz | 90 | 0 | 23 |
| **Pure-Pro:** | | | |
| Pure Pro 35 Shake, all flav., 12 fl.oz | 160 | 0.5 | 5 |
| Pure Pro 50, all flavors, 14.5 fl.oz | 240 | 1.5 | 7 |
| **Maxx Recovery**, all flavors, 18 fl.oz | 400 | 0.5 | 60 |
| **AdvantEDGE** *(EAS)*, | | | |
| Carb Control, av., 11 fl.oz | 105 | 2.5 | 3 |
| **AllSport Hydration:** | | | |
| Regular, all flavors, 20 fl.oz | 150 | 0 | 40 |
| Zero, 20 fl.oz | 0 | 0 | 0 |
| **AMP Energy:** *Per 16 fl.oz Can* | | | |
| **Original** | 220 | 0 | 58 |
| Berry; Pssn'frt; Strawb Limeade | 220 | 0 | 58 |
| Cherry Blast | 120 | 0 | 31 |
| **Boosted**, all flavors | 100 | 0 | 26 |
| **Arizona,** Caution Performance: | | | |
| **Regular,** 11.5 fl.oz | 150 | 0 | 38 |
| **Low Carb,** 11.5 oz | 20 | 0 | 7 |
| **Atkins,** Advantage Shakes, av., 11 fl.oz | 155 | 9 | 4 |
| **Bariatrix,** Proti-Max, | | | |
| Anytime Shakes, av., 8 fl.oz | 100 | 4 | 4 |
| **Bawls Guarana:** | | | |
| Av. all Flavors: 10 fl.oz bottle | 120 | 0 | 30 |
| 16 fl.oz can | 185 | 0 | 46 |
| **Blue Sky,** Blue Energy, 8 fl.oz | 120 | 0 | 29 |
| **BodyArmor,** SuperDrinks, | | | |
| all flavors, 16 fl.oz | 140 | 0 | 36 |
| **Bolthouse:** *Per 8 fl.oz* | | | |
| **Breakfast Smoothies,** | | | |
| Peach/Strawberry Parfait, 8 fl.oz | 190 | 2.5 | 35 |
| **Protein Plus:** Blended Coffee | 190 | 2.5 | 26 |
| Choc.; Mango; Vanilla, av. | 200 | 2 | 30 |
| **Boost** *(Nestle Health Care): Per 8 fl.oz* | | | |
| **Original**, all flavors | 240 | 4 | 41 |
| **Breeze** | 250 | 0 | 54 |
| **Glucose Control**, all flavors | 190 | 7 | 16 |
| **High Protein**, all flavors | 240 | 6 | 33 |
| **Plus**, all flavors | 360 | 14 | 45 |
| **Carnation:** | | | |
| **Breakfast Essentials :** | | | |
| Powder Only: | | | |
| Av. all flav., 1 env., 1.3 oz | 130 | 1 | 27 |
| No Sug. Added, av. , 0.7 oz | 60 | 1 | 12 |
| **Ready To Drink:** Reg., all flav., 8 fl.oz | 240 | 4 | 41 |
| High Protein, average, 8 fl.oz | 220 | 6 | 28 |
| **Celestial Seasoning,** | | | |
| Kombucha, all flavors, 2 oz shot | 30 | 0 | 8 |
| **CeraSport,** EX1, Lime Flavor, 8.5 fl.oz | 20 | 0 | 1 |
| **Champion Lyte,** Sports Drink | 0 | 0 | 0 |

| Champion Nutrition: | C | F | Cb |
|---|---|---|---|
| Heavywt Gainer 900, av., 4 scps, 5.4 oz | 600 | 7 | 102 |
| Pure Whey Plus, av., 1 scoop, 1.2 oz | 130 | 2 | 5 |
| **Clif Shot,** | | | |
| Energy Gel, av. all flavors, 1.2 oz pkt | 105 | 1 | 21 |
| **Cocaine,** Energy, 8.4 fl.oz can | 70 | 0 | 18 |
| **Core Power:** 20g, av. all, 11.5 fl.oz | 150 | 3.5 | 12 |
| 26g, average all flavors, 11.5 fl.oz | 240 | 3.5 | 27 |
| 42g, average all flavors, 14 fl.oz | 240 | 3.5 | 12 |
| **Curves,** Protein Drink, | | | |
| Choc.; Vanilla, 2 scps, 1 oz | 120 | 1 | 12 |
| **CytoSport:** | | | |
| **Muscle Milk:** | | | |
| Powder, all flavors, av., 2 scoops | 310 | 12 | 18 |
| Ready To Drink: Chocolate, 10 fl.oz | 170 | 7 | 8 |
| 17 fl.oz | 340 | 16 | 16 |
| Non Dairy, Chocoalte, 12 fl.oz | 170 | 4 | 13 |
| **EAS** ~ *See AdvantEdge & Myoplex* | | | |
| **Ensure:** *Per Bottle* | | | |
| **Original**, all flavors, 8 fl.oz | 220 | 6 | 33 |
| **Clear**, all flavors, 10 fl.oz | 180 | 0 | 37 |
| **Enlive**, av. all flavors, 8 fl.oz | 350 | 11 | 44 |
| **High Protein** , all flav., 8 fl.oz | 160 | 2 | 19 |
| **Plus**, all flavors, 8 fl.oz bottle | 350 | 11 | 50 |
| **Enterex**, Diabetic, all flavors, 8 fl.oz | 240 | 9 | 27 |
| **Enu**, Nutritional Shakes, av., 11 fl.oz | 485 | 16 | 61 |
| **FRS**, Energy & Endurance, | | | |
| all flavors, 11.5 fl oz | 80 | 0 | 22 |
| **Fruit₂O (Veryfine):** Classic 20 fl.oz | 0 | 0 | 0 |
| Sparkling, 20 fl.oz | 0 | 0 | 1 |
| **Full Throttle:** *Per 16 fl.oz* | | | |
| **Energy:** Citrus; Blue Agave | 220 | 0 | 58 |
| Red Berry | 230 | 0 | 58 |
| **Fuze:** | | | |
| **Blends**, average, 16.9 fl.oz | 185 | 0.5 | 43 |
| **Juice:** Berry Punch, 8 fl.oz | 80 | 0 | 21 |
| Strawb. Lemonade, 8 fl.oz | 100 | 0 | 26 |
| **Gatorade:** | | | |
| **G Series:** *Ready To Drink* | | | |
| Endurance, Thirst Quencher: 12 fl oz | 80 | 0 | 21 |
| 32 fl oz bottle | 215 | 0 | 56 |
| Prime, Sports Fuel, | | | |
| 4 fl oz pouch | 100 | 0 | 25 |
| Recover, | | | |
| Protein Shake, av., 11.2 fl.oz | 270 | 1 | 46 |
| **Genisoy**, Prot. Pdr, Choc.; Van., 1.3 oz | 125 | 0 | 18 |
| **Glaceau:** Smartwater, 8 fl.oz | 0 | 0 | 0 |
| Vitaminwater, all flav., 20 fl.oz | 120 | 0 | 32 |
| **Glucerna,** Shakes, all flavors, 8 fl.oz | 190 | 7 | 23 |

| | C | F | Cb |
|---|---|---|---|
| **GNC:** | | | |
| **Lean Shake:** Powder, all flav., 2 scps | 180 | 2 | 30 |
| Lean Shake 25, Ready To Drink, | | | |
| average all flavors, 14 fl.oz bottle | 170 | 6 | 6 |
| Advanced: Burn, all flavors, 2 scoops | 170 | 0.5 | 11 |
| Tone & Define, Pink Lmnade, 1 scp | 35 | 2.5 | 3 |
| **Pro Performance Powder:** | | | |
| Amplified: Mass XXX, | | | |
| Strawb; Vanilla, 4 level scoops | 750 | 6 | 124 |
| Wheybolic Extr. 60, Choc. Fudge, 1 scp | 100 | 1 | 3 |
| **Golazo:** | | | |
| **Sports Energy:** All flavors, 12 fl.oz | 90 | 0 | 22 |
| Sugar Free, Mango Lime, 12 fl.oz | 10 | 0 | 6 |
| **Sports Hydration,** | | | |
| Mango Lime, 20 fl. oz bottle | 130 | 0 | 33 |
| **Guru,** Energy: Regular, 8 oz can | 80 | 0 | 21 |
| Lite, 12 oz can | 10 | 0 | 3 |
| Water, all flavors, 12 oz can | 0 | 0 | 0 |
| **Hammer,** Gel, av. all, 1.7 Tbsp, 1.2 oz | 85 | 0 | 22 |
| **Hansen's:** Energy Pro, 8 fl.oz | 130 | 0 | 34 |
| Energy Diet Red, 8 fl.oz | 20 | 0 | 6 |
| **Herbalife:** Nutr. Shake, 1 pkt | 90 | 1 | 13 |
| with 8 fl.oz non-fat milk | 170 | 1 | 26 |
| **Hormel:** Protein Powder, 1.2 oz pkt | 130 | 1.5 | 3 |
| Mighty Shakes, all flav., 8.45 fl.oz | 500 | 22 | 54 |
| Vital Quisine, all flavors, 14. fl.oz | 210 | 9 | 8 |
| **Hype:** | | | |
| **Energy:** After Dark, Hype, 8.8 fl.oz | 130 | 0 | 30 |
| MFP, 8.8 fl.oz | 110 | 0 | 25 |
| Up, Ice Berry Max, 8.8 fl.oz | 125 | 0 | 30 |
| **Enlite**, 8.8 fl.oz | 25 | 0 | 4 |
| **Shot**, 3.5 fl.oz | 20 | 0 | 5 |
| **Jarrow:** | | | |
| **Whey Protein:** Unflavored, 0.8 oz | 95 | 2 | 2 |
| Chocolate; Vanilla, 1 oz | 105 | 1 | 6 |
| **Java Monster:** *Per 15 fl.oz Can* | | | |
| **Regular**, average all flavors | 190 | 3 | 33 |
| **Light**, Vanilla | 95 | 3 | 13 |
| **Kellogg's:** | | | |
| **To Go, Breakfast Shakes:** | | | |
| RTD, all flavors, av., 10 fl.oz bottle | 185 | 5 | 29 |
| Shake Mix, all flavors, av., 1 pkt | 130 | 0.5 | 27 |
| **Knudsen:** Recharge, average, 8 fl.oz | 75 | 0 | 18 |
| Simply Nutritious, av. all, 8 fl.oz | 120 | 0 | 30 |
| **Kombucha,** Wonder Drink, 8.4 fl.oz | 60 | 0 | 16 |
| **La Brada:** | | | |
| **Powders, Lean Body:** | | | |
| High Prot. Meal Replacement, 2.8 oz | 330 | 8 | 24 |
| **RTD:** Lean Body, 17 fl.oz | 260 | 9 | 9 |
| On The Go, 14 fl.oz | 180 | 7 | 4 |
| **Liquid Ice:** Black, 8.3 fl.oz | 110 | 0 | 26 |
| Other Flavors, 8.3 fl oz | 120 | 0 | 28 |
| **Liquid Lightning,** | | | |
| Regular, 8.5 fl.oz | 90 | 0 | 22 |

| | C | F | Cb |
|---|---|---|---|
| **Max Velocity:** | | | |
| **Regular:** 8.5 fl.oz can | 130 | 0 | 33 |
| 16 fl.oz can | 240 | 0 | 62 |
| **Sugar Free**, 16 fl.oz can | 15 | 0 | 1 |
| **Met-Rx:** | | | |
| **Protein Plus:** | | | |
| Powder, Choc., 2 scoops | 220 | 1.5 | 7 |
| Ready To Drink 51, av. all, 15 fl.oz | 245 | 2 | 6 |
| **Metabolol:** Endurance, 2 scoop, 1.8 oz | 200 | 5 | 24 |
| GlyProXTS, 1 scoop, 0.7 oz | 30 | 0 | 4 |
| Metabolol II, 2 scoops, 2.3 oz | 260 | 3 | 40 |
| Met Max, mix, 2 scoops, 2.2 oz | 230 | 2.5 | 11 |
| **MLO,** Mus-L Blast, Chocolate, 4 scoops | 570 | 3 | 114 |
| **Monster,** Energy: 16 fl.oz can | 200 | 0 | 54 |
| Lo-Carb, 16 fl.oz | 20 | 0 | 6 |
| M-80, 16 fl.oz | 180 | 0 | 46 |
| Mixxd (with Juice), 16 fl.oz | 220 | 0 | 54 |
| **MRM:** All Natural Whey, 1 scoop, 0.9 oz | 90 | 1 | 2 |
| Low Carb Protein, 1 scoop, 1 .1 oz | 120 | 2.5 | 2 |
| **Muscle Milk** ~ *See Cytosport* | | | |
| **Muscle Tech:** *Dry Powder Only* | | | |
| 100% Ultra Premium, | | | |
| Mass Gainer, 2 scoops, 11.6 oz | 1290 | 4 | 260 |
| Mass-Tech Advantage, | | | |
| Milk Chocolate, 5 scoops, 9 oz | 1000 | 9 | 168 |
| Nitro Tech Lean Muscle, Van., 1.3 oz | 140 | 1.5 | 1 |
| **Myoplex** *(EAS):* | | | |
| **Original Shakes, (RTD):** | | | |
| Average all flavors, 17 fl.oz | 300 | 7 | 19 |
| Strength Formula, 14 fl.oz | 210 | 2.5 | 23 |
| **Powder:** Original Choc. 1 pkt, 2.8 oz | 300 | 6 | 21 |
| Lite, av. all flavors , 1 pkt, 1.9 oz | 180 | 2 | 24 |
| **Nature's Best:** | | | |
| **Carbo Power,** all flavors, 16 fl.oz | 400 | 0 | 100 |
| **Isopure:** Alpine Punch, 20 fl.oz | 260 | 0 | 25 |
| Mass, all flavors, 20 fl.oz | 350 | 0 | 53 |
| Zero Carb, all flavors, 20 fl.oz | 160 | 0 | 0 |
| **JavaPro Ready To Drink**, | | | |
| Coffee, 8 fl.oz | 100 | 1.5 | 5 |
| **Nestle Health Science:** | | | |
| **Diabetisield**, Mixed Berry, 8 fl.oz | 150 | 0 | 30 |
| **No-Fear:** Regular, 16 fl.oz | 260 | 0 | 72 |
| Sugar Free, 16 fl.oz | 20 | 0 | 2 |
| **Noni,** Tahitian, 2 Tbsp | 15 | 0 | 3 |
| **NOS:** | | | |
| **High Performance Energy, CMPLX6** | | | |
| Grape, 16 fl.oz can | 210 | 0 | 54 |
| Av. other flavors, 16 fl.oz | 200 | 0 | 55 |
| Zero, 16 fl.oz | 0 | 0 | 0 |
| **Nutrament** *(Nestle)*, 12 fl.oz | 360 | 10 | 52 |

## Energy/Protein Drinks (Cont)

| | C | F | Cb |
|---|---|---|---|
| **Nutrilite** (Amway): | | | |
| **Body Key Meal Replacement Shakes:** | | | |
| Powder, av. all flavors, 1.2 oz scoop | 110 | 3 | 8 |
| Ready To Drink, all flavors, 11 fl.oz | 140 | 3 | 15 |
| **Optifast** (Nestle): | | | |
| **800:** Shake Mix, 1 pkg | 160 | 3 | 20 |
| Ready To Drink Shakes, 8 fl.oz | 160 | 3 | 20 |
| **HP Shake Mix**, 1 pkg | 200 | 6 | 10 |
| **Optimum Nutrition:** | | | |
| **100%:** Whey, Gold Standard, 1 oz scp | 120 | 1 | 4 |
| Hydro Builder, Choc Shake, 1.9 oz | 180 | 2.5 | 10 |
| Hydro Whey, 1.4 oz scoop | 140 | 1 | 3 |
| **Optisource** (Nestle), | | | |
| Very High Protein Drink, 8 fl.oz | 200 | 6 | 12 |
| **Powerade:** | | | |
| **Sports Drink:** | | | |
| Regular, av. all flav.,12 fl.oz | 80 | 0 | 22 |
| Zero, 12 fl.oz | 0 | 0 | 0 |
| **PowerBar:** | | | |
| Performance Energy Blends, | | | |
| average, 1 pouch | 80 | 0 | 21 |
| Power Gel, av. all flavors, 1.5 oz pkg | 110 | 0 | 27 |
| **Propel,** Purified Water, 12 fl.oz | 0 | 0 | 0 |
| **Protein2O,** av. all flavors, 16.9 fl oz | 70 | 0 | 2 |
| **Radioactive:** | | | |
| Regular: 10.5 oz | 150 | 0 | 37 |
| 16 oz | 220 | 0 | 56 |
| Sugar Free, all sizes | 0 | 0 | 0 |
| **Red Bull:** | | | |
| Energy Drink, all flavors: | | | |
| 8.3 fl.oz | 110 | 0 | 28 |
| 12 fl.oz can | 160 | 0 | 40 |
| Simply Cola, 12 fl.oz | 130 | 0 | 31 |
| Sugar-Free, 8.4 fl.oz | 10 | 0 | 3 |
| Zero Calories, 8.4 fl.oz | 0 | 0 | 0 |
| **Revival,** Soy Mix, unsweetened: | | | |
| Plain, 2 scoops, 0.95 oz | 105 | 1 | 4 |
| Chocolate Day Dream, 1 package | 120 | 2.5 | 7 |
| Strawberry, 1 package | 15 | 2 | 4 |
| **Rhino's,** Energy Drink, | | | |
| all flavors, 100ml | 50 | 0 | 11 |
| **Rip It,** Energy Fuel, Citrus X, 16 fl.oz | 200 | 0 | 52 |
| **Rockstar:** Per 16 fl.oz Can | | | |
| **Energy Drink:** Punched, av. | 270 | 0 | 62 |
| Sugar Free | 20 | 0 | 0 |
| **Rumble,** Supershake, | | | |
| all flavors, 12 fl.oz bottle | 250 | 8 | 28 |
| **Rush:** Per 8.4 fl.oz | | | |
| **Energy Drink:** Regular | 120 | 0 | 32 |
| Sugar Free | 0 | 0 | 0 |
| with Maca, 8 fl.oz | 130 | 0 | 30 |

| | C | F | Cb |
|---|---|---|---|
| **Slim-Fast:** | | | |
| **Meal Replacement Shakes,** | | | |
| Advanced Nutrition, | | | |
| av. all flavors, 11 fl.oz | 180 | 8 | 6 |
| **SoBe:** Per 20 fl.oz Can/Bottle | | | |
| **Citrus Energy Fruit Drink** | 250 | 0 | 64 |
| **Lifewater:** Strawberry Kiwi | 100 | 0 | 26 |
| Coconut Water | 80 | 0 | 21 |
| O-Cal, all flavors | 0 | 0 | 9 |
| Note: Carb figure inlude 7-10g sugar alcohol | | | |
| **Solixir,** Energy Drink, av. all, 12 fl.oz | 55 | 0 | 13 |
| **Special K:** | | | |
| **Protein Shakes,** av. all flavors | 185 | 5 | 23 |
| **Spiru-Tein:** | | | |
| **Energy Meal Shakes Powder:** | | | |
| Chai Latte, 1 scoop, 1.2 oz scoop | 130 | 0 | 16 |
| Av. other flavors, 1.2 oz scoop | 105 | 0 | 13 |
| Gold, Banana Berry Blast, 1.2 oz | 100 | 0 | 19 |
| PureTrition, av., 1.3 oz scoop | 115 | 0.5 | 10 |
| Whey, Cookies & Cream, 1.2 oz scp | 110 | 1 | 10 |
| **Starbucks:** | | | |
| **Refreshers,** av. all flav.,12 fl.oz | 65 | 0 | 19 |
| **Doubleshot Energy** ~ See page 37 | | | |
| **Steaz:** Energy, all flav., 12 fl.oz | 135 | 0 | 35 |
| Zero Calorie, Berry, 12 fl.oz | 0 | 0 | 0 |
| **The Sports Club/LA:** | | | |
| Beachbody Whey Prot. Powder, | | | |
| Chocolate; Vanilla, 2 scoops, 1.4 oz | 130 | 4 | 7 |
| **Twin Lab,** MVP Fuel, all flavors, | | | |
| 1 scoop, 0.5 oz | 25 | 0 | 6 |
| **Venom:** Mojave Rattler, 16 fl.oz | 50 | 0 | 8 |
| Av. other varieties, 16 fl.oz | 235 | 0 | 57 |
| **Verve:** Energy, 8.3 fl.oz can | 80 | 0 | 21 |
| Sugar Free | 5 | 0 | 0.5 |
| **Vital:** | | | |
| **100% Whey Powder**, 1.2 oz packet | 130 | 1.5 | 3 |
| **Protein Nutr. Shakes,** av., 14 fl.oz | 215 | 9 | 10 |
| **Weider:** | | | |
| **100% Whey**, 1 scoop, 1.4 oz | 160 | 3 | 12 |
| **Creatine ATP**, ½ cup, 1.7 oz | 210 | 0 | 37 |
| **Dynamic Weight Gainer**, av., 4.5 oz | 450 | 2 | 96 |
| **Mega Mass 2000**, av., 3.5 oz | 400 | 7 | 62 |
| **Pro Carb**, Ultimate Mass Gainer, | | | |
| 6 scoops, average, 7 oz | 770 | 6 | 161 |
| **Worx,** Energy, | | | |
| Original; Extra Strength, 2 fl.oz | 0 | 0 | 0 |
| **XS** (Quixtar), Energy Drink, 8.4 oz | 10 | 0 | 0 |
| **Zola Acai:** Original Juice, 8 fl.oz | 125 | 2 | 25 |
| Pomegranate, Blueberry, 8 fl.oz | 120 | 2 | 25 |

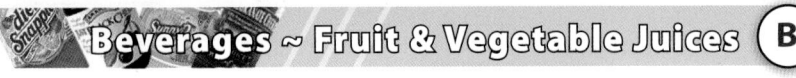
## Quick Guide          **C**  **F**  **Cb**

### Orange Juice
*Average ~ Fresh*

| | C | F | Cb |
|---|---|---|---|
| ½ Cup, 4 fl.oz | 55 | 0 | 13 |
| Small Glass, 6 fl.oz | 85 | 0 | 19 |
| Regular Cup 8 fl.oz | 110 | 0.5 | 26 |
| Regular Glass, 12 fl.oz | 160 | 0.5 | 39 |
| 10 fl.oz Bottle | 140 | 0.5 | 32 |
| 11.5 fl.oz Can | 160 | 0.5 | 37 |
| 16 fl.oz Bottle | 225 | 1 | 52 |
| 20 fl.oz Bottle | 280 | 1 | 64 |

### Juices ~ Generic

*Average All Brands:*

| | C | F | Cb |
|---|---|---|---|
| Aloe Vera Juice, unsweetened, 2 oz | 10 | 0 | 0 |
| Apple Juice: 8 fl.oz | 120 | 0 | 29 |
| 10 fl.oz Bottle | 145 | 0.5 | 36 |
| 16 fl.oz | 235 | 0.5 | 58 |
| Cactus Water, 1 Cup, 8 oz | 25 | 0 | 6 |
| Carrot Juice: Fresh, 6 fl.oz | 35 | 0 | 8 |
| Sweetened, 6 fl.oz | 75 | 0 | 17 |
| Coconut Water, 8 fl.oz | 50 | 0.5 | 9 |
| Cranberry Juice, Cocktail/Blend | 140 | 0 | 34 |
| Fruit Blends, average all, 8 fl.oz | 110 | 0 | 27 |
| Fruit Nectars, average all, 8 fl.oz | 140 | 0 | 36 |
| Grape Juice, 8 fl.oz | 155 | 0 | 38 |
| Grapefruit Juice, 8 fl.oz | 95 | 0 | 22 |
| Lemon/Lime Juice: 1 Tbsp | 5 | 0 | 1 |
| 1 cup, 8 fl.oz | 50 | 0.5 | 16 |
| Concentrate, 1 tsp | 0 | 0 | 0 |
| Noni Juice: | | | |
| Tahitian, 2 Tbsp, 1 fl.oz | 15 | 0 | 3 |
| Tahiti Traders, 1 fl.oz | 20 | 0 | 5 |
| Passion Fruit Juice, Fresh: | | | |
| Purple, 1 cup, 8 fl.oz | 125 | 0 | 34 |
| Yellow, 1 cup, 8 fl.oz | 80 | 1.5 | 14 |
| Papaya/Peach Nectar, av., 8 fl.oz | 140 | 0 | 36 |
| Pear Nectar, 8 fl.oz | 150 | 0 | 40 |
| Pineapple Juice, 8 fl.oz | 130 | 0 | 32 |
| Pomegranate Juice, 8 fl.oz | 160 | 0 | 40 |
| Prune Juice, 8 fl.oz | 180 | 0 | 45 |
| Strawb./Raspberry Juice, 8 fl.oz | 100 | 0 | 23 |
| Tangerine Juice, 8 fl.oz | 105 | 0.5 | 25 |
| Tomato Juice, 8 fl.oz | 40 | 0 | 10 |
| Vegetable Juice, 8 fl.oz | 45 | 0 | 11 |
| Wheat Grass Juice: | | | |
| 1 fl.oz 'Shot' | 10 | 0 | 1.5 |
| 2 fl.oz 'Shot' | 20 | 0 | 3 |

## Quick Guide          **C**  **F**  **Cb**

### Fruit Smoothies (Jamba Juice; Smoothie King)
*Average All Brands*

| | C | F | Cb |
|---|---|---|---|
| **Fruit Only:** 8 fl.oz | 115 | 0.5 | 29 |
| 12 fl.oz | 175 | 1 | 43 |
| 16 fl.oz | 230 | 1 | 58 |
| 24 fl.oz | 350 | 1 | 78 |
| **Fruit + Non-Fat Milk/Soy:** | | | |
| 12 fl.oz | 135 | 0 | 29 |
| 16 fl.oz | 155 | 0 | 37 |
| 24 fl.oz | 265 | 1 | 59 |
| **Fruit + Non-Fat Frozen Yogurt/Sherbet:** | | | |
| 12 fl.oz | 200 | 0.5 | 47 |
| 16 fl.oz | 265 | 1 | 63 |
| 24 fl.oz | 395 | 1.5 | 95 |

### Juice ~ Brands

*Per 8 fl.oz Unless Indicated*

| | C | F | Cb |
|---|---|---|---|
| **Apple & Eve:** | | | |
| **100% Juice**, No Sugar Added: | | | |
| Cherries & Berries; Cranb. Raspb., av. | 120 | 0 | 29 |
| Cranberry Apple | 130 | 0 | 33 |
| Cranberry Pomegranate | 140 | 0 | 34 |
| Fruitables, av. all flavors, 6.75 fl.oz | 60 | 0 | 14 |
| Organic Quenchers, all flav., 6.75 fl.oz | 40 | 0 | 10 |
| **Bolthouse Farms:** *Per 8 fl.oz* | | | |
| **Juice:** 100% Carrot | 70 | 0 | 14 |
| 100% Pomegranate | 150 | 0 | 38 |
| Acai+ 10 Superblend | 120 | 0 | 31 |
| Mango Coconut Squash | 60 | 0 | 15 |
| Orange & Carrot | 100 | 0 | 22 |
| **Fruit Smoothies:** | | | |
| Berry Boost | 120 | 0 | 27 |
| Blue Goodness | 160 | 0 | 34 |
| C-Boost | 110 | 0 | 27 |
| Green Goodness | 130 | 0 | 30 |
| Strawberry Banana | 130 | 0 | 32 |
| **Bright & Early** *(Minute Maid)*, | | | |
| Orange Juice (Chilled/Frozen) | 110 | 0 | 30 |
| **Cactus Cooler,** Orange Pineapple Blast, | | | |
| 12 fl oz can | 150 | 0 | 40 |
| **Campbell's:** | | | |
| **Tomato Juice:** 5.5 fl.oz can | 30 | 0 | 7 |
| 8 fl.oz | 50 | 0 | 10 |

### Juice Brands (Cont) — C F Cb

*Per 8 fl.oz Unless Indicated*

| | C | F | Cb |
|---|---|---|---|
| **Califia Farms:** *Per 10.5 fl.oz* | | | |
| **Agua Fresca:** Mango Chili Lime | 70 | 0 | 17 |
| Pineapple Ginger | 60 | 0 | 15 |
| Watermelon Ginger Lime | 50 | 0 | 13 |
| **Meyer Lemonade** | 100 | 0 | 36 |
| **Ginger Limeade** | 110 | 0 | 32 |
| **Orange Juice** | 110 | 0 | 27 |
| **Tangerine** | 110 | 0 | 25 |
| **Capri Sun:** *Per 6 fl.oz* | | | |
| **100% Juice**, average, | 85 | 0 | 21 |
| **Juice Drinks,** | | | |
| (25% Less Sugar), all flavors | 60 | 0 | 17 |
| **Roarin' Waters**, all flav., 6 fl.oz | 30 | 0 | 8 |
| **Clamato:** *Per 8 fl.oz* | | | |
| Original Tomato Cocktail | 60 | 0 | 12 |
| Picante | 60 | 0 | 13 |
| **Coco Joy,** Coconut Water, 8.4 fl.oz | 30 | 0 | 7 |
| **Coco Libre,** Coconut Water, 11 fl.oz pkg | 60 | 0 | 14 |
| **CocoZia,** Coconut Water: | | | |
| 100% Organic, 11.1 fl.oz pkg | 70 | 0 | 16 |
| Original, 8 fl.oz | 40 | 0 | 10 |
| Chocolate, 8 fl.oz | 60 | 0.5 | 13 |
| **Crystal Geyser:** | | | |
| **Juice Squeeze:** *Per 12 fl.oz Bottle* | | | |
| Blackberry Pomegranate | 170 | 0 | 43 |
| Ruby Grapefruit | 150 | 0 | 36 |
| Average other flavors | 130 | 0 | 32 |
| **Dole:** *Per 8 fl.oz* | | | |
| **Aguas Frescas**, average all flavors | 110 | 0 | 26 |
| **100% Pure**, Chilled or Frozen, av. | 120 | 0 | 28 |
| **Blended Juices**, average all flavors | 120 | 0 | 30 |
| **Florida's Natural:** *Per 8 fl.oz* | | | |
| Apple Juice | 120 | 0 | 29 |
| Cranberry Ruby Red Cocktail | 130 | 0 | 32 |
| Orange, No Pulp | 110 | 0 | 26 |
| 100% Blends: Orange Mango | 110 | 0 | 27 |
| Orange Pineapple | 130 | 0 | 31 |
| Orange Strawberry | 110 | 0 | 26 |
| Ruby Red Grapefruit, Original | 90 | 0 | 22 |
| **Goya:** *Per 12 fl.oz Can* | | | |
| **Nectar:** Guava; Tamarind | 240 | 0 | 59 |
| Mango | 230 | 0 | 56 |
| Papaya; Peach, average | 220 | 0 | 55 |
| Average other varieties | 220 | 0 | 55 |

*Per 8 fl.oz Unless Indicated*

| | C | F | Cb |
|---|---|---|---|
| **Great Value** *(Walmart):* | | | |
| **100% Juice:** *Per 8 fl.oz* | | | |
| Apple | 110 | 0 | 28 |
| Cranberry Pomegranate | 140 | 0 | 35 |
| Grape | 160 | 0 | 40 |
| Orange, all varieties | 110 | 0 | 26 |
| White Grape | 150 | 0 | 38 |
| **Hansen's:** | | | |
| **Juice Box:** *Per 6.75 fl.oz Box* | | | |
| Awesome Apple; Loud Lemonade, av. | 90 | 0 | 23 |
| Burstin Berry; Totally Tropical | 100 | 0 | 24 |
| Strawberry Banana | 110 | 0 | 27 |
| **Junior Juice,** | | | |
| 100% Juice, av. of flavors, | | | |
| 4.23 oz box | 60 | 0 | 16 |
| **Natural,** (64 fl.oz Bottles): *Per 8 fl.oz* | | | |
| Apple | 120 | 0 | 28 |
| Apple Strawberry | 110 | 0 | 27 |
| Cranberry Apple | 110 | 0 | 27 |
| Cranberry Grape | 140 | 0 | 35 |
| Grape | 120 | 0 | 33 |
| White Grape | 140 | 0 | 36 |
| **Hawaii's Own,** Frozen Concentrate, | | | |
| 10% Juice, average all flavors, | | | |
| 8 fl.oz prepared | 105 | 0 | 27 |
| **Hi-C Juice Drinks:** *Per 6.75 fl.oz Box* | | | |
| Flashin' Fruit Punch | 90 | 0 | 25 |
| Orange Lavaburst | 90 | 0 | 25 |
| Poppin' Lemonade | 100 | 0 | 27 |
| **Hood:** *Per 8 fl.oz* | | | |
| Apple | 120 | 0 | 31 |
| Lemonade | 110 | 0 | 29 |
| Orange | 120 | 0 | 30 |
| **Jamba Juice** ~ *See Fast-Foods Section* | | | |
| **Juicy Juice** *(Nestle):* | | | |
| Average all flavors: | | | |
| 4.23 fl.oz box | 60 | 0 | 15 |
| 6.75 fl.oz box | 100 | 0 | 24 |
| **Kerns:** | | | |
| **Nectars:** *Per 11.5 fl.oz Can* | | | |
| Guava; Strawberry | 210 | 0 | 53 |
| Pear; Strawb. Banana, av. | 220 | 0 | 53 |
| Pineapple Coconut | 280 | 8 | 53 |
| **Kool Aid:** *Per 6 fl.oz Containers* | | | |
| **Jammers,** | | | |
| Scary Blackberry; Tropical Punch | 70 | 0 | 19 |
| **L & A:** *Per 8 fl.oz* | | | |
| All Cherry | 180 | 0 | 45 |
| All Cranberry | 60 | 0 | 14 |
| Papaya Delight | 130 | 0 | 32 |
| Pineapple Coconut | 140 | 3 | 28 |

### Juice Brands (Cont)

| | C | F | Cb |
|---|---|---|---|

*Per 8 fl.oz Unless Indicated*

**Lakewood Organic:** *Per 8 fl.oz*

| | C | F | Cb |
|---|---|---|---|
| **Blends:** Acai Amazon Berry | 130 | 1.5 | 29 |
| Blueberry Blend | 120 | 0 | 31 |
| Cranberry Lemonade | 100 | 0 | 24 |
| Lemonade | 100 | 0 | 25 |
| Pineapple Coconut | 190 | 8 | 29 |
| Pomegranate Lemonade | 100 | 0 | 26 |
| Super Kale | 100 | 0 | 24 |
| Super Tomato | 50 | 0 | 14 |
| Super Veggie | 60 | 0 | 12 |
| **Pure:** Apple | 120 | 0 | 30 |
| Beet | 100 | 0 | 23 |
| Blueberry | 110 | 0 | 26 |
| Carrot | 90 | 0 | 21 |
| Pink Grapefruit | 100 | 0 | 24 |
| Prune | 170 | 0 | 41 |
| **Light**, Cranberry | 50 | 0 | 13 |

**Langers:** *Per 8 fl.oz*

| | C | F | Cb |
|---|---|---|---|
| **100% Juice:** All Pomegranate | 140 | 0 | 34 |
| Apple Cider | 120 | 0 | 28 |
| Apple Juice | 120 | 0 | 28 |
| Pineapple Coconut | 140 | 3 | 28 |
| Red/White Grape Juice | 160 | 0 | 40 |
| Strawberry Peach | 120 | 0 | 30 |
| **Juice Cocktails (27% Juice):** | | | |
| Blueberry Cranberry | 135 | 0 | 34 |
| Cranberry | 140 | 0 | 35 |
| Cranberry Grape | 165 | 0 | 41 |
| Cranberry Raspberry | 150 | 0 | 36 |
| Pomegranate, all varieties | 140 | 0 | 34 |
| White Cranberry, all var. | 120 | 0 | 28 |
| **20% Juice**, Strawberry Peach | 120 | 0 | 30 |

**Martinellli's:** *Per 8 fl.oz*

| | C | F | Cb |
|---|---|---|---|
| **Juice**, 100% Apple, all varieties | 140 | 0 | 35 |
| **Sparkling:** Apple Cider | 140 | 0 | 35 |
| Apple-Cranberry | 110 | 0 | 27 |
| Apple Grape | 120 | 0 | 31 |
| Apple-Mango/Pomegranate | 150 | 0 | 38 |
| Apple-Pear/Marionberry, av. | 130 | 0 | 32 |

*Per 8 fl.oz Unless Indicated*

**Minute Maid:**

| | C | F | Cb |
|---|---|---|---|
| **15.2 fl.oz Bottles:** *Per Bottle* | | | |
| Apple Juice | 210 | 0 | 52 |
| Cranb. Apple Raspberry | 230 | 0 | 61 |
| Cranberry Grape | 270 | 0 | 74 |
| Pineapple Orange | 220 | 0 | 55 |
| **Orange Juice,** | | | |
| Pure Squeezed, No Pulp, 8 fl.oz | 110 | 0 | 26 |
| **Coolers**, average all flavors, 6.75 fl.oz | 100 | 0 | 26 |
| **Kid's Juice Boxes,** 100% Juice, | | | |
| Apple White Grape, 6.75 fl.oz | 90 | 0 | 22 |
| **Light Juices:** Orange, 8 fl.oz | 50 | 0 | 13 |
| Average other flavors, 8 fl.oz | 15 | 0 | 3 |
| **Soft Frozen Concentrate,** | | | |
| Limeade, 3 fl.oz tube | 70 | 0 | 19 |

**Mott's:**

| | C | F | Cb |
|---|---|---|---|
| **100% Juice:** | | | |
| Original: Apple, 8 fl.oz | 120 | 0 | 29 |
| Apple White Grape, 6.75 fl.oz | 110 | 0 | 26 |
| Fruit Punch, 4.23 fl.oz | 60 | 0 | 15 |
| Light, Apple, 8 fl.oz | 50 | 0 | 12 |
| **Juice Drink:** | | | |
| Fruit Punch Rush, 8 fl.oz | 60 | 0 | 16 |
| Strawberry Boom, 8 fl.oz | 60 | 0 | 15 |
| Wild Grape Surge, 8 fl.oz | 60 | 0 | 16 |
| **Medleys:** | | | |
| Apple & Carrot, 8 fl.oz | 110 | 0 | 25 |
| Grape & Carrot, 8 fl.oz | 140 | 0 | 33 |
| **Mott's For Tots (47-54% Juice):** | | | |
| 40% Less Sugar: | | | |
| Grape; Apple White Grape, 8 fl.oz | 70 | 0 | 17 |
| Average other flavors, 8 fl.oz | 60 | 0 | 16 |

**Naked Juice:** *Per 8 fl.oz*

| | C | F | Cb |
|---|---|---|---|
| **100% Juice,** No Sugar Added: | | | |
| O-J | 110 | 0 | 27 |
| Orange Mango | 130 | 0 | 31 |
| Pomegranate Blueberry | 150 | 0 | 36 |
| **100% Juice Smoothie,** No Sugar Added: | | | |
| Berry Blast; Strawb. Banana | 130 | 0 | 30 |
| Mighty Mango | 150 | 0 | 36 |
| Orange Carrot | 120 | 0 | 29 |
| Boosted: Acai Machine | 160 | 3 | 31 |
| Blue Machine | 170 | 0 | 40 |
| Green Machine | 140 | 0 | 33 |
| Power-C Machine | 120 | 0 | 29 |
| Red Machine | 170 | 4.5 | 31 |
| **Coconut Water**, Pure, 16.9 fl.oz | 90 | 0.5 | 21 |

### Juice Brands (Cont)

| | **C** | **F** | **Cb** |
|---|---|---|---|

*Per 8 fl.oz Unless Indicated*

**Nantucket Nectars:**
**100% Juice:** *Per 16 fl.oz*

| | C | F | Cb |
|---|---|---|---|
| Peach Orange | 270 | 0 | 64 |
| Pineapple Orange Banana | 290 | 0 | 69 |
| Pomegranate Cherry | 230 | 0 | 57 |
| Premium Orange Juice | 220 | 0 | 51 |
| Pressed Apple | 240 | 0 | 59 |
| **Juice Cocktail**, Cranberry | 270 | 0 | 66 |

**Juice Drinks:** *Per 16 fl.oz*

| | C | F | Cb |
|---|---|---|---|
| Orange Mango | 250 | 0 | 60 |
| Pineapple Orange Guava | 240 | 0 | 58 |
| Pomegranate Pear | 230 | 0 | 57 |
| Red Plum | 250 | 0 | 61 |
| Watermelon Strawberry | 220 | 0 | 55 |
| **Lemonade**, Squeezed | 220 | 0 | 55 |

**Newman's Own:** *Per 8 fl.oz*

| | C | F | Cb |
|---|---|---|---|
| Lemonade, Regular; Pink | 110 | 0 | 27 |
| Limeade | 140 | 0 | 34 |

**Fruit Juice Cocktail:**

| | C | F | Cb |
|---|---|---|---|
| Gorilla Grape | 140 | 0 | 34 |
| Orange Mango Tango | 130 | 0 | 33 |

**Northland:** *Per 8 fl.oz*
**100% Juice:**

| | C | F | Cb |
|---|---|---|---|
| Blueberry Blackberry Acaí | | | |
| Cranb. Blackb./Cherry/Grape | 140 | 0 | 35 |
| Cranberry Cherry | | | |
| Cranberry Raspberry | 110 | 0 | 26 |
| **Superfruits**, Raspb. Pomegr. Goji | 130 | 0 | 32 |

**Ocean Spray:** *Per 8 fl.oz*
**Juice Cocktails:**

| | C | F | Cb |
|---|---|---|---|
| Blueberry; Cranberry | 110 | 0 | 28 |

**100% Juice Blends:**

| | C | F | Cb |
|---|---|---|---|
| Citrus Tangerine Orange | 110 | 0 | 28 |
| Cranberry Concord Grape | 130 | 0 | 33 |
| Cranberry Mango | 120 | 0 | 30 |
| Cranberry Raspberry | 120 | 0 | 30 |

**Juice Drinks:**

| | C | F | Cb |
|---|---|---|---|
| Cran-Apple | 120 | 0 | 31 |
| Cran-Grape | 120 | 0 | 31 |
| Cran-Tangerine | 110 | 0 | 28 |
| **Diet Juice Drinks**, all flavors | 5 | 0 | 2 |
| **Energy**, average all flavors, 10 fl.oz | 35 | 0 | 9 |
| **Light Juice Drinks**, av. all flavors | 50 | 0 | 13 |
| **Sparkling**, av. all flavors, 8.4 fl.oz | 85 | 0 | 21 |
| **Wave**, average all flavors, 8 fl.oz | 80 | 0 | 20 |

*Per 8 fl.oz Unless Indicated*

| | **C** | **F** | **Cb** |
|---|---|---|---|

**Odwalla:**
**100% Juice:** *Per 15.2 fl.oz Bottle*

| | C | F | Cb |
|---|---|---|---|
| Berry Greens | 160 | 0 | 39 |
| Groovin' Greens | 150 | 0 | 37 |
| Orange | 210 | 0 | 47 |

**Smoothies:** *Per 15.2 fl.oz Bottle*

| | C | F | Cb |
|---|---|---|---|
| Citrus C Monster | 240 | 0 | 58 |
| Mango Tango | 260 | 0 | 65 |
| Mo' Beta | 250 | 0 | 59 |
| Original Super Food | 240 | 0 | 58 |
| Red Rhapsody | 210 | 0 | 52 |
| Strawberry C Monster | 240 | 0 | 58 |

**Orange Julius:**
**Originals:** *Per Medium*

| | C | F | Cb |
|---|---|---|---|
| Mango P'apple, 22.2 oz | 450 | 0 | 114 |
| Orange, 17.5 oz | 270 | 0 | 68 |
| Pina Colada, 21 oz | 470 | 7 | 99 |
| Strawberry Banana, 20 oz | 530 | 8 | 114 |
| **Smoothies** ~ *See Fast-Foods Section* | | | |
| **Orangina**, 10 fl.oz bottle | 130 | 0 | 32 |

**Pom Wonderful:**
**100% Juice (8 fl.oz Bottle):**

| | C | F | Cb |
|---|---|---|---|
| Blueberry; Cherry; Pomegranate | 150 | 0 | 37 |

**Juice Blends:** *Per 12 fl.oz Bottle*

| | C | F | Cb |
|---|---|---|---|
| Coconut | 130 | 0 | 32 |
| Hula | 210 | 0 | 52 |
| Mango | 210 | 0 | 51 |

**R.W. Knudsen:** *Per 8 fl.oz*
**Organic, 100% Juice:** Apple

| | C | F | Cb |
|---|---|---|---|
| Organic, 100% Juice: Apple | 120 | 0 | 30 |
| Concord Grape | 150 | 0 | 39 |
| Cranberry Blueberry | 120 | 0 | 31 |

**Natural, 100% Juice:**

| | C | F | Cb |
|---|---|---|---|
| Cranberry Raspberry | 130 | 0 | 32 |
| Mango Peach | 120 | 0 | 30 |
| Papaya | 130 | 0 | 32 |
| Razzleberry | 110 | 0 | 28 |
| Rio Red Grapefruit | 140 | 0 | 34 |

**Just Juice:**

| | C | F | Cb |
|---|---|---|---|
| Just Blueberry | 100 | 0 | 24 |
| Just Black Cherry | 150 | 0 | 36 |
| Just Black Currant | 110 | 0 | 25 |

**Simply Nutritious:** Mega C

| | C | F | Cb |
|---|---|---|---|
| Simply Nutritious: Mega C | 120 | 0 | 30 |
| Average other flavors | 125 | 0 | 31 |

**Sparkling:** Blueberry; Cranberry, av.

| | C | F | Cb |
|---|---|---|---|
| Sparkling: Blueberry; Cranberry, av. | 110 | 0 | 28 |
| Cherry; Pomegranate | 130 | 0 | 32 |
| Organic Pear | 120 | 0 | 31 |

### Juice Brands (Cont)    C   F   Cb

*Per 8 fl.oz Unless Indicated*

**R.W. Knudsen (Cont):**

**Sensible Sippers:** *Per 4.23 fl oz*

| | C | F | Cb |
|---|---|---|---|
| Organic Apple; Fruit Punch | 30 | 0 | 7 |
| Organic Banana/Mixed Berry | 35 | 0 | 9 |
| **Very Veggie**, Original, 8.oz | 60 | 0 | 12 |

**ReaLemon – ReaLime:**

Lemon/Lime Juice (from concentrate):

| | C | F | Cb |
|---|---|---|---|
| 1 teaspoon | 0 | 0 | 0 |
| 2Tbsp, 1 fl.oz | 10 | 0 | 2.5 |

**Santa Cruz:** *Per 8 fl.oz*

**Organic, 100% Juice:**

| | C | F | Cb |
|---|---|---|---|
| Apple Juice; Red Tart Cherry | 120 | 0 | 30 |
| Concord/White Grape | 160 | 0 | 39 |
| Hibiscus Cooler | 100 | 0 | 25 |
| Orange Mango | 120 | 0 | 29 |

**Carbonated Beverages:** *Per 10.5 fl.oz Can*

| | C | F | Cb |
|---|---|---|---|
| Lemon Lime | 130 | 0 | 32 |
| Pomegrante Limeade | 140 | 0 | 36 |
| Average other flavors | 115 | 0 | 29 |

**Lemonade:** Regular; Peach; Mango

| | C | F | Cb |
|---|---|---|---|
| Regular; Peach; Mango | 90 | 0 | 22 |
| Cherry | 100 | 0 | 26 |
| Raspberry; Strawberry, average | 90 | 0 | 24 |

**Simply Orange Juice Company:**

| | C | F | Cb |
|---|---|---|---|
| Lemonade; Limeade | 120 | 0 | 30 |
| Mixed Berry; Fruit Punch; Tropical | 100 | 0 | 26 |
| Orange Juice, with or without pulp | 110 | 0 | 26 |

**Snap•E• Tom,**

| | C | F | Cb |
|---|---|---|---|
| Tomato & Chili Cocktail, 11.5 fl.oz can | 70 | 0 | 15 |

**Snapple:** *Per 16 fl.oz Bottle*

**Juice Drink Blends:**

| | C | F | Cb |
|---|---|---|---|
| Go Bananas; Rasp. Peach, av. | 225 | 0 | 55 |
| Grapeade; Lemonade; Orangeade | 190 | 0 | 46 |
| Fruit Punch | 200 | 0 | 48 |
| **Diet**, Cranberry Raspberry | 20 | 0 | 5 |

**Ssips,** Juice Boxes,

| | C | F | Cb |
|---|---|---|---|
| av. all flavors, 6 fl.oz box | 80 | 0 | 21 |

**Stonyfield Farm:** *Per 10 fl.oz Bottle*

**Smoothies:** Strawb.; Wild Berry

| | C | F | Cb |
|---|---|---|---|
| Strawb.; Wild Berry | 230 | 3 | 39 |
| Peach | 230 | 3 | 42 |
| **6 oz Bottle,** Strawb. Banana | 140 | 2 | 25 |

*Per 8 fl.oz Unless Indicated*    C   F   Cb

**SunnyD:**

**Original:** *Per 64 fl.oz Ctn*

| | C | F | Cb |
|---|---|---|---|
| Orange, all var., 8 fl.oz | 50 | 0 | 12 |

**Blends,** 64 fl.oz Containers,

| | C | F | Cb |
|---|---|---|---|
| average all flavors, 8 fl.oz | 60 | 0 | 15 |

**Baja Juice:** *Per 12 fl.oz Bottles*

| | C | F | Cb |
|---|---|---|---|
| Red Punch | 170 | 0 | 43 |
| Other flavors | 190 | 0 | 46 |

**Chillers:** *Pe 16 fl.oz*

| | C | F | Cb |
|---|---|---|---|
| Blue Raspberry | 110 | 0.5 | 28 |
| Grape | 120 | 0 | 30 |

**Sunsweet:** *Per 8 fl.oz*

**Plum Smart:** Original

| | C | F | Cb |
|---|---|---|---|
| Original | 160 | 0 | 36 |
| Light | 60 | 0 | 15 |

**Prune Juice:** Original

| | C | F | Cb |
|---|---|---|---|
| Original | 180 | 0 | 42 |
| Light | 100 | 0 | 26 |

**Trader Joe's:**

**All Natural Pasteurized,** 32/64.oz Bottle: *Per 8 fl.oz*

| | C | F | Cb |
|---|---|---|---|
| 100% Cranberry | 70 | 0 | 16 |
| Blueberry Pomegranate | 140 | 0 | 34 |
| Just Blueberry | 100 | 0 | 24 |
| Just Pomegranate | 150 | 0 | 37 |
| Mango PassionFruit | 130 | 0 | 32 |
| Omega Orange Carrot | 110 | 0 | 26 |

**Organic,** 32/64.oz Bottle: *Per 8 fl.oz*

| | C | F | Cb |
|---|---|---|---|
| 100% Pomegranate | 140 | 0 | 35 |
| Apple Juice | 120 | 0 | 30 |
| Concord Grape Juice | 160 | 0 | 39 |
| Cranberry | 70 | 0 | 18 |
| Grapefruit Sunset; Lemonade | 120 | 0 | 30 |
| Mango Nectar | 130 | 0 | 32 |
| Pink Lemonade | 130 | 0 | 32 |
| Strawberry Lemonade | 120 | 0 | 29 |
| White Grape Juice | 160 | 0 | 40 |

**Joe's Kids:** *Per 6.75 oz Box*

| | C | F | Cb |
|---|---|---|---|
| From Concentrate: Apple | 90 | 0 | 23 |
| Apple Grape | 100 | 0 | 24 |
| White Grape | 120 | 0 | 30 |
| 10% Juice, Lemonade | 90 | 0 | 22 |

**Sparkling Juices,** 25.4 fl.oz Botle:

| | C | F | Cb |
|---|---|---|---|
| Blueberry, 8 fl.oz | 120 | 0 | 30 |
| Cranberry, 8 fl.oz | 140 | 0 | 35 |
| Pomegranate, 8 fl.oz | 130 | 0 | 31 |

### Juice Brands (Cont)

*Per 8 fl.oz Unless Indicated*    **C**   **F**   **Cb**

| | C | F | Cb |
|---|---|---|---|
| **Tree Top:** | | | |
| **100% Juice Concentrates:** | | | |
| **64 fl.oz Bottle:** *Per 8 fl.oz* | | | |
|   Apple Berry/Grape, average | 125 | 0 | 31 |
|   Apple Cranb.; Blue Pomegranate | 120 | 0 | 30 |
| **11.5 fl.oz Can:** *Per Can* | | | |
|   Apple Berry/Grape, av. | 180 | 0 | 46 |
|   Fruit Punch | 170 | 0 | 42 |
| **6.75 fl.oz Box**, average | 105 | 0 | 26 |
| **Smoothie**, Banana Strawb., 4.5 fl.oz | 100 | 0 | 23 |
| **Tropicana:** *Per 8 fl.oz* | | | |
| **20% Juice**, 15.2 fl.oz Bottle, | | | |
|   Cranberry | 270 | 0 | 67 |
| **Farmstand**, 46 fl.oz bottle, | | | |
|   average all flavors, 8 fl.oz | 120 | 0 | 30 |
| **Pure Premiun:** Orange Juice, 8 fl.oz | 110 | 0 | 26 |
|   OrangeStrawberry, 8 fl.oz | 130 | 0 | 30 |
|   Ruby Red Grapefruit, 8 fl.oz | 90 | 0 | 22 |
| **Trop50**, 50% less sugar, 59 fl.oz bottle, | | | |
|   average all flavors, 8 fl.oz | 50 | 0 | 13 |
| **Trop Twisters**, 59 fl.oz bottle: | | | |
|   Orange Berry Banana Blast | 130 | 0 | 33 |
|   Average other flavors , 8 fl.oz | 110 | 0 | 28 |
| **Tropics**, 59 fl.oz container, | | | |
|   average all flavors, 8 fl.oz | 120 | 0 | 30 |
| **Tru Nopal:** | | | |
| **Cactus Water:** 1 Cup, 8 fl.oz | 25 | 0 | 6 |
|   16.9 fl.oz carton | 50 | 0 | 12 |
| **V8 Juices & Drinks** *(Campbell's):* | | | |
| **Original/Spicy 100% Vegetable Juice:** | | | |
|   5.5 fl.oz can | 35 | 0 | 7 |
|   8 fl.oz cup | 50 | 0 | 10 |
|   11.5 fl.oz can | 70 | 0 | 14 |
|   12 fl.oz bottle | 75 | 0 | 15 |
| **Blends:** Pineapple Passion, 8 fl.oz | 80 | 0 | 19 |
|   Red Radiance, 8 fl.oz | 70 | 0 | 18 |
|   Veggie Greens; Carrot Mango, 8 fl.oz | 60 | 0 | 14 |
| **Infused Water**, all flavors, 16 fl.oz | 30 | 0 | 7 |
| **V-Fusion:** Average all flavors | 115 | 0 | 28 |
|   Light Varieties, av. all flavors | 50 | 0 | 13 |
| **Veryfine:** | | | |
| **100%:** Apple; Orange, 8 fl.oz | 120 | 0 | 29 |
|   Apple Strawb., 11.5 fl.oz can | 170 | 0 | 43 |
| **Vita Coco:** | | | |
| **Coconut Water:** 8 fl.oz | 45 | 0 | 11 |
|   with Orange Juice, 8 fl.oz | 60 | 0 | 15 |

*Per 8 fl.oz Unless Indicated*    **C**   **F**   **Cb**

| | C | F | Cb |
|---|---|---|---|
| **Walnut Acres:** *Per 8 fl.oz* | | | |
| **Organic:** Apple | 110 | 0 | 29 |
|   Apricot; Raspberry | 130 | 0 | 32 |
|   Cherry | 140 | 0 | 34 |
|   Cranberry | 110 | 0 | 26 |
|   Incredible Vegetable | 50 | 0 | 12 |
|   Mango Nectar | 120 | 0 | 29 |
| **Welch's:** *Per 8 fl.oz* | | | |
| **100% Juice:** Concord Grape | 140 | 0 | 36 |
|   Red Grape juice | 160 | 0 | 41 |
|   White Grape | 140 | 0 | 38 |
|   White Grape Cherry/Peach | 140 | 0 | 34 |
| **Essentials Cocktails**, 64 fl.oz Bottles, | | | |
|   average all flavors, 8 fl.oz | 140 | 0 | 35 |
| **Frozen Concentrates,** | | | |
|   100% Juice, Grape; all var., 2 fl oz | 140 | 0 | 39 |
| **Light Juice**, 52 fl.oz Bottle | | | |
|   Concord/White Grape, 8 fl.oz | 45 | 0 | 12 |
| **Sparkling Juice Cocktail:** | | | |
|   Blueberry Grape, 8 fl.oz | 150 | 0 | 38 |
|   Other flavors, 8 fl.oz | 160 | 0 | 40 |
| **Zola:** | | | |
| **Acai:** *Per 12 fl.oz Bottle* | | | |
|   Original | 185 | 3 | 39 |
|   with Blueberry | 180 | 3 | 37 |
|   with Pomegranate | 180 | 3 | 37 |
| **Coconut Water, 17.5 oz Can:** | | | |
|   Original, | 50 | 0 | 13 |
|   Chocolate, 8 fl.oz | 50 | 0 | 12 |
|   Espresso, 8 fl.oz | 60 | 0 | 13 |

**CALORIEKING PORTION WATCH**

| ORANGE JUICE | C | Cb |
|---|---|---|
| **8 fl.oz** | 110 | 26 |
| **16 fl.oz** | 220 | 52 |
| **24 fl.oz** | 330 | 78 |
| **32 fl.oz** | 440 | 104 |

### Quick Guide  C  F  Cb

#### Cow's Milk ~ Average All Brands
**Whole (3.25% fat):**

| | C | F | Cb |
|---|---|---|---|
| 2 Tbsp, 1 fl.oz | 20 | 1 | 1.5 |
| 1 Cup, 8 fl.oz | 150 | 8 | 12 |
| 1 Large Glass, 12 fl.oz | 220 | 12 | 17 |
| 1 Pint, 16 fl.oz | 295 | 16 | 22 |
| 1 Quart, 946 ml | 590 | 32 | 44 |

**Reduced-Fat (2% fat):**

| | | | |
|---|---|---|---|
| 2 Tbsp, 1 fl.oz | 15 | 0.5 | 1.5 |
| 1 Cup, 8 fl.oz | 120 | 5 | 12 |
| 1 Large Glass, 12 fl.oz | 180 | 7.5 | 18 |
| 1 Pint, 16 fl.oz | 245 | 10 | 23 |
| 1 Quart, 946 ml | 490 | 20 | 46 |

**Light/Low-Fat (1% fat):**

| | | | |
|---|---|---|---|
| 2 Tbsp, 1 fl.oz | 13 | 0.3 | 1.5 |
| 1 Cup, 8 fl.oz | 100 | 2.5 | 12 |
| 1 Large Glass, 12 fl.oz | 150 | 4 | 18 |
| 1 Pint, 16 fl.oz | 205 | 5 | 25 |
| 1 Quart, 946 ml | 410 | 10 | 49 |

**Fat Free/Skim (0% fat):**

| | | | |
|---|---|---|---|
| 2 Tbsp, 1 fl.oz | 10 | 0 | 1.5 |
| 1 Cup, 8 fl.oz | 90 | 0.5 | 13 |
| 1 Large Glass, 12 fl.oz | 135 | 0.5 | 19 |
| 1 Pint, 16 fl.oz | 180 | 1 | 26 |

**Half & Half ~** See Page 89

---

### SWITCH & SAVE

**Switch from whole milk to either 2%, 1% or 0% milk and save significant calories.**

*Per 8 oz Cup/Glass*

**WHOLE MILK 3.3% Fat 150 Cals**

| | | |
|---|---|---|
| 2% MILK | 120 Cals | SAVE 30 Cals |
| 1% MILK | 100 Cals | SAVE 50 Cals |
| 0% FAT-FREE | 90 Cals | SAVE 60 Cals |

*Switching to low-fat or fat-free milk also greatly reduces saturated fat.*

---

### Other Milks  C  F  Cb

**Buttermilk:** *Average All Brands*

| | C | F | Cb |
|---|---|---|---|
| Reduced-Fat (2%), 1 cup, 8 fl.oz | 120 | 5 | 10 |
| Low-Fat (1%), 1 cup, 8 fl.oz | 100 | 2.5 | 12 |

**Lactose Free:**
*Lactaid 100:* Whole

| | | | |
|---|---|---|---|
| Whole | 160 | 8 | 13 |
| 2% Reduced-Fat | 130 | 5 | 12 |
| 1% Low-Fat | 110 | 2.5 | 13 |
| Fat Free; Calcium Enriched | 90 | 0 | 13 |

*Smart Balance,*

| | | | |
|---|---|---|---|
| FF + Omega-3s & Vit. E | 100 | 0 | 14 |

**Lower Calorie/Carb Dairy Drinks:** *Per 8 fl.oz Cup*
Calorie Countdown (*Hood*):

| | | | |
|---|---|---|---|
| 2% Reduced-Fat: Plain | 70 | 4.5 | 3 |
| Chocolate | 80 | 4.5 | 6 |
| Fat-Free | 35 | 0 | 4 |

---

### Goat/Sheep Milk, Kefir

**Goat's Milk** (*Meyenberg*):

| | | | |
|---|---|---|---|
| Whole, 1 cup, 8 fl.oz | 140 | 7 | 11 |
| Low-Fat (1%), 8 fl.oz | 100 | 2.5 | 11 |
| Evaporated, reconst., 8 fl.oz | 140 | 8 | 12 |

**Kefir:** *Per 8 fl.oz*
*Lifeway:* Original, Plain

| | | | |
|---|---|---|---|
| Original, Plain | 150 | 8 | 12 |
| Greek, Plain, whole milk | 210 | 14 | 12 |
| Lowfat, average all flavors | 140 | 1.5 | 20 |

*Nancy's:* Plain, low fat

| | | | |
|---|---|---|---|
| Plain, low fat | 140 | 3 | 17 |
| Fruit flavors, average | 205 | 2.5 | 38 |

*Trader Joe's:* Plain, 1%

| | | | |
|---|---|---|---|
| Plain, 1% | 110 | 2.5 | 8 |
| Strawberry | 160 | 2 | 21 |

**Sheep's Milk,** Whole, 1 cup | 265 | 17 | 13 |

---

### Canned & Dried Milk

**Condensed:** Sweetened, 2 T., 1 fl.oz

| | | | |
|---|---|---|---|
| Sweetened, 2 T., 1 fl.oz | 130 | 3 | 22 |
| Low Fat, 2 Tbsp | 120 | 1.5 | 23 |
| Fat-Free, 2 Tbsp | 110 | 0 | 24 |

**Evaporated:** Whole, 2 Tbsp

| | | | |
|---|---|---|---|
| Whole, 2 Tbsp | 40 | 3 | 3 |
| Whole, ½ cup, 4 fl.oz | 170 | 10 | 13 |
| *Carnation:* Low Fat, 2 Tbsp, 1 oz | 25 | 0.5 | 3 |
| ½ cup, 4 fl.oz | 115 | 2.5 | 14 |
| Fat-Free, 2 Tbsp, 1 oz | 25 | 0 | 4 |

**Dried:** Whole, ¼ cup, 1 oz

| | | | |
|---|---|---|---|
| Whole, ¼ cup, 1 oz | 160 | 9 | 12 |
| Skim/Non-Fat, ⅓ cup | 80 | 0 | 12 |
| Made-up, 1 cup, 8 fl.oz | 80 | 0 | 12 |
| Buttermilk (sweet cream): 1 oz | 110 | 2 | 14 |
| Non-Fat, 1 Tbsp | 25 | 0 | 3 |
| *Carnation,* Malted, dry, 3 Tbsp, 0.7 oz | 90 | 2 | 15 |
| *Horlick's,* Malt Powder, dry, 1 oz | 180 | 4 | 27 |

### Soy/Non-Dairy Drinks ~ See Page 49

### Quick Guide

**C  F  Cb**

**Chocolate Milk:**
*Average All Brands:*

| | C | F | Cb |
|---|---|---|---|
| **Whole Milk,** (3.3%): | | | |
| 8 fl.oz cup | 220 | 8 | 29 |
| 1 Pint, 16 fl.oz | 440 | 16 | 58 |
| **Reduced-Fat,** (2%): | | | |
| 8 fl.oz cup | 190 | 5 | 30 |
| 1 Pint, 16 fl.oz | 380 | 10 | 60 |
| **Low-Fat,** (1%): | | | |
| 8 fl.oz cup | 160 | 3 | 26 |
| 1 Pint, 16 fl.oz | 315 | 5 | 52 |

### Flavored Milk ~ Brands

**C  F  Cb**

| | C | F | Cb |
|---|---|---|---|
| **Ready-To-Drink:** *Per 8 fl.oz Cup Unless Indicated* | | | |
| **Albertson's,** Choc Milk | 180 | 2.5 | 29 |
| **Great Value** (Walmart), | | | |
| Low Fat Choc. Milk, 8 oz | 160 | 2.5 | 26 |
| **Hood:** Chocolate | 220 | 8 | 30 |
| Low-Fat (1%), Chocolate | 160 | 2.5 | 28 |
| **Horizon Organic:** | | | |
| Low-Fat: | | | |
| Chocolate with Omega 3 | 150 | 2.5 | 23 |
| Vanilla with Omega 3 | 150 | 2.5 | 22 |
| **Kellogg's:** | | | |
| **To Go, Breakfast Shakes:** *Per 10 fl.oz* | | | |
| Milk Chocolate | 190 | 5 | 29 |
| Strawberry; Vanilla | 180 | 5 | 29 |
| **Mixes,** average all flavors, | | | |
| 1 packet | 130 | 0 | 26 |
| **Kroger,** Simple Truth, | | | |
| Choc Milk, Low-Fat, 1% | 150 | 2.5 | 22 |
| **Land O Lakes:** *Per 8 fl.oz* | | | |
| **Grip 'n Go:** | | | |
| Swiss Chocolate (2% red-fat) | 190 | 5 | 26 |
| Strawberry (whole milk) | 190 | 8 | 22 |
| **Muscle Milk** ~ *See Energy Protein Drinks* | | | |
| **Nesquik:** *Per 8 fl.oz* | | | |
| **Chocolate:** Low Fat | 150 | 2.5 | 24 |
| Average other flavors | 150 | 2.5 | 24 |
| **Chocolate,** No Sugar Added | 100 | 2 | 13 |
| **Prairie Farms:** *Per 8 fl.oz* | | | |
| Chocolate, 2% Reduced Fat | 180 | 5 | 26 |
| Strawberry, 1% Low Fat | 160 | 2.5 | 28 |
| **Ralphs,** | | | |
| Choc., Low-Fat, 8 fl.oz | 210 | 2.5 | 36 |
| **Starbucks** ~*See Page 37* | | | |

### Flavored Milk ~ Brands (Cont)

| | C | F | Cb |
|---|---|---|---|
| **Ready-To-Drink:** | | | |
| **TruMoo:** | | | |
| **Chocolate/Strawberry**: | | | |
| Whole, 8 fl.oz | 220 | 8 | 29 |
| 1% Low-Fat: 8 fl.oz | 140 | 2.5 | 20 |
| 14 fl.oz Bottle | 250 | 5 | 35 |
| Fat-free, 8 fl.oz | 120 | 0 | 20 |
| **High Protein (25g)**: | | | |
| Average all flavors, 14 fl. oz bottle | 410 | 5 | 68 |
| **Yoo-Hoo,** Chocolate,15.5 fl.oz bottle | 230 | 2 | 51 |
| **Bottled Coffee Drinks** ~ *See Page 37* | | | |

### Shakes

| | C | F | Cb |
|---|---|---|---|
| **Arby's:** *Per Medium Size* | | | |
| Chocolate; Jamocha, 16 oz | 570 | 15 | 99 |
| Vanilla, 16 oz | 470 | 15 | 75 |
| **Burger King:** *Per Medium 16 oz* | | | |
| **Hand Spun Shakes:** Chocolate | 760 | 21 | 131 |
| Strawberry | 640 | 15 | 113 |
| Vanilla | 580 | 15 | 98 |
| **Other flavors** ~ *See Fast Food Section* | | | |
| **Denny's:** | | | |
| Chocolate, 16 oz | 860 | 44 | 104 |
| Chocolate Peanut Butter, 17 oz | 1180 | 73 | 146 |
| Oreo, 16 oz | 1180 | 61 | 174 |
| Strawberry, 15 oz | 730 | 33 | 95 |
| Vanilla, 16 oz | 870 | 44 | 107 |
| **Hardees,** all flavors, av., 14 oz | 710 | 33 | 87 |
| **McDonalds,** McCafe Shakes: | | | |
| Chocolate/Strawberry, av.: | | | |
| 12 fl.oz cup | 530 | 16 | 86 |
| 16 fl.oz cup | 635 | 18 | 104 |
| 22 fl.oz cup | 850 | 24 | 141 |
| **Other Restaurants** ~ *See Fast-Foods Section* | | | |

### Smoothies

| | C | F | Cb |
|---|---|---|---|
| **Made Up Ready-To-Drink:** | | | |
| **8 fl. oz Milk/Soy + Fruit:** *Per 12 fl.oz* | | | |
| *Average all flavors:* | | | |
| with Whole Milk | 300 | 8 | 50 |
| + Ice Cream, 1 scoop | 400 | 13 | 62 |
| with Non-Fat Milk | 240 | 0 | 50 |
| **Kroger/Ralph's Smoothies:** *Per 8 fl.oz* | | | |
| Mixed Berry | 210 | 2.5 | 40 |
| Strawberry Banana | 200 | 2.5 | 37 |
| **Freshens; Jamba Juice; TCBY** ~ *See Fast-Foods* | | | |

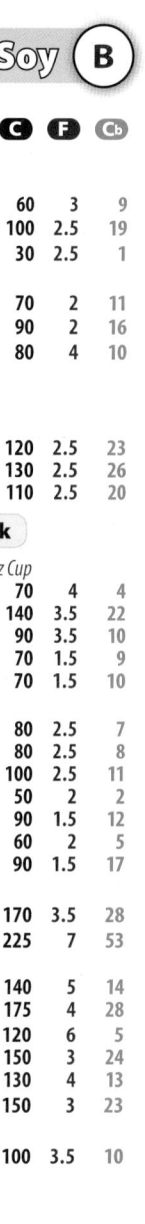

## Nut, Rice & Cereal Drinks

*Per 8 fl.oz Cup Unless Indicated* **C** **F** **Cb**

| | C | F | Cb |
|---|---|---|---|
| **Almond Breeze** (*Blue Diamond*): | | | |
| **Original:** Regular | 60 | 2.5 | 8 |
|   Reduced Sugar | 40 | 2.5 | 4 |
| **Chocolate** | 120 | 3 | 22 |
| **Vanilla** | 80 | 2.5 | 14 |
| **Unsweetened:** Original; Vanilla | 30 | 2.5 | 2 |
|   Chocolate | 40 | 3.5 | 2 |
| **Almond Dream:** *Per 8 oz Cup* | | | |
| **Boosted,** Unsweetened | 120 | 7 | 6 |
| **Enriched,** Unswtnd, Orig. | 50 | 3 | 12 |
| **Amazake,** Oh So Original, | | | |
|   Rice Shake | 150 | 0 | 34 |
| **Better Than Milk:** | | | |
| **Rice Vegan Powder Mix,** | | | |
|   Orig.; Van., 2 Tbsp, 0.7 oz | 70 | 0 | 17 |
| **Cacique,** Horchata Rice Drink | 160 | 3.5 | 31 |
| **Califia Farms:** *Per 8 oz Cup* | | | |
| **Almond Milk:** Original | 70 | 4 | 7 |
|   Unsweetened | 40 | 3.5 | 1 |
|   Vanilla | 50 | 3.5 | 4 |
| **Coconut Almond** | 50 | 4.5 | 1 |
| **Don Jose:** *Per 8 oz Cup* | | | |
| **Cereal Match** | 100 | 3 | 17 |
| **Horchata Rice Drink** | 140 | 4 | 25 |
| **Dream:** *Per 8 fl.oz Cup* | | | |
| **Original:** Boosted | 120 | 7 | 6 |
|   Enriched, unsweetened | 50 | 3.5 | 3 |
|   Ultimate Almond | 150 | 11 | 9 |
|   Usweetened | 130 | 11 | 4 |
| **Pacific:** *Per 8 oz Cup* | | | |
| **Nut Drinks:** | | | |
|   Hazelnut: Original | 110 | 3.5 | 19 |
|     Chocolate | 120 | 5 | 19 |
|   Organic Almond: | | | |
|     Original; Vanilla, av. | 65 | 2.5 | 10 |
|     Chocolate, single serve container | 100 | 3 | 19 |
|   Organic Oat, Original/Vanilla, av. | 130 | 2.5 | 25 |
| **Rice Dream:** *Per 8 fl.oz* | | | |
| **Organic Original Rice:** Classic | 120 | 2.5 | 23 |
|   Vanilla | 130 | 2.5 | 26 |
|   Enriched: Original | 120 | 2.5 | 23 |
|     Unsweetened | 70 | 2.5 | 11 |
|     Chocolate | 160 | 3 | 34 |
| **Horchata,** 8 fl.oz | 160 | 2.5 | 33 |

**Note: Rice/Oat/Nut drinks are very low in protein. Unless enriched with protein (and calcium), they are not suitable for infants as a substitute for milk or calcium-enriched soy drinks.**

## Nut Rice Drinks (Cont)

*Per 8 fl.oz Cup Unless Indicated* **C** **F** **Cb**

| | C | F | Cb |
|---|---|---|---|
| **Silk:** *Per 8 oz Cup* | | | |
| **Almond:** Original | 60 | 3 | 9 |
|   Dark Chocolate | 100 | 2.5 | 19 |
|   Unswt'nd, Orig.; Vanilla | 30 | 2.5 | 1 |
| **Nutchello:** | | | |
|   Caramel, Alm. + Cashews | 70 | 2 | 11 |
|   Rich Dark Choc. +Walnuts | 90 | 2 | 16 |
|   Toasted Coconut + Cashews | 80 | 4 | 10 |
| **Trader Joe's:** *Per 8 oz Cup* | | | |
| **Rice Drinks:** | | | |
|   Unsweetened: | | | |
|     Original, Organic | 120 | 2.5 | 23 |
|     Vanilla | 130 | 2.5 | 26 |
| **WestSoy,** Rice, Plain; Vanilla | 110 | 2.5 | 20 |

## Soy Milk ~ Ready-To-Drink

| | C | F | Cb |
|---|---|---|---|
| **365 Organic** (*Whole Foods*): *Per 8 fl.oz Cup* | | | |
| Original, unsweetened | 70 | 4 | 4 |
| Chocolate | 140 | 3.5 | 22 |
| Vanilla | 90 | 3.5 | 10 |
| **Light:** Original | 70 | 1.5 | 9 |
|   Vanilla | 70 | 1.5 | 10 |
| **8th Continent:** *Per 8 oz Cup* | | | |
|   Original | 80 | 2.5 | 7 |
|   Complete Vanilla | 80 | 2.5 | 8 |
|   Vanilla | 100 | 2.5 | 11 |
|   Light: Original | 50 | 2 | 2 |
|     Chocolate | 90 | 1.5 | 12 |
|     Vanilla | 60 | 2 | 5 |
| **Better Than Milk,** Orig., 8 fl.oz cup | 90 | 1.5 | 17 |
| **Bolthouse Farms:** | | | |
| **Vanilla Chai Tea:** 8 fl.oz cup | 170 | 3.5 | 28 |
|   15.2 fl.oz bottle | 225 | 7 | 53 |
| **Edensoy:** *Per 8 oz Cup* | | | |
| **Organic:** Original | 140 | 5 | 14 |
|   Carob; Chocolate, av. | 175 | 4 | 28 |
|   Unsweetened | 120 | 6 | 5 |
|   Vanilla | 150 | 3 | 24 |
| **Extra:** Original | 130 | 4 | 13 |
|   Vanilla | 150 | 3 | 23 |
| **Great Value** (*Walmart*), | | | |
|   **Vanilla Soy Milk,** 8 fl.oz | 100 | 3.5 | 10 |
| **Kikkoman:** See Pearl (next page) | | | |
| **Odwalla:** See 15.2 fl.oz Bottle | | | |
| **Protein Shakes:** | | | |
|   Strawberry | 300 | 6 | 36 |
|   Vanilla | 370 | 6 | 46 |

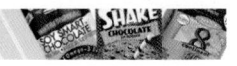

## Soy Milk ~ Ready-To-Drink (Cont)

*Per 8 fl.oz Unless Indicated* **C** **F** **Cb**

| | C | F | Cb |
|---|---|---|---|
| **Pacific:** *Per 8 oz Cup* | | | |
| **Organic,** Original, Unsweetened | 90 | 4.5 | 4 |
| **Select Soy:** Original | 70 | 2.5 | 9 |
| Vanilla | 80 | 2.5 | 11 |
| **Ultra:** Original | 140 | 5 | 12 |
| Vanilla | 140 | 5 | 14 |
| **Pearl** *(Kikkoman): Per 8 oz Cup* | | | |
| Chocolate | 150 | 4.5 | 21 |
| Coffee Flavor | 150 | 4 | 24 |
| Creamy Vanilla | 110 | 3.5 | 11 |
| Original | 110 | 3.5 | 12 |
| Unsweetened | 80 | 2.5 | 6 |
| **Silk:** *Per 8 oz Cup* | | | |
| Original | 110 | 4.5 | 9 |
| Chocolate | 120 | 3 | 21 |
| Vanilla | 100 | 3.5 | 12 |
| Very Vanilla | 130 | 3.5 | 18 |
| Light: Original | 60 | 1.5 | 5 |
| Chocolate | 90 | 1.5 | 16 |
| Vanilla | 70 | 2 | 7 |
| **Organic:** Original | 100 | 4 | 8 |
| Unsweetened | 80 | 4 | 4 |
| **Slim-Fast** ~ *See Page 40* | | | |
| **Soy Dream:** *Per 8 oz Cup* | | | |
| **Enriched:** Original | 100 | 3.5 | 9 |
| Vanilla | 120 | 3.5 | 14 |
| **Shelf Stable:** | | | |
| Classic Vanilla | 140 | 4 | 18 |
| Enriched: Original | 100 | 4 | 8 |
| Chocolate | 150 | 4 | 21 |
| Vanilla | 120 | 4 | 14 |
| **Trader Joe's:** *Per 8 oz Cup* | | | |
| **Soy Milk:** Original | 110 | 2 | 13 |
| Chocolate | 130 | 2.5 | 23 |
| Vanilla | 100 | 2 | 16 |
| **Organic:** Original | 130 | 3 | 17 |
| Chocolate | 120 | 3 | 17 |
| Vanilla | 130 | 3 | 19 |
| **WestSoy:** *Per 8 oz Cup* | | | |
| **Organic Plus,** (25% Less Sugar): | | | |
| Plain | 110 | 4.5 | 11 |
| Vanilla | 110 | 4.5 | 11 |
| **Low-Fat:** Plain | 90 | 2 | 15 |
| Vanilla | 120 | 2 | 23 |
| **Non-Fat:** Plain | 70 | 0 | 10 |
| Vanilla | 80 | 0 | 12 |
| **Unsweetened:** Plain | 90 | 4.5 | 5 |
| Chocolate; Vanilla, av. | 100 | 4.5 | 6 |

## Soy Powder Mix

**C** **F** **Cb**

*1 oz (¼ cup) mix makes 8 fl.oz Cup*

| | C | F | Cb |
|---|---|---|---|
| **Soy Protein Isolate,** dry, 1 oz | 95 | 1 | 2 |
| **Better Than Milk:** | | | |
| Original, 2 Tbsp | 90 | 1.5 | 18 |
| Vanilla, 2 Tbsp | 90 | 1.5 | 18 |
| **Genisoy:** *Per Scoop* | | | |
| **Protein Shake Powder:** | | | |
| Natural, 1 oz | 100 | 0 | 0 |
| Chocolate, 1.2 oz | 120 | 0 | 17 |
| Vanilla, 1.2 oz | 130 | 0 | 18 |
| **Now:** | | | |
| **Soy Protein Isolate:** | | | |
| Plain, ⅓ cup, 0.8 oz | 90 | 0.5 | 0.5 |
| Natural: | | | |
| Chocolate, 1 level scoop, 1.6 oz | 160 | 1.5 | 9 |
| Vanilla, 1 level scoop, 1.6 oz | 180 | 2.5 | 13 |
| **Revival:** *Per Packet* | | | |
| **Unsweetened Shakes:** Plain | 105 | 1 | 4 |
| Chocolate | 120 | 2.5 | 7 |
| Strawberry Banana | 115 | 2 | 4 |
| Strawberry Smile | 115 | 2 | 4 |
| Vanilla Pleasure | 120 | 2 | 6 |
| Average other flavors | 115 | 2 | 4 |
| **Whole Foods:** | | | |
| Chocolate, with Spirulina, 1 oz | 100 | 1 | 10 |
| Vanilla, with Spirulina, 1 oz | 100 | 0 | 11 |

## Coconut Milk Drinks

| | C | F | Cb |
|---|---|---|---|
| **Silk:** *Per 8 fl.oz Cup* | | | |
| **Original** | 80 | 5 | 7 |
| **Unsweetened** | 45 | 4 | 0.5 |
| **Vanilla** | 90 | 5 | 10 |
| **Blends, Almond Coconut:** | | | |
| Original | 50 | 3 | 5 |
| Unsweetned | 35 | 3 | 0.5 |
| **So Delicious:** *Per 8 fl.oz cup* | | | |
| **Original** | 70 | 4.5 | 8 |
| **Chocolate** | 90 | 5 | 13 |
| **Vanilla** | 80 | 4.5 | 10 |
| **Unweetened,** Original | 45 | 4.5 | 2 |
| **Trader Joes:** *Per 8 fl.oz cup* | | | |
| **Unsweetened** | 60 | 5 | 1 |
| **Vanilla** | 90 | 5 | 9 |

(Enriched with calcium + vitamins D & B12)

## Quick Guide

| | C | F | Cb |
|---|---|---|---|
| **Cola:** | | | |
| **Drinks:** *Average all Brands* | | | |
| 8 fl.oz Cup/Can | 100 | 0 | 26 |
| 12 fl.oz Can | 150 | 0 | 39 |
| 16 fl.oz Bottle | 200 | 0 | 52 |
| 20 fl.oz Bottle | 250 | 0 | 65 |
| 24 fl.oz (Pepsi) | 300 | 0 | 84 |
| 1-Liter Bottle (34 fl.oz) | 400 | 0 | 100 |
| 2-Liter Bottle (68 fl.oz) | 800 | 0 | 200 |
| **Other Soda Drinks:** *Per 12 fl.oz, average all brands* | | | |
| Club Soda | 0 | 0 | 0 |
| Cream Soda | 190 | 0 | 48 |
| Ginger Ale | 125 | 0 | 31 |
| Lemonade, Regular/Pink | 180 | 0 | 45 |
| Orange | 180 | 0 | 45 |
| Root Beer | 150 | 0 | 39 |
| Tonic Water | 125 | 0 | 32 |
| **Mineral Water:** Plain | 0 | 0 | 0 |
| Sweetened/flavored | 150 | 0 | 37 |
| with Fruit Juice | 120 | 0 | 30 |
| **Soda Water/Seltzer:** Plain/Diet | 0 | 0 | 0 |
| Sweetened/flavored | 155 | 0 | 39 |
| with Fruit Juice | 160 | 0 | 40 |

## Fountain, Movie Theater & Take-Out

| *Average All Flavors* | C | F | Cb |
|---|---|---|---|
| **Small Cup,** 12 fl.oz: No Ice | 160 | 0 | 40 |
| with ⅓ Ice | 120 | 0 | 30 |
| **Regular,** 16 fl.oz: No Ice | 215 | 0 | 53 |
| with ⅓ Ice | 160 | 0 | 40 |
| **Medium,** 22 fl.oz: No Ice | 295 | 0 | 73 |
| with ⅓ Ice | 220 | 0 | 55 |
| **Large,** 32 fl.oz: No Ice | 430 | 0 | 105 |
| with ⅓ Ice | 320 | 0 | 80 |

*Note: ⅓ Cup of Ice = ¼ Cup Liquid*

## Soft Drink ~ Brands

| *Per 12 fl.oz Unless Indicated* | C | F | Cb |
|---|---|---|---|
| **365 Organic** *(Whole Foods)*, Spritzers, all flavors | 110 | 0 | 28 |
| **A&W:** Root Beer | 170 | 0 | 47 |
| Ten | 10 | 0 | 3 |
| **Albertson's:** | | | |
| Super Chill: Cola | 160 | 0 | 43 |
| Root Beer | 180 | 0 | 48 |
| **Barq's,** Root Beer | 160 | 0 | 45 |
| **Big Red,** Soda, 20 fl.oz | 250 | 0 | 63 |
| **Blue Sky,** Natural Soda, Cola | 160 | 0 | 42 |

## Soft Drink Brands (Cont)

| *Per 12 fl.oz Unless Indicated* | C | F | Cb |
|---|---|---|---|
| **Bubble Up,** Lemon-Lime Soda, 8 fl.oz | 110 | 0 | 28 |
| **Cactus Cooler** | 150 | 0 | 40 |
| **Canada Dry:** *Per 8 fl.oz* | | | |
| Club Soda; Diet Ginger Ale | 0 | 0 | 0 |
| Ginger Ale; Tonic Water, average | 90 | 0 | 25 |
| **Cheerwine** | 150 | 0 | 42 |
| **Coca-Cola:** | | | |
| Classic; Caffeine Free | 140 | 0 | 39 |
| Diet Coke, all varieties | 0 | 0 | 0 |
| Cherry Coke; Vanilla Coke | 150 | 0 | 42 |
| Life | 90 | 0 | 24 |
| **Country Time** *(Dr Pepper/Snapple)*, Lemonade, all varieties, 20 fl.oz | 230 | 0 | 58 |
| **Crush:** *Per 20 fl.oz Bottle* | | | |
| Grape; Orange | 270 | 0 | 72 |
| Peach; Pineapple, average | 315 | 0 | 85 |
| Strawberry | 290 | 0 | 77 |
| **Dad's:** Orange Cream Soda | 180 | 0 | 46 |
| Root Beer | 165 | 0 | 41 |
| **Diet Rite,** Pure Zero | 0 | 0 | 0 |
| **Dr Pepper:** *Per 12 fl.oz Can* | | | |
| Regular | 150 | 0 | 40 |
| Cherry | 160 | 0 | 43 |
| Ten | 10 | 0 | 3 |
| **Fanta:** Orange | 160 | 0 | 45 |
| Other flavors | 180 | 0 | 48 |
| **Fresca,** all flavors | 0 | 0 | 0 |
| **GuS,** average all flavors | 95 | 0 | 23 |
| **Hansen's:** *Per 12 fl.oz* | | | |
| Natural Cane Sugar: | | | |
| Creamy Root Beer | 160 | 0 | 43 |
| Original Cola | 160 | 0 | 41 |
| Pomegranate | 130 | 0 | 35 |
| Diet, all flavors | 0 | 0 | 0 |
| **Hawaiian Punch:** *Per 12 fl.oz Can* | | | |
| Aloha Morning, 40% less sugar, all flavors | 90 | 0 | 20 |
| Maizin Melon Mix; Wild Purple Splash | 165 | 0 | 44 |
| Average other flavors | 100 | 0 | 27 |
| **Henry Weinhard's:** Root Beer | 170 | 0 | 43 |
| Orange/Vanilla Cream, av. | 180 | 0 | 44 |
| **Hires,** Root Beer | 170 | 0 | 46 |
| **IBC:** Root Beer | 160 | 0 | 44 |
| Cream Soda; Black Cherry | 180 | 0 | 48 |
| **Icee:** Coca-Cola; Orange Fanta | 100 | 0 | 27 |
| Lemon Lime Fanta | 90 | 0 | 24 |
| Minute Maid, Raspberry Lemonade | 100 | 0 | 27 |
| **Jarritos,** all flavors, 8 fl.oz | 110 | 0 | 28 |
| **Jelly Belly,** all flavors | 180 | 0 | 42 |
| **Jolt,** Cola | 150 | 0 | 41 |

## Soft Drink Brands (Cont)

| Per 12 fl.oz Unless Indicated | C | F | Cb |
|---|---|---|---|
| **Jones Soda:** | | | |
| Regular, all flavors, 12 fl.oz | 170 | 0 | 42 |
| Stripped, all flavors, 12 fl.oz | 30 | 0 | 8 |
| Zilch, sugar free, 12 fl.oz | 0 | 0 | 0 |
| **Kool Aid,** Bursts, av. 6.75 fl.oz | 35 | 0 | 9 |
| **Mello Yello,** Regular | 170 | 0 | 47 |
| **Mountain Dew:** All flavors | 170 | 0 | 46 |
| Diet varieties | 0 | 0 | 0 |
| Dewshine, 12 fl.oz | 160 | 0 | 42 |
| Black Label, 16 fl.oz | 210 | 0 | 54 |
| **Mug,** Root Beer | 160 | 0 | 43 |
| **Natural Brew:** Chai Cola | 170 | 0 | 41 |
| Draft Root Beer | 170 | 0 | 43 |
| Outrageous Ginger Ale | 180 | 0 | 44 |
| Vanilla Cream Soda | 160 | 0 | 39 |
| **Nehi,** Peach | 190 | 0 | 51 |
| **Pepsi:** Per 12 fl.oz | | | |
| Regular; Caffeine Free | 150 | 0 | 41 |
| Diet Pepsi; Jazz; Pepsi One | 0 | 0 | 0 |
| Pepsi Next | 60 | 0 | 16 |
| Pepsi True: 7.5 fl.oz can | 60 | 0 | 17 |
| 12 fl.oz can | 100 | 0 | 27 |
| **Perrier,** Carbonated Water | 0 | 0 | 0 |
| **Pibb,** Xtra | 140 | 0 | 39 |
| **RC Cola:** Regular | 160 | 0 | 43 |
| Ten | 10 | 0 | 3 |
| **Reed's,** Ginger Brew, | | | |
| all varieties | 145 | 0 | 38 |
| **7•UP:** Lemon Lime; Cherry | 140 | 0 | 39 |
| Diet flavors | 0 | 0 | 0 |
| Ten, Lemon Lime | 10 | 0 | 3 |
| **Safeway:** Per 8 fl.oz | | | |
| Refreshe: Cola; Lemon Lime, av | 110 | 0 | 28 |
| Grape | 140 | 0 | 36 |
| Mtn Breeze; Strawberry | 120 | 0 | 30 |
| Refreshe Ice, all flavors, 17 fl.oz | 0 | 0 | 0 |
| **Santa Cruz:** Or. Mango, 10.5 fl.oz | 120 | 0 | 29 |
| Raspberry Lemonade, 10.5 fl.oz | 100 | 0 | 26 |
| Average other varieties, 10.5 fl.oz | 135 | 0 | 33 |
| **Schweppes:** Ginger Ale | 120 | 0 | 33 |
| Tonic Water | 130 | 0 | 33 |
| **Shasta:** Cream Soda | 190 | 0 | 47 |
| Cherry Cola | 180 | 0 | 45 |
| Club Soda; Diet, all flavors | 0 | 0 | 0 |
| Dr. Shasta | 150 | 0 | 38 |
| Ginger Ale | 130 | 0 | 33 |
| Tiki Punch; Pineapple; Orange | 200 | 0 | 50 |
| Average other flavors | 170 | 0 | 41 |
| **Sierra Mist,** Lemon Lime | 120 | 0 | 30 |
| **Sprite:** Regular, 12 fl.oz | 140 | 0 | 38 |
| Zero | 0 | 0 | 0 |

| Per 12 fl.oz Unless Indicated | C | F | Cb |
|---|---|---|---|
| **Squirt,** Ruby Red | 170 | 0 | 45 |
| **Stewarts:** Root Beer | 160 | 0 | 41 |
| Grape; Orange 'n Cream | 190 | 0 | 48 |
| **Sun Drop:** Citrus Soda, 20 fl.oz | 290 | 0 | 76 |
| Diet Citrus Soda | 10 | 0 | 1 |
| **Sunkist:** Orange | 170 | 0 | 44 |
| **Ten,** Orange, 12 fl.oz | 10 | 0 | 2 |
| **Surge,** 16 fl.oz | 230 | 0 | 62 |
| **TAB** | 0 | 0 | 0 |
| **Tampico:** Per 12 fl.oz | | | |
| **Punch:** Blue Raspberry | 45 | 0 | 21 |
| Pineapple Coconut | 105 | 0 | 25 |
| Average other flavors | 90 | 0 | 21 |
| **Soda,** all flavors, 12 fl.oz | 180 | 0 | 42 |
| **Thomas Kemper:** Per 12 fl.oz | | | |
| Black Cherry | 170 | 0 | 44 |
| Ginger Ale; Vanilla Cream | 150 | 0 | 36 |
| Root Beer | 160 | 0 | 41 |
| **Trader Joe's:** | | | |
| **Sparkling:** | | | |
| French Berry Lemonade: | | | |
| 1 cup, 8 fl.oz | 130 | 0 | 31 |
| 1 bottle, 33.8 fl.oz | 520 | 0 | 124 |
| Lime Ade: 1 cup, 8 fl.oz | 110 | 0 | 28 |
| 1 bottle, 33.8 fl.oz | 440 | 0 | 108 |
| Pink Lemonade: 1 cup, 8 fl.oz | 130 | 0 | 31 |
| 1 Bottle, 33.8 fl.oz | 520 | 0 | 124 |
| **Vernors,** Ginger Soda, 20 fl.oz | 240 | 0 | 65 |
| **Virgil's,** Root Beer | 160 | 0 | 42 |
| **Walgreens:** Per 20 fl.oz | | | |
| Orchard Grape Soda | 300 | 0 | 84 |
| Cola; Zesty Lemon Lime, av. | 225 | 0 | 65 |
| Root Beer | 225 | 0 | 75 |
| **Zevia,** all flavors | 0 | 0 | 4 |
| (Contains between 4-7g Erythritol) | | | |

## Powdered Soft Drink Mixes

| Per 8 fl.oz Prepared, Unless Indicated | C | F | Cb |
|---|---|---|---|
| **Country Time:** | | | |
| Lemonade; Pink Lemonade | 60 | 0 | 16 |
| Strawberry Lemonade | 80 | 0 | 19 |
| **Crystal Light** (Kraft): | | | |
| Fruit Drinks, all flavors, ½ tsp | 5 | 0 | 0 |
| Pure Fitness, average all flavors, 1 pkt | 15 | 0 | 4 |
| **Flavor Aid,** ⅛ package | 0 | 0 | 0 |
| **Kool-Aid,** sweetened, 0.6 oz | 60 | 0 | 16 |
| **Tang,** Regular, 2 Tbsp, 1 oz | 90 | 0 | 24 |

### Quick Guide  **C  F  Cb**

**Teas**

**Regular:** Bag, Loose or Instant

| | | | |
|---|---|---|---|
| Brewed, 1 cup, 8 fl.oz | 2 | 0 | 0.5 |
| (Add extra for sugar/milk) | | | |
| **Herbal:** All flav., av., 1 cup | 2 | 0 | 0.5 |
| *Bigelow*, all flavors | 0 | 0 | 0 |
| *Celestial Seasonings*, all flavors | 0 | 0 | 0 |
| **Bubble Milk Tea,** w/ Pearls, 8 fl.oz | 175 | 0 | 41 |
| **Chai Tea,** 2 Tbsp | 120 | 3.5 | 21 |
| **Starbucks** ~ *See Fast-Foods Section* | | | |

**Iced Tea**

*Average All Brands*

| | | | |
|---|---|---|---|
| **Sweetened:** 8 fl.oz cup | 90 | 0 | 22 |
| 12 fl.oz glass/can | 140 | 0 | 35 |
| 16 fl.oz bottle | 180 | 0 | 45 |
| 20 fl.oz bottle | 225 | 0 | 55 |
| **Unsweetened,** 8 fl.oz | 0 | 0 | 0 |

### Iced Tea Mixes

*Per 8 fl.oz Made-Up*

**4C Iced Tea:**

| | | | |
|---|---|---|---|
| Average all flavors, 0.67 oz | 70 | 0 | 18 |
| Totally Light, all flavors | 0 | 0 | 0 |
| **Crystal Light,** sugar free | 5 | 0 | 0 |
| **Lipton:** | | | |
| **Sweetened:** Lemon | 70 | 0 | 18 |
| Mango; Peach | 80 | 0 | 19 |
| Unsweetened | 0 | 0 | 0 |
| Diet, all varieties | 5 | 0 | 1 |

### Bottled & Canned Teas

| | | | |
|---|---|---|---|
| **Arizona:** *Per 8 fl.oz* | | | |
| **Black:** Cranberry | 80 | 0 | 22 |
| Sweet | 90 | 0 | 23 |
| with Ginseng | 60 | 0 | 15 |
| **Green Tea,** average all flavors | 70 | 0 | 18 |
| **Bigelow:** *Per 8 fl.oz* | | | |
| Green Tea, average all flavors | 60 | 0 | 15 |
| Half & Half Tea, Lemonade | 70 | 0 | 16 |
| Unsweetened Tea | 0 | 0 | 0 |
| **Fuze,** Iced Lemon | 70 | 0 | 19 |
| **Gold Peak,** Lemon, 12 fl.oz | 120 | 0 | 30 |
| **Honest Tea:** *Per 16 fl.oz Bottle* | | | |
| Just Black/Green | 0 | 0 | 0 |
| Assam Black | 35 | 0 | 9 |
| Community/Jasmin | | | |

### Bottled & Canned Teas (Cont)

**Lipton:**  **C  F  Cb**

**Iced Tea:** *Per 20 fl.oz Unless Indicated*

| | | | |
|---|---|---|---|
| Citrus Green Tea | 120 | 0 | 33 |
| Diet, all flavors | 0 | 0 | 0 |
| Half & Half | 120 | 0 | 31 |
| Lemon | 120 | 0 | 32 |
| Peach | 120 | 0 | 30 |
| Sparkling: Peach | 70 | 0 | 18 |
| Diet | 0 | 0 | 0 |
| Sweet Iced Tea, 8 fl.oz | 80 | 0 | 23 |
| White Tea, with Raspberry, 16.9 fl.oz | 110 | 0 | 29 |

**Nestea:**

**Iced Tea,** with Lemon:

| | | | |
|---|---|---|---|
| 8 fl.oz | 50 | 0 | 12 |
| 20 fl.oz bottle | 125 | 0 | 30 |
| **Diet,** Green/Lemon | 0 | 0 | 0 |

**POM:**

**Antioxidant Super Tea:** *Per 12 fl.oz*

Pomegranate:

| | | | |
|---|---|---|---|
| Lemonade Tea | 140 | 0 | 35 |
| Peach Passion White Tea | 130 | 0 | 32 |
| Sweet Tea | 120 | 0 | 30 |
| Honey Green Tea | 130 | 0 | 35 |
| **Snapple:** *Per 16 fl.oz* | | | |
| Green Tea | 120 | 0 | 31 |
| Diet Green Tea | 0 | 0 | 0 |
| Lemon/ Raspberry Tea | 150 | 0 | 37 |
| Diet Lemon/Raspberry Tea | 10 | 0 | 1 |
| **SnapTea:** Lemon | 120 | 0 | 31 |
| Peach Green Tea | 120 | 0 | 31 |
| Sweet Tea | 130 | 0 | 34 |
| **SoBe,** Elixir, Green Tea, 20 fl.oz | 200 | 0 | 52 |
| **Ssips,** Lemon Iced, 6.fl.oz | 70 | 0 | 18 |
| **Steaz,** Green Tea, | | | |
| av. all flavors, 16 fl.oz | 80 | 0 | 20 |
| **Tampico,** Iced Tea, | | | |
| average all flavors, 12 fl.oz | 135 | 0 | 35 |
| **Tazo,** Org. Iced Black Tea, 13.8 fl oz | 60 | 0 | 15 |
| **TeaZazz:** Original; Peach, 20 fl.oz | 50 | 0 | 12 |
| Green Tea Lemon, 20 fl.oz | 60 | 0 | 17 |
| **Trader Joe's:** *Per 8 fl.oz* | | | |
| Organic Tea & Lemonade | 100 | 0 | 25 |
| Pomegranate Green Tea | 60 | 0 | 15 |
| **Turkey Hill:** Iced Tea, 16 fl.oz | 180 | 0 | 42 |
| Peach Tea, 16 fl.oz | 200 | 0 | 46 |
| Green Tea, Mango | 180 | 0 | 42 |
| **365 Organic** *(Whole Foods):* | | | |
| Unsweetened: Black Tea | 0 | 0 | 0 |
| Green Tea | 0 | 0 | 0 |

Note: Most breads have similar calories on a weight basis. However, volume may vary.

For example, 1 oz of bread may equal 1 slice regular bread or 2 slices of a lighter bread. It is best to weigh bread used and calculate using: 1 oz bread = 70 calories, 14g carb.

### Quick Guide  **C** **F** **Cb**

#### Bread

**White or Wheat:** *Average Per Slice*

| | C | F | Cb |
|---|---|---|---|
| **Thin or Light,** 0.75 oz | 50 | 0.5 | 9 |
| **Sandwich slice,** 1 oz | 70 | 1 | 12 |
| **Thick or Large,** 1.5 oz | 105 | 1.5 | 18 |
| **Thick,** 2 oz | 140 | 2 | 23 |
| **Extra Thick,** 3 oz | 210 | 3 | 35 |
| **Whole Loaf:** 16 oz | 1120 | 15 | 185 |
| 24 oz Loaf | 1680 | 24 | 280 |

**Multi Grain/Whole Grain:** *Per Slice*

| | C | F | Cb |
|---|---|---|---|
| **Sandwich Slice,** 1 oz | 75 | 1.5 | 12 |
| **Thick Slice,** 2 oz | 150 | 2.5 | 25 |

**Toast:** *Based on same counts as White/Wheat as above*

**1 Slice (1 oz fresh):**

| | C | F | Cb |
|---|---|---|---|
| with 1 tsp butter/margarine | 105 | 5 | 12 |
| with 1 tsp "light" butter/marg. | 90 | 3.5 | 12 |
| with 2 tsp butter/margarine | 140 | 9 | 12 |
| with 2 tsp "light" butter/marg. | 110 | 6 | 12 |

### Breads

*Per Slice Unless Indicated*

| | C | F | Cb |
|---|---|---|---|
| **12-Grain,** 1.5 oz | 110 | 1.5 | 22 |
| **Bran style/Dark,** 1 oz | 70 | 1 | 14 |
| **Buttermilk,** average, 1.5 oz | 110 | 1 | 22 |
| **Challah,** 0.75 oz | 85 | 1.5 | 17 |
| **Chapati,** 1 oz | 110 | 3 | 18 |
| **Ciabatta,** 2 oz | 130 | 1 | 26 |
| **Cornbread,** average, 3 oz | 220 | 6 | 37 |
| **Cracked Wheat Sourdough,** 1.5 oz | 130 | 0.5 | 27 |
| **Croissants ~** *See Page 134* | | | |
| **Crustless Bread,** regular, slice, 0.75 oz | 40 | 0.5 | 8.5 |
| **Crusts Only,** regular slice, 0.25 oz | 30 | 0 | 7 |
| **English Toasting,** 2 oz | 140 | 1.5 | 27 |
| **Flax & Grain,** 1.5 oz | 120 | 3 | 19 |
| **Foccacia:** Plain, 2 oz serve | 150 | 2.5 | 28 |
| Cheese & Garlic; Pesto, 2 oz serve | 160 | 6 | 21 |
| Tomato & Olive, 2 oz serve | 150 | 5 | 21 |

### Breads (Cont)  **C** **F** **Cb**

*Per Slice Unless Indicated*

| | C | F | Cb |
|---|---|---|---|
| **French Stick/Baguette,** 1 oz | 70 | 1 | 15 |
| **French Toast:** Slices, 1.5 oz | 140 | 2 | 26 |
| *Aunt Jemima,* Sticks, av., 2 oz | 110 | 2 | 18 |
| **Garlic Bread/Toast:** | | | |
| Small slice + 1 tsp spread, 0.75 oz | 80 | 5 | 7 |
| Medium slice + 2 tsp spread, 1.5 oz | 160 | 10 | 14 |
| Thick slice + 3 tsp spread, 1.8 oz | 220 | 14 | 20 |
| *Pepperidge Farm,* 1 slice, 1.4 oz | 160 | 10 | 15 |
| **Hawaiian Sweet Bread,** 1.5 oz | 110 | 2 | 19 |
| **Hemp Bread,** 1.2 oz | 95 | 2 | 12 |
| **Italian Bread,** 2 oz | 140 | 1 | 28 |
| **Lower Carb,** (higher protein/fiber), average all brands, 1 oz | 60 | 1.5 | 9 |
| **MultiGrain,** 1.5 oz | 100 | 2 | 21 |
| **Naan Flatbread,** 2 oz | 160 | 3.5 | 29 |
| **Nut/Health Nut,** 1.35 oz | 90 | 1.5 | 18 |
| **Oatmeal/Oatbran Bread,** 1.5 oz | 90 | 0.5 | 19 |
| **Pita,** average all types: | | | |
| Small (4" diam), 1 oz | 90 | 0 | 18 |
| Large (6½" diam), 2 oz | 140 | 1.5 | 27 |
| Extra Large (9" diam), 4 oz | 300 | 1.5 | 60 |
| **Popovers,** (1), without butter | 130 | 2 | 18 |
| **Pumpernickel:** | | | |
| Cocktail/Party size | 30 | 0.5 | 6 |
| Large slice, 1.35 oz | 80 | 0 | 15 |
| **Raisin Bread,** 1 oz | 80 | 1 | 15 |
| **Rye:** 1 thin slice, av., 1 oz | 80 | 1 | 14 |
| 1 thick slice, 2 oz | 150 | 2 | 25 |
| Cocktail size, 0.4 oz | 25 | 0.5 | 4 |
| **Sandwich Pockets,** 2 oz | 140 | 1.5 | 27 |
| **Sourdough:** Regular, 1.5 oz | 120 | 1 | 25 |
| French Style, 1 oz | 75 | 0 | 14 |
| **Spelt,** 1.6 oz | 130 | 1 | 26 |
| **Sprouted 7-Grain,** 1.5 oz | 110 | 0.5 | 18 |
| **Squaw,** 1.1 oz | 85 | 0.5 | 13 |
| **Tacos/Tortillas ~** *See Page 172* | | | |
| **Turkish/Middle Eastern,** 1 oz | 80 | 1.5 | 16 |
| **Wheat-Free Breads:** Spelt, 1.6 oz | 130 | 1 | 26 |
| Rice, with Fruit Juice, 1.5 oz | 110 | 2 | 21 |
| Healthseed Rye, 1.6 oz | 90 | 1 | 20 |
| Millet, 1.5 oz | 100 | 1 | 20 |

## Bread ~ Brands

| | C | F | Cb |
|---|---|---|---|

*Per Slice Unless Indicated*

**Ener-G,** Gluten-Free Breads:
Brown Rice Loaf,

| | C | F | Cb |
|---|---|---|---|
| Regular, 1.3 oz | 100 | 3 | 16 |
| High Fiber Loaf, 1.4oz | 90 | 4.5 | 16 |
| Tapioca, regular, sliced, 1 oz | 80 | 3 | 11 |

**Ezekiel:**

| | C | F | Cb |
|---|---|---|---|
| Sprouted: 7 Sprouted Grains, 1.2 oz | 80 | 0.5 | 15 |
| Sesame, 1.2 oz | 80 | 0.5 | 14 |
| Whole Grain, 1.3 oz | 80 | 0.5 | 15 |

**Francisco International:**
Extra Sourdough Loaf,

| | C | F | Cb |
|---|---|---|---|
| 1 slice, 1.7 oz | 130 | 1 | 24 |
| French, 2 slices, 1.6 oz | 120 | 1 | 22 |
| Sourdough Sliced Bread, 2 sl., 1.4 oz | 110 | 1 | 22 |

**Oroweat:**

| | C | F | Cb |
|---|---|---|---|
| 3 Seed Oatnut, 1.34 oz | 120 | 3 | 18 |
| 100% Whole Wheat, 1.34 oz | 90 | 1 | 16 |
| Country Buttermilk, 1.34 oz | 100 | 1 | 20 |
| Extra Grainy, 17 Grains & Seeds, 1.2 oz | 110 | 2.5 | 18 |

**Pepperidge Farm:**

| | C | F | Cb |
|---|---|---|---|
| 100% Whole Wheat | 110 | 2 | 20 |
| 15 Grain | 110 | 2 | 20 |
| Farmhouse, Hearty White | 110 | 1.5 | 22 |
| Italian, with Sesame Seeds | 90 | 1.5 | 17 |
| Light Style, av. all varieties | 135 | 1 | 27 |

**Frozen Breads:**
Garlic Bread:

| | C | F | Cb |
|---|---|---|---|
| Original | 180 | 8 | 21 |
| Five Cheese | 200 | 10 | 20 |
| Texas Toast: Cheddar | 160 | 9 | 16 |
| Garlic | 150 | 8 | 15 |

| | C | F | Cb |
|---|---|---|---|
| **Roman Meal:** Orig. Multigr., 2 slices | 110 | 1.5 | 21 |
| Honey Oat Bran, 1.5 oz | 110 | 1.5 | 20 |
| **Sara Lee:** Honey Wheat, 1 oz | 70 | 0.5 | 13 |
| 100% Whole Wheat, 1 oz | 60 | 1 | 12 |
| Cracked Wheat, 1 oz | 80 | 0.5 | 15 |

**Schwan's,** Frozen:

| | C | F | Cb |
|---|---|---|---|
| Cheese Stuffed Breadsticks, 1.7 oz | 130 | 5 | 15 |
| French Baguette, ¼ loaf, 1.7 oz | 120 | 0 | 25 |
| **Trader Joe's:** Gourmet White, 1.5 oz | 120 | 3.5 | 19 |
| Soft 10 Grain, 1.5 oz | 90 | 1.5 | 16 |
| Sprouted Rye, 1.2 oz | 90 | 1 | 15 |

## Biscuits, Bread Rolls & Buns

**Biscuits:** *Average, 2½" diameter*

| | C | F | Cb |
|---|---|---|---|

Plain/Butter Milk:

| | C | F | Cb |
|---|---|---|---|
| Prepared from Recipe | 210 | 10 | 27 |
| Refrig. Dough, Baked | 95 | 4 | 13 |
| Brown 'n Serve, av., 1 oz | 70 | 1 | 13 |

Refrigerated Dough:
*Pillsbury,* Buttermilk Biscuit,

| | C | F | Cb |
|---|---|---|---|
| (3), 2.25 oz | 150 | 2 | 30 |

**Buns:**

| | C | F | Cb |
|---|---|---|---|
| Frankfurter/Hot Dog: 1.25 oz | 110 | 1.5 | 21 |
| 1.5 oz | 130 | 2 | 25 |
| Hamburger: Regular, 1.5 oz | 110 | 1.5 | 22 |
| Large, 3 oz | 210 | 3 | 40 |
| Hoagie/Submarine, Plain, 2.3 oz | 200 | 1 | 38 |

**Rolls:**

| | C | F | Cb |
|---|---|---|---|
| Ciabatta Roll, 3.5 oz | 230 | 4 | 41 |
| Crescent Roll, Original, 1 oz | 100 | 6 | 11 |

Dinner:

| | C | F | Cb |
|---|---|---|---|
| 1 small, 1 oz | 90 | 1.5 | 17 |
| 1 medium (3" diam),1.5 oz | 110 | 1 | 23 |
| French: 1 med, 1.3 oz | 110 | 1.5 | 22 |
| 1 large, 3 oz | 230 | 2.5 | 42 |

Kaiser:

| | C | F | Cb |
|---|---|---|---|
| Small, 2 oz | 200 | 2.5 | 35 |
| Large, 3.5 oz | 350 | 4 | 61 |
| Plain, 6", average all, 2.5 oz | 200 | 1 | 38 |
| Sourdough, 1.3 oz | 110 | 1 | 21 |
| Wheat Rolls: Small, 1.2 oz | 100 | 1 | 17 |
| Medium, 1.8 oz | 130 | 1.5 | 23 |
| Large, 3.5 oz | 260 | 3 | 46 |

## Breadsticks, Croutons

**Breadsticks:**

| | C | F | Cb |
|---|---|---|---|
| Salt Sticks, plain, 1 oz | 110 | 1 | 20 |
| Fresh baked (1), 2 oz | 180 | 2.5 | 34 |
| *Stella D'oro:* Original (1) | 45 | 1 | 7 |
| Sesame (1) | 50 | 2 | 7 |
| **Croutons:** Seasoned, 2 Tbsp, 0.3 oz | 35 | 1.5 | 4 |
| *Pepp. Farm,* Zesty Italian, 6 croutons | 30 | 1 | 5 |

## Bread Products

**Bread Crumbs,** dry:

| | C | F | Cb |
|---|---|---|---|
| Plain or seasoned: 1 oz | 110 | 1.5 | 20 |
| 1 cup, 3.5 oz | 385 | 5 | 70 |
| **Corn Flake Crumbs,** 1 oz | 120 | 0 | 29 |
| **Graham Cracker Crumbs** *(Keebler)*,1 oz | 110 | 2.5 | 20 |

**Bread Dough,** average:

| | C | F | Cb |
|---|---|---|---|
| Frozen, 1 slice, 2 oz | 140 | 2 | 26 |
| Refrigerated: French, 1" sl. | 60 | 1 | 13 |
| Wheat; White, 1" slice | 80 | 2 | 14 |
| **Coating Mixes,** av., 2 Tbsp., 1 oz | 100 | 0.5 | 20 |
| **Stuffing:** Dry mix, average all,1 oz | 110 | 1 | 10 |
| Prepared, ½ cup, 4 oz | 180 | 9 | 22 |

## Quick Guide · C · F · Cb

### Bagels
*Average All Brands*

**Plain/Onion:**

| | C | F | Cb |
|---|---|---|---|
| 1 mini/bagelette, 1 oz | 65 | 0.5 | 13 |
| 1 small bagel, 2 oz | 145 | 1 | 29 |
| 1 medium bagel, 3 oz | 220 | 1.5 | 43 |
| 1 large bagel, 4 oz | 290 | 2 | 57 |
| **Bagel Chips,** 1 oz | 130 | 4.5 | 19 |
| **Pizza Bagel Bites** (*Bagel Bites*), average all varieties. 4 pieces, 3 oz | 190 | 5.5 | 27 |
| **Bagel Crisps** (*New York Style*), average all varieties, 6 crisps, 1 oz | 130 | 5 | 17 |
| **Bagel Thins** (*Thomas'*), 1, 1.5 oz | 110 | 1 | 25 |

### Bagel ~ Brands

*Per Bagel*

| | C | F | Cb |
|---|---|---|---|
| **Bubba's:** Plain; Onion, average | 240 | 2 | 48 |
| Blueberry | 150 | 0.5 | 32 |
| Cinnamon Raisin | 250 | 1.5 | 51 |
| **Costco Bakery:** Plain | 330 | 1.5 | 70 |
| Cinnamon Raisin | 340 | 1.5 | 73 |
| Whole Grain | 300 | 5 | 56 |
| **Lender's,** Fresh, NY Style: | | | |
| Plain, 3.3 oz | 240 | 2 | 46 |
| Blueberry, 2 oz | 150 | 0.5 | 32 |
| Whole Grain, 3.3 oz | 250 | 1.5 | 49 |
| Whole Wheat, 3.3 oz | 210 | 1.5 | 41 |
| **Panera Bread:** Plain | 290 | 1.5 | 58 |
| Cinnamon & Raisin Swirl, 3.8 oz | 320 | 2 | 66 |
| Everything, 4 oz | 300 | 2 | 58 |
| Whole Grain, 4.3 oz | 350 | 2.5 | 68 |
| **Sara Lee:** Mini, average, 1.3 oz | 100 | 0.5 | 20 |
| Plain, 3.4 oz | 260 | 1 | 52 |
| Blueberry, 3.4 oz | 260 | 1 | 54 |
| Cinnamon Raisin, 3.7 oz | 260 | 0.5 | 54 |
| Everything, 3.4 oz | 270 | 3 | 50 |
| Onion, 3.4 oz | 260 | 1 | 53 |
| **Western,** The Alternatives, av., 2 oz | 120 | 0.5 | 29 |

### Bagel Spreads

**Cream Cheese:**

| | C | F | Cb |
|---|---|---|---|
| Plain: 2 Tbsp, 1 oz | 100 | 9 | 1 |
| 2 oz mini-tub | 200 | 18 | 2 |
| Reduced Fat: 2 Tbsp, 1 oz | 60 | 5 | 2 |
| 2 oz mini-tub | 120 | 10 | 4 |
| **Flavors:** Lox, 1 oz | 90 | 8 | 2 |
| Honey Nut, 1 oz | 80 | 7 | 4 |
| Strawberry, 1 oz | 90 | 7 | 5 |
| Sundried Tomato, 1 oz | 80 | 7 | 2 |
| Vegetable, 1 oz | 90 | 8 | 2 |

### English Muffins · C · F · Cb
*Average All Brands*

| | C | F | Cb |
|---|---|---|---|
| **Plain/Whole Wheat:** Regular, 2 oz | 135 | 1.5 | 26 |
| Heavier, 2.5 oz | 155 | 2 | 31 |
| Super Size, 3.2 oz | 190 | 2 | 38 |
| **Raisin-Cinnamon,** 2.2 oz | 150 | 1 | 30 |

Note: Actual weight of packaged muffins can be 10-15% heavier than stated net weight.

### Rice Cakes

| | C | F | Cb |
|---|---|---|---|
| Regular size (1), average, 0.3 oz | 35 | 0.5 | 7.5 |
| **Hain,** Mini, Mild Cheddar (10) | 70 | 2.5 | 11 |
| **Lundberg,** all varieties, av., 0.4 oz | 70 | 0.5 | 14 |
| **Quaker,** Apple Cinn., 0.5 oz | 50 | 0 | 11 |

### Tortillas & Shells

**Tortillas:** *Per Tortilla*

Corn Flour:

| | C | F | Cb |
|---|---|---|---|
| White/Yellow: 6", 1 oz | 55 | 1 | 11 |
| 7", 1.2 oz | 75 | 1 | 14 |
| Wheat Flour: | | | |
| 6", 1.2 oz | 100 | 3 | 16 |
| 8", 1.4 oz | 130 | 4 | 20 |
| 10", 2.3 oz | 200 | 6 | 31 |

**Shells:** *Per Shell, without Fillings*

Corn Taco Shells:

| | C | F | Cb |
|---|---|---|---|
| Mini, 3", 0.2 oz | 25 | 1 | 3 |
| Medium, 5", 0.5 oz | 60 | 2.5 | 8 |
| Large, 6½", 0.7 oz | 100 | 4.5 | 13 |
| Salad Shell, 10" | 310 | 17 | 34 |
| **Tostada Shells,** fried: | | | |
| White Corn, 5½" diam., 0.4 oz | 55 | 2.5 | 8 |
| Yellow Corn, 5½" diam., 0.5 oz | 80 | 3.5 | 11 |
| **Sopes,** 1 shell, 4" 2 oz | 110 | 1.5 | 23 |
| **La Tortilla Factory:** | | | |
| **100 Calorie,** Whole Wheat, 2 oz | 100 | 1.5 | 24 |
| **Hand Made Style:** | | | |
| Flour, 1.7 oz | 150 | 5 | 21 |
| Green Chile, 1.4 oz | 50 | 1 | 14 |
| **Low Carb High Fiber,** Trad. Flour, 1.2 oz | 70 | 2.5 | 15 |
| **Traditional,** Flour, Soft Taco Size, 1.2 oz | 130 | 3.5 | 18 |
| **Whole Wheat,** Low Carb High Fiber, Original; Garlic & Herb, 1.3 oz | 50 | 2 | 10 |
| **Mission Foods:** | | | |
| **Corn,** Yellow/White, Super Soft: | | | |
| Regular size, 2 Tortillas, 1.7 oz | 100 | 1.5 | 20 |
| Super size (1), 1.1 oz | 70 | 1 | 13 |
| **Flour:** Super Soft, 1 Tortilla, 1.8 oz | 170 | 6 | 24 |
| Homestyle, 1 Tortilla, 2.2 oz | 190 | 6 | 29 |

## Quick Guide

C F Cb

### Cooked Cereals

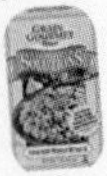

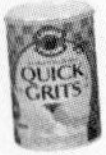

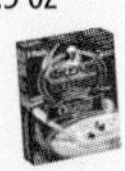

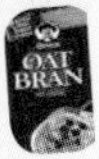

| | C | F | Cb |
|---|---|---|---|
| **Barley,** pearled, cooked, 1 cup | 195 | 0.5 | 44 |
| **Buckwheat Groats,** roasted: | | | |
| Dry, ½ cup, 3 oz | 285 | 2 | 61 |
| Cooked, 1 cup, 6 oz | 155 | 1 | 34 |
| **Bulgur:** Dry, ½ cup, 2.5 oz | 240 | 1 | 53 |
| Cooked, 1 cup, 6.5 oz | 150 | 0.5 | 34 |
| **Corn/Hominy Grits:** | | | |
| Dry: Regular, ¼ cup, 1.4 oz | 140 | 0.5 | 32 |
| Instant: 0.8 oz packet | 75 | 0 | 18 |
| w/ Imitation Bacon Bits, 1 oz | 100 | 0.5 | 22 |
| Cooked, ¾ cup, 6.5 oz | 110 | 0.5 | 23 |
| **Cream of Rice,** cooked, ¾ cup, 6.5 oz | 95 | 0 | 21 |
| **Cream of Wheat:** | | | |
| Cooked: Regular, ¾ cup, 6.5 oz | 95 | 0.5 | 20 |
| Instant, ¾ cup, 6.5 oz | 105 | 0.5 | 21 |
| Quick, ¾ cup, 6.5 oz | 100 | 0.5 | 22 |
| **Farina,** cooked, ¾ cup, 6 oz | 95 | 0.5 | 19 |
| **Millet,** dry, ¼ cup, 1.8 oz | 190 | 2 | 36 |
| **Oat Bran:** Raw, ⅓ cup, 1 oz | 70 | 2 | 19 |
| Cooked, ½ cup, 3.8 oz | 45 | 1 | 13 |
| **Oatmeal:** | | | |
| Dry: Regular, ⅓ cup, 1 oz | 100 | 1.5 | 18 |
| Instant: Regular, average, 1 oz | 105 | 1.5 | 18 |
| Flavored, average, 1.5 oz | 165 | 2 | 34 |
| Cooked: Regular, ¾ cup, 6 oz | 125 | 2.5 | 21 |
| 1 cup, 8 oz | 165 | 3.5 | 28 |
| **Whole Wheat,** cooked, ¾ cup, 6.5 oz | 115 | 0.5 | 25 |

### Brans, Wheat Germ, Add-Ons

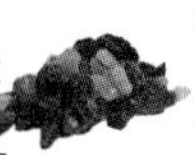

| | C | F | Cb |
|---|---|---|---|
| **Bee Pollen Granules,** 1 Tbsp, 0.3 oz | 25 | 1 | 2 |
| **Bran:** | | | |
| **Oat Bran:** Raw, 1 Tbsp, 0.2 oz | 20 | 0.5 | 3 |
| ⅓ cup, 1 oz | 100 | 2 | 17 |
| **Rice Bran:** Raw, 1 Tbsp, 0.2 oz | 15 | 1 | 2.5 |
| ¼ cup, 1 oz | 95 | 6 | 15 |
| **Fruit:** Dried, average, 1 oz | 70 | 0 | 18 |
| Banana, ½ medium | 55 | 0 | 14 |
| Prunes in Syrup (5), 3 oz | 90 | 0 | 23 |
| **Honey,** 1 Tbsp, 0.75 oz | 65 | 0 | 17 |
| **Lecithin Granules,** 1 Tbsp, 0.4 oz | 55 | 4 | 0.5 |
| **Nuts:** Almonds (6), 0.3 oz | 40 | 4 | 1.5 |
| **Psyllium Husks,** 1 Tbsp, 0.2 oz | 10 | 0 | 4 |
| **Wheat,** unprocessed, 1 Tbsp | 5 | 0 | 2 |
| **Wheat Germ:** Raw, 1 Tbsp, 0.3 oz | 25 | 0.5 | 4 |
| ¼ cup, 1 oz | 105 | 3 | 15 |

## Hot/Cooked Cereals ~ Brands

*Per Serving, Dry Mix only* C F Cb

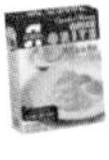

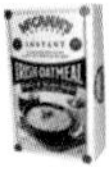

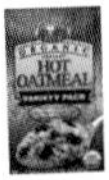

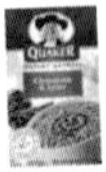

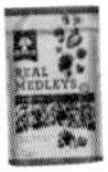

| | C | F | Cb |
|---|---|---|---|
| **Albers,** | | | |
| Quick Grits, ¼ cup, 1.4 oz | 140 | 0.5 | 31 |
| **B&G:** | | | |
| **Cream of Wheat Instant:** | | | |
| Original, 1 oz | 100 | 0 | 19 |
| Cinn. Swirl, Maple Br. Sugar, 1.3 oz | 130 | 0 | 29 |
| **Bobs Red Mill:** | | | |
| **10 Grain,** ¼ cup, 1.5 oz | 130 | 1 | 26 |
| **Mighty Taste Hot Cereal,** 1.4 oz | 150 | 1.5 | 31 |
| **Oats Groats,** ¼ cup, 1.6 oz | 170 | 3 | 31 |
| **Dr. McDougall's:** *without Sugar* | | | |
| **Chia Berry Superfood,** 2.5 oz | 190 | 4.5 | 34 |
| **Cranberry Almond & Grains,** 3 oz | 260 | 4 | 47 |
| **Maple,** 2.5 oz | 270 | 3.5 | 55 |
| **Mighty Omega Superfood,** 2.6 oz | 240 | 7 | 38 |
| **Great Value** *(Walmart):* | | | |
| **Instant Oatmeal:** | | | |
| Maple & Brown Sugar, 1.5 oz pkg | 160 | 2 | 33 |
| Peaches & Cream, 1.2 oz pkg | 130 | 2.5 | 27 |
| **McCann's:** | | | |
| **Instant Irish Oatmeal:** | | | |
| Regular, 1 oz package | 100 | 2 | 19 |
| Apple & Cinn., 1.3 oz | 130 | 1.5 | 27 |
| Maple & Brown Sugar, 1.5 oz | 160 | 2 | 32 |
| **Malt-O-Meal:** Original; Choc., 1.2 oz | 130 | 0.5 | 27 |
| Maple Brown Sugar, ¼ cup | 170 | 0 | 37 |
| **Natures Path:** | | | |
| **Oatmeal:** Flax Plus, 1 oz | 110 | 1.5 | 23 |
| Apple Cinnamon, 1.7 oz | 210 | 2.5 | 40 |
| Maple Nut, 1.7 oz | 210 | 4 | 38 |
| **NutriSystem,** | | | |
| Oatmeal, Apple Cinnamon, 1 pkt | 130 | 1.5 | 26 |
| **Quaker:** | | | |
| **Instant Grits,** av. all flavors, 1 oz | 100 | 1 | 22 |
| **Quick Grits,** Original, ¼ cup, 1.3 oz | 130 | 0.5 | 29 |
| **Instant Oatmeal:** | | | |
| Original, Organic 1 oz | 100 | 2 | 19 |
| Maple & Brown Sugar, | 160 | 2 | 32 |
| Peaches & Cream, 1.3 oz | 130 | 2 | 27 |
| **Old Fash'nd/Quick Oats,** ½ c., 1.4 oz | 150 | 3 | 27 |
| **Real Medleys:** | | | |
| Blueberry Hazelnut, 2.5 oz | 270 | 7 | 49 |
| Summer Berry, 2.5 oz | 250 | 3 | 51 |
| Av. other varieties, 2.6 oz | 290 | 8 | 49 |
| **Supergrains,** av. all flavors, 2.5 oz | 275 | 8 | 49 |
| **Wegmans:** | | | |
| **Instant Oatmeal:** Orig., 1.4 oz pkt | 150 | 2.5 | 27 |
| Maple & Brown Sugar, 1.5 oz pkt | 160 | 2 | 32 |

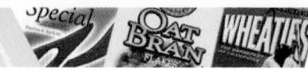

## Quick Guide | **C** | **F** | **Cb**

### Cold Cereals
*Average All Brands*

| | C | F | Cb |
|---|---|---|---|
| Bran Flakes, ¾ cup, 1 oz | 95 | 0.5 | 24 |
| Corn Flakes, 1 cup, 1 oz | 100 | 0 | 22 |
| Frosted Flakes, ¾ cup, 1 oz | 110 | 0 | 27 |
| Granola, 100% Nat., ½ cup, 1.7 oz | 205 | 6 | 35 |
| Oat Bran Cereal, ½ cup, 1.5 oz | 145 | 3 | 25 |
| Puffed Rice, 1 cup. 0.5 oz | 55 | 0 | 13 |
| Puffed Wheat, 1 cup, 0.5 oz | 45 | 0 | 10 |
| Raisin Bran, ½ cup, 1 oz | 90 | 0.5 | 22 |
| Rice Crisps, 1 cup, 1 oz | 105 | 0.5 | 24 |
| Shredded Wheat, 1 biscuit, 1 oz | 85 | 0.5 | 20 |
| Wheat Flakes, ¾ cup, 1 oz | 105 | 1 | 24 |

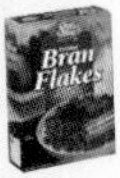

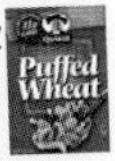

**Breakfast/Cereal Bars** ~ *See Page 31*

### Ready-To-Eat Cereal ~ Brands

**Arrowhead Mills:**

| | C | F | Cb |
|---|---|---|---|
| **Flakes:** Amaranth, 1.2 oz | 140 | 2 | 26 |
| Kamut, 1 oz | 120 | 1 | 25 |
| Oat Bran, 1.2 oz | 140 | 2.5 | 24 |
| Spelt, 1 oz | 120 | 1 | 24 |
| Sprouted Wheat Berry & Quinoa, 1.5 oz | 100 | 1 | 22 |
| **Breadshop Granola,** | | | |
| Blueberry 'n Cream, ½ cup, 1.8 oz | 210 | 6 | 36 |
| **Puffed:** Corn, 0.5 oz | 60 | 1 | 12 |
| Kamut, 0.5 oz | 50 | 0 | 11 |
| Millet, 0.5 oz | 60 | 0.5 | 11 |
| Rice, 0.5 oz | 60 | 0 | 14 |
| Wheat, 0.5 oz | 60 | 0 | 12 |
| **Shredded Wheat:** | | | |
| Bite Size: | | | |
| Regular, 1.7 oz | 190 | 1 | 38 |
| Sweetened, 1.8 oz | 200 | 1 | 42 |

**Back to Nature:** *Per ½ Cup*

| | C | F | Cb |
|---|---|---|---|
| **Granola:** Apple Blueberry, 1.8 oz | 190 | 2.5 | 37 |
| Banana Walnut, 1.8 oz | 200 | 5 | 36 |
| Chocolate Delight, 1.8 oz | 200 | 5 | 36 |
| Classic, 1.8 oz | 200 | 2.5 | 38 |
| Cranberry Pecan, 1.6 oz | 180 | 5 | 34 |
| Orange Chia Crunch, 1.8 oz | 200 | 4 | 37 |
| Sunflower & Pumpkin Seed, 1.8 oz | 210 | 7 | 31 |
| Vanilla Almond Agave, 1.8 oz | 200 | 6 | 34 |

**Barbara's Bakery:**
**Classics, Organic & Sweetened:**

| | C | F | Cb |
|---|---|---|---|
| Brown Rice Crisps, 1 oz | 120 | 1 | 25 |
| Corn Flakes, 1 cup, 1 oz | 110 | 1 | 25 |
| Honest O's, Original, 1 oz | 120 | 2 | 24 |

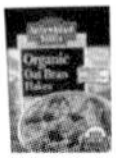

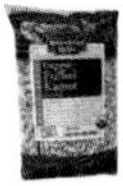

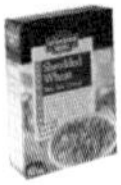

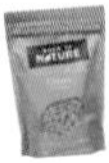

**Barbara's Bakery (Cont):** | **C** | **F** | **Cb**

**High Fiber:**

| | C | F | Cb |
|---|---|---|---|
| Original, 12 oz | 180 | 1.5 | 42 |
| Cranberry, 2 oz | 190 | 1.5 | 42 |
| **Morning Oat Crunch:** | | | |
| Original, 2 oz | 210 | 2 | 44 |
| Cinnamon, 2 oz | 230 | 3 | 43 |
| Van. Almond,; Blueb. Burst, 2 oz | 220 | 3 | 42 |
| **Puffins:** | | | |
| Original, ¾ cup, 1 oz | 90 | 1 | 23 |
| Cinnamon, ⅔ cup, 1 oz | 90 | 1 | 26 |
| Multigrain, ¾ cup, 1 oz | 110 | 0 | 25 |
| PB/PB & Choc., av., ¾ cup, 1 oz | 110 | 2 | 24 |
| **Snackanimals,** av. all varieties, 1 oz | 110 | 0.5 | 26 |
| **Shredded Wheat,** 2 biscuits, 1.4 oz | 140 | 1 | 31 |
| **Spoonfuls,** Multigrain, ¾ cup, 1 oz | 120 | 1.5 | 24 |
| **Squarefuls,** Multigrain, 1 cup, 1.9 oz | 200 | 1 | 47 |

**Bear Naked, Granola:**

| | C | F | Cb |
|---|---|---|---|
| **Fruit & Nutty,** ¼ cup, 1 oz | 140 | 6 | 20 |
| **Original Cinn.,** ¼ cup, 1 oz | 140 | 6 | 15 |
| **Triple Berry,** ¼ cup, 1 oz | 120 | 2 | 23 |
| **Vanilla Almond,** ¼ cup, 1 oz | 120 | 2.5 | 22 |

**Bob's Red Mill,**

| | C | F | Cb |
|---|---|---|---|
| **Muesli,** Old Country, ¼ cup, 1 oz | 110 | 3 | 21 |

**Cascadian Farm:**

| | C | F | Cb |
|---|---|---|---|
| **Buzz Crunch,** 1 cup, 2.1 oz | 230 | 3 | 47 |
| **Cinn. Crunch,** ¾ cup, 1 oz | 110 | 2.5 | 22 |
| **Graham Crunch,** ¾ cup, 1 oz | 110 | 2 | 23 |
| **Granola:** Ancient Grains, 2 oz | 240 | 6 | 41 |
| French Vanilla Almond, 2 oz | 250 | 7 | 42 |
| Oats & Honey, 2.2 oz | 260 | 7 | 46 |
| **Honey Nut O's,** 1 oz | 110 | 1 | 25 |
| **Multi Grain Squares,** | | | |
| 1 cup, 1.9 oz | 210 | 1 | 44 |
| **Raisin Bran,** 1 cup, 1.8 oz | 180 | 1 | 41 |

**EnviroKidz:** *Per 1 oz*

| | C | F | Cb |
|---|---|---|---|
| **Amazon Frosted Flakes,** 1 oz | 120 | 0 | 26 |
| **Gorilla Munch,** 1 oz | 120 | 1 | 26 |
| **Leapin' Lemurs,** 1 oz | 120 | 1.5 | 25 |
| **Panda Puffs,** 1 oz | 130 | 3.5 | 23 |

**Erewhon:**

| | C | F | Cb |
|---|---|---|---|
| **Corn Flakes,** 1 cup, 1.2 oz | 130 | 0 | 30 |
| **Crispy Brown Rice,** | | | |
| Original/Cinnamon, av. 1 cup, 1 oz | 110 | 0.5 | 25 |
| **Harvest Medley,** 1 cup, 1 oz | 110 | 1 | 24 |
| **Honey Rice Twice,** ¾ cup, 1 oz | 120 | 0 | 26 |
| **Simply Vanilla Granola,** | | | |
| ¾ cup, 2 oz | 240 | 6 | 41 |

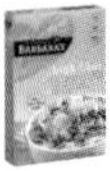

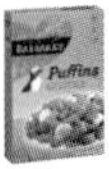

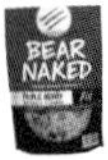

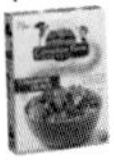

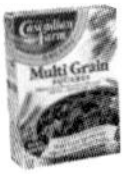

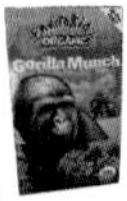

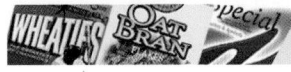

## Ready-To-Eat Cereal (Cont)

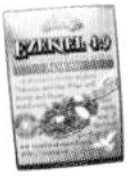

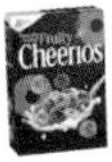

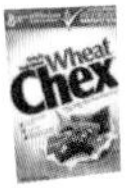

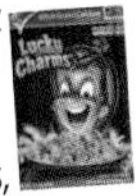

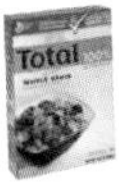

### Ezekiel 4.9:

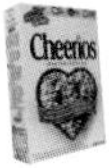

**Sprouted Whole Grain Cereals:**

| | C | F | Cb |
|---|---|---|---|
| Original, ½ cup, 2 oz | 190 | 1 | 40 |
| Almond, ½ cup, 2 oz | 200 | 3 | 38 |
| Cinnamon Raisin, 2 oz | 190 | 1 | 41 |
| Golden Flax, ½ cup, 2 oz | 180 | 2.5 | 37 |

### General Mills:

**Cheerios:** *Per ¾ Cup Unless Indicated*

| | C | F | Cb |
|---|---|---|---|
| Original, 1 cup, 1 oz | 100 | 2 | 20 |
| Ancient Grains, ¾ c., 1 oz | 110 | 2 | 22 |
| Apple Cinn., ¾ cup, 1 oz | 120 | 1.5 | 24 |
| Chocolate, av.,¾ cup, 1 oz | 100 | 1.5 | 22 |
| Frosted, ¾ cup, 1 oz | 100 | 1.5 | 22 |
| Fruity, Nat Flav., ¾ c., 1 oz | 100 | 1.5 | 23 |
| Honey Nut, ¾ cup, 1 oz | 110 | 1.5 | 22 |
| Multigrain, Regular, 1 c., 1oz | 110 | 1.5 | 24 |
| Protein: Cinn. Almond, 1¼ c., 2 oz | 220 | 4.5 | 40 |
| Oats & Honey, 1¼ cups, 2 oz | 210 | 2.5 | 41 |
| **Chex:** Corn, 1 cup, 1 oz | 120 | 0.5 | 26 |
| Chocolate, ¾ cup, 1 oz | 130 | 2.5 | 26 |
| Honey Nut, ¾ cup, 1 oz | 120 | 0.5 | 28 |
| Rice, 1 cup, 1 oz | 100 | 0.5 | 23 |
| Vanilla, ¾ cup, 1 oz | 120 | 2 | 25 |
| Wheat, ¾ cup, 1.7 oz | 160 | 1 | 39 |
| **Fiber One:** Original, ½ cup, 1 oz | 60 | 1 | 25 |
| Honey Clusters, 1 cup, 1.8 oz | 170 | 1.5 | 44 |
| Nutty Clusters & Almonds, 2 oz | 190 | 3.5 | 44 |
| Protein, av. all flavors, 1 cup, 2 oz | 215 | 5 | 41 |
| Raisin Bran Clusters, 1 cup, 2 oz | 170 | 1 | 46 |
| **Kix:** Original, 1¼ cups, 1 oz | 110 | 1 | 25 |
| Berry Berry; Honey, 1¼ cup, 1.2 oz | 120 | 1.5 | 28 |
| **Lucky Charms,** all varieties, average, ¾ cup, 1 oz | 110 | 1.5 | 23 |
| **Monsters,** Count Chocula, ¾ cup, 1 oz | 100 | 1.5 | 23 |
| **Tiny Toast,** all flavors, ¾ c.up, 1 oz | 120 | 3 | 22 |
| **Toast Crunch:** Chocolate, ¾ c., 1oz | 130 | 4 | 24 |
| Cinnamon, ¾ c., 1 oz | 130 | 3 | 25 |
| Peanut Butter, ¾ cup, 1 oz | 120 | 3 | 23 |
| **Total:** Original, ¾ cup, 1 oz | 100 | 0.5 | 23 |
| Raisin Bran, 1 cup, 2 oz | 160 | 1 | 40 |
| **Trix,** 1 cup, 1 oz | 130 | 1.5 | 27 |
| **Wheaties,** Original, 1 oz | 100 | 0.5 | 23 |

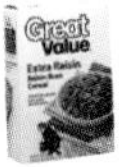

### Great Value *(Walmart):*

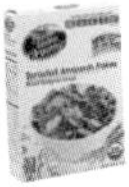

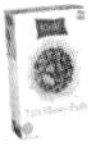

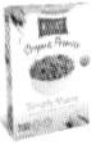

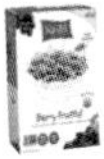

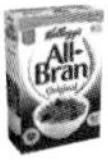

| | C | F | Cb |
|---|---|---|---|
| Apple Blasts, 1 cup, 1.2 oz | 120 | 0 | 29 |
| Crunch Honey Oats, with Almonds, ¾ cup, 1 oz | 130 | 1.5 | 26 |
| Extra Raisin Raisin Bran, 1 cup, 2 oz | 200 | 1 | 43 |
| Frosted Shredded Wheat, 1.9 oz | 180 | 1 | 42 |
| Fruit Spins, 1 cup, 1 oz | 110 | 1 | 25 |

### Health Valley:

| | C | F | Cb |
|---|---|---|---|
| Crunch-Ems!, Rice, 1¼ cups, 1 oz | 110 | 0 | 26 |
| **Organic Flakes:** | | | |
| Oat Bran, 1 cup, 1.8 oz | 190 | 1.5 | 39 |
| Sprouted Amaranth, 1¼ cups, 2 oz | 210 | 2 | 43 |

### Heartland:

| | C | F | Cb |
|---|---|---|---|
| **Granola:** Original, ½ cup, 2 oz | 240 | 6 | 41 |
| Fruit & Nut, ½ cup, 1.8 oz | 210 | 6 | 34 |
| Harvest Spice, ½ cup, 1.8 oz | 210 | 5 | 37 |
| Low-Fat with Raisin, ½ cup, 1.8 oz | 200 | 3 | 40 |

### Hershey's, Cookies 'n' Creme, 1 oz

| | C | F | Cb |
|---|---|---|---|
| | 110 | 3 | 21 |

### Kashi:

| | C | F | Cb |
|---|---|---|---|
| **7 Whole Grain:** Flakes, 1 c., 1.8 oz | 170 | 0.5 | 41 |
| Honey Puffs, 1 cup, 1 oz | 110 | 1 | 26 |
| Nuggets, ½ cup, 2 oz | 210 | 1.5 | 46 |
| Puffs, 1 cup, 0.7 oz | 100 | 1 | 22 |
| **GoLEAN:** Original, 1¼ cups, 2 oz | 180 | 2 | 40 |
| Crunch!: Original, ¾ cup, 2 oz | 190 | 3 | 38 |
| Honey Almond Flax, ⅔ cup, 2 oz | 200 | 5 | 35 |
| Vanilla Pepitas, 1 cup, 2 oz | 230 | 6 | 37 |

### Heart to Heart:

| | C | F | Cb |
|---|---|---|---|
| Honey Toasted Oat, ¾ cup, 1.2 oz | 120 | 1.5 | 26 |
| Oat Flakes & Blueb. Clusters, 1 c., 2 oz | 200 | 2.5 | 42 |
| Warm Cinnamon Oat, ¾ cup, 1.2 oz | 120 | 1.5 | 26 |

### Organic Corn:

| | C | F | Cb |
|---|---|---|---|
| Indigo Morning, ¾ cup | 100 | 1 | 22 |
| Simply Maize, ¾ cup, 1 oz | 100 | 1 | 23 |

### Organic Promise:

| | C | F | Cb |
|---|---|---|---|
| Sprouted Grains, 1¼cups, 2 oz | 190 | 1 | 45 |
| Sweet Potato Sunshine, 1cup 1.8 oz | 180 | 1 | 43 |

### Wheat Biscuit

| | C | F | Cb |
|---|---|---|---|
| Berry Fruitful, 1.8 oz | 170 | 0.5 | 42 |
| Dark Cocoa Karma, 1.95 oz | 180 | 1 | 42 |

### Kellogg's:

**All-Bran:**

| | C | F | Cb |
|---|---|---|---|
| Original, ½ cup, 1 oz | 80 | 1 | 23 |
| Bran Buds, ⅓ cup, 1 oz | 80 | 1 | 24 |
| Compl. Wheat Flakes, 1 oz | 90 | 0.5 | 24 |
| **Apple Jacks,** 1 cup, 1 oz | 100 | 1 | 25 |
| **Cinnabon,** 1 cup, 1 oz | 120 | 2 | 25 |

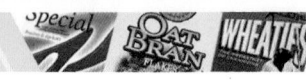

## Ready-To-Eat Cereal (Cont)

| | C | F | Cb |
|---|---|---|---|
| **Kellogg's (Cont):** | | | |
| **Corn Flakes,** Orig., 1 c., 1 oz | 100 | 0 | 24 |
| **Cracklin' Oat Bran,** | | | |
| ¾ cup, 1.8 oz | 200 | 7 | 34 |
| **Crispix,** Original, 1 cup, 1 oz | 110 | 0 | 25 |
| **Crunchy Nut,** Golden Nut Flakes, | | | |
| ¾ cup, 1 oz | 120 | 1 | 26 |
| **Froot Loops:** Original, 1 cup, 1 oz | 110 | 1 | 26 |
| Marshmallow, 1 cup, 1 oz | 110 | 1 | 26 |
| **Frosted Flakes:** | | | |
| Original, ¾ cup, 1 oz | 110 | 0 | 26 |
| with Marshmallows, 1 oz | 110 | 0 | 26 |
| **Honey Smacks,** ¾ cup, 1 oz | 100 | 0.5 | 24 |
| **Krave:** | | | |
| Chocolate, ¾ cup, 1.1 oz | 120 | 3.5 | 24 |
| Double Choc., ¾ c., 1.1 oz | 120 | 3.5 | 23 |
| **Mini-Wheats, Frosted:** | | | |
| Big Bites (7), 2 oz | 200 | 1 | 49 |
| Bite Size, Orig. (21), 2 oz | 190 | 1 | 46 |
| Crunch, 1 cup, 2 oz | 200 | 2 | 44 |
| Little Bites: Orig., 1 c., 2 oz | 200 | 1 | 47 |
| Chocolate, 1 cup, 2 oz | 200 | 2 | 46 |
| Touch of Fruit In Middle, | | | |
| Raspberry (24), 2 oz | 190 | 1 | 45 |
| **Mini Wheats,** unfrosted, | | | |
| Bite Size (30), 2 oz | 190 | 1 | 45 |
| **Mueslix,** ⅔ cup, 2 oz | 200 | 3 | 41 |
| **Origins:** | | | |
| Ancient Grains, ¾ cup, 1.1 oz | 110 | 0.5 | 26 |
| Fruit & Nut, ¾ cup, 1.7 oz | 190 | 4 | 38 |
| Granola, av., ½ cup, 1.8 oz | 200 | 3.5 | 38 |
| Muesli, ½ cup, 1.8 oz | 180 | 4 | 34 |
| **Product 19,** 1 cup, 1 oz | 110 | 0 | 25 |
| **Raisin Bran:** Reg., 1 cup, 2 oz | 190 | 1 | 46 |
| Crunch, 1 cup, 2 oz | 190 | 1 | 45 |
| **Rice Krispies:** | | | |
| Original, 1¼ cups, 1.2 oz | 130 | 0 | 29 |
| Frosted, ¾ cup, 1 oz | 120 | 0 | 27 |
| Treats, ¾ cup, 1 oz | 120 | 1 | 26 |
| **Smart Start,** | | | |
| Original Antioxidants, 1 cup, 1.8 oz | 190 | 1 | 43 |
| **Special K:** | | | |
| Chocolate Almond, ⅔ cup, 1 oz | 110 | 1.5 | 23 |
| Cinnamon Pecan, ¾ cup, 1.1 oz | 110 | 2 | 24 |
| Granola, Touch of Honey, | | | |
| Low Fat, ½ cup, 1.8 oz | 190 | 3 | 39 |
| Oats & Honey, ¾ cup, 1 oz | 100 | 0.5 | 25 |
| Protein, average, ¾ cup, 1.1 oz | 115 | 1 | 21 |
| Vanilla Almond, ¾ cup | 110 | 1.5 | 25 |

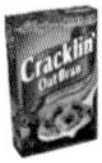

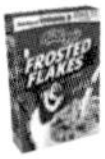

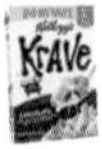

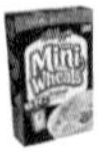

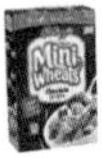

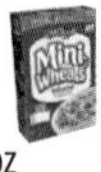

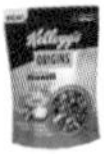

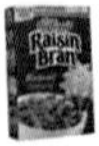

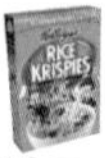

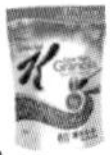

| | C | F | Cb |
|---|---|---|---|
| **Malt-O-Meal:** | | | |
| **Apple Zings,** 1 cup, 1.2 oz | 130 | 1 | 30 |
| **Cocoa Dyno-Bites,** ¾ c. | 120 | 1 | 26 |
| **Coco Roos,** ¾ cup, 1 oz | 120 | 1.5 | 26 |
| **Frosted Flakes,** ¾ cup, 1 oz | 120 | 0 | 28 |
| **Frosted Mini Spooners,** 1 cup | 190 | 1 | 45 |
| **Golden Puffs,** ¾ cup, 1 oz | 100 | 0 | 24 |
| **Honey Nut Scooters,** | | | |
| 1 cup, 1 oz | 120 | 1.5 | 24 |
| **Raisin Bran,** 1 cup, 2 oz | 220 | 1.5 | 45 |
| **Nature's Path:** | | | |
| **Flax Plus:** Flakes, 1 oz | 110 | 1.5 | 23 |
| Maple Pecan Crunch, ¾ cup | 220 | 7 | 38 |
| Pumpkin Raisin Crunch, ¾ c. | 210 | 4.5 | 40 |
| Raisin Bran, 2 oz | 190 | 2.5 | 41 |
| **Heritage Flakes,** 1 oz | 120 | 1 | 24 |
| **Honey'd Corn Flakes,** | | | |
| ¾ cup, 1 oz | 120 | 0 | 27 |
| **Kamut Puffs,** 1 cup, 0.5 oz | 50 | 0 | 11 |
| **Multigrain Oatbran Flakes,** | | | |
| ¾ cup, 1 oz | 110 | 1 | 24 |
| **Qi'a,** all varieties, av., 2Tbsp, 1 oz | 135 | 6.5 | 14 |
| **Optimum Power,** | | | |
| Blueberry Cinnamon Flax, 1 oz | 120 | 1.5 | 25 |
| **New England Natural Bakers:** | | | |
| **Organic/Granola:** (11-12 oz Pouches) | | | |
| Antioxidants Granola, ½ cup, 1.9 oz | 230 | 6 | 37 |
| Cinn. Raisin Muesli, unsw'd, ⅔ c., 2 oz | 260 | 10 | 35 |
| Gluten-Free Crispy Fruit, ⅔ c., 2 oz | 250 | 9 | 39 |
| Omega Hemp & Flax, ½ cup, 1.8 oz | 240 | 10 | 33 |
| Granola Clusters, av. ⅔ cup, 2 oz | 250 | 8 | 38 |
| Hi Protein: 5-Seed, unsw'd, ½ c., 2 oz | 270 | 14 | 28 |
| Blueb. Harvest, ⅔ cup, 2.1 oz | 260 | 10 | 35 |
| **NutriSystem:** *Per Package* | | | |
| **Apple Cinnamon Oatmeal** | 130 | 1.5 | 26 |
| **Granola Cereal** | 150 | 3 | 28 |
| **NutriFlakes** | 110 | 1 | 23 |
| **Sweetened O's** | 110 | 0 | 22 |
| **Peace:** | | | |
| **Clusters & Flakes:** | | | |
| Cherry /Vanilla Almond, 2 oz | 240 | 6 | 42 |
| Av. other varieties, 2 oz | 235 | 5 | 43 |
| Low Fat, Wild Berry, 2 oz | 220 | 3 | 44 |
| **Crispy Rice & Flakes,** | | | |
| Blueberry Pomegranate, 2 oz | 240 | 6 | 41 |
| **Granola:** Coconut Craze, 2 oz | 270 | 12 | 37 |
| Average other varieties, 2 oz | 245 | 7 | 40 |

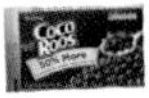

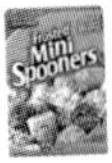

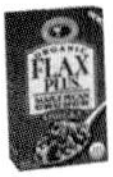

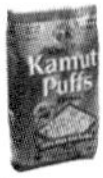

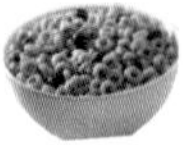

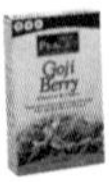

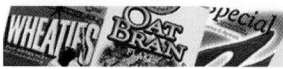

## Ready-To-Eat Cereal ~ Brands (Cont)

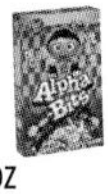

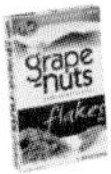

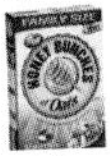

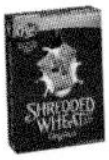

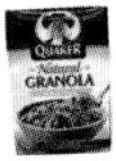

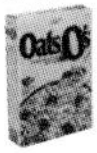

**Post:**
| | C | F | Cb |
|---|---|---|---|
| **Alpha Bits**, 1 cup, 1 oz | 120 | 1.5 | 24 |
| **Bran Flakes**, ¾ cup, 1 oz | 100 | 0.5 | 24 |
| **Good Mornings**, average, 1 oz | 120 | 1.5 | 25 |
| **Grape-Nuts:** Original, 2 oz | 210 | 1 | 47 |
| Fit, ⅔ cup, 2 oz | 230 | 4 | 41 |
| Flakes, ¾ cup, 1 oz | 110 | 1 | 24 |
| **Great Grains:** | | | |
| Banana Nut Crunch, 1 cup, 2 oz | 230 | 5 | 42 |
| Cranb. Alm. Crunch, 1cup, 2 oz | 210 | 3.5 | 41 |
| Prot. Blend, Hon., Oats & Seeds, 2 oz | 220 | 5 | 37 |
| **Honey Bunches of Oats:** | | | |
| Almond/Honey Crunch, av., 1.2 oz | 130 | 1.5 | 27 |
| Chocolate, 1.2 oz | 130 | 1.5 | 27 |
| Granola Protein Choc., 1.8 oz | 220 | 6 | 31 |
| Real Fruit Var., av., 1.1 oz | 120 | 2 | 26 |
| Roasted, 1.1 oz | 120 | 1.5 | 25 |
| With Almonds, ¾ cup, 1 oz | 130 | 2.5 | 26 |
| **Honeycomb**, Original, 1½ cups, 1 oz | 130 | 1 | 28 |
| **Pebbles**, average all varieties, ¾ cup, 1 oz | 115 | 1 | 24 |
| **Raisin Bran**, 1 cup, 2 oz | 190 | 1 | 47 |
| **Selects**, Blueberry Morning, 1¼ cups, 2 oz | 220 | 3 | 45 |
| **Shredded Wheat**, Spoon Size: | | | |
| Original, 1.7 oz | 170 | 1 | 40 |
| Honey Nut, 2.1 oz | 220 | 2 | 49 |
| **Waffle Crisp**, 1 cup, 1 oz | 120 | 1.5 | 25 |
| **Quaker:** | | | |
| **King Vitaman**, 1½ cups, 1 oz | 120 | 1 | 26 |
| **Life**, all types, ¾ cup, 1 oz | 120 | 1.5 | 25 |
| **Natural Granola:** | | | |
| Apple Cranberry Almond, 1.7 oz | 200 | 5 | 37 |
| Oats, Honey, & Alm., ½ cup, 1.7 oz | 200 | 6 | 35 |
| **Oatmeal Squares**, all varieties, 2 oz | 210 | 2.5 | 44 |
| **Quisps**, 1 cup 1 oz | 100 | 1.5 | 23 |
| **Stop & Shop:** | | | |
| **Fiber Select**, ½ cup, 1 oz | 50 | 0.5 | 23 |
| **Granola**, Oats & Honey, ½ c., 1.8 oz | 230 | 9 | 31 |
| **Oats & O's**, 1 cup, 1.1 oz | 110 | 1.5 | 22 |
| **Raisin Bran**, 1 cup, 2 oz | 190 | 1 | 46 |
| **Shredded Wheat**, Bite Size, 1 c., 1.5 oz | 140 | 1 | 33 |
| **Sweet Home Farm:** | | | |
| **Blueberry**, w/Flax, ¾ cup, 2 oz | 250 | 8 | 40 |
| **Cinnamon**, w/Raisins, ½ c., 1.8 oz | 200 | 3 | 43 |
| **French Vanilla**, w/Alm., ⅔ c., 2 oz | 250 | 8 | 40 |
| **Honey Nut**, w/Alm., ½ c., 2 oz | 260 | 10 | 37 |
| **Maple Pecan**, w/Syrup, ½ c., 2 oz | 250 | 8 | 40 |
| **Pumpkin Flax**, ⅔ cup, 2 oz | 240 | 9 | 37 |

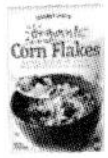

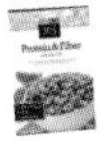

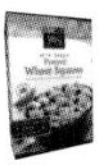

**Trader Joe's:**
| | C | F | Cb |
|---|---|---|---|
| **Bran Flakes**, ¾ cup, 1 oz | 100 | 0.5 | 24 |
| **Clusters:** Raisin Bran, 1 cup, 2 oz | 190 | 3 | 41 |
| Super Nutty Toffee, ¾ cup, 2 oz | 250 | 9 | 38 |
| Vanilla Almond, ⅔ cup, 2 oz | 220 | 8 | 34 |
| Av. other Flavors, 1 c., 2 oz | 230 | 8 | 40 |
| **Cornflakes**, 1 cup, 1 oz | 110 | 0 | 26 |
| **Crisp Rice Cereal**, 1 c., 1 oz | 120 | 0 | 26 |
| **Frosted Flakes**, ¾ c., 1 oz | 110 | 0 | 24 |
| **High Fiber Cereal:** Reg., ⅔ cup, 1 oz | 80 | 0.5 | 23 |
| Fruit & Nut, Multigrain, ⅔ c., 1 oz | 90 | 1.5 | 25 |
| **Granola:** Gluten Free, ¾ cup, 2 oz | 60 | 12 | 35 |
| Low Fat, av., ¾ cup, 2 oz | 210 | 3 | 44 |
| Org., Apple/Mango, av., ⅔ cup, 2 oz | 240 | 8 | 37 |
| **Joe's O's**, 1 cup, 1 oz | 110 | 2 | 20 |
| **Just The Clusters**, av., ⅔ cup, 2 oz | 240 | 9 | 36 |
| **O's**, av. all flavours, ¾ - 1 cup, 1 oz | 120 | 2 | 24 |
| **Oatmeal (Instant):** Per 40g Pkt | | | |
| Ancient Grains | 160 | 6 | 24 |
| Mango; Maple & Brown Sugar, av. | 160 | 2 | 32 |
| Unsweetened | 160 | 3.5 | 27 |
| **Oatmeal Complete:** Plain, 40g pkt | 170 | 3 | 29 |
| Maple Brown Sugar, 40g pkt | 210 | 3 | 38 |
| **Raisin Bran:** Regular, 1 cup, 1 oz | 170 | 1 | 44 |
| Clusters, 1 cup, 2 oz | 190 | 3 | 41 |
| w/ Pomegr. Blue. Flakes/Clusters, 1 c. | 210 | 2 | 44 |
| **Shredded Wheat**, 1 cup, 1.7 oz | 180 | 1 | 38 |
| **Toasted Oatmeal Flakes**, ¾ c.,1 oz | 110 | 1 | 23 |
| **Udi's:** | | | |
| **Granola:** Orig.; Cranb., ¼ c., 1 oz | 140 | 6 | 21 |
| All Naturel; Vanilla, av., ¼ cup, 1 oz | 120 | 4 | 19 |
| **Uncle Sam:** Original, ¾ cup, 2 oz | 190 | 5 | 38 |
| Raisin Bran, 1 cup, 2 oz | 190 | 1 | 42 |
| **Weetabix**, 2 biscuits, 1.3 oz | 130 | 1 | 29 |
| **Wegmans:** | | | |
| **Cinnamon Muffin Squares**, 1 oz | 130 | 3.5 | 24 |
| **Cinnamon Oat Crisps**, 1 oz | 120 | 1 | 26 |
| **Chocolaty Rice Crisps**, 1 oz | 120 | 1 | 26 |
| **Crunchy Raisin Bran**, 1 cup, 1.8 oz | 190 | 1 | 44 |
| **Granola**, ½ cup | 230 | 9 | 31 |
| **Peanut Butter Corn Crunch**, 1 oz | 110 | 2.5 | 20 |
| **Shredded Wheat**, 1 cup, 2 oz | 190 | 1 | 45 |
| **Whole Foods 365:** | | | |
| **Corn Flakes**, 1 cup, 1 oz | 110 | 0 | 26 |
| **Frosted Flakes**, 1 oz | 110 | 0 | 27 |
| **Honey Flakes & Oat Clusters**, ¾ cup, 1 oz | 120 | 1 | 25 |
| **Protein & Fiber Crunch**, 1.8 oz | 190 | 11 | 33 |
| **Raisin Bran**, 1 cup, 2 oz | 180 | 1 | 44 |
| **Wheat Squares:** | | | |
| Bite Sized, 1.7 oz | 180 | 1 | 38 |
| Frosted, 1 cup, 1.9 oz | 210 | 1 | 45 |

### Ready-to-Eat  **C** **F** **Cb**

*Per Piece/Slice*

| | C | F | Cb |
|---|---|---|---|
| **Angel Food**, Plain: without oil, 2 oz | 145 | 0 | 33 |
| with oil, 2 oz | 145 | 1 | 27 |
| with Cream Frosting | 255 | 7 | 45 |
| **Almond Croissant**, 5 oz | 620 | 35 | 67 |
| **Apple Danish**, 5 oz | 450 | 18 | 67 |
| **Apple Pie** ~ *See Pies/Tarts Page 134* | | | |
| **Baklava**, 1½" square, 1.75 oz | 200 | 10 | 27 |
| **Banana Cake**, with Butter Cream, 2 oz | 230 | 9 | 37 |
| **Banana Walnut Cake**, 3 oz | 270 | 11 | 40 |
| **Bear Claw**, 4.5 oz | 540 | 24 | 71 |
| **Black Forest**, 3 oz | 345 | 11 | 59 |
| **Brownie**: Small, 2" Square, 1 oz | 130 | 8 | 14 |
| Large, 3 oz | 390 | 24 | 42 |
| **Bundt Cakes**, average all types: | | | |
| 3 oz slice | 300 | 13 | 42 |
| Mini-Bundt, 5 oz | 500 | 22 | 70 |
| **Cannoli's**: Mini, 1 oz | 85 | 3 | 11 |
| Regular, 2.5 oz | 215 | 8 | 28 |
| **Carrot Cake**: Plain, 3 oz | 300 | 16 | 37 |
| with Cream Cheese Frosting | 400 | 22 | 48 |
| **Cheesecake**: | | | |
| Small serving, 3 oz | 240 | 13 | 26 |
| Large serving, 5 oz | 400 | 21 | 44 |
| with Low-Fat Cheese/Fruit, 3 oz | 170 | 4 | 28 |
| *Denny's*, NY Style, 5oz | 510 | 34 | 43 |
| **Chocolate Cake**: | | | |
| with Chocolate Frosting, 4 oz | 415 | 18 | 62 |
| without Frosting, ¹⁄₁₂ of 9", 3.5 oz | 340 | 14 | 51 |
| **Chocolate Croissant**, 4.25 oz | 470 | 26 | 54 |
| **Chocolate Eclair**, w/ custard, 3.5 oz | 260 | 16 | 24 |
| **Chocolate Fudge Cake**, 3 oz | 270 | 12 | 40 |
| **Chocolate Meringue**, 2.5 oz | 320 | 13 | 48 |
| **Churros**, 1 stick, 1.5 oz | 165 | 8 | 21 |
| **Cinnamon Crumb Cake**, 2.5 oz | 260 | 9 | 40 |
| **Cinnamon Rolls**: Small, 2 oz | 220 | 8 | 34 |
| Regular, 4 oz | 440 | 16 | 68 |
| Large, 6 oz | 660 | 24 | 102 |
| **Brands** ~ *See Page 67* | | | |
| **Coffee Cake**, 2 oz | 180 | 6 | 30 |
| **Concha**: Small, 2 oz | 240 | 9 | 33 |
| Large (5" diameter), 5.5 oz | 615 | 23 | 85 |
| **Cream Puff**, custard filled, 4.6 oz | 335 | 20 | 30 |
| **Cream Horn**, 3 oz | 210 | 5 | 36 |
| **Crumble Coffee Cake**, 4.5 oz | 500 | 25 | 65 |
| **Danish Pastries**: | | | |
| Small, 2.5 oz | 250 | 14 | 25 |
| Large, 5 oz | 500 | 28 | 50 |
| **Donuts** ~ *See Page 66* | | | |
| **Eclair**, Chocolate, custard filled, 3.5 oz | 260 | 16 | 24 |
| **Fig Bars**, average | 160 | 3 | 31 |

### Ready-to-Eat (Cont)  **C** **F** **Cb**

*Per Piece/Slice*

| | C | F | Cb |
|---|---|---|---|
| **Fruit Cake**, Dark/Light, 2 oz | 185 | 5 | 34 |
| **Fudge Nut Brownie**, 3.5 oz | 380 | 18 | 54 |
| **Gingerbread**, from mix, 3" square | 210 | 4 | 41 |
| **Honey Bun**, 2.7 oz | 310 | 15 | 39 |
| **Jelly Roll**, ½ roll, 1.8 oz | 150 | 2 | 32 |
| **Key Lime Pie**, 4.3 oz | 400 | 25 | 41 |
| **Kringles**: Almond; Pecan, average | 205 | 12 | 24 |
| Blueberry: Cherry; Raspberry, av. | 165 | 8 | 24 |
| **Lady Finger**, 3 oz | 310 | 4.5 | 59 |
| **Lemon Cake**, 4 oz | 440 | 24 | 49 |
| **Lemon Poppy Seed Creme**, 1.6 oz | 180 | 9 | 23 |
| **Marble Cake**, 4 oz | 430 | 23 | 50 |
| **Mississippi Mud Pie**, 4 oz | 480 | 22 | 67 |
| **Mud Cake**, 4.5 oz | 380 | 20 | 44 |
| **Muffins** ~ *See Page 67* | | | |
| **Palmier Cookie**, large, 4.5 oz | 490 | 25 | 62 |
| **Pineapple Upside Down Cake**, | | | |
| 2.5 oz | 230 | 9 | 36 |
| **Peach Melba**, 3.5 oz | 300 | 8 | 52 |
| **Pecan Sticky Roll**, 6.5 oz | 690 | 22 | 91 |
| **Pecan Twirls**, 1.3 oz | 170 | 7 | 26 |
| **Pies & Tarts** ~ *See Page 134* | | | |
| **Pound Cakes**: Iced Lemon, 3.5 oz | 360 | 17 | 50 |
| Marble, 3.75 oz | 350 | 13 | 53 |
| **Raspberry Rugulah**, | | | |
| 1.2 oz | 110 | 9 | 7 |
| **Scone**, fruit, 2 oz | 200 | 9 | 30 |
| **Sponge Cake**: Plain, 2.5 oz | 220 | 10 | 33 |
| with Chocolate Frosting | 290 | 12 | 45 |
| with Cream & Strawberry Jam | 390 | 12 | 69 |
| **Starbucks Cakes** ~ *Page 244* | | | |
| **Strawberry Creme Cake**, 4.7 oz | 400 | 27 | 33 |
| **Strudel Bites**, 0.75 oz | 60 | 2.5 | 9 |
| **Strudel**, fruit, av., 4.5 oz | 300 | 17 | 32 |
| **Swiss Rolls**, 1 oz | 135 | 6 | 19 |
| **Tiramisu**, 4.5 oz | 440 | 22 | 34 |
| **Turnovers**, fruit, average, 3 oz | 290 | 15 | 35 |

### Cupcakes

*Average all Varieties*

| | C | F | Cb |
|---|---|---|---|
| **Regular**: | | | |
| Cake only, 1.5 oz | 140 | 5.5 | 20 |
| Cake + Icing, 2.5 oz | 260 | 13 | 34 |
| **Large**: (Muffin Size): | | | |
| Cake only, 2.5 oz | 235 | 9 | 34 |
| Cake + Icing, 5 oz | 520 | 27 | 67 |
| **Mini**, (2-Bite): | | | |
| Cake only, 0.4 oz | 40 | 1.5 | 5.5 |
| Cake + Icing, 1 oz | 110 | 5.5 | 13 |
| **Icing Only**: Per 1 oz | 115 | 7 | 13 |
| Thick/Tall amount, 2.5 oz | 290 | 17 | 32 |

## Cakes ~ Brands | C | F | Cb |

### Albertson's Bakery:
**Ring Cakes:** *Per ⅛ Cake*

| | C | F | Cb |
|---|---|---|---|
| Angel Food, 2 oz | 160 | 0 | 36 |
| Butter; Chocolate, av., 3 oz | 305 | 15 | 39 |

**Cake Slices:** *Per Slice Unless Indicated*

| | | | |
|---|---|---|---|
| Banana Nut Loaf 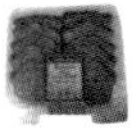 | 330 | 17 | 39 |
| Butter Creme | 110 | 6 | 20 |
| Creme Cake (2), 3.2 oz | 300 | 12 | 43 |
| Cinnamon Streusel (2), 3.2 oz | 350 | 18 | 43 |

### Bimbo Bakery:
**Concha**, Vanilla, 2 oz | 260 | 11 | 35

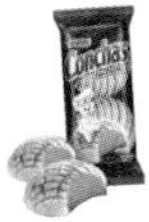

**Pound Cakes:** *Per Slice*

| | | | |
|---|---|---|---|
| Panquecitos, 1.8 oz | 170 | 4.5 | 29 |
| Pecan, 2.3 oz | 260 | 11 | 36 |
| Raisin, 2.3 oz | 240 | 9 | 38 |

### Bon Appetit Bakery:
**Banana Bread**, 4 oz | 440 | 25 | 49

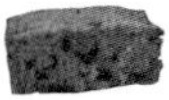

**Cream Cheese Cake**,

| | | | |
|---|---|---|---|
| 4 oz slice | 430 | 24 | 49 |

**Danish:** Apple (1), 5 oz | 210 | 11 | 25

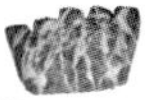

| | | | |
|---|---|---|---|
| Bear Claw (1), 5 oz | 240 | 13 | 27 |
| Cheese & Berries (1), 5 oz | 250 | 14 | 26 |
| Vienna Cream (1), 5 oz | 240 | 14 | 27 |

**Slices:** Cheesecake, 4 oz | 430 | 24 | 49

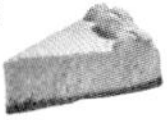

| | | | |
|---|---|---|---|
| Lemon Cake, 4 oz | 430 | 24 | 49 |
| Marble Cake, 4 oz | 430 | 24 | 50 |

**Walnut Brownie**, 3.5 oz | 380 | 18 | 54

**Cheesecake Factory** ~ *See Fast-Foods Section*

### Entenmann's: *Per Slice*
**Crumb Cakes:** All Butter French, 1.8 oz | 210 | 10 | 29

| | | | |
|---|---|---|---|
| Cheese-Filled, 2 oz | 200 | 10 | 25 |
| Chocolate, ⅛ oz | 270 | 12 | 39 |

**Danish:** Pecan Twist, ⅙ cake | 260 | 16 | 27

| | | | |
|---|---|---|---|
| Raspberry Twist, 2 oz | 220 | 11 | 29 |
| Walnut Twist, ⅙ cake 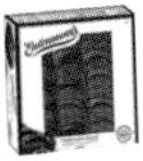 | 260 | 15 | 26 |

**Dessert Cakes:**

| | | | |
|---|---|---|---|
| Chocolate Fudge, 2.3 oz | 240 | 10 | 37 |
| Lemon/Louisiana Crunch, 3 oz | 330 | 14 | 49 |
| Strawberry Iced Cake, ⅙ cake | 350 | 17 | 47 |

**Loaf Cakes:** Chocolate, ⅙ loaf | 190 | 8 | 29

| | | | |
|---|---|---|---|
| Cinnamon Crunch, ⅙ loaf | 270 | 14 | 33 |

### Glenny's:
**100 Calorie:**

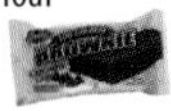

| | | | |
|---|---|---|---|
| Blondie, Choc. Chip, 1.5 oz | 100 | 4 | 15 |
| Brownies: Chocolate Chip, 1.5 oz | 100 | 4 | 12 |
| Peanut Butter, 1.5 oz | 100 | 4 | 15 |

**Muffins/Sweet Rolls ~ See Page 67**

### Great American Cookies: | C | F | Cb |
**Cookie Cakes:** *Per Slice*

| | | | |
|---|---|---|---|
| By the Slice, 4.5 oz 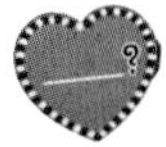 | 580 | 27 | 83 |
| Heart Shaped, 3.5 oz | 440 | 21 | 64 |
| M&M, 4 oz | 500 | 24 | 73 |

### Great Value (Walmart):

| | | | |
|---|---|---|---|
| Chocolate Cup Cake, (1), 1.8 oz | 170 | 5 | 31 |
| Devil's Food Cake, (1), 1.4 oz | 160 | 7 | 23 |
| Snack Cakes: Fudge Swirl, (1), 1.3oz | 165 | 8 | 23 |
| Choc./Lemon Snack Cake, 1 oz | 120 | 6 | 18 |
| Swiss Roll Snack Cake (1), 1 oz | 120 | 5 | 17 |

### Hostess:
**Cup Cakes:**

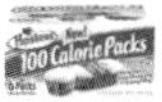

| | | | |
|---|---|---|---|
| 100 Calorie Packs, av., 3 minicakes | 100 | 2.5 | 21 |
| 8 Pack, Chocolate, 1 cake, 1.5 oz | 160 | 6 | 26 |

| | | | |
|---|---|---|---|
| Ding Dongs, (1) | 165 | 9 | 22 |
| Ho Hos, (1) 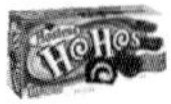 | 120 | 5 | 18 |

**Twinkies:**

| | | | |
|---|---|---|---|
| Original; Banana, av., (1) 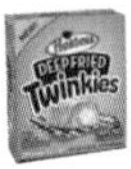 | 140 | 5 | 24 |
| Deep Fried: Original (1) | 220 | 9 | 32 |
| Chocolate (1) | 220 | 8 | 36 |
| Zingers, (2) | 250 | 9 | 41 |

**Donettes ~** *Page 66*

### Little Debbie:

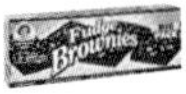

| | | | |
|---|---|---|---|
| Brownie, Fudge (1) | 300 | 13 | 43 |
| Choc. Chip Cake, 2 oz | 300 | 14 | 42 |
| Choc. Cup Cake, Creme Filled (1) | 430 | 17 | 65 |
| Cocoa Cremes, (1), 1.5 oz 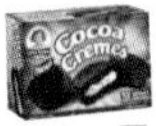 | 170 | 8 | 24 |
| Devil Cremes ,(1), 1.7 oz | 260 | 11 | 38 |
| Devil Squares, (2), 2.2 oz | 260 | 11 | 38 |
| Fancy Cakes, (2) 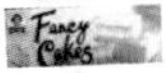 | 310 | 15 | 43 |
| Frosted Fudge Cake, 1.5 oz | 190 | 9 | 27 |
| Roll, Boston Creme, 2.2 oz | 270 | 12 | 40 |
| Zebra Cake, (2), 2.5 oz 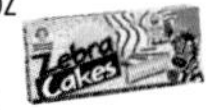 | 320 | 14 | 48 |

### Ne-Mo's:
**Breads:** Banana, 4 oz | 460 | 23 | 57

| | | | |
|---|---|---|---|
| Carrot, 4 oz | 450 | 22 | 56 |
| Cheese Coffee Cake, 4 oz | 460 | 21 | 62 |
| Wild Blueberry Bread, 4 oz | 430 | 20 | 58 |

**Brookie**, (1), 1.5 oz | 160 | 7 | 26

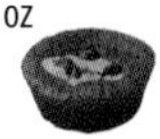

**Bundt:** Chocolate, 4 oz | 380 | 14 | 62

| | | | |
|---|---|---|---|
| Coconut Pineapple, 4 oz 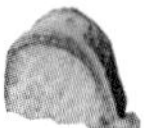 | 410 | 18 | 60 |
| Key Lime, 4 oz | 440 | 18 | 67 |
| Orange Dreamswirl | 440 | 18 | 67 |

**Cake Squares:** Carrot, 3.6 oz | 390 | 21 | 47

| | | | |
|---|---|---|---|
| Banana; Chocolate, av, 3 oz | 300 | 12 | 45 |

**Crumble Cake:** Blueberry (1), 4 oz | 390 | 17 | 54

| | | | |
|---|---|---|---|
| Cinnamon Streusel (1), 4 oz | 420 | 18 | 59 |
| Lemon Rasp. (1), 4 oz | 400 | 19 | 55 |

### Cakes ~ Brands (Cont)

| | C | F | Cb |
|---|---|---|---|
| **Pepperidge Farm:** | | | |
| **3-Layer Cakes:** *Per ⅛ Cake* | | | |
| Chocolate Fudge | 240 | 13 | 32 |
| Coconut | 250 | 12 | 34 |
| Key Lime; Vanilla | 240 | 12 | 34 |
| Average other varieties | 240 | 11 | 33 |
| **Turnovers (Frozen):** | | | |
| Apple; Cherry (1) | 260 | 13 | 31 |
| Chocolate (1) | 350 | 22 | 35 |
| Peach; Raspberry (1) | 270 | 13 | 34 |
| **Pop Tarts** *(Kellogg's):* | | | |
| Fruit/Frosted/Unfrosted, av. | 200 | 5 | 36 |
| Gone Nutty, | | | |
| average all varieties, 1.8 oz | 200 | 6 | 35 |
| **Safeway Select,** | | | |
| Molten Chocolate Lava Cake, 4.5 oz | 440 | 26 | 50 |
| **Sara Lee:** | | | |
| **Carrot Cake**, ⅙ cake | 340 | 18 | 41 |
| **Cheesecakes:** | | | |
| Classic: French, 4.7 oz slice | 410 | 26 | 38 |
| Strawberry, 4.3 oz slice | 320 | 18 | 37 |
| New York Style, 5 oz slice | 480 | 29 | 48 |
| Limited Edition, | | | |
| NY Style, Chocolate, 5 oz slice | 500 | 29 | 55 |
| Original Cream: | | | |
| Cherry, 4.8 oz slice | 320 | 11 | 50 |
| Classic, 4.3 oz slice | 340 | 18 | 38 |
| Strawberry, 4.7 oz slice | 330 | 12 | 51 |
| **Coffee Cake**, Butter Streusel, ⅙ cake | 190 | 9 | 24 |
| **Pound Cakes:** | | | |
| All Butter, 1.9 oz slice | 260 | 9 | 42 |
| Lemon, 2.7 oz slice | 270 | 9 | 42 |
| Individual Slices: | | | |
| All Butter, 1 oz | 100 | 3 | 15 |
| Double Choc., 1.8 oz | 180 | 7 | 28 |
| Lemon, 1 oz | 100 | 3.5 | 15 |
| Original, 1.6 oz | 160 | 5 | 25 |
| **Smart Ones** *(Weight Watchers):* | | | |
| **Smart Delights:** *Per Sundae* | | | |
| Chocolate Chip Cookie Dough | 140 | 3 | 26 |
| Peanut Butter Cup | 130 | 3 | 23 |
| Strawberry Shortcake | 120 | 4 | 19 |
| **Special K,** | | | |
| Pastry Crisps, all varieties, (2), 1 oz | 100 | 2 | 20 |

| | C | F | Cb |
|---|---|---|---|
| **Tastykake:** | | | |
| **Choc Cupcakes:** | | | |
| Choc. Koffee Kake, 2.1 oz | 240 | 9 | 37 |
| Cream Filled, 2.1 oz | 220 | 8 | 34 |
| Banana Pudding, 2 oz | 180 | 6 | 31 |
| **Kandy Kake:** | | | |
| Lemon Flavored, 2 oz | 290 | 16 | 34 |
| Peanut Butter, 1.4 oz | 190 | 11 | 19 |
| **Krimpets**,Spice Kake Cake, (2) | 220 | 7 | 37 |
| **Mini Cupcakes**, Koffee Kake (3) | 180 | 8 | 25 |
| **Toaster Strudel** *(Pillsbury): Per 2 oz* | | | |
| **Boston Cream Pie** | 180 | 7 | 26 |
| **Cream Cheese**, | | | |
| average all varieties | 180 | 9 | 26 |
| **Fruit flavors**, all var. | 180 | 7 | 27 |
| **Trader Joe's:** | | | |
| **Bakery Fresh:** | | | |
| Apricot Almond Tart, | | | |
| 4 oz slice | 450 | 24 | 56 |
| Cheesecake Brownie Bites (1) | 110 | 7 | 9 |
| Chocolate Ganache Cake, 3 oz slice | 390 | 22 | 44 |
| Flourless Chocolate Cake, | | | |
| 1 slice, 2 oz | 260 | 17 | 23 |
| Lemon Cake, 3.3oz slice | 350 | 19 | 43 |
| Mini Carrot Cake, 5 oz | 450 | 19 | 68 |
| Whoopie Pie (1), 2.5 oz | 350 | 14 | 54 |
| Bread Cake: | | | |
| Banana Bonanza, 2.6 oz slice | 250 | 9 | 39 |
| Pumpkin Nut, 2.6 oz slice | 270 | 10 | 43 |
| Walnut Streusel Coffee, 2 oz slice | 180 | 8 | 25 |
| Zucchini Carrot, 2 oz slice | 200 | 7 | 32 |
| Loaf Cake: | | | |
| Cranberry Pumpkin, 2 oz slice | 140 | 2 | 30 |
| Pumpkin Nut, 2.6 oz slice | 270 | 10 | 43 |
| **Frozen:** | | | |
| Apple Raspberry Turnover, 3.2 oz | 280 | 14 | 34 |
| Chocolate Dilemma Cheesecake: | | | |
| Plain, 3.5 oz | 320 | 19 | 30 |
| Choc. Chip; Triple Choc, av., 3.5 oz | 345 | 20 | 35 |
| Tuxedo, 3.5 oz | 320 | 17 | 34 |
| Choc Lava Cake (1), 4 oz | 360 | 23 | 40 |
| Karat Cake, 3 oz slice | 320 | 19 | 37 |
| N.Y. Style Cheesecake, 4.5 oz slice | 400 | 28 | 32 |
| Tiramisu Torte, 3.2 oz slice | 230 | 12 | 24 |
| Tarts: | | | |
| Pear, 3.5 oz slice | 250 | 9 | 39 |
| Raspberry, 5 oz slice | 290 | 10 | 51 |
| Wild Blueberry, 3.5 oz slice | 260 | 6 | 52 |

### Cakes ~ Mixes

| | C | F | Cb |
|---|---|---|---|

*Prepared as Directed*

**Arrowhead Mills:**
**Brownie Mix:**

| | C | F | Cb |
|---|---|---|---|
| Regular, 1/20 package, 1 oz | 150 | 7 | 21 |
| Gluten Free, Fudge Brownie | | | |
| 1/20 package, 1 oz | 160 | 8 | 21 |

**Cake Mix:**

| | | | |
|---|---|---|---|
| Chocolate, organic, 1/12 pkg., 1.5 oz | 260 | 11 | 39 |
| Vanilla, 1/12 package, 1.8 oz | 260 | 10 | 39 |

**Betty Crocker:** *Prepared as Directed*
**Brownie Mix:**

| | | | |
|---|---|---|---|
| Dark Choc. Fudge, 1/20 pkg | 160 | 6.5 | 24 |
| Fudge, 1/20 package | 170 | 8 | 23 |
| Low-Fat Fudge, 1/18 pkg | 140 | 3 | 28 |
| Gluten Free, Chocolate, 1/16 pkg | 150 | 5 | 24 |
| Premium: | | | |
| Chocolate Chunk, 1/16 pkg | 170 | 7 | 26 |
| Original Supreme, 1/16 package | 190 | 8 | 27 |
| P'nut Butter; Walnut, av., 1/16 pkg | 170 | 7 | 24 |
| Triple Chunk, 1/16 package | 180 | 7 | 28 |
| Ultimate Fudge, 1/16 package | 170 | 6.5 | 26 |

**Gluten Free Cake Mix:**

| | | | |
|---|---|---|---|
| Devils Food, 1/10 Pkg | 260 | 12 | 36 |
| Yellow, 1/10 Pkg | 260 | 11 | 37 |

**SuperMoiste Cake Mixes:** *Per 1/10 Package*

| | | | |
|---|---|---|---|
| Butter Recipe Yellow | 240 | 9 | 36 |
| Carrot | 310 | 18 | 35 |
| Cherry Chip | 280 | 14 | 36 |
| Devil's Food; French Vanilla | 280 | 14 | 35 |
| French Vanilla | 280 | 14 | 35 |
| Lemon | 280 | 14 | 36 |
| Milk Chocolate | 250 | 10 | 35 |
| Triple Chocolate Fudge | 280 | 14 | 34 |

If using No-Cholesterol Recipe, deduct 40 cals and 4g fat.

**Dessert Bars:** Reeses, 1 oz mix

| | | | |
|---|---|---|---|
| | 180 | 12 | 20 |
| Sunkist Lemon, 1 oz mix | 140 | 4.5 | 24 |

**Duncan Hines:**
**Brownie Mix:** *Per 1/20 Pkg Unless Indicated*

| | | | |
|---|---|---|---|
| Decadent, Caramel Turtle, 1/16 pkg | 150 | 7 | 23 |
| Premium: Dark Chocolate | 140 | 6 | 21 |
| Milk Chocolate | 160 | 8 | 21 |

**Cake Mix,**

| | | | |
|---|---|---|---|
| Classic, Dark Choc. Fudge, 1/12 pkg | 220 | 11 | 28 |

**Decadent:** *Per 1/12 Package*

| | | | |
|---|---|---|---|
| Classic Carrot | 260 | 10 | 39 |
| German Chocolate | 290 | 14 | 37 |

*Prepared as Directed*

**Duncan Hines (Cont):**
**Signature:** *Per 1/2 Pkg*

| | C | F | Cb |
|---|---|---|---|
| Banana Supreme | 270 | 12 | 36 |
| French Vanilla; German Choc., av. | 270 | 12 | 34 |
| Red Velvet | 250 | 12 | 33 |

**Jell-O:**
**No Bake Cheesecake:**

| | | | |
|---|---|---|---|
| Cherry, 1/9 pkg, 2.4 oz | 290 | 11 | 48 |
| Real Cheesecake, 1/8 pkg, 2.1 oz | 220 | 5 | 40 |

**Krusteaz:**

| | | | |
|---|---|---|---|
| Cinn. Swirl Crumb Cake, 2½x2" pce | 210 | 5 | 39 |
| Lemon; Key Lime Bar, 2" bar | 140 | 3 | 26 |

**Pillsbury:**
**Brownies, Premium Mix:** *Dry Mix Only*

| | | | |
|---|---|---|---|
| Caramel Swirl, 1/12 pkg, 1.2 oz | 120 | 1 | 28 |
| Cheesecake Swirl, 1/15 pkg, 1 oz | 110 | 1.5 | 25 |
| Chocolate Extreme, 1/15 pkg, 1 oz | 120 | 2 | 24 |
| Double Chocolate, 1/16 pkg, 1 oz | 100 | 0.5 | 24 |

**Cakes:**

| | | | |
|---|---|---|---|
| Funfetti: Bold Purple 1/6 pkg, 1.4 oz | 140 | 1.5 | 32 |
| Neon Yellow, 1/6 pkg, 1.4 oz | 140 | 1.5 | 21 |
| Moist Supreme: Per 1/10 Pkg, Dry Mix Only | | | |
| Classic White/Yellow, 1.5 oz | 160 | 1.5 | 35 |
| Devils Food, 1.5 oz | 160 | 2 | 35 |

### Cake Frostings

**Betty Crocker:**
**Rich & Creamy,**

| | C | F | Cb |
|---|---|---|---|
| average all flavors, 2 Tbsp, 1.2 oz | 135 | 5 | 22 |
| **Whipped,** av. all flavors., 2 T., 0.9 oz | 100 | 4.5 | 15 |
| **Cool Whip,** Original, 2 Tbsp, 0.3 oz | 25 | 1.5 | 2 |

**Duncan Hines:**

| | | | |
|---|---|---|---|
| **Creamy Homestyle,** av. all flav., 2T. | 140 | 6 | 23 |
| **Whipped,** av. all flavors, 3 Tbsp | 150 | 7 | 21 |

**Pillsbury:** *Per 2 Tbsp*
**Creamy Supreme:**

| | | | |
|---|---|---|---|
| Choc Fudge; Milk Choc., | | | |
| average, 1.2 oz | 130 | 6 | 21 |
| Classic White; Vanilla, 1.2 oz | 140 | 5 | 22 |
| **Fluffy,** av. all flavors, 2 Tbsp, 0.8 oz | 100 | 5 | 14 |
| **Funfetti,** av. all flavors, 2 Tbsp,1.2 oz | 140 | 5 | 23 |
| **Sugar Free,** average, 2 Tbsp, 1.1 oz | 100 | 6 | 16 |

### Quick Guide    C   F   Cb

**Donuts**

*Average All Brands*

| | C | F | Cb |
|---|---|---|---|
| **Cake:** Plain, 1.8 oz | 205 | 12 | 23 |
| Chocolate Iced, 2 oz | 255 | 14 | 29 |
| Sugared, 0.8 oz | 205 | 10 | 29 |
| **Non-Cake,** Glazed, 2 oz | 225 | 11 | 29 |

**Croissant-Donuts**

(Includes Cronuts/Frissants)

*Average all Brands*

| | C | F | Cb |
|---|---|---|---|
| Cream-filled, 3.5 oz | 430 | 26 | 45 |
| Custard-filled, 3.5 oz | 360 | 19 | 45 |

**Extra Listings** ~ *See CalorieKing.com*

*(Cronut is a trademark of Dominique Ansel Bakery, New York)*

### Donuts ~ Brands

**Albertson's:**
**Donut Holes:**

| | C | F | Cb |
|---|---|---|---|
| Glazed Old Fashioned (4) | 240 | 12 | 31 |
| Powdered Sugar (4) | 210 | 12 | 24 |
| **Gem Donuts:** Plain Cake (3) | 190 | 12 | 20 |
| Cinnamon Sugar (3) | 240 | 15 | 23 |
| Glazed (1) | 140 | 6 | 21 |

**Bon Appetit:**
**Mini Donuts:**

| | C | F | Cb |
|---|---|---|---|
| Chocolate (4) | 270 | 16 | 29 |
| Crumb (4) | 240 | 12 | 32 |
| Powdered (4) | 250 | 12 | 34 |

**Dunkin' Donuts:**

| | C | F | Cb |
|---|---|---|---|
| **Apple Crumb** | 320 | 15 | 43 |
| **Apple N' Spice** | 260 | 14 | 29 |
| **Barvarian Kreme** | 270 | 15 | 31 |
| **Blueberry Butternut** | 420 | 17 | 60 |
| **Blueberry Crumb Cake** | 380 | 18 | 50 |
| **Boston Kreme** | 300 | 16 | 37 |
| **Chocolate Frosted Cake** | 350 | 19 | 40 |
| **Chocolate Headliight** | 330 | 18 | 39 |
| **Choc. Peanut Butter Flav. Cream** | 360 | 19 | 44 |
| **Glazed Chocolate** | 340 | 19 | 38 |
| **Jelly Filled** | 270 | 14 | 32 |
| **Powdered** | 320 | 19 | 33 |
| **Vanilla Creme** | 330 | 20 | 35 |

**Extra Listings** ~ *See Fast Food Section*

### Donuts ~ Brands (Cont)    C   F   Cb

**Entenmann's:**
**8 Pack:** *Per Donut*

| | C | F | Cb |
|---|---|---|---|
| Chocolate Lovers, 2 oz | 300 | 20 | 31 |
| Crumb, 2 oz | 250 | 12 | 36 |
| Frosted Devil's, 2.4 oz | 310 | 18 | 36 |
| Rich Frosted, 2 oz | 300 | 20 | 30 |

**Pop'ems:**

| | C | F | Cb |
|---|---|---|---|
| Frosted (4), 2 oz | 320 | 23 | 28 |
| Powdered (4), 1.8 oz | 230 | 13 | 28 |

**Hostess:**

| | C | F | Cb |
|---|---|---|---|
| **Mini Donettes:** Crumb, 6-pack, 4 oz | 430 | 18 | 63 |
| Frosted, 6-pack, 3 oz | 360 | 22 | 38 |
| Powdered, 6-pack, 3 oz | 340 | 17 | 43 |

**Krispy Kreme:**

| | C | F | Cb |
|---|---|---|---|
| **Apple Fritter**, 3.5 oz | 390 | 20 | 50 |
| **Baseball Donut**, 2.2 oz | 280 | 15 | 34 |
| Chocolate: Iced Cake, 2.2 oz | 280 | 16 | 32 |
| Iced Custard Filled, 3.5 oz | 350 | 22 | 35 |
| Iced Glazed Cruller, 2.5 oz | 300 | 18 | 34 |
| Iced Glazed, 2.3 | 240 | 12 | 32 |
| Iced Kreme Filled, 3 oz | 340 | 17 | 42 |
| Iced Glazed w/ Sprinkles, 2.3 oz | 250 | 12 | 34 |
| **Cinnamon Twist**, 2 oz | 230 | 12 | 30 |
| **Glazed Cruller**, 2 oz | 250 | 17 | 23 |
| **Glazed Doughnut Holes:** | | | |
| Original (5) | 200 | 9 | 27 |
| Blueberry (4) | 180 | 10 | 22 |
| Chocolate Cake (4) | 180 | 10 | 21 |
| **Glazed Kreme Filled**, 3 oz | 370 | 23 | 38 |
| **Maple Iced Glazed**, 2.3 oz | 230 | 11 | 31 |
| **New York Cheesecake**, 3.3 oz | 400 | 26 | 37 |
| **Original Glazed**, 1.7 oz | 190 | 11 | 21 |
| **Powdered Cake**, 2.3 oz | 260 | 16 | 26 |
| **Traditional Cake**, 2 oz | 230 | 15 | 20 |

**Little Debbie,**

| | C | F | Cb |
|---|---|---|---|
| Donut Sticks, 1.9 oz | 270 | 16 | 29 |

**Tastykake:**

| | C | F | Cb |
|---|---|---|---|
| **Cinnamon**, 1.8 oz | 210 | 11 | 26 |
| **Mini:** Coated, 3 oz | 380 | 22 | 42 |
| Powdered Sugar (6), 2.5 oz | 280 | 13 | 37 |

## Quick Guide   **C  F  Cb**

### Muffins: Ready-To-Eat
**Average All Brands**

| | C | F | Cb |
|---|---|---|---|
| Small, 1 oz | 90 | 3.5 | 14 |
| Medium, 2 oz | 185 | 6.5 | 28 |
| Large, 3 oz | 275 | 10 | 42 |
| Extra Large, 4 oz | 365 | 13 | 57 |
| Giant, 6 oz | 550 | 20 | 84 |
| Super Size, 8 oz | 730 | 27 | 112 |

### Muffins Ready-To-Eat ~ Brands

**Albertsons:**

| | C | F | Cb |
|---|---|---|---|
| **Minis:** Banana Nut (2) | 200 | 12 | 20 |
| Blueberry (2) | 180 | 10 | 21 |
| Honey Raisin Bran (2) | 170 | 7 | 24 |
| **Entenmann's,** | | | |
| Blueberry; Choc. Chip; Corn (1) | 190 | 9 | 26 |
| **Garden Lites:** Chocolate (1), 2 oz | 120 | 4 | 21 |
| Banana Choc Chip (1), 2 oz | 120 | 3 | 23 |
| Blueberry (1), 2 oz | 120 | 2 | 25 |
| Av. other flavors (1), 1 oz | 70 | 2 | 13 |
| **Great Value** (Walmart): | | | |
| **Double Banana Filled**, (1), 4 oz | 360 | 16 | 52 |
| **Double Blueberry Filled**, (1), 4 oz | 430 | 16 | 65 |
| **Triple Chocolate Filled**, (1), 4 oz | 420 | 18 | 61 |
| **Little Debbie:** Banana Nut (1), 1.9 oz | 210 | 9 | 30 |
| Blueberry (1), 1.9 oz | 190 | 8 | 27 |
| Chocolate Chip (1), 1.9 oz | 210 | 9 | 28 |
| **My Favorite Muffin:** Per 6 oz Muffin | | | |
| **Banana Nut** | 585 | 33 | 63 |
| **Blueberry** | 505 | 24 | 66 |
| **Boston Cream Pie** | 530 | 21 | 78 |
| **Chocolate Chip** | 635 | 33 | 81 |
| **Lemon Poppyseed** | 605 | 30 | 75 |
| **Otis Spunkmeyer:** | | | |
| **Banana Nut**, 4 oz | 440 | 22 | 58 |
| **Choc. Chip**, 4 oz | 460 | 24 | 58 |
| **Wild Blueberry**, 4 oz | 400 | 16 | 58 |
| **Starbucks** ~ See Fast-Foods Section | | | |
| **Trader Joe's:** Per Muffin | | | |
| **Apple Cranberry**, 4.8 oz | 220 | 5 | 38 |
| **Banana Chocolate Chip**, 4 oz | 400 | 18 | 57 |
| **Carrot**, 4 oz | 320 | 11 | 52 |
| **Triple Berry**, 4 oz | 310 | 11 | 49 |
| **Vitalicious:** | | | |
| **VitaTops:** Average all varieties, 2 oz | 100 | 1.5 | 25 |
| Sugar free, av. all varieties, 2 oz | 100 | 3 | 25 |
| **Weight Watchers,** | | | |
| Blueb.; Double Choc, av., 2.5 oz | 185 | 2.5 | 42 |

## Muffin Mixes   **C  F  Cb**

*Per Muffin, Prepared*

| | C | F | Cb |
|---|---|---|---|
| **Betty Crocker:** Banana Nut | 170 | 8 | 22 |
| Cinnamon Streusel | 180 | 8 | 26 |
| Wild Blueberry | 160 | 6.5 | 24 |
| Pouch Mix: | | | |
| Banana Nut | 120 | 3 | 22 |
| Blueberry; Triple Berry | 120 | 2.5 | 23 |
| Chocolate Chip | 130 | 3.5 | 22 |
| **Fiber One,** | | | |
| Apple Cinnamon; Blueberry, av. | 160 | 6 | 29 |
| **Krusteaz:** | | | |
| Choc Chunk | 260 | 13 | 33 |
| Lemon Poppyseed | 170 | 4 | 31 |
| Oat Bran | 180 | 4.5 | 32 |
| **Trader Joe's**, Triple Berry | 150 | 2 | 28 |

## Sweet Rolls & Buns

Note: It is best to weigh for accuracy as actual weight can be 10-50% higher than label weight·
*Per Sweet Roll or Bun Unless Indicated*

| | C | F | Cb |
|---|---|---|---|
| **Bimbo,** Bimbolete, 2.2 oz | 250 | 10 | 36 |
| **Bon Appetit,** | | | |
| Cinnamon Roll, 2.5 oz | 230 | 8 | 34 |
| **Cinnabon:** Classic | 880 | 37 | 127 |
| Caramel Pecanbon | 1080 | 51 | 146 |
| **Cloverhill Bakery,** | | | |
| Jumbo Glazed Honey Bun, 4.8 oz | 600 | 35 | 64 |
| **Entenmann's,** Cinn. Swirl Bun, 3 oz | 320 | 14 | 44 |
| **Little Debbie:** | | | |
| **Honey Bun:** 2.3 oz | 280 | 16 | 32 |
| 4 oz | 480 | 26 | 56 |
| with Chocolate Icing, 2 oz | 310 | 20 | 29 |
| with White Icing, 4 oz | 490 | 25 | 60 |
| **Pecan Spinwheels**, 1 oz | 100 | 3.5 | 17 |
| **McDonald's,** Cinnamon Melts, 4 oz | 460 | 19 | 66 |
| **Pillsbury:** | | | |
| **Sweet Rolls,** Refrigerated: Per Roll Unless Indicated | | | |
| Cinnamon, w/ Icing, all varieties | 140 | 5 | 23 |
| Reduced Fat | 130 | 3 | 24 |
| Orange Flavored, with Icing, 1.7 oz | 160 | 5 | 26 |
| Twists, Flaky Cinnamon, with Icing | 160 | 7 | 23 |
| **Grands,** Refrigerated: Per Roll | | | |
| Cinnabon: Cinnamon Roll, | | | |
| with Cream Cheese Icing | 300 | 7 | 54 |
| Caramel Rolls, with Icing, 3.5 oz | 300 | 8 | 53 |
| Flaky Supreme Cinnamon Roll, | | | |
| with Icing, 3.5 oz | 360 | 17 | 47 |
| **7-Eleven:** Iced Honey Bun, 6 oz | 820 | 58 | 68 |
| Glazed Honey Bun, 5 oz | 620 | 35 | 70 |
| **Sara Lee,** Cinnamon Roll, 2.4 oz | 260 | 12 | 33 |

## Quick Guide

|  | C | F | Cb |
|---|---|---|---|
| **Chocolate:** | | | |
| ***Average All Brands*** | | | |
| **Milk Chocolate**, regular: | | | |
|   **Plain/Nuts/Fruit,** average, 1 oz | 150 | 9 | 17 |
|   1.5 oz Bar | 230 | 13 | 25 |
|   2 oz Bar | 305 | 17 | 34 |
|   4 oz Block | 610 | 34 | 68 |
|   8 oz Block | 1220 | 68 | 136 |
|   1 Pound, 16 oz | 2440 | 136 | 272 |
| **Dark/White Chocolate:** 1 oz | 155 | 9 | 17 |
|   *Hershey's,* Sugar Free, 5 pieces | 110 | 13 | 24 |
| **Milk Chocolate-Coated:** | | | |
|   Almonds, 5-6, 1 oz | 150 | 10 | 15 |
|   Cherry Cordial Centers, 2 pcs, 1 oz | 145 | 6 | 21 |
|   Clusters, Nut, 3 pieces, 1.2 oz | 210 | 14 | 20 |
|   Coffee Beans, 1.4 oz | 220 | 13 | 22 |
|   Macadamias, 10 pieces, 1.4 oz | 220 | 16 | 21 |
|   Mints, 1 medium, 0.5 oz | 55 | 1 | 11 |
|   Nougat & Caramel, 1 oz | 150 | 9 | 15 |
|   Peanuts, 12 medium, 1 oz | 145 | 10 | 14 |
|   Raisins, 28 medium, 1 oz | 110 | 4 | 19 |
| **Baking Chocolate:** | | | |
|   *Baker's,* Bittersweet, 1 oz | 140 | 12 | 14 |
|   Semi-sweet, 1 oz | 140 | 9 | 16 |
|   *Nestle,* Chips: Dark, 1 Tbsp. 0.5 oz | 70 | 5 | 3 |
|   Semi-Sweet, 1 Tbsp. 0.5oz | 70 | 4 | 9 |
|   Unsweetened, 1 oz | 140 | 14 | 8 |
| **Carob**, Plain, 1 oz | 155 | 9 | 16 |

## Candy ~ Brands & Generic

*Per Piece/Serving*

|  | C | F | Cb |
|---|---|---|---|
| **3 Musketeers:** Orig., 1 bar, 1.9 oz | 240 | 7 | 42 |
|   2 To Go, 1.7 oz Bar | 200 | 6 | 36 |
|   Fun Size, 3 bars, 1.6 oz | 190 | 6 | 34 |
|   Minis, 7 pieces, 1.4 oz | 170 | 5 | 32 |
| **100 Grand:** 1.5 oz bar | 190 | 8 | 30 |
|   Snack Size (1), 0.8 oz | 95 | 4 | 15 |
|   Super Size, 2.8 oz | 360 | 14 | 58 |
| **Abba Zabba,** 2 oz bar | 250 | 5 | 48 |
| **After Dinner Mints,** 1 small | 25 | 1.5 | 3 |
| **After Eight Mint,** each | 35 | 1.5 | 4 |
| **Airhead,** 1 bar, 0.5 oz | 60 | 1 | 14 |
| **Almond Joy:** 2 bars, 1.6 oz | 220 | 13 | 26 |
|   King Size, 4 bars, 3.2 oz | 440 | 26 | 53 |
|   Snack Size, 0.6 oz bar | 80 | 4.5 | 10 |
|   Pieces (46), 1.4 oz | 200 | 10 | 27 |

*Per Piece/Serving*

|  | C | F | Cb |
|---|---|---|---|
| **Almond Roca,** 3 pieces, 1.3 oz | 200 | 15 | 17 |
| **Almond:** Sugar-coated (15), 1.4 oz | 190 | 7 | 27 |
|   Jordan, 15 pieces, 1.4 oz | 180 | 8 | 28 |
| **Almond Clusters:** | | | |
|   *True North,* 1 oz | 170 | 12 | 9 |
|   *Trader Joe's,* 1.2 oz | 190 | 14 | 13 |
| **Altoids,** 3 pieces | 10 | 0 | 2 |
| **Andes,** Thins (8), av. all var., 1.4 oz | 205 | 13 | 22 |
| **Anthon Berg:** | | | |
|   Creamy Mint (4), 1.4 oz | 180 | 6 | 31 |
|   Marzipan with Plum, in Madeira | 120 | 6 | 14 |
| **Atomic Fireball,** 1 piece, 0.3 oz | 35 | 0 | 9 |
| **Baby Ruth:** King Size, 3.5 oz bar | 500 | 24 | 66 |
|   2 oz bar | 280 | 14 | 39 |
|   Fun size, 2 bars | 170 | 8 | 24 |
|   Minis, 4 bars | 210 | 11 | 28 |
| **Baci** *(Perugina),* | | | |
|   1 piece, 0.5 oz | 75 | 6 | 7 |
| **Baskin-Robbins:** Sugar Candy, 3 pcs | 60 | 1 | 12 |
|   Sugar Free, 4 pieces, average, 0.6 oz | 40 | 1 | 16 |
|   *Note: Carb includes 16g sugar alcohol* | | | |
| **Big Hunk,** 2 oz Bar | 230 | 3 | 47 |
| **Bit-O-Honey:** 1.7 oz bar | 180 | 3.5 | 39 |
|   Chews, 6 pieces, 1.4 oz | 150 | 3 | 32 |
| **Bliss** *(Hershey's):* | | | |
|   Milk/Dark Choc./Caramel, 6 pieces | 120 | 14 | 25 |
|   Meltaway Centers: | | | |
|     Milk Chocolate, 6 pieces | 220 | 15 | 24 |
|     Raspberry, 6 pieces | 220 | 14 | 24 |
| **Blow Pops,** each, 0.6 oz | 60 | 0 | 17 |
| **Bon Bons,** 3 pieces | 65 | 0 | 15 |
| **Boston Baked Beans,** (11), 0.5 oz | 70 | 2 | 11 |
| **Brach's:** | | | |
|   Almond Supremes (10) | 200 | 14 | 20 |
|   Bridge Mix (15), 1.4 oz | 190 | 10 | 26 |
|   Double Dippers (15), 1.4 oz | 210 | 14 | 22 |
|   Gummi Bears (14), 1.4 oz | 130 | 0 | 30 |
|   Lemon Drops, Sugar Free, 4 pieces | 35 | 0 | 17 |
|   *Note: Carb figures include 17g Sugar Alcohol* | | | |
|   Mandarin/Orange Slices (3), 1.6 oz | 150 | 0 | 37 |
|   Maple Nut Goodies (8), 1.5 oz | 190 | 9 | 27 |
|   Milk Maid Crmls (4), 1.3 oz | 150 | 4 | 25 |
|   Peanut Cluster (3), 1.4 oz | 210 | 15 | 20 |
| **Breath Savers,** all varieties, each | 5 | 0 | 2 |
| **Bubble Gum** — See Page 75 | | | |
| **Bulls Eyes,** 3 pieces, 1.2 oz | 130 | 3 | 23 |
| **Buncha Crunch:** ⅓ cup, 1.4 oz | 180 | 9 | 25 |
|   Movie Box, 3.2 oz | 450 | 20 | 65 |
| **Burnt Peanuts,** (31), 1.4 oz | 170 | 6 | 29 |

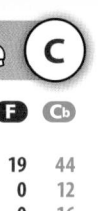

## Candy ~ Brands & Generic (Cont)

| Per Piece/Serving | C | F | Cb |
|---|---|---|---|
| **Butterfinger:** 2 oz bar | 270 | 11 | 43 |
| King Size (3 bars), 3.5 oz | 480 | 18 | 75 |
| Fun Size, (1), 0.8 oz | 100 | 4 | 15 |
| Giant, (Pieces in Choc.), ¼ bar, 1 oz | 150 | 8 | 21 |
| Miniatures: | | | |
| 1 piece, 0.4 oz | 45 | 2 | 8 |
| 4 pieces, 1.4 oz | 180 | 8 | 32 |
| Crisp Bar: Original, 2 oz bar | 270 | 11 | 43 |
| King Size, 3 pieces, 2 oz | 310 | 17 | 38 |
| Minis, 2 bars, 1.4 oz | 210 | 11 | 25 |
| Snackerz: | | | |
| Single, 1.3 oz | 170 | 8 | 23 |
| Fun Size, 2 pcs, 1.2 oz | 150 | 7 | 21 |
| King Size, 10 pcs, 1.4 oz | 190 | 8 | 25 |
| **Butter Mints,** 7 pieces, 0.5 oz | 50 | 0 | 12 |
| **Butterscotch:** 3 pieces | 60 | 0 | 15 |
| Discs (Walgreens), 3 pieces, 0.6 oz | 70 | 0 | 17 |
| **Cadbury:** Caramello Bar, 1.6 oz | 220 | 10 | 29 |
| Caramel Egg, 1.2 oz | 170 | 8 | 22 |
| Dairy Milk Bar, 7 pcs, 1.4 oz | 200 | 11 | 23 |
| Mini Eggs (Candy), 12 pcs, 1.4 oz | 190 | 8 | 28 |
| **Candy Apple**, medium, 6.5 oz | 280 | 0 | 60 |
| **Candy Cane**, medium, 5", 0.5 oz | 40 | 0 | 14 |
| **Candy Corn**, 20 pieces, 1.4 oz | 150 | 0 | 38 |
| **Candy Jar Mix** (Jewel), 3 pcs, 0.6 oz | 60 | 0 | 14 |
| **Candy Necklace** (Smarties), (1), 0.8 oz | 90 | 0.5 | 20 |
| **Caramels:** Each, 0.4 oz | 40 | 1 | 8 |
| Chocolate, each, 0.3 oz | 25 | 0.3 | 6 |
| Creams (3), 1.3 oz | 130 | 3 | 23 |
| **Caramel Popcorn,** ⅔ cup | 150 | 6 | 23 |
| **Cella's,** | | | |
| Milk Choc. Cherries, 3 pcs, 1.5 oz | 160 | 6 | 27 |
| **Certs,** Breath Mints, 1 piece | 5 | 0 | 2 |
| **Charleston Chew:** | | | |
| Chocolate Bar (1), 1.4 oz | 160 | 4.5 | 30 |
| Mini Bars, 13 pieces | 190 | 6 | 34 |
| **Charms:** Blow Pop | 60 | 0 | 17 |
| Flat Pop, 0.5 oz | 50 | 0 | 14 |
| **Chew-ets,** Peanut Chews, Original (4), 1.6 oz | 230 | 12 | 29 |
| **Chewz,** 1 roll, 1 oz | 120 | 1 | 28 |
| **Chick O Stick,** 2 oz | 240 | 9 | 42 |

| Per Piece/Serving | C | F | Cb |
|---|---|---|---|
| **Chunky Bar (Nestlé)** | | | |
| King Size, 2.5 oz | 340 | 19 | 44 |
| **Chupa Chups,** 1 Pop | 50 | 0 | 12 |
| **Cinn. Buttons** (Walgreens), 3 pieces | 60 | 0 | 16 |
| **Cinnamon Disks** (Walmart), 3 pieces | 70 | 0 | 18 |
| **Circus Peanuts** (Spangler), 6 pieces, 1.3 oz | 165 | 0 | 41 |
| **CocoaVia,** Orig., 0.8 oz | 100 | 6 | 12 |
| **Coconut Stacks,** (8) | 320 | 16 | 46 |
| **Coffee Go,** Candy, (4) | 60 | 1 | 12 |
| **Conversation Hearts** (Necco): | | | |
| Small (40), 1.4 oz | 160 | 0 | 39 |
| 1 large | 10 | 0 | 3 |
| **Cookie Dough Bites,** 1.4 oz | 200 | 10 | 27 |
| **Cote d'Or:** Dark 86% Coca, 4 pcs | 270 | 22 | 14 |
| Dark, 70%, Orange, 3.5 oz | 575 | 46 | 34 |
| Dark, Raspberry, 3.5 oz | 580 | 46 | 34 |
| Milk, Intense, 3.5 oz | 575 | 40 | 45 |
| **Cotton Candy,** 1 oz | 110 | 0 | 28 |
| **Cough Drops** ~ See Page 75 | | | |
| **Cracker Jack,** ½ cup, 1 oz | 120 | 2 | 23 |
| **Creme Savers:** | | | |
| 3 pieces, 0.5 oz | 60 | 1 | 11 |
| Sugar-Free, 3 pieces | 30 | 1 | 8 |
| **Crisped Rice,** Choc Chip, 1 bar, 1 oz | 115 | 4 | 20 |
| **Crows,** 11 pieces, 1.4 oz | 130 | 0 | 33 |
| **Crunch Bar** ~ See Nestle | | | |
| **Dots,** 11 dots, 1.4 oz | 130 | 0 | 33 |
| **Double Dip Stick,** 1 stick | 15 | 0.5 | 3 |
| **Dove:** | | | |
| **Milk Choc:** Singles Bar, 1.4 oz | 220 | 13 | 24 |
| Large Tablet Bar, 9 pcs, 1.5 oz | 230 | 13 | 25 |
| Choc. Cov. Almonds, 13 pcs, 1.4 oz | 220 | 15 | 19 |
| Promises: Milk Choc., 1 pce, 0.3 oz | 45 | 2.5 | 5 |
| w/ Caramel, 1 piece, 0.3 oz | 40 | 2 | 5 |
| w/ Peanut Butter, 1 pce, 0.3 oz | 45 | 3 | 4 |
| Swirls, all var., 9 pieces 1.5 oz | 230 | 14 | 25 |
| **Dark Choc:** Singles Bar, 1.3 oz | 220 | 13 | 24 |
| Large Tablet Bar, 9 pcs, 1.5 oz | 220 | 14 | 25 |
| Choc. Cov. Almds, 13 pcs, 1.4 oz | 210 | 15 | 19 |
| Promises, Almond, 1 piece, 0.3 oz | 40 | 3 | 4 |
| Swirls, Raspberry, 9 pcs, 1.4 oz | 220 | 14 | 24 |
| **Sugar Free,** all flav., 5 pcs, 1.4 oz | 195 | 15 | 21 |
| **Dum Dum Pops** (Spangler), 1 pop | 25 | 0 | 7 |
| **Drops** (Hershey's): | | | |
| Cookies 'n' Creme, 14 pieces, 1.5 oz | 210 | 11 | 26 |
| Milk Chocolate, 15 pieces, 1.4 oz | 200 | 12 | 25 |

## Candy ~ Brands & Generic (Cont)

| Per Piece/Serving | C | F | Cb |
|---|---|---|---|
| **English Toffee**, 1 piece, 0.4 oz | 70 | 4 | 6 |
| **5th Avenue:** 2 oz bar | 260 | 12 | 38 |
| King Size, 3.5 oz | 440 | 20 | 64 |
| **Fannie May:** | | | |
| Mint Meltaway (1) | 230 | 15 | 24 |
| Pixie (1), 1.5 oz | 210 | 12 | 24 |
| Trinidad (1), 1.5 oz | 200 | 12 | 23 |
| **Fast Break (Reese's):** 2 oz bar | 260 | 12 | 35 |
| 3.5 oz bar | 460 | 22 | 62 |
| **Ferrero Rocher:** 1 piece | 75 | 5 | 5 |
| 3 pieces, 1.3 oz | 220 | 16 | 16 |
| Rondnoir, 3 pieces, 1 oz | 180 | 13 | 14 |
| **Fifty 50 Snack Bars:** | | | |
| **Milk Chocolate:** 5 pieces, 1 oz | 135 | 11 | 14 |
| Almond, 5 pieces, 1 oz | 135 | 12 | 14 |
| Crunch Bar, 7 pcs, 1 oz | 140 | 12 | 16 |
| **Dark Chocolate,** 5 pieces, 1 oz | 120 | 11 | 15 |
| *Note: Carb figures include 9-12g Sugar Alcohol* | | | |
| **Fluffy Stuff** (Charms), | | | |
| Cotton Candy, 1.4 oz | 150 | 0 | 40 |
| **Fondant:** Choc-coated, 1.2 oz | 125 | 3 | 27 |
| Mint, 1 oz | 105 | 0 | 25 |
| **Fran's:** Gold Bar, Almond (1) | 250 | 14 | 27 |
| GoldBite, Almond (1) | 120 | 7 | 13 |
| **Fruit Drops,** (1), ¼ oz | 20 | 0 | 4 |
| **Fruit Gems** (Sunkist), (4), 1.4 oz | 130 | 0 | 33 |
| **Fruit Leathers,** average, 0.5 oz | 50 | 0.5 | 12 |
| **Fruit Pastilles** (Rowntree), 1 roll | 185 | 0 | 45 |
| **Fruit Roll-Ups** (Betty Crocker/Sunkist), | | | |
| 1 roll, 0.5 oz | 50 | 1 | 12 |
| **Fruit Runts** (Walgreens), | | | |
| 12 pieces | 60 | 0 | 14 |
| **Fruit Flavored Shapes** (Betty Crocker), | | | |
| all varieties, 0.8 oz | 80 | 0 | 19 |
| **Fudge:** | | | |
| Chocolate; Mint, 1 oz | 130 | 8 | 14 |
| P'nut Butter & Choc., 1 oz | 130 | 8 | 13 |
| *Brevin's:* Cashew, 1 oz | 195 | 9 | 28 |
| Triple Decker, 1 oz | 165 | 7 | 25 |
| **Ghirardelli:** | | | |
| **3 oz Bars:** Dark Choc., 4 squares | 220 | 17 | 23 |
| Filled, P'nut Butter, 4 squares | 250 | 17 | 22 |
| Intense Dark Bars, | | | |
| Ev'ng Dream, 3 pcs | 190 | 15 | 20 |
| **Squares:** | | | |
| Dark Choc., (4), 1.5 oz | 210 | 16 | 23 |
| Milk & Caramel (3), 1.5 oz | 220 | 12 | 27 |
| Sea Salt Escape (4), 1.5 oz | 210 | 15 | 24 |

| Per Piece/Serving | C | F | Cb |
|---|---|---|---|
| **Godiva:** | | | |
| **Bars:** Milk/Dark, av., 1.5 oz | 230 | 14 | 26 |
| Extra Dark: 75%, 1.5 oz | 230 | 17 | 18 |
| 85%, 1.4 oz | 260 | 21 | 14 |
| **Chocoiste:** Dk Choc. Cherries (12) | 190 | 7 | 30 |
| Milk Chocolate Cashews (14) | 230 | 15 | 19 |
| **Hearts:** Dark Ganache (4) | 200 | 12 | 23 |
| Milk Praline (4) | 220 | 13 | 23 |
| **Go Lightly:** | | | |
| Assorted Toffee, 5 pieces, 1 oz | 85 | 2 | 24 |
| Fruit Chews, 5 pieces, 1 oz | 95 | 2 | 26 |
| Hard Candy, Assorted (4), 0.5 oz | 45 | 0 | 15 |
| *Note: Carb figures include 15-25g sugar alcohol* | | | |
| **Goobers Peanuts,** 1 package, 1.4 oz | 200 | 13 | 21 |
| **Good & Plenty** (Hershey's), (33), 1.4 oz | 140 | 0 | 35 |
| **GooGoo Clusters,** 1 piece, 1.8 oz | 240 | 12 | 30 |
| **Gum** ~ *See Page 75* | | | |
| **Gum Drops:** 1 small, 0.1 oz | 15 | 0 | 3 |
| 5 pieces, 0.5 oz | 75 | 0 | 15 |
| **Gummi** (Shur Fine): | | | |
| Bears (15), 1.4 oz | 130 | 0 | 29 |
| Chewy Sweet Tarts (4) | 160 | 0 | 36 |
| Worms (9), 1.5 oz | 140 | 0 | 31 |
| **Guylian:** | | | |
| **Bars:** Dark Chocolate (3), 1 oz | 150 | 12 | 11 |
| Milk Choc. w/ Hazelnuts (3),1 oz | 170 | 11 | 15 |
| **No Sugar Added Bars:** | | | |
| Milk Chocolate, 3 squares | 150 | 11 | 16 |
| 54% Cocoa, Dark Choc., 3 sqrs. | 140 | 11 | 16 |
| **Seashells:** | | | |
| Bar, 1.4 oz | 210 | 13 | 21 |
| Boxed, Originals (1), 0.4 oz | 60 | 4 | 6 |
| Truffles, (1), 0.4 oz | 70 | 5.5 | 5 |
| **Heath:** Original (1), 1.4 oz | 210 | 13 | 24 |
| King Size, 2.8 oz | 410 | 22 | 49 |
| Snack Size, 3 pieces, 1.5 oz | 230 | 14 | 27 |
| **Hershey's:** | | | |
| **Cookies 'n' Creme,** 1.6 oz Bar | 220 | 12 | 26 |
| **Milk Chocolate:** | | | |
| Bars: 1.6 oz | 210 | 13 | 26 |
| with Almonds, 1 bar, 1.4 oz | 210 | 14 | 21 |
| King Size, 1 Bar, 2.5 oz | 370 | 22 | 44 |
| Kisses, 9 pieces, av., 1.4 oz | 200 | 12 | 25 |
| Nuggets: 4 pieces, 1.4 oz | 200 | 13 | 20 |
| w/ Toffee & Alm., 4 pcs, 1.3 oz | 200 | 13 | 21 |
| **Extra Dark Choc.,** 4 pcs, 1.4 oz | 180 | 14 | 21 |
| **Simple Pleasures,** 6 pcs, av. | 180 | 8 | 29 |
| **Special Dark Choc.,** 1.5 oz bar | 190 | 12 | 25 |
| **Sugar Free Choc.,** 5 pieces, 1.4 oz | 160 | 13 | 24 |

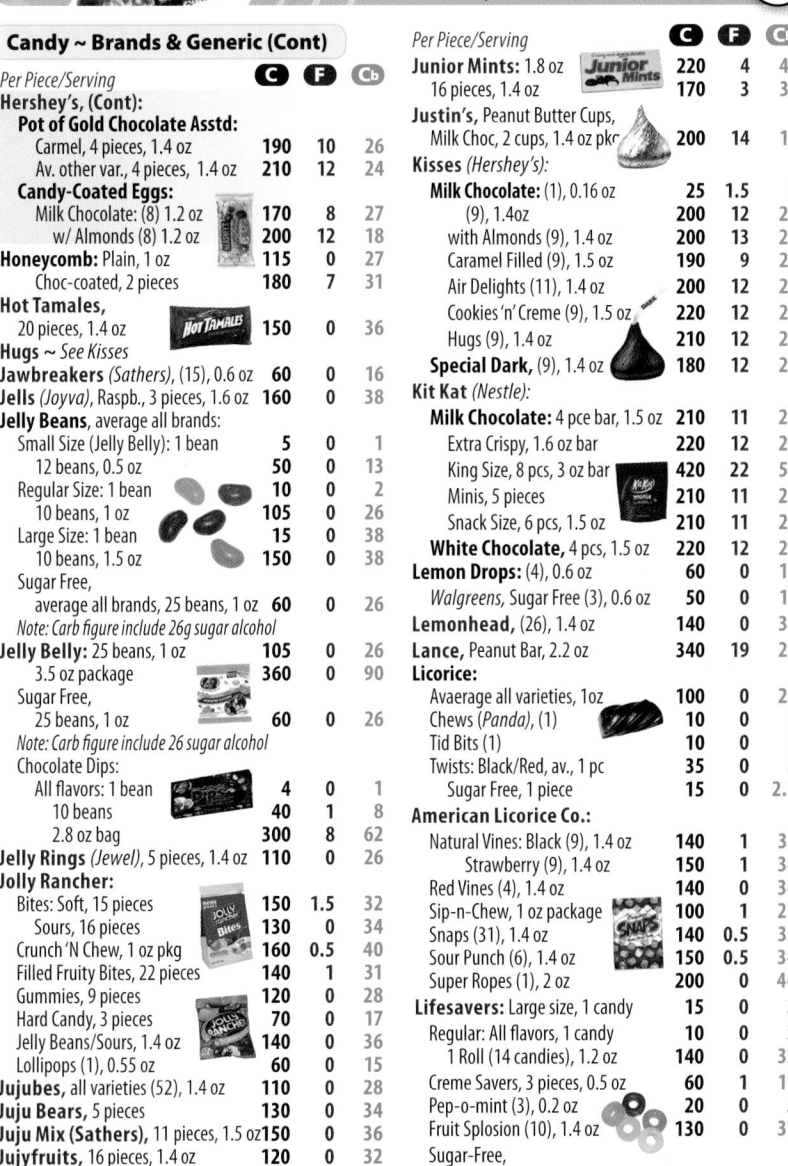

### Candy ~ Brands & Generic (Cont)

*Per Piece/Serving*    **Ⓒ** **Ⓕ** **Cb**

**Hershey's, (Cont):**
**Pot of Gold Chocolate Asstd:**

| | C | F | Cb |
|---|---|---|---|
| Carmel, 4 pieces, 1.4 oz | **190** | **10** | **26** |
| Av. other var., 4 pieces, 1.4 oz | **210** | **12** | **24** |

**Candy-Coated Eggs:**

| | C | F | Cb |
|---|---|---|---|
| Milk Chocolate: (8) 1.2 oz | **170** | **8** | **27** |
| w/ Almonds (8) 1.2 oz | **200** | **12** | **18** |
| **Honeycomb:** Plain, 1 oz | **115** | **0** | **27** |
| Choc-coated, 2 pieces | **180** | **7** | **31** |
| **Hot Tamales,** 20 pieces, 1.4 oz | **150** | **0** | **36** |
| **Hugs ~ See Kisses** | | | |
| **Jawbreakers** *(Sathers)*, (15), 0.6 oz | **60** | **0** | **16** |
| **Jells** *(Joyva)*, Raspb., 3 pieces, 1.6 oz | **160** | **0** | **38** |

**Jelly Beans**, average all brands:

| | C | F | Cb |
|---|---|---|---|
| Small Size (Jelly Belly): 1 bean | **5** | **0** | **1** |
| 12 beans, 0.5 oz | **50** | **0** | **13** |
| Regular Size: 1 bean | **10** | **0** | **2** |
| 10 beans, 1 oz | **105** | **0** | **26** |
| Large Size: 1 bean | **15** | **0** | **38** |
| 10 beans, 1.5 oz | **150** | **0** | **38** |
| Sugar Free, | | | |
| average all brands, 25 beans, 1 oz | **60** | **0** | **26** |

*Note: Carb figure include 26g sugar alcohol*

| | C | F | Cb |
|---|---|---|---|
| **Jelly Belly:** 25 beans, 1 oz | **105** | **0** | **26** |
| 3.5 oz package | **360** | **0** | **90** |
| Sugar Free, | | | |
| 25 beans, 1 oz | **60** | **0** | **26** |

*Note: Carb figure include 26 sugar alcohol*

Chocolate Dips:

| | C | F | Cb |
|---|---|---|---|
| All flavors: 1 bean | **4** | **0** | **1** |
| 10 beans | **40** | **1** | **8** |
| 2.8 oz bag | **300** | **8** | **62** |
| **Jelly Rings** *(Jewel)*, 5 pieces, 1.4 oz | **110** | **0** | **26** |

**Jolly Rancher:**

| | C | F | Cb |
|---|---|---|---|
| Bites: Soft, 15 pieces | **150** | **1.5** | **32** |
| Sours, 16 pieces | **130** | **0** | **34** |
| Crunch 'N Chew, 1 oz pkg | **160** | **0.5** | **40** |
| Filled Fruity Bites, 22 pieces | **140** | **1** | **31** |
| Gummies, 9 pieces | **120** | **0** | **28** |
| Hard Candy, 3 pieces | **70** | **0** | **17** |
| Jelly Beans/Sours, 1.4 oz | **140** | **0** | **36** |
| Lollipops (1), 0.55 oz | **60** | **0** | **15** |
| **Jujubes,** all varieties (52), 1.4 oz | **110** | **0** | **28** |
| **Juju Bears,** 5 pieces | **130** | **0** | **34** |
| **Juju Mix (Sathers),** 11 pieces, 1.5 oz | **150** | **0** | **36** |
| **Jujyfruits,** 16 pieces, 1.4 oz | **120** | **0** | **32** |
| **Junior Caramels:** 13 pieces, 1.5 oz | **190** | **6** | **33** |
| Mini, 2 boxes, 1 oz | **130** | **4** | **23** |

*Per Piece/Serving*    **Ⓒ** **Ⓕ** **Cb**

| | C | F | Cb |
|---|---|---|---|
| **Junior Mints:** 1.8 oz | **220** | **4** | **45** |
| 16 pieces, 1.4 oz | **170** | **3** | **35** |
| **Justin's,** Peanut Butter Cups, | | | |
| Milk Choc, 2 cups, 1.4 oz pkg | **200** | **14** | **18** |

**Kisses** *(Hershey's):*

| | C | F | Cb |
|---|---|---|---|
| **Milk Chocolate:** (1), 0.16 oz | **25** | **1.5** | **3** |
| (9), 1.4 oz | **200** | **12** | **25** |
| with Almonds (9), 1.4 oz | **200** | **13** | **22** |
| Caramel Filled (9), 1.5 oz | **190** | **9** | **27** |
| Air Delights (11), 1.4 oz | **200** | **12** | **24** |
| Cookies 'n' Creme (9), 1.5 oz | **220** | **12** | **26** |
| Hugs (9), 1.4 oz | **210** | **12** | **24** |
| **Special Dark,** (9), 1.4 oz | **180** | **12** | **25** |

**Kit Kat** *(Nestle):*

| | C | F | Cb |
|---|---|---|---|
| **Milk Chocolate:** 4 pce bar, 1.5 oz | **210** | **11** | **28** |
| Extra Crispy, 1.6 oz bar | **220** | **12** | **29** |
| King Size, 8 pcs, 3 oz bar | **420** | **22** | **56** |
| Minis, 5 pieces | **210** | **11** | **28** |
| Snack Size, 6 pcs, 1.5 oz | **210** | **11** | **27** |
| **White Chocolate,** 4 pcs, 1.5 oz | **220** | **12** | **26** |
| **Lemon Drops:** (4), 0.6 oz | **60** | **0** | **16** |
| *Walgreens,* Sugar Free (3), 0.6 oz | **50** | **0** | **17** |
| **Lemonhead,** (26), 1.4 oz | **140** | **0** | **36** |
| **Lance,** Peanut Bar, 2.2 oz | **340** | **19** | **29** |

**Licorice:**

| | C | F | Cb |
|---|---|---|---|
| Avaerage all varieties, 1oz | **100** | **0** | **25** |
| Chews *(Panda)*, (1) | **10** | **0** | **3** |
| Tid Bits (1) | **10** | **0** | **2** |
| Twists: Black/Red, av., 1 pc | **35** | **0** | **8** |
| Sugar Free, 1 piece | **15** | **0** | **2.5** |

**American Licorice Co.:**

| | C | F | Cb |
|---|---|---|---|
| Natural Vines: Black (9), 1.4 oz | **140** | **1** | **33** |
| Strawberry (9), 1.4 oz | **150** | **1** | **34** |
| Red Vines (4), 1.4 oz | **140** | **0** | **34** |
| Sip-n-Chew, 1 oz package | **100** | **1** | **23** |
| Snaps (31), 1.4 oz | **140** | **0.5** | **33** |
| Sour Punch (6), 1.4 oz | **150** | **0.5** | **34** |
| Super Ropes (1), 2 oz | **200** | **0** | **46** |

**Lifesavers:**

| | C | F | Cb |
|---|---|---|---|
| Large size, 1 candy | **15** | **0** | **3** |
| Regular: All flavors, 1 candy | **10** | **0** | **3** |
| 1 Roll (14 candies), 1.2 oz | **140** | **0** | **35** |
| Creme Savers, 3 pieces, 0.5 oz | **60** | **1** | **11** |
| Pep-o-mint (3), 0.2 oz | **20** | **0** | **5** |
| Fruit Splosion (10), 1.4 oz | **130** | **0** | **31** |
| Sugar-Free, | | | |
| Pep-O-Mint (4), 0.5 0z | **35** | **0** | **14** |

*Note: Carb figure includes 14g sugar alcohol*

## Candy ~ Brands & Generic (Cont)

*Per Piece/Serving* **C F Cb**

| | C | F | Cb |
|---|---|---|---|
| Lik-m-aid *(Nestle)*, Fun Dip, 1 package | 50 | 0 | 13 |
| Lindt: Lindor Truffles (1), average | 75 | 6 | 5 |
| **Swiss Milk Chocolate Bars:** | | | |
| 70% Cocoa, 4 pieces | 220 | 17 | 13 |
| Classic, with Hazelnuts, 10 pieces | 230 | 16 | 20 |
| Raspberry filled, 7 pieces | 200 | 10 | 25 |
| **Dark Choc. Truffles,** | | | |
| with filling, 7 pieces | 240 | 18 | 18 |
| **Lollipops:** Mini, 0.3 oz | 25 | 0 | 6 |
| Small, 0.5 oz | 50 | 0 | 12 |
| Medium, 1 oz | 100 | 0 | 25 |
| Giant (4" diam), 7 oz | 790 | 0 | 198 |
| **M & M's:** | | | |
| **Dark Chocolate:** 1.5 oz package | 210 | 10 | 29 |
| Peanuts, 1.5 oz | 220 | 12 | 25 |
| **Milk Chocolate:** 28 piece, 1 oz | 145 | 6.5 | 21 |
| 1.5 oz package | 210 | 9 | 30 |
| 1.7 oz package | 240 | 10 | 34 |
| Almond Choc., 1.5 oz | 220 | 12 | 25 |
| Minis, 1 tube, 1 oz | 150 | 7 | 21 |
| **Peanut:** 28 pieces, 1 oz | 155 | 8 | 17 |
| 1.75 oz pkg | 250 | 13 | 30 |
| **Peanut Butter,** 1.6 oz pkg | 240 | 14 | 26 |
| **Premiums:** Chocolate Trio, 1.5 oz | 230 | 14 | 25 |
| Mint Thrills, 1.5 oz | 240 | 14 | 25 |
| **Pretzels,** ½ pkg, 1.4 oz | 180 | 6 | 29 |
| **Snack Mix,** av. ⅓ cup, 1.5 oz | 200 | 9 | 25 |
| Mamba Sours, Fruit Chews, | | | |
| 6 pieces, 1 oz | 100 | 1 | 22 |
| **Marshmallow Egg,** 1 egg, 1 oz | 120 | 3 | 22 |
| **Mary Jane** *(Necco)*, 5 pieces, 1.4 oz | 160 | 3.5 | 32 |
| **Marshmallows:** Firm/Soft, 1 oz | 90 | 0 | 23 |
| Regular size, 4 pieces, 1 oz | 100 | 0 | 24 |
| Mini-Marshmallow, ⅔ cup, 1 oz | 95 | 0 | 24 |
| *Joyva,* Choc-coated Twists | 95 | 2 | 10 |
| *Fluff,* 2 Tbsp, 0.6 oz | 60 | 0 | 15 |
| *Kraft:* Creme, 0.5 oz | 45 | 0 | 11 |
| Funmallows, ⅔ cup, 1 oz | 100 | 0 | 24 |
| Jet-Puffed, 5 pieces, 1 oz | 100 | 0 | 24 |
| Mini, 1 oz | 90 | 0 | 23 |
| **Marzipan,** 2 Tbsp, 1.4 oz | 160 | 4 | 29 |
| **Mauna Loa,** Mountains, 4 pcs | 230 | 17 | 21 |
| **Mexican Hats,** (7), 1.4 oz | 120 | 0 | 30 |
| **Mentos:** Regular | 10 | 0 | 3 |
| Sugar Free | 5 | 0 | 2 |
| **Mike & Ike:** | | | |
| Original: 2.1 oz package | 220 | 0 | 55 |
| 23 pieces, 1.4 oz | 140 | 0 | 36 |
| **Milk Duds,** 1 box, 1.8 oz | 230 | 8 | 38 |

*Per Piece/Serving* **C F Cb**

| | C | F | Cb |
|---|---|---|---|
| **Milky Way** *(Mars)*: | | | |
| **Bars:** Single, 2 oz | 240 | 9 | 37 |
| Fun Size, 2 bars, 1.2 oz | 160 | 6 | 24 |
| To Go, 1.8 oz | 230 | 9 | 36 |
| Minis, 5 pieces, 1.5 oz | 190 | 7 | 30 |
| Midnight Bars: 1.8 oz | 230 | 8 | 36 |
| Minis, 5 pieces, 1.4 oz | 190 | 7 | 30 |
| Simply Caramel, 1.9 oz | 250 | 11 | 37 |
| **Mints:** Uncoated, 3 pieces | 70 | 0 | 17 |
| 1 mint, medium | 7 | 0 | 1 |
| 1 large mint | 15 | 0 | 3 |
| **Mon Cheri** *(Ferrero)*, 4 pieces, 2 oz | 260 | 18 | 20 |
| **Mounds:** 1.75 oz bar | 240 | 13 | 28 |
| King Size, 4 pieces, 3.5 oz | 480 | 26 | 56 |
| Snack Size, 1 piece, 0.6 oz | 80 | 4.5 | 10 |
| **Mr Goodbar:** 1.8 oz bar | 250 | 17 | 26 |
| King Size, 2.6 oz bar | 380 | 26 | 38 |
| **Munch Bar,** 1.4 oz | 220 | 15 | 24 |
| **Necco,** Candy Wafers (40), 2 oz | 220 | 0 | 56 |
| **Nestle, Crunch:** Orig.,1.6 oz bar | 220 | 11 | 30 |
| Fun Size, 3 bars, 1.4 oz | 180 | 9 | 26 |
| Miniatures, 4 bars, 1.4 oz | 200 | 10 | 27 |
| Buncha Crunch, ⅓ cup, 1.2 oz | 180 | 9 | 25 |
| Crunch Crisp, 1.8 oz | 240 | 13 | 32 |
| **Newman's Own:** | | | |
| **Milk Choc.:** Caramel Cups (3) | 160 | 8 | 21 |
| Peanut Butter Cups (3) | 180 | 12 | 17 |
| **Dark Choc.:** Caramel Cups (3) | 160 | 9 | 20 |
| Peanut Butter Cups (3) | 180 | 13 | 16 |
| **Nips,** all varieties, 2 pieces, 0.5 oz | 60 | 2 | 11 |
| **Nougat:** 3 pieces, 1.5 oz | 170 | 1 | 39 |
| Chocolate Covered, 1 oz | 125 | 4 | 22 |
| **Nuggets** ~ *See Hershey's* | | | |
| **Nutrageous Bar** *(Reese's)*, 1.8 oz | 260 | 16 | 28 |
| **Oh Henry!:** Fun Size, 0.9 oz | 120 | 5 | 16 |
| 1.8 oz bar | 230 | 11 | 33 |
| **Orange Slices:** | | | |
| *Jewel,* 3 pieces, 1.5 oz | 140 | 0 | 35 |
| *Walgreens,* 4 pieces, 1.6 oz | 160 | 0 | 39 |
| **Pastel Mints** *(Walgreens)*, 20 pieces | 60 | 0 | 14 |
| **PayDay Bar:** 1.8 oz bar | 240 | 13 | 27 |
| King Size, 3.5 oz bar | 440 | 24 | 50 |
| Snack Size, 0.7 oz | 90 | 5 | 10 |
| Avalanche, 1.8 oz bar | 250 | 13 | 29 |
| **Peanut Bar** *(Planter's)*, 1.6 oz | 240 | 14 | 21 |
| **Peanut Butter Cups** ~ *See Reese's; Newman's Own* | | | |
| **Peanut Brittle:** 1 piece, 1.5 oz | 190 | 5 | 32 |
| Sugar Free *(Russell Stover)*, | | | |
| 4 pieces, 1.3 oz | 140 | 10 | 24 |

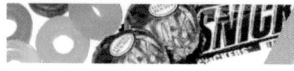

## Candy ~ Brands & Generic (Cont)

*Per Piece/Serving*

| | C | F | Cb |
|---|---|---|---|
| **Peanuts,** choc-covered, 14 pieces | 230 | 14 | 23 |
| **Pearson's,** Mint Patties, (5), 1.3 oz | 150 | 2.5 | 31 |
| **Peppermints:** 7 small, 0.5 oz | 60 | 0 | 15 |
| Brach's, Star Brites (3) | 60 | 0 | 16 |
| **Pez,** 1 roll | 35 | 0 | 9 |
| **Planters,** | | | |
| Double Peanut Bar, 1.6 oz | 240 | 14 | 21 |
| **Pop Rocks,** 0.4 oz package | 35 | 0 | 9 |
| **Pot of Gold** (Hershey's): | | | |
| Assortment: Caramel, 4 pieces | 190 | 10 | 25 |
| Nut, 4 pieces | 210 | 13 | 23 |
| **Pretzels:** Choc-covered, Mini (6) | 200 | 9 | 25 |
| White Choc Bites (23), 1.4 oz | 200 | 9 | 25 |
| **Pretzel Flipz** (Nestlé), 8 pieces, 1 oz | 130 | 5 | 20 |
| **Raisinets:** | | | |
| Milk Choc: 1.58 oz pkg | 190 | 8 | 32 |
| Movie Pack, 3.5 oz | 380 | 16 | 64 |
| Dark Chocolate, ¼ cup, 1.6 oz | 180 | 8 | 32 |
| **Reese's:** | | | |
| **Clusters,** 3 pieces, 1.5 oz | 220 | 12 | 24 |
| **Crispy Crunchy Bar:** 1.7 oz | 260 | 18 | 22 |
| 2 pieces, 1.2 oz | 170 | 10 | 19 |
| King Size, 3 oz | 480 | 32 | 40 |
| **Fast Break,** 2 oz bar | 260 | 12 | 35 |
| **P'nut Butter Chips,** 0.5 oz | 80 | 4 | 8 |
| **P'nut Butter Cups:** | | | |
| Milk Choc: (2), 1.5 oz | 210 | 13 | 24 |
| Miniatures (5), 1.5 oz | 220 | 13 | 26 |
| Minis (11) | 200 | 12 | 23 |
| Big Cup (1), 1.4 oz | 200 | 12 | 22 |
| Sugar Free, Minis (5), 1.4 oz | 180 | 13 | 27 |
| **Dark Chocolate (2),** 1.5 oz | 210 | 14 | 23 |
| **Pieces,** Peanut Butter (51) | 200 | 9 | 25 |
| **Sticks:** 1.5 oz pkg | 220 | 13 | 23 |
| King Size, 3 oz pkg | 440 | 26 | 46 |
| Snack Size (1), 0.6 oz | 90 | 5 | 9 |
| **Snacksters,** 1 package, 0.8 oz | 100 | 4 | 14 |
| **Whipps,** 1.5 oz | 230 | 9 | 37 |
| **Rice Krispies Treats** (Kellogg's), | | | |
| 1 bar, average all varieties, 0.8 oz | 95 | 2.5 | 17 |
| **Riesen,** Choc. Chew, 4 pieces, 1.3 oz | 170 | 6 | 28 |
| **Rocky Road,** Milk/Dark, 1.8 oz bar | 240 | 11 | 34 |
| **Roca Thins,** 3 pieces, av. all varieties | 210 | 14 | 24 |
| **Rolo:** Regular, all varieties, 1.7 oz roll | 220 | 10 | 23 |
| Mini Chews, Caramel in milk choc. (11) | 190 | 9 | 26 |
| **Root Beer Barrels,** (3), 0.6 oz | 60 | 0 | 17 |

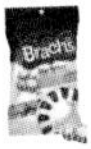

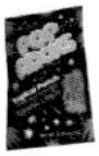

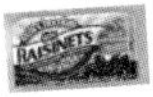

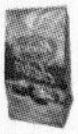

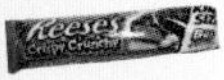

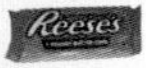

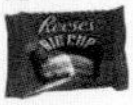

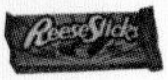

*Per Piece/Serving*

| | C | F | Cb |
|---|---|---|---|
| **Russell Stover Candy:** | | | |
| **Boxed Chocolates Choc. Coated:** | | | |
| Assorted (2), 1.2 oz | 150 | 7 | 22 |
| Cherry Cordials (3), 0.4 oz | 150 | 5 | 25 |
| Dairy Crm Caramels (2), 1.2 oz | 160 | 7 | 22 |
| Elegant Collection (3), 1.6 oz | 210 | 10 | 25 |
| French Choc. Mints (4), 1.4 oz | 220 | 13 | 22 |
| Nut, Chewy & Crisp Centers (2) | 160 | 8 | 21 |
| **Sugar Free:** | | | |
| Ass'td Hard Candies (3), 1.6 oz | 210 | 16 | 24 |
| Bags: Caramel (3), 1.3 oz | 180 | 8 | 25 |
| Coconut (3), 1.5 oz | 160 | 10 | 28 |
| Mint Patty (3), 1.5 oz | 180 | 12 | 26 |
| Peanut Butter Cups (2), 1.2 oz | 160 | 12 | 17 |
| Pecan Delight (2), 1.2 oz | 160 | 12 | 19 |
| Note: Carbohydrate figures include sugar alcohol | | | |
| **Salt Water Taffy** (Brach's), (5) | 170 | 2.5 | 36 |
| **Seashells** (Guylian), (4), 1.6 oz | 260 | 17 | 24 |
| **See's Candies:** | | | |
| Almond Royal (5) | 190 | 13 | 18 |
| Butterscotch Chews (5) | 210 | 12 | 27 |
| Krispy's: Caffe Latte (5) | 180 | 8 | 27 |
| Mint (5) | 170 | 8 | 27 |
| Little Pops: | | | |
| Butterscotch (4), 0.5 oz | 60 | 2 | 12 |
| Chocolate (4), 0.5 oz | 60 | 3 | 10 |
| Vanilla (4), 0.5 oz | 50 | 2 | 9 |
| Lollypops, average, 0.7 oz | 90 | 3 | 17 |
| Milk Molasses Chips ( 6), 1.4 oz | 180 | 8 | 27 |
| Milk Peppermints, 2 pieces, 1.3 oz | 150 | 4 | 28 |
| Peanut Brittle Bar, 1 oz | 150 | 10 | 15 |
| P'nut Butter Patties (2), 1.2 oz | 170 | 10 | 16 |
| Peppermint Twists (3) | 60 | 0 | 15 |
| Toffee-ettes, 3 pcs | 270 | 21 | 18 |
| **Sugar Free:** Dark Bar, 1.5 oz | 180 | 16 | 24 |
| Dark Walnut Clusters (4), 1.5 oz | 230 | 21 | 17 |
| Peanut Brittle, 1.5 oz | 170 | 14 | 17 |
| **Skinny Cow:** | | | |
| Dreamy Clusters, all var., 1 pouch | 120 | 6 | 20 |
| Heavenly Crips, all varieties, 1 bar | 110 | 6 | 14 |
| **Skittles:** Original, 2 oz | 230 | 2.5 | 52 |
| Sour, 1.8 oz | 200 | 2 | 44 |
| Tropical; Wild Berry, 2.2 oz | 250 | 2.5 | 56 |
| Fun Size, 1 bag, 0.5 oz | 60 | 1 | 14 |
| Tear & Share, 4 oz bag | 420 | 4.5 | 93 |
| **Skor,** Toffee Bar (1), 1.4 oz | 200 | 12 | 25 |
| **Smarties:** Candy Rolls (1), 0.3 oz | 25 | 0 | 6 |
| Giant, 1 roll, 1 oz | 100 | 0 | 25 |

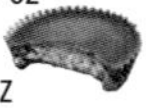

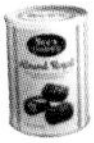

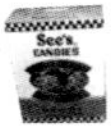

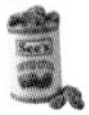

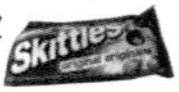

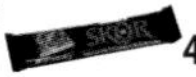

## Candy ~ Brands & Generic (Cont)

*Per Piece/Serving*

| | C | F | Cb |
|---|---|---|---|
| **Snickers:** | | | |
| **Milk Chocolate:** | | | |
| 1.9 oz bar | 250 | 12 | 33 |
| Fun Size, 2 bars, 1.2 oz | 160 | 8 | 21 |
| To Go Bar, 1.6 oz | 220 | 10 | 29 |
| Almond Bar, 1.8 oz | 230 | 11 | 32 |
| P'nut Butter Squared, 2 bars, 1.8 oz | 250 | 13 | 30 |
| Miniatures: (4) | 170 | 8 | 22 |
| Sugar Free, 5 pcs | 180 | 13 | 27 |
| **Dark Chocolate Bar,** 1.8 oz | 250 | 12 | 31 |
| **Sno Caps,** ¼ cup, 1.4 oz | 180 | 8 | 30 |
| **Soft 'N Chewy,** Butter Toffee, 1 piece | 30 | 0.5 | 5 |
| **Sorbee,** Crystal Light Hard Candy, 4 pieces | 25 | 0 | 13 |
| *Note: Carb figures include Isomalt which has fewer calories than sugar.* | | | |
| **Sour Patch:** Kids, average, 2 oz | 210 | 0 | 52 |
| Extreme, 1.8 oz | 190 | 0 | 47 |
| **Spearmint Leaves:** | | | |
| *Jewel,* 5 pieces, 1.4 oz | 140 | 0 | 35 |
| *Walgreens,* 4 pieces, 1.6 oz | 160 | 0 | 39 |
| **Spree Candies:** Original, 15 pieces | 50 | 0 | 13 |
| Chewy, 8 pieces | 60 | 0 | 13 |
| **Starburst:** | | | |
| Candy Canes, 0.5 oz | 70 | 0 | 18 |
| Fruit Chews: Original (1) | 20 | 0.5 | 4 |
| 8 pieces, 1.4 oz | 160 | 3.5 | 33 |
| Gummibursts, 9 pieces, 1.4 oz | 130 | 0 | 31 |
| Jellybeans, 1.5 oz | 150 | 0 | 37 |
| **Starlight Mints,** 3 pieces, 0.5 oz | 60 | 0 | 15 |
| **Suckers** *(Walgreens),* 1 piece, 0.4 oz | 45 | 0 | 11 |
| **Sugar Babies,** Original, 1.6 oz | 160 | 1.5 | 37 |
| **Sugar Coated Peanuts,** 1 oz | 120 | 8 | 10 |
| **Sunbursts Sunflowers** *(Kimmie):* | | | |
| Choco Rocks Milk, 1.4 oz | 210 | 10 | 27 |
| Kettle Corn Nuggets, 1.4 oz | 200 | 9 | 29 |
| Sunburst Milk, 1.4 oz | 210 | 11 | 23 |
| **Swedish Fish,** 7 pieces, 1.5 oz | 150 | 0 | 38 |
| **SweeTARTS:** | | | |
| Orig., 8 pieces, 0.5 oz | 50 | 0 | 13 |
| Mini Chewy, 23 pieces, 0.5 oz | 50 | 0.5 | 12 |
| **Symphony** *(Hershey's):* | | | |
| **Milk Choc:** 1.5 oz bar | 220 | 14 | 23 |
| Large Block: 5 pieces, 1.4 oz | 200 | 12 | 22 |
| w/ Alm. & Toffee, 5 pcs, 1.3 oz | 200 | 13 | 21 |

*Per Piece/Serving*

| | C | F | Cb |
|---|---|---|---|
| **Taffy,** | | | |
| Fruit Chews, 1 piece | 20 | 0.5 | 4 |
| **Take 5** *(Hershey's):* Orig., 1.5oz | 200 | 11 | 25 |
| King Size, 2.3 oz | 300 | 16 | 37 |
| Snack Size, 2 pcs, 1 oz | 150 | 8 | 19 |
| **3 Musketeers:** | | | |
| Original, 1.9 oz | 240 | 7 | 42 |
| 2 To Go, 1 bar, 1.6 oz | 200 | 6 | 35 |
| Fun Size, 3 bars, 1.6 oz | 190 | 6 | 34 |
| Minis, 7 pieces, 1.4 oz | 170 | 5 | 32 |
| **Tang-a-Roos,** 1 roll | 25 | 0 | 6 |
| **Terry's:** Chocolate Orange (5), 1.5 oz | 230 | 12 | 27 |
| Dark Chocolate Orange (5), 1.5 oz | 240 | 13 | 28 |
| **Tic Tac:** all varieties, 1 piece | 2 | 0 | 0 |
| **Toblerone:** 1.3 oz bar | 190 | 10 | 22 |
| 1.8 oz bar | 270 | 15 | 31 |
| 3.5 oz bar | 540 | 30 | 63 |
| 5.3 oz Package, 5 pieces, 1.5 oz | 230 | 13 | 27 |
| **Toffees,** Regular, 1 oz | 160 | 9 | 18 |
| **Tootsie Pops,** (1), 0.6 oz | 60 | 0 | 15 |
| **Tootsie Roll:** 2.3 oz roll | 245 | 2 | 55 |
| Midgees, 1.4 oz | 140 | 3 | 28 |
| **Truffles:** Reg., 1 piece, 0.4 oz | 60 | 4 | 6 |
| Large *(Godiva),* 0.8 oz | 110 | 6.5 | 12 |
| Extra Large *(J.Schmidt),* 1.5 oz | 220 | 13 | 24 |
| **Turtles:** Original, 1 piece, 0.6 oz | 85 | 5 | 10 |
| Sugar Free, 1 piece, 0.4 oz | 50 | 3.5 | 7 |
| **Twists,** Licorice; Strawb., sugar free, 7 pieces, 1.4 oz | 90 | 0 | 25 |
| **Twix:** | | | |
| **Caramel:** 2 cookies, 1.8 oz | 250 | 12 | 34 |
| Fun Size, 2 cookies, 1.7 oz | 250 | 14 | 27 |
| 4 To Go, 1 cookie, 0.8 oz | 110 | 5 | 15 |
| 6 To Go, 1 cookie, 0.5 oz | 80 | 4 | 11 |
| Minis, 3 pieces, 1 oz | 150 | 7 | 20 |
| **Peanut Butter:** | | | |
| Single, 2 cookies, 1.7 oz | 250 | 14 | 27 |
| 4 to Go, 1 cookie, 0.8 oz | 250 | 12 | 34 |
| **Twizzlers:** Cherry Bites (17), 1.4 oz | 140 | 0.5 | 32 |
| Cherry Nibs, 29 pieces, 1.4 oz | 140 | 1 | 32 |
| **Pull 'n' Peel,** Cherry, 1 piece, 1.2 oz | 110 | 0.5 | 26 |
| **Twists Strawb.,** 1.3 oz | 120 | 0.5 | 29 |
| **U-No Bar,** 1.5 oz | 250 | 17 | 22 |
| **Weight Watchers** *(Whitman's):* | | | |
| Caramel Medallions (3) | 160 | 9 | 24 |
| Coconut (3) | 150 | 9 | 23 |
| English Toffee Squares (3) | 150 | 9 | 21 |
| Mint Patties (3) | 150 | 9 | 23 |
| Peanut Butter Cups (4) | 180 | 8 | 31 |
| Pecan Crowns (3) | 160 | 10 | 24 |

## Candy ~ Brands & Generic (Cont)

| Per Piece/Serving | C | F | Cb |
|---|---|---|---|
| **Werther's:** | | | |
| Hard Candy: Original (3), 0.5 oz | 70 | 1.5 | 14 |
| Sugar-Free Original (5) | 40 | 1.5 | 15 |
| *Note: Carb figure includes 14g sugar alcohol* | | | |
| Soft, Chocolate Caramel (4), 1.4 oz | 190 | 8 | 28 |
| **Whatchamacallit:** 1.5 oz Bar | 230 | 12 | 28 |
| King Size Bar, 2.5 oz | 370 | 20 | 45 |
| **Whitman's, Boxed Chocolates:** | | | |
| Sampler (4), 1.6 oz | 220 | 12 | 27 |
| 12 oz Box, 3 pieces, 1.2 oz | 170 | 9 | 21 |
| Reserve, 7 oz Box, 2 pieces, 1.2 oz | 160 | 9 | 21 |
| Sugar Free, 10 oz Box, 3 pcs, 1.5 oz | 190 | 13 | 25 |
| **Whoppers,** av. all varieties, 18 pcs | 190 | 7 | 31 |
| **Wonka:** | | | |
| Bar (1), 2.5 oz | 360 | 19 | 49 |
| Exceptional Bars, average, 4 pieces | 200 | 13 | 23 |
| Gobstopper, 9 pieces, 0.5 oz | 60 | 0 | 14 |
| **Laffy Taffy:** Ropes, all var., 0.8 oz | 80 | 1.5 | 18 |
| Stretchy & Tangy, all var., 1.5 oz | 150 | 3.5 | 29 |
| Nerds, Giant, Chewy, 1.8 oz package | 180 | 0 | 42 |
| **Yogurt Candy,** | | | |
| Coated Raisins, 27 pieces, 1.4 oz | 180 | 8 | 28 |
| **York:** Mints, (3) | 10 | 0 | 3 |
| Peppermint Pattie, reg, 1.4 oz | 140 | 2.5 | 31 |
| Pieces (50) | 170 | 8 | 28 |
| ***Zagnut,*** 1.75 oz bar | 220 | 9 | 35 |
| **Zero Bar:** 1.8 oz bar | 230 | 8 | 37 |
| King Size, 3.5 oz | 400 | 14 | 68 |

## Gum

| Per Piece | C | F | Cb |
|---|---|---|---|
| ***Bazooka*** | 15 | 0 | 4 |
| ***Beechies*** | 6 | 0 | 2 |
| ***Big League Chews*** | 10 | 0 | 2 |
| ***Bubble Yum:*** Original | 25 | 0 | 6 |
| Sugarless | 10 | 0 | 3 |
| Candilicious | 30 | 0 | 2 |
| ***Carefree,*** Sugarless/Regular | 5 | 0 | 2 |
| ***Chiclet*** | 5 | 0 | 1 |
| ***Dentyne*** | 5 | 0 | 0.5 |
| ***Double Bubble Ball*** | 20 | 0 | 5 |
| ***Estee,*** Bubble/Regular | 5 | 0 | 2 |
| ***Extra*** (Wrigley's), Sugar-Free | 5 | 0 | 2 |
| ***Freshen-Up*** | 10 | 0 | 3 |
| ***Hubba Bubba:*** Regular | 25 | 0 | 6 |
| Sugar-free, average | 14 | 0 | 0.5 |
| ***Ice Breakers*** | 5 | 0 | 2 |
| ***Jolt Gum*** | 5 | 0 | 2 |
| ***Super Bubble*** | 15 | 0 | 4 |
| ***Trident,*** Orig.; White | 5 | 0 | 1 |
| ***Wrigley's,*** all flavors | 10 | 0 | 2 |

## Carob Candy

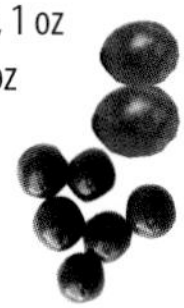

| | C | F | Cb |
|---|---|---|---|
| *Per Piece/Serving* | | | |
| **Carob**, Plain/Natural, 1 oz | 155 | 9 | 15 |
| **Carob Coated:** Raisins, 1 oz | 130 | 8 | 15 |
| Almonds/Peanuts, 1 oz | 150 | 10 | 14 |
| Caramels, 1 oz | 110 | 4 | 18 |
| Dates, 1 oz | 125 | 5 | 20 |
| Malt Balls, 1 oz | 135 | 8 | 15 |
| Soybeans | 145 | 9 | 16 |
| Trail/Party Mix, 1 oz | 150 | 9 | 15 |

## Cough Drops

| Per Drop/Piece | C | F | Cb |
|---|---|---|---|
| **Beech Nut,** 1 drop | 10 | 0 | 2 |
| **CVS,** Honey Lemon Cough Drops | 15 | 0 | 4 |
| **Diabetic Tussin** | 0 | 0 | 0 |
| **Halls, Defense Vitamin C:** Regular | 15 | 0 | 4 |
| Sugar Free | 5 | 0 | 3 |
| Fruit Breezers | 15 | 0 | 4 |
| Menthol Drops: Regular | 15 | 0 | 4 |
| Sugar Free | 5 | 0 | 4 |
| Plus | 20 | 0 | 5 |
| **Listerine** *(Amer. Chicle)*, Lozenge | 10 | 0 | 2 |
| **Luden's,** Throat Drops: Reg., all var. | 10 | 0 | 2 |
| Sugar Free | 0 | 0 | 0 |
| **Pine Bros,** Cough Drops | 10 | 0 | 2 |
| **Ricola,** Cough Drops: | | | |
| Natural Herbs | 10 | 0 | 3 |
| Sugar-Free Lemon Mint | 0 | 0 | 1 |
| **Rolaids,** Sodium Free | 5 | 0 | 1 |
| **Sathers,** Peppermint Lozenges | 15 | 0 | 3 |
| **Sucrets** *(Beecham)*, Lozenges | 10 | 0 | 2.5 |
| **Wintergreen,** Lozenges | 15 | 0 | 3 |

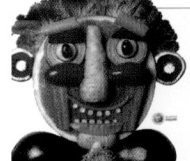

*Eat at least 5 servings of fruit and vegetables every day . . . and Enjoy Better Health!*

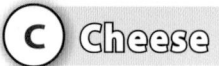

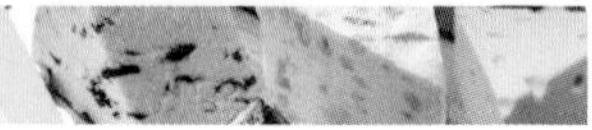

# C Cheese

## Quick Guide    C   F   Cb

### Firm/Hard Cheeses
**American, Cheddar, Jack, Swiss:**
**Average All Brands**
**Regular Cheese:**

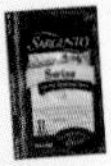

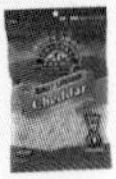

| | C | F | Cb |
|---|---|---|---|
| Thin Deli slice, 0.8 oz | 80 | 6 | 0.5 |
| 1 oz slice/piece | 110 | 9 | 0.5 |
| 8 oz package | 880 | 72 | 3 |
| **Cubes:** 1" cube, 0.6 oz | 70 | 5.5 | 0.5 |
| 1¼" cube, 1 oz | 115 | 9 | 0.5 |
| **Diced,** 1 cup, 4.5 oz | 510 | 41 | 3 |
| **Melted,** ¼ cup, 2 oz | 245 | 20 | 1 |
| **Shredded:** ¼ cup, 1 oz | 110 | 9 | 0.5 |
| 1 cup, 4 oz | 440 | 36 | 2 |

## Cheese & Cheese Products

*Per 1 oz Unless Indicated*

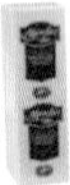

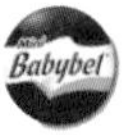

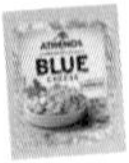

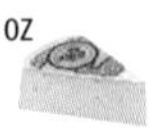

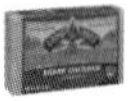

| | C | F | Cb |
|---|---|---|---|
| **Almond** (*Lisanatti*), Chunks, average | 50 | 1 | 3 |
| **American:** | | | |
| Regular: 1 slice, 1 oz | 105 | 9 | 0.5 |
| *Kraft,* Regular, 0.67 oz slice | 60 | 4.5 | 0 |
| *Land O'Lakes,* 0.67 oz slice | 70 | 4 | 2 |
| Reduced Fat: | | | |
| *Alpine Lace,* Yellow/White, 0.8 oz | 90 | 6 | 2 |
| *Borden,* 1 slice, 0.8 oz | 50 | 3 | 2 |
| *Kraft,* 2% Milk, 0.67 oz | 45 | 2.5 | 1 |
| *Land O Lakes,* 2% Milk, 1 oz | 90 | 6 | 2 |
| **Babybel** (*Laughing Cow*), Mini: | | | |
| Original (1), 0.8 oz | 70 | 6 | 0 |
| Light (1), 0.8 oz | 50 | 3 | 0 |
| Bonbel (1), 0.8 oz | 70 | 6 | 0 |
| Light Original (1), 0.8 oz | 50 | 3 | 0 |
| Gouda (1), 0.8 oz | 80 | 6 | 0 |
| **Blue/Bleu:** *Average all Brands* | | | |
| Crumbled, ¼ cup, 1 oz | 100 | 8 | 0 |
| Light, 0.8 oz | 35 | 1.5 | 2 |
| **Brie:** Average, 1 oz | 95 | 8 | 0 |
| *Alouette,* | | | |
| Baby Brie Wedge, 1 oz | 110 | 10 | 1 |
| **Camembert,** 1 oz | 85 | 7 | 0 |
| **Caraway,** 1 oz | 105 | 8 | 1 |
| **Castello,** 1 oz | 120 | 12 | 0 |
| **Cheddar:** | | | |
| Regular: Medium/Sharp, av., 1 oz | 110 | 9 | 1 |
| Shredded, ¼ cup, 1 oz | 110 | 9 | 1 |
| *Cracker Barrel:* Extra Sharp, 1 oz | 110 | 10 | 0 |
| Sharp, Shreds, 1 oz | 110 | 9 | 1 |

## Cheese & Cheese Products (Cont)

*Per 1 oz Unless Indicated*

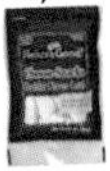

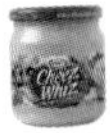

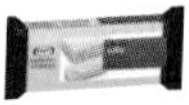

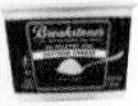

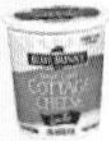

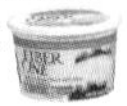

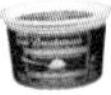

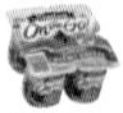

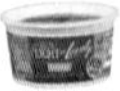

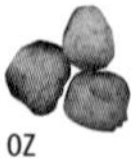

| | C | F | Cb |
|---|---|---|---|
| **Cheddar (Cont):** | | | |
| Reduced Fat, 2% Milk, Shredded, | | | |
| *Kraft,* 1 oz | 80 | 6 | 1 |
| Curds, Cheddar Cheese, | | | |
| *Heluva Good!,* 1 oz | 110 | 9 | 0 |
| **Cheese Curds** ~ *See Cottage Cheese* | | | |
| **Cheese Logs** (*Kaukauna*), average | 100 | 7 | 4 |
| **Cheese Whiz:** | | | |
| Original, 2 Tbsp, 1 oz | 90 | 7 | 4 |
| Light, 2 Tbsp, 1 oz | 80 | 3.5 | 6 |
| Salsa Con Queso, | | | |
| 2 Tbsp, 1 oz | 90 | 7 | 4 |
| **Cheshire,** 1 oz | 110 | 9 | 1.5 |
| **Colby,** Regular, 1 oz | 110 | 8 | 0 |
| **Colby-Jack:** | | | |
| Big Slice, 0.8 oz | 90 | 7 | 0 |
| **Cottage Cheese (Curds):** *Average All Brands* | | | |
| Creamed (4% milk fat): | | | |
| 2 Tbsp, 1 oz | 30 | 1 | 1.5 |
| ½ cup, 4 oz | 110 | 5 | 4 |
| with fruit, ½ cup, 4 oz | 115 | 4 | 5 |
| Reduced-Fat (2%): 2 Tbsp, 1 oz | 25 | 0.5 | 1 |
| ½ cup, 4 oz | 100 | 3 | 4 |
| Low-Fat (1%): 2 Tbsp, 1 oz | 20 | 0.5 | 1 |
| ½ cup, 4 oz | 80 | 1 | 3 |
| Fat-Free/Non-Fat: 2 T., 1 oz | 20 | 0 | 1 |
| ½ cup, 4 oz | 80 | 0 | 5 |
| **Cottage Cheese (Curds):** *Brands* | | | |
| *Fiber One,* 1% Fat, ½ c., 4 oz | 80 | 2 | 8 |
| *Friendship:* | | | |
| 1% Low-Fat with Pineapple, 4 oz | 120 | 1 | 16 |
| Nonfat with Pineapple, ½ cup, 4 oz | 110 | 0 | 17 |
| Pot Style, 2%, ½ cup, 4 oz | 90 | 2.5 | 3 |
| *Hood,* Low Fat, 4 oz | 90 | 1 | 5 |
| *Knudsen/Breakstone's:* | | | |
| Free, Non-Fat, ½ cup, 4 oz | 70 | 0 | 7 |
| 2% Milk Fat, ½ cup, 4 oz | 100 | 2.5 | 6 |
| On the Go!, | | | |
| Low-Fat, 4 oz carton | 90 | 2.5 | 6 |
| *Lactaid,* Low-Fat, ½ cup, 4 oz | 80 | 1 | 7 |
| *Light n' Lively:* | | | |
| Fat-Free, ½ cup, 4.4 oz | 80 | 0 | 8 |
| Low-Fat, ½ cup, 4.4 oz | 80 | 1.5 | 6 |
| Breaded & Fried: | | | |
| *A&W,* 5 oz | 570 | 40 | 27 |
| *Culver's,* Wisconsin, 5.3 oz | 510 | 25 | 51 |

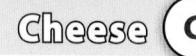
## Cheese & Cheese Products (Cont)

*Per 1 oz Unless Indicated*  C  F  Cb

**Cream Cheese:** *Average All Brands*

| | C | F | Cb |
|---|---|---|---|
| Regular/Soft: | | | |
| 2 Tbsp, 1 oz | 95 | 10 | 1 |
| 3 oz package | 290 | 29 | 3.5 |
| 8 oz package | 780 | 78 | 9 |
| Light, Plain, 1 oz | 60 | 4.5 | 2.5 |
| Fat-Free, Plain, 1 oz | 30 | 0 | 2 |
| **Easy Cheese** (Kraft), | | | |
| American, 2 Tbsp, 1.2 oz | 90 | 6 | 2 |
| **Edam**, 1 oz | 100 | 8 | 0.5 |
| **Farmer**, Low-Fat, 1 oz | 40 | 2.5 | 0 |
| **Feta:** Regular, 1 oz | 75 | 6 | 1 |
| Crumbled, ½ cup, 2.5 oz | 190 | 15 | 3 |
| *Athenos*, Reduced-Fat, | | | |
| 1 oz | 60 | 4 | 1 |
| **Fontina**, 2 Tbsp, 1 oz | 110 | 9 | 0.5 |
| **Galaxy,** Cheese Substitute: | | | |
| Grated Parmesan Flavor, 2 tsp, 0.2 oz | 15 | 0 | 0 |
| Rice, Mozzarella flavor, 1 sl., 0.6 oz | 40 | 2.5 | 0.5 |
| Veggy, all varieties, 1 slice, 0.5 oz | 40 | 2.5 | 0.5 |
| **Goat's Milk Cheese:** | | | |
| Chevre: Original, 2 Tbsp | 75 | 6 | 0.5 |
| Semi-Soft, 1 oz | 100 | 8.5 | 1 |
| Hard, 1 oz | 130 | 10 | 0.5 |
| *Chavrie:* Regular, 2 Tbsp, 1 oz | 50 | 3.5 | 1 |
| Caramelized Onion, 2 Tbsp | 50 | 3 | 4 |
| Logs, average all varieties, 1 oz | 80 | 7 | 3 |
| Gjetost, fresh, 1 oz | 130 | 8 | 12 |
| Myzithra, grated, 1 oz | 80 | 4 | 2 |
| **Gorgonzola**, 1 oz | 100 | 8 | 0.5 |
| **Galbani,** Dolcelatte, 1 oz | 95 | 8 | 1 |
| **Gouda**, 1 oz slice | 100 | 8 | 0.5 |
| **Gruyere**, 1 oz | 115 | 9 | 1 |
| **Handi-Snacks** (Kraft): | | | |
| Breadsticks 'n Cheez Single, 1 oz | 110 | 4.5 | 14 |
| Ritz Crackers 'n Cheez Dip, 1 oz | 100 | 6 | 11 |
| **Havarti** (Land O'Lakes), 0.8 oz | 80 | 7 | 0 |
| **Italian Pasta Blend** (Sargento), 1 oz | 90 | 6 | 3 |
| **Jarlsberg:** Average, 1 oz | 100 | 8 | 0 |
| Reduced Fat, shredded, 1 oz | 70 | 3.5 | 0 |
| **Labneh**, (Lebanese Cream Chse), 1.8 oz | 70 | 4 | 4 |

## Cheese & Cheese Products (Cont)

*Per 1 oz Unless Indicated*  C  F  Cb

| | C | F | Cb |
|---|---|---|---|
| **Laughing Cow,** Wedges: | | | |
| Original Creamy Swiss (1) | 50 | 4 | 1 |
| Light Varieties, av., (1) | 35 | 2 | 2 |
| **Lifetime,** Cholesterol Reducing, | | | |
| Low Fat, all varieties, 1 Slice, 1 oz | 45 | 1.5 | 1 |
| **Limburger**, 1 oz | 95 | 8 | 0 |
| **Mascarpone**, av., 1 oz | 125 | 13 | 0.5 |
| **Mexican:** | | | |
| *Cacique:* Asadero, sliced | 70 | 5 | 1 |
| Cotija | 100 | 8 | 0 |
| Enchilado; Manchego | 90 | 7 | 0 |
| Panela | 80 | 6 | 0 |
| Queso Fresco | 80 | 6 | 0 |
| Queso Quesadilla | 90 | 7 | 0 |
| Ranchero | 80 | 6 | 0 |
| *Chi-Chi's,* Salsa Con Quéso, Mild | 45 | 3 | 4 |
| *El Mexicano:* Asadero, Regular | 90 | 7 | 0 |
| Cotija, Regular | 110 | 9 | 0 |
| *Kraft,* Mexican Four Cheese; Taco, | | | |
| Shredded, | 100 | 8 | 1 |
| *Sargento,* 4 Cheese Mexican | 110 | 9 | 1 |
| *Supremo:* Quéso Chihuahua, 1 oz | 100 | 8 | 0 |
| Quéso Oaxaca | 80 | 5 | 1 |
| **Monterey Jack:** | | | |
| Regular, shredded, 1 oz | 100 | 8 | 1 |
| *Alpine Lace,* Co-Jack, 1 oz | 70 | 5 | 0 |
| *Kraft,* 1 oz | 100 | 8 | 1 |
| **Mozzarella:** | | | |
| Regular: Average 1 oz | 85 | 6.5 | 0.5 |
| *Land O'Lakes/Polly-O:* | | | |
| Slice, average, 1 oz | 90 | 6 | 1 |
| Shredded, 1 oz | 90 | 6 | 1 |
| Fat-Free, | | | |
| *Kraft,* Shredded, 1 oz | 45 | 0 | 1 |
| Light: | | | |
| *Kraft,* 2% Milk Fat, Reduced Fat | 70 | 5 | 1 |
| *Polly-O Lite,* Shredded, 1 oz | 60 | 2.5 | 1 |
| Part Skim: | | | |
| *Borden/Kraft,* Shredded | 80 | 5 | 2 |
| *Kraft,* String | 80 | 6 | 0 |
| **Muenster:** | | | |
| Regular, 1 oz | 105 | 9 | 0.5 |
| Low-Fat, 1 oz | 85 | 5 | 1 |

## Cheese & Cheese Products (Cont)

*Per 1 oz Unless Indicated*

| | C | F | Cb |
|---|---|---|---|
| **Parmesan:** | | | |
| Fresh/Block, Dry, 1 oz | 110 | 7.5 | 1 |
| Grated (Packaged): 1 Tbsp | 20 | 1.5 | 0 |
| 1 oz | 120 | 8 | 1 |
| ½ cup, 1.8 oz | 215 | 14 | 2 |
| *Kraft*, Reduced-Fat Topping, 1 Tbsp | 20 | 1 | 2 |
| ***Philadelphia:*** | | | |
| **Cream Cheese:** Original, 2 T. 1 oz | 100 | 9 | 1 |
| 3 oz package | 300 | 27 | 3 |
| Regular, 1 oz | 90 | 9 | 2 |
| **Creme,** Cooking, av. all var., ¼ cup | 110 | 9 | 4 |
| **Flavored:** | | | |
| Blueberry, 1 oz | 80 | 6 | 5 |
| Honey Nut; Strawberry, av., 1 oz | 80 | 7 | 5 |
| Garden Vegetable, 1 oz | 80 | 7 | 2 |
| Salmon, 1 oz | 70 | 7 | 1 |
| **Light,** Plain, 1 oz | 70 | 5 | 2 |
| **⅓ Less Fat:** Plain, 2 T., 1 oz | 70 | 6 | 2 |
| Garden Veggie; Chive & On., 1 oz | 70 | 5 | 2 |
| Neufchatel, 2 T., 1 oz | 70 | 6 | 1 |
| **Fat-Free,** Plain, 1 oz | 30 | 0 | 2 |
| **Indulgence:** | | | |
| Milk/White Chocolate: | | | |
| 1 Tbsp, 0.6 oz | 60 | 3.5 | 6 |
| Mini Tub, 1.3 oz | 125 | 7 | 13 |
| 8 oz container | 800 | 47 | 80 |
| Dark Chocolate, 1 T., 0.6 oz | 55 | 3.5 | 6 |
| **Spread:** Regular, 1 oz | 80 | 7 | 2 |
| Flavors, average, 1.2 oz | 80 | 6 | 5 |
| **Whipped:** | | | |
| Regular, 0.8 oz | 60 | 5 | 2 |
| Mixed Berry, 0.7 oz | 70 | 5 | 3 |
| **Pizza Four Cheese,** shredded, | | | |
| *Kraft/Sargento*, Regular, av., 1 oz | 90 | 7 | 1 |
| **Port de Salut,** 1 oz | 100 | 8 | 0 |
| **Port Wine** (*Kaukauna/WisPride*): | | | |
| 8 oz Tub: Average, 1 oz | 85 | 7 | 3 |
| Lite, 2 Tbsp, average, 1 oz | 60 | 3 | 5 |
| Ball, 1 oz | 100 | 6 | 4 |
| Log, 1 oz | 100 | 7 | 4 |
| **Provolone:** Regular, 1 oz | 100 | 7.5 | 0.5 |
| *Alpine Lace*, Reduced-Fat, 0.8 oz | 60 | 4.5 | 0 |
| *Sargento*, Deli Style 1 slice, 0.67 oz | 50 | 3 | 0 |
| **Pub** (*Rondele*), average all varieties | 75 | 7 | 1 |
| **Quark:** 40% fat | 45 | 3 | 1 |
| 20% fat | 30 | 1.5 | 1 |
| Skim/Non-Fat | 20 | 0 | 1.5 |
| **Queso:** | | | |
| *Anejo/Asadero/Blanco*, 1 oz | 105 | 9 | 1 |
| *Chichuahua/De Papa*, 1 oz | 110 | 9 | 2 |
| **Rice Cheese Chunks** (*Lisanatti*), | | | |
| average, 1 oz | 60 | 3 | 2 |
| **Swiss** (*Lifetime*), Fat Free, 1 oz | 40 | 0 | 1 |

## Cheese & Cheese Products (Cont)

*Per 1 oz Unless Indicated*

| | C | F | Cb |
|---|---|---|---|
| **Ricotta Cheese:** | | | |
| Whole Milk: 1 oz | 50 | 3.5 | 1 |
| ½ cup, 4.5 oz | 215 | 16 | 4 |
| Part Skim: 1 oz | 40 | 2 | 1.5 |
| ½ cup, 4.5 oz | 170 | 10 | 6 |
| Light/Low-Fat: 1 oz | 25 | 1 | 1.5 |
| ½ cup, 4.5 oz | 125 | 5 | 6 |
| Fat-Free, ½ cup, 4.5 oz | 100 | 0 | 10 |
| Baked Ricotta, 2 oz | 130 | 9 | 3 |
| **Romano:** Block/Loaf | 110 | 8 | 1 |
| Grated: 1 oz | 120 | 9 | 1 |
| 1 Tbsp, 0.2 oz | 20 | 1.5 | 0 |
| **Roquefort,** 1 oz | 105 | 9 | 0.5 |
| **Sheep's Milk,** (Manchego), | | | |
| *Trader Joes/Wegman's*, 1 oz | 120 | 10 | 0 |
| **Soy Cheese:** | | | |
| *Trader Joe's*, Cheddar flavor, 0.7 oz | 45 | 2 | 3 |
| *Soy Kaas:* Cheddar, 1 oz | 50 | 2 | 8 |
| Monterey Jack, 1 oz | 60 | 4 | 0 |
| *Soy Sation*, Chunks, | | | |
| all varieties, 1 oz | 60 | 3 | 2 |
| **Smoked Cheddar,** average, 1 oz | 110 | 10 | 0 |
| **Stilton,** average, 1 oz | 110 | 10 | 0 |
| **String:** | | | |
| Regular, average all brands | 80 | 6 | 0.5 |
| *Kraft*, Twist-Ums & String-ums, | | | |
| Super Long, 1 stick, 1.1 oz | 90 | 6 | 1 |
| Light/Lite: | | | |
| *Frigo*, String | 60 | 2.5 | 0.5 |
| *Polly-O*, String, | | | |
| 2% Red-Fat, 0.8 oz | 60 | 2.5 | 0 |
| *Sargento:* 1 piece, 0.8 oz | 50 | 2.5 | 1 |
| Part Skim, 0.9 oz | 70 | 4.5 | 1 |
| **Swiss:** Regular, 1 oz | 110 | 8 | 1.5 |
| *Alpine Lace*, Reduced-Fat, 0.8 oz | 70 | 4.5 | 1 |
| *Kraft Singles*, 2% Milk, 0.67 oz | 45 | 2.5 | 2 |
| **Tilsit,** 1 oz | 100 | 7.5 | 0.5 |
| **Tybo,** 1 oz | 100 | 7 | 0.5 |
| **Tofutti,** Better Than Cream Cheese, | | | |
| all varieties, 1 oz | 85 | 5 | 9 |
| **Velveeta** (*Kraft*): | | | |
| Original, 1 oz | 80 | 5 | 3 |
| Reduced Fat, 2% Milk, 1 oz | 60 | 3 | 4 |
| Extra Thick, 1.2 oz | 100 | 7 | 3 |
| Mexican: Hot, 1 oz | 90 | 6 | 3 |
| Mild, 1 oz | 80 | 6 | 3 |

## Dips/Spreads    **C** **F** **Cb**

*Per 2 Tbsp, 1 oz, Unless Indicated*

**Average All Brands**

| | C | F | Cb |
|---|---|---|---|
| Avocado/Guacamole | 45 | 4 | 2 |
| Baba Ghanoush (Eggplant/Sesame) | 70 | 6 | 2 |
| Cheese Fondue, ½ cup, 4 oz | 260 | 15 | 4 |
| French Onion Dip | 60 | 4.5 | 3 |
| Hummus: 2 Tbsp | 50 | 1 | 5 |
|    ½ cup, 4.5 oz | 220 | 4.5 | 23 |
| Tzatziki (Cucumber/Yogurt) | 30 | 2.5 | 2 |
| **Clearman's,** Original Spread | 150 | 16 | 0 |
| **De La Casa,** 5 Layer Party Dip | 45 | 2.5 | 4 |

**Fritos:** *Per 2 Tbsp*

**Dips:**

| | C | F | Cb |
|---|---|---|---|
|    Bean; Hot Bean w/ Jalap. | 35 | 1 | 5 |
|    French Onion | 60 | 5 | 3 |
|    Jalapeno Cheddar Cheese | 40 | 2.5 | 3 |

**Guiltless Gourmet,**

| | C | F | Cb |
|---|---|---|---|
|    Black Bean/Spicy Black Bean Dip | 40 | 0 | 7 |

**Heluva Good Cheese,**

| | C | F | Cb |
|---|---|---|---|
|    French Onion Dip, 2 Tbsp | 50 | 4.5 | 2 |

**Hidden Valley,**

| | C | F | Cb |
|---|---|---|---|
|    For Everything Topping, av. | 130 | 14 | 3 |

**Kaukauna** *(Wisconsin)*:
Spreadable Cheddar:

| | C | F | Cb |
|---|---|---|---|
|    Sharp/Smokey Cheddar | 80 | 6 | 3 |
|    Cheese Balls, all varieties | 100 | 6 | 4 |
|    Cheese Logs, all varieties | 100 | 7 | 4 |

**Kemps:** *Per 2 Tbsp*

**Dips:**

| | C | F | Cb |
|---|---|---|---|
|    French Onion | 60 | 5 | 2 |
|    Ranch Style | 60 | 5 | 2 |
|    Top The Tater, | | | |
|     Taco Fiesta; Veggie Ranch, av. | 60 | 5 | 3 |

**Kroger,** Dips, all varieties | 60 | 5 | 3

**Kraft:** *Per 2 Tbsp*

**Dips:**

| | C | F | Cb |
|---|---|---|---|
| Average all varieties | 60 | 5 | 3 |
|    Cheez Whiz: Orig., 1.2 oz | 90 | 7 | 4 |
|     Light | 80 | 3.5 | 6 |
|    Old English Spread, 2 Tbsp, 1.2 oz | 90 | 8 | 0 |
|    Salsa Con Queso | 90 | 7 | 4 |

**Spreads:** Olive & Pimento, 1.2 oz | 70 | 6 | 3

| | C | F | Cb |
|---|---|---|---|
|    Old English Sharp; Roka Blue, av | 85 | 8 | 2 |

**Marzetti:** *Per 2 Tbsp*

**Dips:**

| | C | F | Cb |
|---|---|---|---|
| Choc Fruit, 1.4 oz | 110 | 1 | 25 |
|    Caramel, fat free, 1.4 oz | 110 | 0 | 26 |
|    Veggie: Dill, Light, 1 oz | 60 | 5 | 4 |

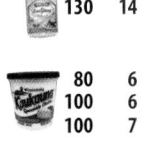

| | C | F | Cb |
|---|---|---|---|
|     Ranch, 1 oz | 110 | 12 | 2 |
|     Light Ranch, 1 oz | 60 | 5 | 4 |

## Dips/Spreads (Cont)    **C** **F** **Cb**

*Per 2 Tbsp, 1 oz, Unless Indicated*

**Marie's:**

| | C | F | Cb |
|---|---|---|---|
| **Dips:** Buttermilk Ranch; Crmy Dill. av. | 90 | 10 | 2 |
|    Guacamole | 40 | 3 | 3 |

**Naturally Fresh:** *Per 2 Tbsp*

| | C | F | Cb |
|---|---|---|---|
| **Dips:** Chocolate | 90 | 0 | 23 |
|    Cream Cheese Strawb. | 90 | 3 | 15 |
|    Caramel | 100 | 4 | 16 |

**Old Dutch:**

| | C | F | Cb |
|---|---|---|---|
| **Dips:** French Onion, 1 oz | 50 | 3 | 5 |
|    Mild Cheddar, 1 oz | 40 | 3 | 2 |
|    Nacho Cheese: 1 oz | 35 | 2.5 | 2 |
|     Microwave variety ,1 oz | 80 | 6 | 3 |

**Old El Paso:** *Per 2 Tbsp*

| | C | F | Cb |
|---|---|---|---|
| **Dips:** Cheese & Salsa, 1.2 oz | 40 | 3 | 3 |
|    Thick N' Chunky Salsa | 10 | 0 | 2 |

**Price's:** *Per 2 Tbsp*

| | C | F | Cb |
|---|---|---|---|
| **Dips:** Pimiento Cheese | 90 | 7 | 4 |
|    Light Pimiento | 50 | 3 | 3 |
|    Zesty Jalapeno | 80 | 7 | 3 |

**Stop & Shop:** *Per 2 Tbsp*

| | C | F | Cb |
|---|---|---|---|
| **Dips:** Veggie | 100 | 10 | 3 |
|    Sour Cream French Onion | 60 | 4.5 | 2 |

**TGI Fridays,**

| | C | F | Cb |
|---|---|---|---|
|    Spinach, Cheese & Artichoke Dip, 1 oz | 30 | 2 | 2 |

**Toby's,** Orig. Tofu Spread, 2 Tbsp | 80 | 8 | 2

**Tostitos:**

| | C | F | Cb |
|---|---|---|---|
| **Dips:** Bean Dip, 1 oz | 35 | 1 | 5 |
|    French Onion, 2Tbsp | 60 | 5 | 3 |
|    Mild Cheddar, 2 Tbsp | 40 | 3 | 3 |

**Wise:** *Per 2 Tbsp*

| | C | F | Cb |
|---|---|---|---|
| **Dips:** French Onion, 1.2 oz | 60 | 5 | 3 |
|    Spinach, 1.2 oz | 50 | 4 | 3 |

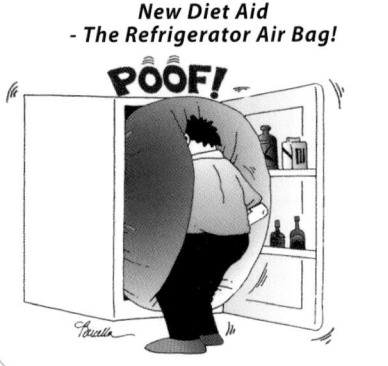

*New Diet Aid - The Refrigerator Air Bag!*

POOF!

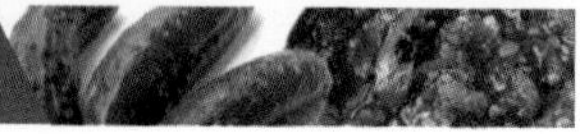

# C  Condiments ◆ Salsa

## Condiments, Sauces    C   F   Cb

### Average of Brands & Homemade

| | C | F | Cb |
|---|---|---|---|
| **Apple Sauce:** | | | |
| Sweetened, ¼ cup, 2.5 oz | 55 | 0 | 13 |
| Unsweetened, ¼ cup, 2 oz | 25 | 0 | 7 |
| **Barbecue Sauce:** | | | |
| Regular, av. all flavors, 2 Tbsp, 1 oz | 40 | 0 | 10 |
| *Bull's Eye*, Original, 1 oz | 60 | 0 | 14 |
| **Bearnaise Sauce**, ¼ cup, 2.5 oz | 190 | 19 | 5 |
| **Buffalo Wing Sce:** Hon. Mustard, 1 T. | 40 | 3 | 3 |
| Average other varieties, 1 Tbsp | 25 | 2 | 2 |
| **Cheese**, h/made, ¼ cup, 2.5 oz | 150 | 10 | 12 |
| **Chef-Mate**, Hot Dog, ¼ cup | 70 | 2.5 | 9 |
| **Chili Sauce** *(Heinz)*, 1 Tbsp | 20 | 0 | 5 |
| **Cocktail Sauce:** ¼ cup | 110 | 0 | 15 |
| *Walden Farms*, Fat-Free, 1 Tbsp | 0 | 0 | 0 |
| **Cranberry Sauce**, av. all varieties: 2 T. | 45 | 0 | 11 |
| ¼ cup, 2.5 oz | 110 | 0 | 27 |
| **Demi Glaze Gold**, 2 tsp | 30 | 0.5 | 3 |
| **Honey Mustard** *(French's)*, 2 Tbsp | 60 | 0.5 | 12 |
| **Horseradish:** 1 tsp | 2 | 0 | 0 |
| *Kraft*, 1 tsp | 15 | 1.5 | 1 |
| **Ketchup:** Regular, 1 Tbsp | 15 | 0 | 4 |
| *Heinz:* Reduced Sugar, 1 Tbsp | 5 | 0 | 1 |
| Simply Heinz, 1 Tbsp | 20 | 0 | 5 |
| **Mole:** | | | |
| *Dona Maria*, av. all varieties., 2 T. | 150 | 10 | 10 |
| *Rogelio Bueno*, 2 Tbsp, 1 oz | 160 | 11 | 12 |
| **Mushroom Sce**, ½ cup, 2 oz | 50 | 2 | 5 |
| **Mustard**, average, 1 tsp | 5 | 0 | 0.5 |
| **Pesto Sauce**, ¼ cup, 2 oz | 270 | 28 | 2 |
| **Pizza Sauce**, ¼ cup, 2 oz | 30 | 0 | 6 |
| **Seafood Cocktail Sce**, ¼ cup | 60 | 0 | 15 |
| **Soy Sauce:** Average all, 1 Tbsp | 10 | 0 | 1 |
| *Kikkoman*, Lite Soy, 1 Tbsp | 10 | 0 | 1 |
| **Spaghetti Sce**, ½ cup, 4.5 oz | 135 | 6 | 19 |
| **Steak Sauce:** | | | |
| *Kraft*, A1, 1 Tbsp, 0.5 oz | 15 | 0 | 3 |
| *Lea & Perrins*, 1 Tbsp, 0.5 oz | 20 | 0 | 5 |
| **Strawb. Puree Sauce**, Unsweet., 2 T. | 10 | 0 | 2 |
| **Sweet & Sour Sauce:** | | | |
| *Contadina*, 1.2 oz | 40 | 1 | 8 |
| *Kraft*, 1 Tbsp | 60 | 0 | 13 |
| **Tabasco Sauce**, 1 tsp | 2 | 0 | 0 |
| **Taco Sauce**, average all, 2 Tbsp, 1 oz | 10 | 0 | 1 |
| **Tartar Sauce:** *(Heinz)*, 2 Tbsp, 1 oz | 120 | 11 | 4 |
| *Hellmann's*, Regular, 2 Tbsp, 1 oz | 80 | 7 | 4 |
| *McCormick*, Fat-Free, 2 Tbsp, 1 oz | 30 | 0 | 7 |
| **Teriyaki Sauce** *(Kikkoman)*, 1 T., 0.5 oz | 15 | 0 | 2 |
| **Vinegar**, White or Wine, 2 T. | 4 | 0 | 1 |
| **White Sauce**, ½ cup, 5 oz | 130 | 7 | 10 |
| **Worcestershire Sauce**, 1 tsp | 5 | 0 | 1 |

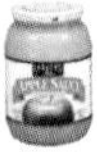

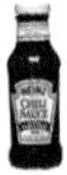

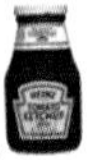

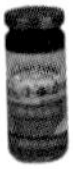

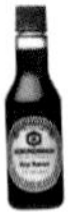

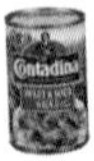

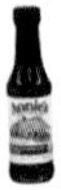

## Pickles & Relish    C   F   Cb

### Average All Brands

| | C | F | Cb |
|---|---|---|---|
| **Bread & Butter Pickles**, 4 sl.,1 oz | 25 | 0 | 6 |
| **Chutney**, 2 Tbsp, 1.25 oz | 50 | 0.5 | 11 |
| **Dill Pickles:** | | | |
| Slices, 4 slices, 1 oz | 4 | 0 | 1 |
| 1 large, (3¾"x 1¼" diam.), 2.25 oz | 12 | 0 | 3 |
| Extra large (4"x 1¾" diam.), 5 oz | 30 | 0 | 6 |
| Halves: Small, 1 oz | 3 | 0 | 0.5 |
| Large, 2.5 oz | 8 | 0 | 2 |
| **Gherkins**, sweet, 1 medium, 1 oz | 30 | 0 | 7 |
| **Green Chiles**, chopped, 2 Tbsp | 5 | 0 | 1 |
| **Horseradish**, 1 Tbsp | 10 | 0 | 2 |
| **Jalapenos**, pickled (2), 2 oz | 10 | 0.5 | 2 |
| **Jalapeno Relish**, 1 Tbsp, 0.5 oz | 5 | 0 | 1 |
| **Mustard**, av. all brands, 1 tsp | 5 | 0 | 0.5 |
| **Peppers**, Hot/Mild (1), 1.5 oz | 20 | 0 | 4 |
| **Pickled:** Beets, ½ cup, 4 oz | 75 | 0 | 19 |
| Cocktail Onion, 1 onion | 2 | 0 | 0 |
| Red Cabbage, ½ cup, 3 oz | 65 | 0 | 15 |
| **Pickles:** Sweet, 2 Tbsp, 1 oz | 35 | 0 | 8 |
| Large (3"x ¾ diam.),1.25 oz | 40 | 0 | 10 |
| Pickle in a Pouch, 1 large | 12 | 0 | 3 |
| **Relishes:** | | | |
| Cranberry-Orange, 1 Tbsp | 30 | 0 | 7 |
| Hot Dog *(Heinz)*, 1 T., 0.5 oz | 17 | 0 | 3 |
| S'wich Spread, 1 tsp | 20 | 1 | 5 |
| Sweet Pickle, 1 Tbsp, 0.5 oz | 20 | 0 | 5 |
| Sweet Cauliflower, 1 oz | 35 | 0 | 8 |
| Sugar Free Relish, 1 tsp | 5 | 0 | 1 |
| Sweet Gherkins (2), 1 oz | 5 | 0 | 1 |
| **Sauerkraut,** | | | |
| Drained, 1 cup, 5 oz | 25 | 0 | 6 |

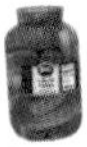

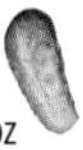

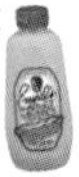

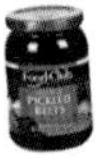

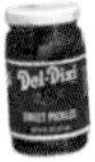

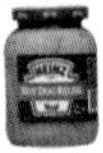

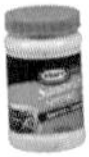

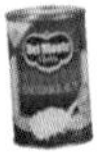

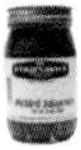

## Salsa

### Average all Types:

| | C | F | Cb |
|---|---|---|---|
| Regular, w/out oil, 2 T., 1 oz | 15 | 0 | 3.5 |
| Made with oil, 2 Tbsp, 1 oz | 40 | 3 | 8 |
| **La Victoria**, 2 Tbsp, 1 oz | 10 | 0 | 2 |
| **Old El Paso**, 1 Tbsp, 1 oz | 10 | 0 | 3 |
| **TGI Friday's**, 1.2 oz | 15 | 0 | 4 |

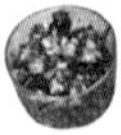

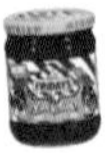

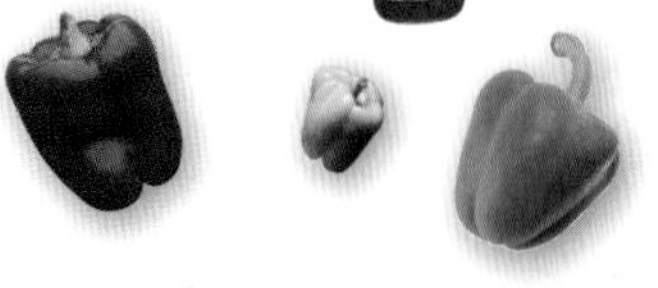

### Quick Guide  **C** **F** **Cb**

#### Cookies:
**Average All Brands:** *Per Cookie*

| | | C | F | Cb |
|---|---|---|---|---|
| **Biscotti:** Small, 0.5 oz | | 70 | 3 | 10 |
| Regular, 1 oz | | 140 | 6.5 | 18 |
| **Chocolate Chip:** | | | | |
| Small/Thin, 0.5 oz | | 70 | 3.5 | 9 |
| Regular, 1 oz | | 140 | 7 | 18 |
| Large (*Mrs Fields*), 3 oz | | 350 | 17 | 45 |
| Extra Large, 4 oz | | 555 | 28 | 73 |
| **Oatmeal/Oatmeal Raisin:** | | | | |
| Small/Thin, 0.5 oz | | 65 | 2.5 | 10 |
| Regular, 1 oz | | 130 | 5 | 20 |
| Large (*Mrs Fields*), 2.5 oz | | 330 | 14 | 44 |
| Extra Large, 4 oz | | 510 | 20 | 78 |
| **Peanut Butter:** | | | | |
| Small/Thin, 0.5 oz | | 70 | 3.5 | 9 |
| Regular, 1 oz | | 135 | 7 | 17 |
| Large (*Mrs Fields*), 2.5 oz | | 330 | 17 | 41 |
| Extra Large, 4 oz | | 540 | 27 | 67 |
| **Low-Fat Cookies:** | | | | |
| Choc Chip (Low-Fat), (1), 0.5 oz | | 65 | 2 | 10 |
| Oatmeal Raisin (Fat-Free), (1), 1 oz | | 95 | 0.5 | 22 |
| Peanut Butter (Low-Fat), (1), 1 oz | | 105 | 5 | 15 |

### Quick Guide

#### Crackers
**Average All Brands:** *Per Cracker Unless Indicated*

| | C | F | Cb |
|---|---|---|---|
| **Cheese Crackers:** | | | |
| Plain: 1" square | 5 | 0 | 0.5 |
| Bag, single serving, 1 oz | 140 | 7 | 16 |
| Cheese/P'nut Butter filled | 30 | 1.5 | 4 |
| **Crispbread**, Rye | 35 | 0 | 8 |
| **Grahams**, 2½" square | 30 | 0.5 | 5 |
| **Melba Toast**, Plain, 1 piece | 20 | 0 | 4 |
| **Matzo**, Plain, 1 oz | 110 | 0.5 | 23 |
| **Oyster/Soup**, ½ cup | 95 | 2 | 17 |
| **Rice:** 1 crackers | 70 | 1.5 | 11 |
| Oriental Style, 1 oz | 130 | 3.5 | 23 |
| **Saltines**, 5 crackers | 65 | 2 | 11 |
| **Snack-type**, 1 round cracker | 15 | 1 | 2 |
| **Soda Crackers** (*Saltine*), 2 | 25 | 1 | 4.5 |
| **Water Cracker** (*Carr's*), Original | 15 | 0.5 | 2.5 |
| **Wheat:** | | | |
| Wheat Thins | 10 | 0.5 | 1.5 |
| Cheese/Peanut Butter filled | 35 | 2 | 4 |

### Cookies & Crackers ~ Brands

*Per Cookie/Cracker, Unless indicated*  **C** **F** **Cb**

| | C | F | Cb |
|---|---|---|---|
| **Albertsons:** | | | |
| Animal Crackers (6), 1 oz | 130 | 3.5 | 22 |
| **Chocolate Chip:** | | | |
| Original (3), 1 oz | 150 | 7 | 20 |
| Chewy (2), 1 oz | 130 | 6 | 18 |
| Chunky (1), 0.5 oz | 80 | 3.5 | 10 |
| **Chocolate S'wich Cremes:** (3) 1 oz | 150 | 6 | 25 |
| Double Filled (2), 1 oz | 140 | 6 | 22 |
| Fudge Graham (3), 1 oz | 140 | 7 | 18 |
| Fudge Wafer (3), 1 oz | 140 | 8 | 18 |
| Fudge Marshmallow Ring | 120 | 5 | 19 |
| Pinwheels, Chocolate Marshmallow | 120 | 5 | 20 |
| Vanilla Wafers (9), 1 oz | 140 | 4 | 25 |
| **Graham:** Cinnamon (2) | 150 | 3 | 28 |
| Honey (2), 1 oz | 140 | 2 | 28 |
| **Annie's:** | | | |
| **Bunny Grahams:** | | | |
| Chocolate; Choc Chip, 1 oz | 130 | 4.5 | 21 |
| Cinnamon; Honey, 1 oz | 140 | 4.5 | 23 |
| Friends, 1 oz | 130 | 4.5 | 22 |
| Gluten Free: Cocoa & Vanilla, 1 oz | 120 | 3.5 | 22 |
| SnickerDoodles, 1 oz | 130 | 4 | 21 |
| **Cheddar Bunnies:** | | | |
| Regular: | | | |
| 1 oz Snack Pack | 130 | 6 | 18 |
| 7.5 oz Box | 1050 | 45 | 145 |
| Extra Cheesy, 1 oz | 150 | 7 | 18 |
| White Cheddar; Whole Wheat, 1 oz | 150 | 7 | 19 |
| **Arnott's:** Original Tim Tams (2) | 190 | 10 | 24 |
| Pack of 0 cookies | 950 | 50 | 120 |
| **Austin:** | | | |
| **Sandwich Crackers:** *Per Package* | | | |
| Cheese: with Cheddar Cheese | 190 | 10 | 23 |
| with Peanut Butter | 190 | 10 | 23 |
| Grilled Cheese, 1.4 oz | 190 | 9 | 24 |
| Toasty, with Peanut Butter | 190 | 9 | 23 |
| Zoo Animals (16), 1 oz | 130 | 2 | 25 |
| **Barbara's Bakery:** | | | |
| **Fig Bars:** Raspberry, 1.4 oz | 120 | 0 | 27 |
| Wheat/Multigrain | 110 | 0.5 | 26 |
| **Snackimals:** | | | |
| Choc Chip, 1 oz | 120 | 4 | 19 |
| Double Chocolate, 1 oz | 140 | 4.5 | 23 |
| Vanilla, 1 oz | 110 | 4 | 17 |
| **Bear Naked:** | | | |
| **Soft-Baked Granola,** | | | |
| Double Choc.; Fruit & Nut, av. | 130 | 6 | 19 |

## Cookies & Crackers ~ Brands (Cont)

*Per Cookie/Cracker, Unless Indicated* **C** **F** **Cb**

**BelVita** *(Nabisco):*

**Breakfast Biscuits:**

| | C | F | Cb |
|---|---|---|---|
| Crunchy, 1 pack (4 biscuits), average | 230 | 8 | 36 |
| Soft Baked, 1 biscuit, average | 190 | 7 | 32 |
| **Bites**, (46), 1.8 oz | 230 | 8 | 36 |

**Blue Diamond:**

| | C | F | Cb |
|---|---|---|---|
| **Artisan Nut Thins** , (13), av. all var. | 130 | 3.5 | 22 |
| **Nut Thins**, (17), average all varieties | 130 | 3 | 23 |

**Brent & Sam's:**

**Natural:** *Per 2 Cookies*

| | C | F | Cb |
|---|---|---|---|
| Chocolate Chip Pecan | 130 | 7 | 14 |
| Key Lime White Chocolate | 120 | 6 | 16 |
| Triple Chocolate Bliss, 1 oz | 120 | 6 | 16 |

**Soft & Chewy:** *Per 1 Cookie*

| | C | F | Cb |
|---|---|---|---|
| Choc Chunk | 130 | 5 | 20 |
| Oatmeal Raisin | 140 | 6 | 20 |
| Snickerdoodle | 130 | 4 | 21 |

| | C | F | Cb |
|---|---|---|---|
| **Carr's:** Rstd Garlic & Herbs (4) | 50 | 1 | 10 |
| Rosemary Crackers(4) | 70 | 2.5 | 11 |
| Whole Wheat Crackers (2) | 80 | 3.5 | 11 |

**Cheez•It** ~ *See Sunshine, Page 87*

**Chips Ahoy!** ~ *See Nabisco, Page 85*

**Country Choice:**

**Sandwich Cremes,**

| | C | F | Cb |
|---|---|---|---|
| all varieties, 2 pieces | 130 | 5 | 19 |

**Snacking:**

| | C | F | Cb |
|---|---|---|---|
| Ginger Snaps (5); Vanilla Wafers (7) | 140 | 5 | 22 |
| Iced Oatmeal (4) | 120 | 4 | 21 |

**Dr. Kracker:**

| | C | F | Cb |
|---|---|---|---|
| **Crispbread:** Klassic 3 Seed (1) | 100 | 4 | 15 |
| Pumpkin Seed Cheddar (1) | 110 | 5 | 15 |
| **Snackers**, Pumpkin Seed Cheddar (8) | 125 | 5 | 13 |

**Erin Baker's:**

**Original Breakfast:** *Per 3 oz*

| | C | F | Cb |
|---|---|---|---|
| Banana Walnut | 300 | 8 | 53 |
| Peanut Butter | 320 | 11 | 48 |

**Minis:** *Per 1 oz Cookie*

| | C | F | Cb |
|---|---|---|---|
| Peanut Butter | 100 | 3.5 | 16 |
| Dble Chocolate; Oatmeal Raisin, av. | 100 | 2.5 | 18 |

**Famous Amos:**

**Bite Size:** Choc. Chip,

| | C | F | Cb |
|---|---|---|---|
| 4 Cookies, 1 oz | 150 | 7 | 20 |
| Choc. Chip & Pecans (4) | 150 | 8 | 18 |
| Sandwich, Creme Filled, | | | |
| Choc.; Vanilla, 3 cookies, 1 oz | 170 | 7 | 25 |

*Per Cookie/Cracker, Unless Indicated* **C** **F** **Cb**

**Fig Newtons** ~ *See Nabisco, Page 85*

**Fifty50:**

| | C | F | Cb |
|---|---|---|---|
| **Butter**, (4) | 190 | 9 | 24 |
| **Average other varieties**, (4) | 165 | 9 | 22 |
| **Wafers**, average all varieties, (6) | 160 | 9 | 22 |

**Gamesa:**

| | C | F | Cb |
|---|---|---|---|
| **Animalitos**, 14 cookies, 1 oz | 110 | 1 | 25 |
| **Arcoiris Marshmallow**, | | | |
| 2 oz pkg, 6 cookies | 220 | 5 | 38 |
| **Chocolatines Marshmallow**, | | | |
| 2 cookies, 1 oz | 130 | 5 | 18 |
| **Chokis**, Chocolate Chip, 1.4 oz pkg | 190 | 9 | 27 |
| **Emperador:** Cream Cookie Sandwich | | | |
| Lemon Creme, 1 pkg, 6 cookies | 270 | 8 | 45 |
| Av. other flavors, 1 pkg, 6 cookies | 360 | 12 | 57 |
| **Fruitbars**, average, 1 cookie, 1 oz | 110 | 4.5 | 18 |
| **Giro**, 3 cookies, 1 oz | 140 | 6 | 20 |
| **Mamut**, Choc Marshmallow, | | | |
| 1 cookie, 1 oz | 130 | 5 | 19 |
| **Marias**, 8 cookies, 1 oz | 120 | 2 | 24 |
| **Sugar Wafers**, (3), average, 1.2 oz | 160 | 7 | 25 |

**Girl Scouts Cookies:**

| | C | F | Cb |
|---|---|---|---|
| **Caramel DeLites/Samoas**, (2) | 130 | 6 | 19 |
| **Do-si-dos**, (3) | 160 | 7 | 22 |
| **Peanut Butter Patties**, (2) | 130 | 8 | 14 |
| **Savannah Smiles**, (5) | 140 | 5 | 23 |

**Goya:**

| | C | F | Cb |
|---|---|---|---|
| **Lady Fingers** , 3 cookies | 65 | 0.5 | 13 |
| **Maria**, 5 cookies, 1 oz | 130 | 3 | 24 |
| **Wafers**, average all flavors, | | | |
| 4 wafers, 1 oz | 150 | 7 | 20 |

**Grandma's:**

**Homestyle:** *Per Cookie*

| | C | F | Cb |
|---|---|---|---|
| Chocolate Brownie | 190 | 8 | 27 |
| Chocolate Chip | 200 | 10 | 25 |
| Oatmeal Raisin | 180 | 7 | 26 |
| Peanut Butter | 190 | 10 | 22 |

**Sandwich Cremes:**

| | C | F | Cb |
|---|---|---|---|
| Peanut Butter (5) | 200 | 9 | 25 |
| Vanilla (5) | 190 | 9 | 27 |
| Mini's, Vanilla Flavored (9) | 150 | 7 | 22 |

### Cookies & Crackers ~ Brands (Cont)

*Per Cookie/Cracker, Unless Indicated* **C** **F** **Cb**

**Great American Cookies:**

| | C | F | Cb |
|---|---|---|---|
| Chewy Choc. Supreme | 200 | 9 | 29 |
| Chewy Pecan Supreme | 230 | 12 | 31 |
| Double Fudge with Reese's | 230 | 11 | 33 |
| Original, w/ Reese's or M&M's | 240 | 12 | 31 |
| Peanut Butter w/ M&M's | 250 | 14 | 29 |
| White Chunk Macadamia | 250 | 14 | 30 |
| **Double Doozies:** | | | |
| Original, 5.3 oz | 690 | 34 | 94 |
| M&M Big Bite, 2.5 oz | 340 | 17 | 46 |
| **Cookie Cakes:** | | | |
| 16", 3.5 oz | 460 | 22 | 67 |
| 16" M&M, 4 oz | 500 | 24 | 73 |
| Heart Shaped, 3.5 oz | 440 | 21 | 64 |

**Great Value** *(Walmart): Per Cookie Unless Indicated*

| | C | F | Cb |
|---|---|---|---|
| Caramel Coconut Fudge | 130 | 6 | 18 |
| Chocolate Chip: Chewy | 120 | 5 | 17 |
| Chunky | 150 | 7 | 21 |
| Classic | 160 | 7 | 23 |
| Dble Filled Switch Aroos, | | | |
| Choc. & Vanilla | 150 | 6 | 21 |
| Fudge Marshmallow | 120 | 5 | 19 |
| Oatmeal Cream Pie | 170 | 8 | 24 |
| Pecan Shortbread, 2 cookies | 150 | 8 | 17 |
| Soft Cookies, Fudge & Cream | 150 | 6 | 22 |
| Twist & Shout, Chocolate; Vanilla | 160 | 6 | 25 |
| **Crackers:** | | | |
| Buttery Rounds: Baked, (5) | 80 | 4.5 | 10 |
| Reduced Fat, (5) | 70 | 2 | 11 |
| Cheese Crackers, 1 oz | 150 | 8 | 18 |

**Joseph's:**

**Sugar Free:** *Per 4 Cookies*

| | C | F | Cb |
|---|---|---|---|
| Almond; Chocolate Walnut, average | 95 | 4 | 14 |
| Chocolate Chip; Pecan Choc. Chip, av. | 95 | 5 | 14 |
| Average other varieties | 95 | 4 | 15 |

*Note: Carb figures include 6 grams Maltitol*

**Kashi:** *Per Cookie*

| | C | F | Cb |
|---|---|---|---|
| Chocolate Almond Butter | 130 | 5 | 19 |
| Oatmeal: Dark Chocolate | 130 | 5 | 20 |
| Raisin Flax | 120 | 4.5 | 20 |
| **Crackers:** | | | |
| Original 7 Grain ,(15) | 120 | 3.5 | 20 |
| Fire Roasted Veggie, (15) | 120 | 3.5 | 20 |
| **Pita Crisps:** | | | |
| Original 7 Grain with Salt (10), 1 oz | 110 | 2.5 | 21 |
| Garlic Pesto (10), 1 oz | 110 | 2.5 | 21 |

*Per Cookie/Cracker, Unless Indicated* **C** **F** **Cb**

**Keebler:**

**Animals:**

| | C | F | Cb |
|---|---|---|---|
| Crackers: 8 Crackers, 1 oz | 130 | 4 | 22 |
| Variety Pak, 1.4 oz | 180 | 6 | 30 |
| Frosted Cookies: 7 pcs, 1 oz | 145 | 6.5 | 20 |
| Variety Pak, 1.4 oz | 200 | 10 | 28 |
| Iced Cookies: 6pcs, 1 oz | 130 | 4 | 20 |
| Variety Pak, 1.4 oz | 180 | 6 | 30 |
| **Chips Deluxe:** Original (2) | 160 | 8 | 19 |
| Chocolate Lovers (2) | 170 | 9 | 20 |
| Coconut (2) | 160 | 9 | 18 |
| Peanut Butter Cups (2) | 170 | 9 | 19 |
| Soft & Chewy (2) | 140 | 6 | 21 |
| **Rainbow:** | | | |
| Triple Choc. Chip wih M&M's (2) | 160 | 8 | 20 |
| Choc Chip Minis, with M&M's, | | | |
| 5 cookies, 1 oz | 140 | 7 | 19 |
| Danish Wedding, (4) | 140 | 7 | 19 |
| **E.L. Fudge:** Original (2) | 180 | 7 | 25 |
| Double Stuffed (2) | 180 | 9 | 24 |
| **Fudge Shoppe:** | | | |
| Deluxe Grahams (3) | 140 | 7 | 18 |
| **Fudge Sticks:** | | | |
| Original (3) | 150 | 8 | 20 |
| Jumbo (1) | 160 | 8 | 21 |
| Jumbo Peanut Butter (1) | 170 | 9 | 19 |
| **Fudge Stripes:** | | | |
| Original (2) | 140 | 6 | 19 |
| Mini Original, 1.4 oz pkg | 200 | 9 | 27 |
| Dark Chocolate (3) | 150 | 7 | 22 |
| Grasshopper (4) | 140 | 7 | 20 |
| S'mores Peanut Butter (1) | 130 | 6 | 17 |
| Gripz, Chips Deluxe, 0.9 oz pouch | 120 | 5 | 18 |
| Oatmeal, (2), average all varieties | 140 | 6 | 20 |
| **Sandies Cookies:** | | | |
| Dark Choc. Almond; Pecan Shtbrd, av. | 170 | 10 | 19 |
| Pecan Shortbread (2) | 170 | 10 | 18 |
| **Vienna Fingers:** | | | |
| Creme Filled (2) | 150 | 6 | 23 |
| Reduced Fat (2) | 140 | 4.5 | 24 |
| **Wafers:** Vanilla (8) | 140 | 5 | 22 |
| Mini Vanilla (18) | 140 | 5 | 22 |

*continued next page...*

## Cookies & Crackers ~ Brands (Cont)

*Per Cookie/Cracker, Unless Indicated* **C F Cb**

**Keebler (Cont):**

**Crackers:**

| | C | F | Cb |
|---|---|---|---|
| **Club:** Original (4) | 70 | 3 | 9 |
| Reduced Fat (5) | 70 | 2 | 12 |
| **Grahams:** Original (8) | 120 | 3.5 | 22 |
| Honey (8) | 140 | 4.5 | 23 |
| **Town House:** Original (5) | 90 | 5 | 9 |
| Reduced Fat (6) | 60 | 1.5 | 12 |
| **Kraft,** Macaroni & Cheese Crackers, | | | |
| av. all varieties, 1. oz | 150 | 7 | 18 |
| **Kroger:** | | | |
| **Chip Mates:** Orig. (3), 1.5 oz | 150 | 7 | 22 |
| Chunky (2), 1 oz | 120 | 6 | 17 |
| Peanut Butter (2), 1 oz | 120 | 7 | 15 |
| White Chip (2), 1 oz | 120 | 6 | 16 |
| **Chocolate Sandwich:** | | | |
| Original (3), 1.2 oz | 150 | 6 | 24 |
| Double Filled (2), 1 oz | 140 | 6 | 22 |
| Olde Southern Pecan Shortbread (2) | 150 | 9 | 16 |
| Vanilla Wafers (7) | 130 | 3.5 | 23 |
| **Crackers:** | | | |
| **Grahams,** Orig.; Honey, (4) | 120 | 3 | 20 |
| **Saltines,** Original (5), 0.5oz | 60 | 1.5 | 10 |
| **Lance:** | | | |
| **6 Pack:** *Per Pack of 6 Cookies* | | | |
| Choc-O-Lunch/Van-O-Lunch, av. | 225 | 9 | 34 |
| Nekot, Peanut Butter | 240 | 11 | 32 |
| **Crackers:** | | | |
| **Cracker Sandwiches:** *Per 6 Crackers* | | | |
| Malt, with Peanut Butter Filling | 180 | 8 | 20 |
| Nip Chee, Cheddar Cheese | 190 | 9 | 24 |
| Toastchee, | | | |
| Peanut Butter | 210 | 10 | 25 |
| Toasty, Peanut Butter | 210 | 10 | 25 |
| Wholegrain, Cheddar Cheese | 200 | 9 | 26 |
| **Little Debbie:** | | | |
| Apple Oatmeal Pies (1) | 140 | 4.5 | 24 |
| Chocolate Chip Cream Pie (1) | 150 | 6 | 23 |
| Cookie Wreaths (1) | 100 | 5 | 12 |
| Marshmallow Puffs | 150 | 5 | 25 |
| Oatmeal Creme Pie (1) | 170 | 7 | 26 |
| Star Crunch(1) | 150 | 6 | 22 |

**Lu:**

| | C | F | Cb |
|---|---|---|---|
| Petit Beurre (1), 1.2 oz | 140 | 4 | 24 |
| Petit Ecolier, av. all var., (1), 0.9 oz | 130 | 6 | 17 |
| Pim's, Raspberry (1), 0.9 oz | 100 | 3 | 16 |
| **Manischewitz:** | | | |
| **Crackers:** | | | |
| **Tam Tams:** Original (10) | 120 | 4.5 | 17 |
| Everything; Garlic (1), av. | 140 | 5 | 19 |
| **Mary's Gone Crackers:** | | | |
| Chocolate Chip (2) | 130 | 6 | 19 |
| Ginger Snaps (3) | 140 | 5 | 23 |
| **Crackers:** | | | |
| Super Seed varieties (12) | 150 | 7 | 18 |
| Other varieties (13) | 140 | 5 | 21 |
| **Miss Meringue:** | | | |
| **Madeleines:** | | | |
| Traditional (2), 1.2 oz | 160 | 9 | 19 |
| Traditional & Dipped (2), 1.2 oz | 160 | 9 | 18 |
| **Meringue Classiques:** | | | |
| Cappuccino (4), 1 oz | 110 | 0 | 26 |
| Mint Choc. Chip (4), 1 oz | 120 | 1.5 | 25 |
| Triple Chocolate (4), 1 oz | 120 | 1.5 | 25 |
| Vanilla Rainbow/Van. (4), 1 oz | 110 | 0 | 27 |
| **Meringue Minis,** Low Fat: | | | |
| Mini: Choc. Chip (12), 1 oz | 130 | 1.5 | 26 |
| Mint Choc. Chip (12), 1 oz | 120 | 1.5 | 26 |
| **Meringue Minis,** Fat Free: | | | |
| Chocolate (12), 1 oz | 110 | 0 | 26 |
| Vanilla; Rainbow Vanilla (13), 1 oz | 110 | 0 | 27 |
| **Mother's:** | | | |
| **Chocolate Chip,** (4), 1 oz | 150 | 7 | 20 |
| **Circus Animal,** (7), 1 oz | 150 | 7 | 21 |
| **Coconut Cocadas,** (5), 1.2 oz | 160 | 8 | 21 |
| **Double Fudge,** (2), 1.3 oz | 190 | 8 | 27 |
| **Iced Oatmeal,** (4), 1.2 oz | 150 | 6 | 23 |
| **Peanut Butter Gauchos,** (2), 1.3 oz | 190 | 9 | 26 |
| **Taffy; Vanilla Cream,** (2), av., 1.3 oz | 195 | 9 | 27 |

**Mrs Fields Cookies** ~ See Page 219

## Cookies & Crackers ~ Brands (Cont)

*Per Cookie/Cracker, Unless Indicated* **C** **F** **Cb**

**Nabisco Cookies:**

**Chips Ahoy!,** Chocolate Chip:

| | C | F | Cb |
|---|---|---|---|
| 100 Calorie Pack, Thin Crisps, Baked, (6), 0.8 oz | 100 | 3 | 18 |
| Original: | | | |
| 2 cookies, 1.1 oz | 160 | 8 | 22 |
| Single Serve, 1.4 oz | 190 | 9 | 27 |
| Mini Choc. Chips: 1.1 oz | 150 | 7 | 21 |
| 3 oz Package | 450 | 21 | 63 |
| Go-Pak, 3.5 oz | 525 | 25 | 74 |
| Reduced Fat (2), 1.2 oz | 150 | 6 | 24 |
| Candy Blasts (2),1.2 oz | 180 | 9 | 22 |
| Chewy: Regular (2), 1.1 oz | 140 | 6 | 21 |
| Chewy (2), 1.1 oz | 150 | 7 | 21 |
| Chunky, Choc. Chunk (2), 1.2 oz | 160 | 8 | 20 |
| Made with Reeses PB Cups, 1.1 oz | 160 | 9 | 18 |

**Lorna Doone:**

| | C | F | Cb |
|---|---|---|---|
| 100 Calorie Pack, Shortbread Cookie Crisps (6), 0.7 oz | 100 | 3 | 16 |
| Shorbread: 1 oz cookie | 140 | 6 | 19 |
| 1.5 oz cookie | 210 | 10 | 28 |
| **Mallomars** (1), 1 oz | 120 | 5 | 18 |

**Newtons:**

| | C | F | Cb |
|---|---|---|---|
| **100% Whole Grain:** | | | |
| Blueberry (2), 1 oz | 100 | 1.5 | 22 |
| Other varieties (2), 1 0z | 100 | 1.5 | 21 |
| **Original Fig:** 2 cookies, 1 oz | 110 | 2 | 22 |
| Fat-Free, 2 cookies, 1 oz | 100 | 0 | 23 |
| **Fruit Thins,** Crispy (3), all var., 1 oz | 140 | 5 | 21 |

**Nilla Wafers:**

| | C | F | Cb |
|---|---|---|---|
| 8 wafers, 1 oz | 140 | 6 | 21 |
| Reduced-Fat (8), 1 oz | 120 | 2 | 24 |

**Nutter Butter,** Peanut Butter Sandwich:

| | C | F | Cb |
|---|---|---|---|
| 16 oz package, 1 cookie 1 oz | 130 | 5 | 20 |
| 4.8 oz package, 2 cookies, 0.9 oz | 120 | 5 | 17 |
| 1.9 oz package, 4 cookies | 250 | 10 | 37 |
| **Bites,** Go-Paks!, 3.5 oz pkg | 490 | 21 | 73 |

**Oreo, Chocolate/Golden:** *Average All fillings*

| | C | F | Cb |
|---|---|---|---|
| 100 Calorie Pack, Thin Crisps (6) | 100 | 2 | 19 |
| Original: 1 cookie | 55 | 2.5 | 8 |
| 3 cookies, 1.2 oz | 160 | 7 | 25 |
| Single Serve pkg (6), 2 oz | 270 | 11 | 41 |

*Per Cookie/Cracker, Unless Indicated* **C** **F** **Cb**

**Nabisco (Cont):**

**Original Continued:**

| | C | F | Cb |
|---|---|---|---|
| Reduced Fat (3), 1.2 oz | 150 | 5 | 27 |
| Sugar Free, 1 cookie | 50 | 2.5 | 5 |
| Mini Bite: Bite Size (9), 1 oz | 130 | 6 | 21 |
| Go-Paks, 3.5 oz | 455 | 21 | 74 |

**Oreo, Choc./Golden (Cont):** *Average All Fillings*

| | C | F | Cb |
|---|---|---|---|
| Double Stuf: 2 cookies, 1 oz | 140 | 7 | 21 |
| Single Serve, 1.5 oz | 210 | 10 | 30 |
| Fudge Cremes: 1 cookie | 60 | 3 | 8 |
| 3 cookies | 180 | 9 | 24 |
| Triple Double Chcolate (1), 0.75 oz | 100 | 5 | 15 |

**Teddy Grahams, 10 oz Box:**

| | C | F | Cb |
|---|---|---|---|
| Snacks: Honey (24), 1 oz | 120 | 4 | 21 |
| Chocolate; Cinnamon (24), 1 oz | 130 | 4 | 22 |

**Nabisco Crackers:**

**Barnum's Animals:**

| | C | F | Cb |
|---|---|---|---|
| 8 crackers, 1 oz Pack | 120 | 3.5 | 22 |
| Snack Saks, 1.2 oz Pack | 140 | 4 | 24 |

**Cheese Nips:**

| | C | F | Cb |
|---|---|---|---|
| Cheddar: 19 pieces, 1 oz | 140 | 6 | 19 |
| Mini, Despicable Me, 1 oz Pack | 130 | 4 | 19 |

**Honey Maid:**

| | C | F | Cb |
|---|---|---|---|
| Grahamfuls, S'Mores; PB & Choc. 0.9 oz pkg, av. | 115 | 4 | 18 |
| Grahams (8), average all var., 1 oz | 130 | 3 | 24 |

**Premium:**

| | C | F | Cb |
|---|---|---|---|
| Saltine: Original, 5 crackers, 0.5 oz | 70 | 1.5 | 12 |
| Unsalted Tops (5), 0.5 oz | 70 | 1.5 | 13 |
| Rounds: Original (6), 0.5 oz | 60 | 1.5 | 12 |
| Wholegrain (6), 0.5 oz | 60 | 1.5 | 11 |

**Triscuit:**

| | C | F | Cb |
|---|---|---|---|
| Original (6 ), 1 oz | 120 | 4 | 20 |
| Reduced Fat (7), 1.1 oz | 110 | 2.5 | 21 |
| Brown Rice & Wheat, average all varieties (6) | 130 | 3 | 22 |

**Wheat Thins:** *Per 9 oz Box*

| | C | F | Cb |
|---|---|---|---|
| Original (16), 1.1 oz | 140 | 5 | 22 |
| Reduced Fat (16), 1 oz | 130 | 3 | 22 |
| Av. other flav. (14), 1.1 oz | 140 | 5 | 21 |
| Multigrain (14), 1.1 oz | 130 | 4 | 22 |
| Popped, av. all flavors, 24 pcs | 125 | 3 | 23 |

*Per Cookie/Cracker, Unless Indicated* **C** **F** **Cb**

**Nana's:** *Per Cookie*

| | C | F | Cb |
|---|---|---|---|
| Choc. Chip; Oatmeal Raisin, av. | 410 | 17 | 59 |
| Coconut Chip; Peanut Butter, av. | 370 | 18 | 50 |
| Maple Syrup; Orange Cream | 260 | 14 | 32 |
| **Gluten Free:** Choc. Crunch | 360 | 12 | 62 |
| Ginger | 360 | 10 | 64 |
| Lemon | 360 | 14 | 60 |
| **Bites,** Oatmeal; P'Nut Butter, av., | 125 | 6 | 18 |
| **Cookie Bars,** average | 150 | 6 | 23 |

**Newman's Own Organics:**

| | C | F | Cb |
|---|---|---|---|
| **Alphabet:** Chocolate (10) | 110 | 3 | 21 |
| Other varieties (10) | 120 | 3 | 21 |
| **Chocolate Cups:** Milk/Dark: | | | |
| Peanut Butter (3), average | 180 | 13 | 17 |
| Dark Chocolate Peppermint (3) | 180 | 11 | 19 |
| **Double Choc Chip,** 5 cookies | 150 | 8 | 22 |
| **Family Recipe,** Ginger Snaps, 5 cookies, 1 oz | 130 | 3.5 | 24 |

**Fig Newman's:**

| | C | F | Cb |
|---|---|---|---|
| Fat-Free, 2 cookies | 100 | 0 | 24 |
| Low-Fat, 2 cookies | 110 | 1.5 | 23 |
| Wheat/Dairy-Free, 2 cookies | 110 | 1.5 | 23 |
| **Ginger Snaps,** 5 cookies | 130 | 3.5 | 24 |
| **Newman-O's:** Original (2) | 130 | 5 | 20 |
| Choc.,; Hint O Mint Creme, av., (2) | 130 | 5 | 20 |
| Peanut Butter, 2 cookies | 120 | 5 | 18 |

**Nonni's:**

**Biscotti:**

| | C | F | Cb |
|---|---|---|---|
| Original; Decadence, average, 1 piece, 0.8 oz | 95 | 4 | 15 |
| Average other varieties, (1), 0.8 oz | 110 | 4 | 17 |
| Bites: Almond Dark Chocolate (3) | 120 | 6 | 16 |
| Berry Almond (3) | 110 | 4 | 18 |
| Double Choc. Salted Caramel (3) | 110 | 4 | 18 |

**Oreo Cookies** ~ *See Nabisco, Page 85*

**Payaso:**

| | C | F | Cb |
|---|---|---|---|
| **Animalitos,** 19 pieces | 120 | 1.5 | 23 |
| **Marias,** (8), 1 oz | 120 | 2.5 | 22 |
| **Orejitas Finas,** (4) | 100 | 5 | 13 |

**Pepperidge Farm:**

**Cookies:**

**American Collection:** *Per Cookie*

| | C | F | Cb |
|---|---|---|---|
| Chesapeake, Dark Chocolate Pecan | 130 | 7 | 16 |
| Lexington, Milk Chocolate, Toffee Almond | 130 | 6 | 17 |
| Nantucket: Dark Chocolate | 130 | 6 | 18 |
| Double | 140 | 7 | 19 |
| Sausalito, Milk Choc. Macadamia | 130 | 7 | 17 |
| Tahoe, White Choc. Macadamia | 130 | 7 | 17 |

*Per Cookie/Cracker, Unless Indicated* **C** **F** **Cb**

**Pepperidge Farm (Cont):**

| | C | F | Cb |
|---|---|---|---|
| **Brussels** (3) | 150 | 7 | 20 |
| **Geneva** (3) | 160 | 9 | 19 |
| **Milano:** Milk Chocolate (3) | 170 | 9 | 21 |
| Double Chocolate (2) | 140 | 8 | 17 |
| Mint; Orange; Raspb. (2) | 130 | 7 | 16 |
| Melts, Boston Cream Pie (2) | 150 | 8 | 18 |
| Slices (3), av. all varieties | 150 | 8 | 18 |
| **Pirouettes,** (2), av. all var. | 120 | 5 | 19 |

**Sweeet & Simple**

| | C | F | Cb |
|---|---|---|---|
| Brown Butter Rum (3) | 130 | 6 | 18 |
| **Tahiti,** Coconut (2) | 170 | 10 | 17 |

**Crackers:**

| | C | F | Cb |
|---|---|---|---|
| **Cracker Trio (3)** | 60 | 2 | 9 |
| **Golden Butter (4)** | 70 | 2 | 10 |

**Goldfish (30 oz Cartons):** *Per 55 pieces*

| | C | F | Cb |
|---|---|---|---|
| Cheddar; Cheddar Colors | 140 | 5 | 20 |
| Wholegrain | 140 | 5 | 19 |
| Flavor Blasted Xtra Chedda | 140 | 5 | 19 |
| **Harvest Wheat (4)** | 100 | 4 | 14 |

**Ritz:**

| | C | F | Cb |
|---|---|---|---|
| **Originals:** Orig., (5), 0.5 oz | 80 | 4.5 | 10 |
| Reduced Fat (5), 0.5 oz | 70 | 2 | 11 |
| Bacon; Garlic Butter (5), 0.5 oz | 80 | 4 | 10 |
| Whole Wheat (5), 0.5 oz | 70 | 1.5 | 10 |

**Toasted Chips:**

| | C | F | Cb |
|---|---|---|---|
| Original (14), 1 oz | 130 | 4.5 | 19 |
| Cheddar; Sour Cream & Onion, (14), 1 oz | 135 | 6 | 19 |

**Safeway Select:**

| | C | F | Cb |
|---|---|---|---|
| **Homestyle,** Oatmeal Raisin, 1 oz | 130 | 6 | 18 |
| **Indulgent:** Double Choc Chunk, 1 oz | 130 | 7 | 18 |
| Milk Chocolate Macadamia Nut, 1 oz | 140 | 8 | 17 |

**Gourmet Sandwich Cremes:**

| | C | F | Cb |
|---|---|---|---|
| Maple Creme (2), 1 oz | 170 | 7 | 25 |
| Raspberry Swirl (2), 1 oz | 130 | 5 | 20 |
| Strawberry Swirl (2), 1 oz | 130 | 6 | 19 |

**Sedano's:**

| | C | F | Cb |
|---|---|---|---|
| **Cinnamon,** 5 cookies | 160 | 6 | 24 |
| **Maria,** 5 cookies, 1 oz | 120 | 3 | 22 |

**Shar Gluten Free** ~ *See CalorieKing.com*

### Cookies & Crackers ~ Brands (Cont)

*Per Cookie/Cracker, Unless Indicated*

| | C | F | Cb |
|---|---|---|---|
| **Special K:** *Per 1 oz Serving* | | | |
| **Crackers,** Parm. Sesame Quinoa (14) | 130 | 4.5 | 21 |
| **Cracker Chips,** all varieties | 120 | 4 | 22 |
| **Popcorn Chips,** White Cheddar( 25) | 120 | 3 | 22 |
| **Stella D'Oro:** | | | |
| Breakfast Treats (1), av. all var. | 90 | 3 | 15 |
| Margherite: Chocolate (2) | 130 | 6 | 19 |
| Vanilla (2) | 120 | 4 | 20 |
| Roman Egg Biscuits, 1 oz | 130 | 4.5 | 19 |
| Swiss Fudge (3) | 170 | 9 | 22 |
| **Toast & Sponge:** | | | |
| Almond Toast (2) | 100 | 2 | 20 |
| Anisette Sponge (3) | 90 | 1 | 18 |
| Anisette Toast (3), 1 oz | 130 | 1 | 27 |
| **Streit's:** | | | |
| **Flavored Wafers:** | | | |
| Chocolate (3) | 160 | 9 | 19 |
| Vanilla (3) | 160 | 9 | 19 |
| **Sunshine:** | | | |
| **Cheez-It Snack:** | | | |
| Average all varieties, 1 oz | 150 | 8 | 17 |
| 1.25 oz bag | 180 | 9 | 20 |
| **Big,** all varieties, 1 oz | 150 | 8 | 17 |
| **Reduced Fat,** all varieties,1 oz | 130 | 4.5 | 20 |
| **Extra Toast,** 1 oz | 150 | 8 | 17 |
| **Grooves,** Sharp White Chedd., 1 oz | 140 | 6 | 19 |
| **Trader Joe's:** | | | |
| 100 Calorie Packs, average | 100 | 2.5 | 18 |
| Almond Windmill (2), 1 oz | 140 | 6 | 18 |
| Charmingly Chewy Choc Chip (2), 1 oz | 130 | 5 | 20 |
| Cherry Granola (2), 1 oz | 110 | 4 | 18 |
| **Chocolate Chip:** Small (4), 1 oz | 140 | 7 | 18 |
| Large, singles, 1.7 oz | 280 | 14 | 35 |
| Vegan (1), 1 oz | 130 | 6 | 18 |
| Caramel Cashew (3), 1 oz | 140 | 7 | 16 |
| Crispy Crunchy Choc Chip (12) | 150 | 9 | 19 |
| Crispy Oatmeal Choc Chip (12) | 150 | 7 | 19 |
| Dark Choc Chunks with almonds (3) | 140 | 7 | 17 |
| Dunkers: Chocolate Chip (2), 1.2 oz | 160 | 7 | 21 |
| Choc. Coated Choc. Chip (2), 1.3 oz | 190 | 9 | 25 |

*Per Cookie/Cracker, Unless Indicated*

| | C | F | Cb |
|---|---|---|---|
| **Trader Joe's: (Cont):** | | | |
| Ginger Snaps, Gluten Free (5), 1 oz | 140 | 6 | 21 |
| Highbrow Chocolate (2) | 140 | 7 | 17 |
| Joe Joe's S'wich Cremes, | | | |
| Choc./ Vanilla (2), 1 oz | 130 | 6 | 19 |
| Macarons A La Parisienne (2) | 90 | 3 | 10 |
| Meringues, Vanilla (4) | 110 | 0 | 27 |
| Oatmeal Raisin, 1.8 oz | 270 | 12 | 35 |
| Pecan S'thrn Style (4), 1 oz | 150 | 9 | 15 |
| **Thins:** Meyer Lemon (9) | 130 | 4.5 | 22 |
| Toasted Coconut (8) | 130 | 4.5 | 22 |
| Triple Choc Chunk, 1 oz | 140 | 7 | 20 |
| Ultimate Vanilla Wafers (5) | 120 | 6 | 15 |
| Way More Chocolate Chip (3) | 160 | 11 | 14 |
| **Crackers,** Water (4) | 60 | 1 | 12 |
| **Triscuits** ~ *See Page 85* | | | |
| **Voortman:** | | | |
| **Classics:** Coconut (1) | 100 | 5 | 10 |
| Chunky Chip (1) | 100 | 4.5 | 14 |
| **Sugar Free:** Oatmeal Flaxseed (1) | 80 | 4 | 12 |
| Shortbread Swirls (1) | 100 | 6 | 12 |
| *Note: Carb figures include 4g of sugar alcohols* | | | |
| **Wafers,** Vanilla (1) | 140 | 6 | 20 |
| **Whole Foods (365 Organic):** | | | |
| Choc Chip (2), 1 oz | 150 | 7 | 21 |
| Classic Fig Bars (2), 1.3 oz | 140 | 2.5 | 27 |
| Lemon Wafers (7), 1 oz | 110 | 3 | 19 |
| Oatmeal (2), 1 oz | 130 | 4.5 | 20 |
| S'wich Cremes; Sugar (2), average | 130 | 5 | 20 |

### Cookie ~ Mixes

*Prepared as Directed*

| | C | F | Cb |
|---|---|---|---|
| **Betty Crocker:** | | | |
| **Pouch Mix:** *Per 2 Cookies* | | | |
| Double Choc. Chunk; P'nut Butter, av. | 140 | 6 | 21 |
| Walnut Chocolate Chip | 170 | 9 | 20 |
| Average other varieties | 145 | 6 | 22 |

## Thaw, Bake & Serve   C  F  Cb

*Per Cookie/Cracker Unless Indicated*

**Pillsbury Cookies:**

**Refrigerated Cookie Dough:** *Per Cookie*

| | C | F | Cb |
|---|---|---|---|
| Chocolate Chip Cookie | 130 | 6 | 18 |
| Peanut Butter | 120 | 5 | 17 |
| Sugar, Regular | 120 | 5 | 18 |

**Ready To Bake:**

| | C | F | Cb |
|---|---|---|---|
| Big Deluxe Classics: | | | |
| Chocolate Chip (1) | 160 | 7 | 23 |
| Oatmeal Raisin (1) | 150 | 5 | 24 |
| Peanut Butter Cup (1) | 160 | 7 | 22 |
| White Chunk Macadamia (1) | 170 | 8 | 22 |
| Simply Cookies: Choc. Chip (1) | 150 | 7 | 20 |
| Peanut Butter (1) | 140 | 6 | 19 |
| Chocolate Chip (2) | 160 | 7 | 23 |
| Choc. Chunk & Chip (2) | 160 | 7 | 24 |
| Holiday Cookies, Sugar, | | | |
| average all shapes, (2) | 120 | 6 | 15 |
| Oatmeal Chocolate Chip (2) | 160 | 7 | 24 |

**Refrigerated Sweet Buns/Rolls~** *See Page 67*

**Toll House (Nestle):**

**Refrigerated Dough Bars:** *Per Cookie*

| | C | F | Cb |
|---|---|---|---|
| Chocolate Chip | 90 | 4 | 11 |
| Chocolate Peppermint | 90 | 4.5 | 12 |
| Hot Cocoa | 80 | 3.5 | 12 |
| Oatmeal Raisin | 80 | 3 | 12 |
| P'B Chocolate Chip | 80 | 4.5 | 10 |
| Walnut Chocolate Chip | 90 | 4.5 | 11 |

**Ultimates Refrigerated Dough:** *Per Cookie*

| | C | F | Cb |
|---|---|---|---|
| Chocolate Chip Lovers | 180 | 9 | 23 |
| Chocolate Pecan Deluxe | 190 | 10 | 22 |
| Choc. P'nut Butter Deluxe | 180 | 9 | 23 |
| Dark Chocolate Delight | 160 | 8 | 21 |
| Pecan Turtle Delight | 160 | 7 | 23 |

## Crispbreads   C  F  Cb

*Per Crispbread Unless Indicated*

**Finn Crisp:**

| | C | F | Cb |
|---|---|---|---|
| **Classic:** Traditional Rye | 40 | 0.5 | 7 |
| Hi-Fibre | 40 | 0.5 | 7 |
| **Round:** Original | 45 | 0.5 | 8 |
| Sesame | 50 | 1 | 8 |
| **Thin Crisps,** Original | 20 | 0 | 4 |
| **New York Flatbread Crisps,** | | | |
| Sesame, 0.4 oz | 50 | 1.5 | 8 |
| **Ry-Krisp:** Natural (2) | 50 | 0 | 11 |
| Seasoned (2) | 60 | 1 | 11 |
| Sesame (2) | 60 | 1.5 | 10 |

**Ryvita:**

| | C | F | Cb |
|---|---|---|---|
| **Crackerbreads,** Original; Wholegrain | 20 | 0 | 4 |
| **Crispbreads,** Original; Dark | 35 | 0 | 6.5 |

**WASA:**

| | C | F | Cb |
|---|---|---|---|
| Crisp'n Light 7 Grain (3) | 60 | 0 | 13 |
| Fiber (1), 0.35 oz | 40 | 1 | 7 |
| Hearty, 0.5 oz | 60 | 0 | 12 |
| Light Rye (2), 0.5 oz | 60 | 0 | 14 |
| Whole Grain, 0.5 oz | 50 | 0 | 11 |

## Matzos

**Manischewitz:**

| | C | F | Cb |
|---|---|---|---|
| **Matzos:** Egg'n Onion, 1 oz | 80 | 0.5 | 17 |
| Thin Salted/Tea, average, 0.9 oz | 95 | 0 | 20 |
| Whole Wheat, 1 oz | 110 | 1 | 21 |
| Yolk Free, 1.2 oz | 100 | 0 | 20 |

**Crackers:**

| | C | F | Cb |
|---|---|---|---|
| **Tam Tam:** Original (10), 1 oz | 110 | 4 | 16 |
| Everything; Onion (10), 1 oz | 140 | 5 | 19 |
| Rye (10), 1 oz | 110 | 4 | 16 |

**Streit's:**

| | C | F | Cb |
|---|---|---|---|
| Mediterranean Matzos, | | | |
| 1 Matzo, 1 oz | 90 | 0.5 | 18 |
| Unsalted Matzos, | | | |
| 1 Matzo, 1 oz | 100 | 0 | 23 |

## Quick Guide  **C**  **F**  **Cb**

### Cream
**Average All Brands**
**Half & Half Cream:**

| | C | F | Cb |
|---|---|---|---|
| 1 Tbsp, 0.5 oz | 20 | 1.5 | 0.5 |
| 2 Tbsp, 1 oz | 40 | 3 | 1 |
| ¼ cup, 2 oz | 80 | 6 | 2 |
| **Light:** Coffee/table (20% fat): 1 Tbsp | 30 | 3 | 0.5 |
| 2 Tbsp, 1 oz | 60 | 6 | 0.5 |

**Sour Cream:**

| | C | F | Cb |
|---|---|---|---|
| **Regular:** 1 Tbsp, 0.5 oz | 25 | 2.5 | 1 |
| 1 cup, 8 oz | 445 | 45 | 7 |
| **Low-Fat/Light:** 1 Tbsp, 0.5 oz | 20 | 1.5 | 1 |
| 2 Tbsp, 1 oz | 40 | 3 | 2 |
| **Fat-Free:** Av., 2 Tbsp, 1 oz | 20 | 0 | 4.5 |
| *Hood,* 2 Tbsp, 1 oz | 25 | 0 | 4 |
| *Knudsen,* 2 Tbsp, 1 oz | 30 | 0 | 5 |
| *Kroger,* 2 Tbsp, 1 oz | 20 | 0 | 3 |
| *Naturally Yours; Oak Farm,* 2 Tbsp | 20 | 0 | 3 |

**Sour Cream Substitute:**

| | C | F | Cb |
|---|---|---|---|
| *Albertson's,* 2 Tbsp, 1 oz | 60 | 5 | 2 |
| *Tofutti,* Sour Supreme, 2 Tbsp, 1 oz | 85 | 5 | 9 |

**Whipping Cream:**
**Heavy,** (37% fat):

| | C | F | Cb |
|---|---|---|---|
| 1 Tbsp fluid/2 Tbsp whipped | 50 | 5.5 | 0.5 |
| ¼ cup whipped | 105 | 11 | 1 |
| ½ cup fluid/1 cup whipped | 410 | 44 | 3.5 |
| **Light,** (30% fat): | | | |
| 1 Tbsp fluid/2 Tbsp whipped | 45 | 4.5 | 0.5 |
| ½ cup fluid/1 cup whipped | 350 | 37 | 3.5 |

### Coconut Cream/Milk

**Coconut Cream,** (Canned):

| | C | F | Cb |
|---|---|---|---|
| **Plain/unsweetened:** 2 Tbsp, 1 oz | 75 | 6.5 | 3 |
| ½ cup, 4 oz | 285 | 26 | 12 |
| **Sweetened:** | | | |
| *Coco Lopez:* 1 oz | 130 | 5 | 21 |
| ½ cup, 4 oz | 520 | 20 | 84 |
| **Coconut Milk:** (Canned): | | | |
| *Thai Kitchen:* Lite, ⅓ cup, 2 fl.oz | 50 | 4.5 | 1 |
| Premium/Organic, 2 fl.oz | 115 | 10 | 4 |
| Unsweetened, ⅓ cup | 140 | 14 | 3 |
| **Coconut Water,** (Center), 1 cup | 45 | 0.5 | 9 |

### Whipped Toppings

**Average All Brands**

| | C | F | Cb |
|---|---|---|---|
| **Cream (Pressurized):** 2 Tbsp | 20 | 1.5 | 1 |
| ¼ cup | 40 | 3.5 | 2 |
| **Cream Topping,** Lite, 2 Tbsp | 20 | 1 | 3 |

## Whipped Toppings (Cont)

**Kraft:**  **C**  **F**  **Cb**

| | C | F | Cb |
|---|---|---|---|
| **Cool Whip:** Regular, Original, ⅓ oz | 25 | 1.5 | 2 |
| Extra Creamy, 2 Tbsp | 25 | 2 | 2 |
| Lite, 2 Tbsp, ¼ oz | 20 | 1 | 3 |
| Free, 2 Tbsp, 0.3 oz | 20 | 0 | 3 |
| Seasons Delight, Fr. Vanilla, 0.3 oz | 25 | 1.5 | 2 |
| **Dream Whip,** 2 Tbsp | 10 | 0 | 2 |

**Reddi-wip:**

| | C | F | Cb |
|---|---|---|---|
| **Original,** 2 Tbsp, 0.3 oz | 15 | 1 | 1 |
| **Extra Creamy,** 2 Tbsp, 0.3 oz | 15 | 1 | 1 |
| **Fat-Free,** 2 Tbsp, 0.3 oz | 5 | 0 | 1 |
| **Chocolate,** 2 Tbsp, 0.3 oz | 15 | 1 | 1 |

### Creamers (Non-Dairy)

**Powder:**
**Coffee-Mate/Cremora/N-Rich:**

| | C | F | Cb |
|---|---|---|---|
| **Original:** Unsweetened, 1 tsp | 10 | 0.5 | 1 |
| 1 heaping tsp | 25 | 2 | 2 |
| Lite, 1 tsp | 10 | 0 | 2 |
| Sweetened, 4 tsp | 60 | 2.5 | 9 |
| Flavors: Av., 4 tsp | 60 | 3 | 9 |
| Fat-Free, average, 4 tsp | 50 | 0 | 11 |

**Liquid/Refrigerated:**
*Per Tablespoon*

| | C | F | Cb |
|---|---|---|---|
| **Baileys,** Coffee Creamer, all flavors, 1 Tbsp, 15ml | 25 | 0.5 | 5 |
| **Califia Farms,** all flavors, 1 Tbsp | 15 | 0 | 4 |
| **Coffee-Mate:** *Per Tablespoon* | | | |
| **Flavors:** Average all flavors | 35 | 1.5 | 5 |
| Fat-Free, all flavors | 25 | 0 | 5 |
| Sugar free, all flavors | 15 | 1 | 2 |
| **Unflavored:** Original | 20 | 1 | 2 |
| Fat-Free | 10 | 0 | 1 |
| Low-Fat | 10 | 0.5 | 2 |
| **Natural Bliss,** all flavors | 35 | 1.5 | 5 |
| **Hood,** Country Creamer, 1 Tbsp | 20 | 1.5 | 2 |
| **International Delight:** *Per Tbsp* | | | |
| **American/Classic/Coffee House:** | | | |
| Regular, all flavors | 35 | 1.5 | 6 |
| Fat-Free, all flavors | 30 | 0 | 7 |
| Fat-Free, Sugar-Free, all flav. | 15 | 0 | 3 |
| **Kroger:** *Per Tbsp* | | | |
| **Coffee Creamers:** Original | 20 | 1 | 3 |
| Caramel Vanilla; Hazelnut | 35 | 1.5 | 6 |
| Fat-free, Hazelnut | 30 | 0 | 6 |
| **Silk:** Almond, Vanilla | 20 | 1 | 3 |
| Soy: Original | 20 | 1.5 | 2 |
| Hazelnut | 30 | 1.5 | 4 |

# D Desserts ~ Puddings ◆ Gelatin

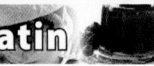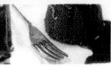

## Ready-To-Serve

| | C | F | Cb |
|---|---|---|---|
| **Hunt's:** | | | |
| **Snack Pack Puddings:** | | | |
| **3.3 oz Container:** | | | |
| Butterscotch; Tapioca | 110 | 2.5 | 21 |
| Chocolate/ Chocolate Fudge | 120 | 3 | 21 |
| Vanilla | 100 | 2.5 | 20 |
| Fat Free: Chocolate | 90 | 0 | 20 |
| Tapioca | 80 | 0 | 19 |
| Sugar Free: Chocolate | 70 | 3 | 14 |
| Caramel; Vanilla | 60 | 3 | 10 |
| **Juicy Gels:** Lemon Lime, 5.5 oz | 150 | 0 | 38 |
| Strawberry, 5.5 oz | 170 | 0 | 41 |
| Sugar Free, Cherry, 3.25 oz | 10 | 0 | 2 |
| **Jell-O** *(Kraft)*: | | | |
| **Gelatin,** av. all flavors, 3.4 oz | 70 | 0 | 17 |
| **Puddings & Mousse, 4 Pack:** | | | |
| Pudding Snacks, av. all flav., 3.9 oz | 110 | 1.5 | 23 |
| Mix Ins, Turtle Sundae, 3.4 oz | 150 | 6 | 23 |
| Pudding, Tapioca, 3.9 oz | 100 | 1.5 | 24 |
| Rice, Cinnamon/Vanilla, 3.6 oz | 110 | 3 | 20 |
| Temptations, Dble Choc. Pie, 3.4 oz | 110 | 3.5 | 18 |
| **Fat Free Puddings, 4 Pack:** | | | |
| Chocolate, 3.9 oz | 100 | 0 | 22 |
| Tapioca Pudding, 3.9 oz | 100 | 0 | 22 |
| **Red. Calorie Puddings, 4 Pack:** | | | |
| Boston Cream Pie, 3.6 oz | 60 | 1 | 10 |
| Chocolate, 3.6 oz | 60 | 1.5 | 13 |
| **Kozy Shack:** | | | |
| **Flan,** Creme Caramel, 1 cup, 4 oz | 160 | 4 | 28 |
| **Gluten Free Puddings:** | | | |
| Chocolate, 4.6 oz | 140 | 2.5 | 27 |
| Cinnamon Raisin, 4.6 oz | 140 | 2.5 | 26 |
| French Vanilla Rice, 4.6 oz | 140 | 2.5 | 24 |
| Original Rice, 4.6 oz | 130 | 2.5 | 24 |
| Tapioca, 4.6 oz | 130 | 2 | 25 |
| **Simply Well Puddings:** | | | |
| Chocolate, 4 oz | 90 | 2.5 | 13 |
| Rice; Tapioca, 4 oz | 90 | 1.5 | 14 |
| **Kroger:** *Per Container* | | | |
| **Puddings:** *Per 3.5 oz* | | | |
| Butterscotch | 110 | 2 | 22 |
| Chocolate | 110 | 2.5 | 21 |
| **Swiss Miss:** | | | |
| **Puddings:** *Per 4 oz Cup* | | | |
| Classic Butterscotch | 130 | 3.5 | 22 |
| Creamy : Milk Choc. | 150 | 3.5 | 27 |
| Vanilla | 140 | 3.5 | 24 |
| Old Fashioned Tapioca | 140 | 3.5 | 24 |
| Sugar Free: Chocolate | 70 | 3.5 | 15 |
| Vanilla | 60 | 3 | 11 |

## Homemade Puddings

| | C | F | Cb |
|---|---|---|---|
| Apple Tapioca, ½ cup | 150 | 0 | 32 |
| Bread Pudding, ½ cup | 250 | 8 | 40 |
| Blancmange, ½ cup | 140 | 5 | 19 |
| Chocolate, ½ cup | 190 | 6 | 30 |
| Crème Brûlée, ½ cup | 400 | 35 | 16 |
| Plum Pudding, 2 oz | 170 | 3 | 32 |
| Rice with Raisins, ½ cup | 200 | 4 | 38 |
| Sponge Pudding, 3.5 oz | 340 | 16 | 45 |
| Tapioca Cream, ½ cup | 110 | 4 | 15 |
| Trifle, ½ cup | 180 | 7 | 26 |

## Custards

| | C | F | Cb |
|---|---|---|---|
| **Custard Mix** *(Jello/Royal Flan)*, average: | | | |
| Dry, ¼ of 2.9 oz package, 0.7 oz | 80 | 0 | 19 |
| Prepared: Whole milk, ½ cup | 155 | 4 | 25 |
| 2% milk, ½ cup | 140 | 2.5 | 25 |
| Non-Fat milk, ½ cup | 125 | 0 | 25 |
| **Home Made Egg Custard:** | | | |
| With Whole Milk, ½ cup | 170 | 8 | 18 |
| With 2% Milk, ½ cup | 155 | 6.5 | 18 |

## Gelatin • Parfait • Jell-O

| | C | F | Cb |
|---|---|---|---|
| **Jell-O:** | | | |
| **Gelatin Dessert Mix:** *Dry Mix Only* | | | |
| All flavors, 0.8 oz | 80 | 0 | 19 |
| Sugar free, all flavors, 0.3 oz | 10 | 0 | 0 |
| **Instant Pudding & Pie Filling:** *Dry Mix Only* | | | |
| Chocolate/Fudge, 1 oz | 100 | 0 | 25 |
| Devil's Food, 1 oz | 140 | 0 | 25 |
| Oreo, | | | |
| Cookies 'N Cream, 1 oz | 120 | 1 | 28 |
| White Chocolate, 0.8 oz | 90 | 0 | 23 |
| Sugar free, Fat-Free: | | | |
| Chocolate var., 0.3 oz | 35 | 0 | 8 |
| Other flavors, 0.3 oz | 25 | 0 | 6 |
| **No Bake Dessert Mix:** *Dry Mix Only* | | | |
| Cheesecake: Real, 2 oz | 290 | 15 | 39 |
| Cherry, 2.2 oz | 210 | 3.5 | 42 |
| Strawberry, 2.4 oz | 200 | 3.5 | 42 |
| Oreo, 2 oz | 280 | 8 | 48 |
| Peanut Butter Cup, 2 oz | 290 | 15 | 39 |
| Pumpkin Style Pie, 1.2 oz | 130 | 1.5 | 29 |
| **Ida Mae,** Strawberry Parfait | 90 | 2 | 18 |
| **Reser's,** Parfaits, av. all flavors, 3.9 oz | 100 | 2 | 19 |

## Meringues

| | C | F | Cb |
|---|---|---|---|
| Meringue Swirl, ½ cup | 50 | 0 | 8 |
| Meringue Shell, 1 oz | 100 | 0 | 16 |

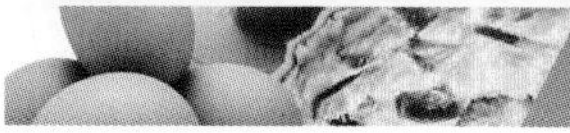

## Chicken Eggs

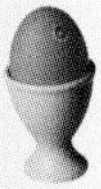

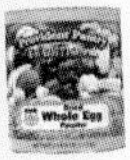

**C F Cb**

**Fresh Eggs:**
**Raw:**

| | C | F | Cb |
|---|---|---|---|
| Small | 55 | 4 | 0 |
| Medium | 65 | 4 | 0 |
| Large | 70 | 5 | 0 |
| Extra Large | 80 | 5.5 | 0 |
| Jumbo | 90 | 6 | 0 |
| **Egg Yolk,** 1 extra large | 55 | 4.5 | 0 |
| **Egg White,** 1 extra large | 17 | 0 | 0 |

**Dried Egg Powder:**

| | C | F | Cb |
|---|---|---|---|
| **Whole Egg:** ¼ cup, 1 oz | 170 | 12 | 0 |
| 1 Tbsp | 30 | 2 | 0 |
| **Egg White,** ¼ cup, 1 oz | 105 | 0 | 0 |
| **Egg Yolk,** ¼ cup, 1 oz | 195 | 18 | 0 |

## Egg Substitutes

*¼ Cup (Equivalent to 1 Egg) ~ Zero Cholesterol*

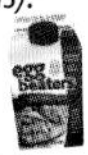

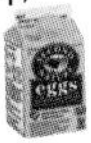

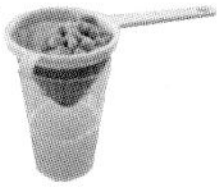

| | C | F | Cb |
|---|---|---|---|
| **All Whites** (Crystal Farms), 1.6 oz | 25 | 0 | 0 |
| **Better 'n Eggs** (Crystal Farms): | | | |
| Regular, ¼ cup, 2 oz | 30 | 0 | 1 |
| **Egg Beaters** (ConAgra): | | | |
| Regular, 3 Tbsp, 1.6 oz | 25 | 0 | 1 |
| Southwestern Style, 3 Tbsp, 1.6 oz | 20 | 0 | 1 |
| Three Cheese, 3 Tbsp, 1.6 oz | 25 | 0.5 | 1 |
| **Egg Replacer** (Ener-g), 1.5 tsp, | 15 | 0 | 4 |
| **Eggs** (Second Nature), | | | |
| Egg Whites, Fat-Free, ¼ cup, 2 fl.oz | 35 | 0 | 1 |
| **Egg Substitute** (Albertson's), ¼ cup | 30 | 0 | 1 |
| **Naturegg** (Burnbrae Farms), | | | |
| Simply Egg White, ¼ cup, 2 oz | 30 | 0 | 1 |
| **Vegan Egg Substitute:** | | | |
| **Aquafaba,** ¼ cup, 2 oz | 10 | 0 | 2 |

*Liquid from cooked/canned beans or chickpeas. Replaces eggs and egg whites in recipes.*
*Extra Info: www.aquafaba.com*

## Other Eggs

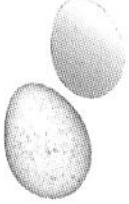

| | C | F | Cb |
|---|---|---|---|
| Duck, 1 large, 2.5 oz | 130 | 9.5 | 0 |
| Goose, 1 large, 5 oz | 280 | 19 | 0 |
| Quail, 3 eggs, 1 oz | 42 | 3 | 0 |
| Turkey, 1 large, 3 oz | 135 | 9.5 | 0 |
| Turtle, 1 egg, 1.75 oz | 75 | 5 | 0 |

## Omega-3 Fat Enriched

| | C | F | Cb |
|---|---|---|---|
| **Egg·Land's Best,** 1 large | 60 | 4 | 0 |
| **Horizon Organic,** 1 large | 70 | 4.5 | 1 |

*Note: Cholesterol content is the same as regular eggs.*

## Cooked Eggs

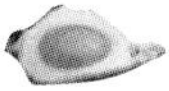

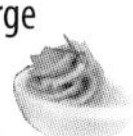

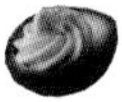

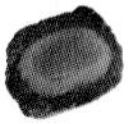

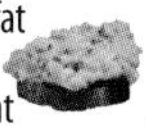

**C F Cb**

| | C | F | Cb |
|---|---|---|---|
| **Boiled Egg:** *Same as Raw Egg* | | | |
| **Hard-Cooked,** Small, peeled | 65 | 4 | 0 |
| **Fried Egg:** | | | |
| With fat: 1 large egg | 105 | 9 | 0.5 |
| 2 small eggs | 175 | 13 | 1 |
| No fat/nonstick pan, 1 large | 75 | 5 | 0.5 |
| **Deviled Egg,** 2 halves | 145 | 13 | 0.5 |
| **Eggs Benedict,** (2), | | | |
| on Toast or English Muffin | 860 | 56 | 25 |
| **Eggs Florentine,** (2), | | | |
| on Toast or English Muffin | 890 | 59 | 25 |
| **Pickled Egg,** 1 large | 80 | 5.5 | 0 |
| **Poached Egg,** 1 large | 65 | 4 | 0 |
| **Quiche** (Homemade): | | | |
| Egg & Bacon, 1 slice, 5.3 oz | 580 | 43 | 27 |
| Ham & Cheese, 1 slice, 5.3 oz | 475 | 33 | 29 |
| **Scotch Egg,** 1 egg | 300 | 21 | 16 |
| **Scrambled Eggs:** | | | |
| 1 large egg: | | | |
| With 1 Tbsp milk + 1 tsp fat | 120 | 9 | 1 |
| With 1 Tbsp skim milk/no fat | 85 | 5.5 | 1 |
| 2 large eggs: | | | |
| With 2 Tbsp milk + 2 tsp fat | 260 | 20 | 2 |
| With 2 Tbsp skim milk, w/o fat | 180 | 11 | 2 |

## Omelets

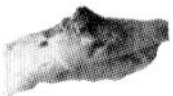

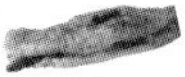

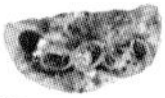

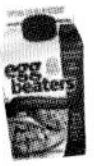

| | C | F | Cb |
|---|---|---|---|
| **1 Egg:** | | | |
| Plain (with 1 tsp fat) | 125 | 10 | 0.5 |
| With: ½ oz cheese | 175 | 15 | 0.5 |
| ½ oz cheese + ½ oz ham | 200 | 16 | 0.5 |
| **2 Eggs:** | | | |
| Plain (with 2 tsp fat) | 250 | 20 | 1 |
| With: 1 oz cheese | 360 | 29 | 2 |
| 1 oz cheese + 1 oz ham | 410 | 32 | 2 |
| **3 Eggs:** | | | |
| Plain (with 1 Tbsp fat) | 360 | 29 | 1.5 |
| With: 2 oz cheese | 580 | 47 | 2.5 |
| 2 oz cheese + 2 oz ham | 680 | 53 | 2.5 |
| **Extras,** Tomato/Onion/Veggies, 2 oz | 20 | 0 | 4.5 |
| **Egg Substitute** (EggBeaters): | | | |
| 2 eggs (½ cup) + 1 tsp fat | 100 | 4 | 2 |
| 3 eggs (¾ cup) + 2 tsp fat | 160 | 8 | 3 |
| Extras: 1 oz Cheese | 110 | 9 | 1 |
| 1 oz Ham | 50 | 3 | 1 |

## Egg Nog

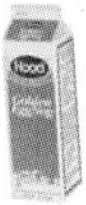

*Average all Brands,*

| | C | F | Cb |
|---|---|---|---|
| ½ cup, 4 oz | 170 | 9.5 | 17 |
| **Borden,** Regular, 4 fl.oz | 160 | 8 | 18 |
| **Hood,** Golden, ½ cup, 4 fl.oz | 180 | 9 | 22 |
| **Horizon/Hood,** Light/Low-Fat, | 140 | 4 | 22 |

## Breakfast Sides | **C** | **F** | **Cb**

| | C | F | Cb |
|---|---|---|---|
| **Toast:** | | | |
| Plain, 1 thick slice | 85 | 1 | 13 |
| With: 2 tsp butter/marg. | 155 | 9 | 13 |
| 3 tsp/1 Tbsp fat | 190 | 13 | 13 |
| **English Muffin:** | | | |
| Plain, 2 oz | 130 | 1 | 26 |
| With 3 tsp fat | 230 | 12 | 26 |
| **Bacon,** 2 strips | 70 | 5 | 0 |
| **Ham,** lean, 2 oz | 100 | 3 | 0 |
| **Hash Brown:** | | | |
| ½ cup, 3 oz | 125 | 6.5 | 14 |
| 1 cup serving, 6 oz | 250 | 13 | 28 |
| **Sausages,** 2 oz link | 180 | 16 | 1.5 |

## Frozen Egg Breakfasts

| | C | F | Cb |
|---|---|---|---|
| **Jimmy Dean:** | | | |
| **Breakfast Sandwich:** *Per Sandwich* | | | |
| Biscuit, Sausage, Egg & Cheese | 410 | 29 | 26 |
| Croissant, Egg, Red Peppers, Onions | | | |
| & Jack Cheese | 290 | 16 | 27 |
| Muffin, Meat Lovers | 480 | 34 | 26 |
| **Omelets:** *Per Omelet* | | | |
| Three Cheese | 290 | 23 | 4 |
| Ham & Cheese | 250 | 19 | 4 |
| **MorningStar Farms,** | | | |
| **Breakfast Sandwich,** | | | |
| Sausage, Egg & Cheese | 220 | 10 | 20 |
| **Pillsbury:** | | | |
| **Toaster Scrambles:** Bacon | 190 | 10 | 18 |
| Bacon & Sausage | 180 | 11 | 18 |
| Ham | 180 | 10 | 17 |
| **Red Baron:** | | | |
| **Biscuit Scrambles:** | | | |
| Bacon (1), 5.85 oz | 440 | 21 | 47 |
| Sausage (1), 5.85 oz | 430 | 20 | 47 |
| **Frozen Pancake/Waffles ~** *See Page 132* | | | |
| **Toaster Pastries ~** *See Page 64* | | | |

## Frozen Egg Rolls

| | C | F | Cb |
|---|---|---|---|
| **Kahiki:** *Each, without sauce* | | | |
| Chicken, 2.3 oz | 150 | 4 | 25 |
| Vegetable, 2.3 oz | 150 | 3 | 26 |
| **Lotus Restaurant:** | | | |
| Imperial, Chicken/Pork (1) | 160 | 6.5 | 24 |
| Vegetarian (1) | 120 | 5 | 20 |
| **Pagoda Express:** *Each, with Sauce* | | | |
| Chicken | 160 | 4 | 24 |
| Pork | 180 | 7 | 23 |
| Pork & Shrimp | 180 | 7 | 23 |
| Vegetable | 140 | 4 | 24 |

## Fast-Foods/Restaurants | **C** | **F** | **Cb**

| | C | F | Cb |
|---|---|---|---|
| **Arby's,** | | | |
| Bacon, Egg & Cheese Croissant | 440 | 27 | 29 |
| **Au Bon Pain,** 2 Egg on Plain Bagel | 390 | 11 | 51 |
| **Bob Evans:** | | | |
| **Omelets:** | | | |
| Border Scramble | 680 | 49 | 15 |
| Western | 490 | 34 | 5 |
| **Bojangles:** Egg & Cheese Biscuit | 410 | 24 | 38 |
| Bacon, Egg & Cheese Biscuit | 460 | 28 | 38 |
| **Bruegger's:** | | | |
| **Bagel:** With Egg & Cheese, 6.8 oz | 430 | 18 | 63 |
| With Egg, Cheese & Sausage, 8.3 oz | 590 | 34 | 63 |
| **Burger King:** | | | |
| **Egg-Normous Burrito** | 310 | 19 | 22 |
| **Croissan'wich:** | | | |
| Bacon, Egg & Cheese | 340 | 18 | 30 |
| Ham, Egg & Cheese | 340 | 16 | 31 |
| King, with Double Sausage | 700 | 51 | 31 |
| **Carl's Jr:** | | | |
| **Burrito:** Bacon & Egg | 570 | 34 | 38 |
| Big Country | 680 | 41 | 52 |
| Loaded Breakfast | 790 | 50 | 53 |
| Steak & Egg | 650 | 36 | 44 |
| **Chick-fil-A,** Chicken, Egg & Cheese, | | | |
| on Sunflower Multigrain Bagel | 480 | 20 | 48 |
| **Del Taco,** Egg & Cheese Burrito | 430 | 21 | 38 |
| **Denny's:** *With Hashbrowns, Without Bread* | | | |
| **Omelette:** | | | |
| Ultimate | 830 | 66 | 25 |
| Veggie, Loaded | 600 | 43 | 25 |
| **Dunkin Donuts:** | | | |
| **Bagel,** Ham, Egg & Cheese | 440 | 8 | 67 |
| **Croissant,** Bacon, Egg & Cheese | 490 | 29 | 40 |
| **Eat 'N Park:** | | | |
| **Omelette:** | | | |
| Ham & Cheese | 535 | 35 | 5 |
| Meat Lovers | 725 | 55 | 4 |
| **Hardee's:** | | | |
| **Biscuit:** Loaded Omelet | 490 | 28 | 40 |
| Sausage & Egg | 560 | 37 | 39 |
| **IHOP:** 3 Eggs, Scrambled | 330 | 26 | 3 |
| Omelette, Spinach & Mushroom | 890 | 70 | 20 |
| **Jack in the Box:** | | | |
| **Biscuit:** Bacon, Egg & Cheese | 410 | 25 | 26 |
| Sausage, Egg & Cheese | 535 | 38 | 27 |
| **McDonald's:** | | | |
| **Biscuit,** Bacon, Egg & Cheese, regular | 440 | 24 | 37 |
| **McMuffin,** Egg | 290 | 12 | 29 |
| **Whataburger,** Breakfast Platter, | | | |
| with Bacon | 620 | 40 | 36 |

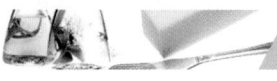

## Quick Guide  C F Cb

### Butter
*Average All Brands*

| | C | F | Cb |
|---|---|---|---|
| **Regular:** 1 tsp, 0.2 oz | 35 | 4 | 0 |
| 1 Tbsp, 0.5 oz | 100 | 11 | 0 |
| 2 Tbsp, 1 oz | 205 | 23 | 0 |
| 1 Stick, ½ cup, 4 oz | 810 | 92 | 0 |
| 1 Pound, 2 cups, 16 oz | 3255 | 368 | 0 |
| **Light:** Regular, 40% Fat | | | |
| 1 tsp, 0.2 oz | 30 | 3 | 0 |
| 1 Tbsp, 0.5 oz | 70 | 7.5 | 0 |
| 2 Tbsp, 1 oz | 140 | 15 | 0 |
| **Whipped Butter:** Regular | | | |
| 1 tsp, 0.1 oz | 20 | 2.5 | 0 |
| 1 Tbsp, 0.3 oz | 65 | 7.5 | 0 |
| 1 Stick, 2.7 oz | 545 | 62 | 0 |
| **Whipped Light Butter** (Land O Lakes): | | | |
| 1 tsp, 0.15 oz | 15 | 1.5 | 0 |
| 1 Tbsp, 0.4 oz | 45 | 5 | 0 |
| 2 Tbsp, 0.8 oz | 90 | 10 | 0 |
| **Unsalted** ~ *Same as Salted* | | | |

### Flavored Butter/Spreads

*Average All Brands*

| | C | F | Cb |
|---|---|---|---|
| **Honey Butter,** (60% Fat): | | | |
| 1 Tbsp, 0.5 oz | 90 | 8 | 4 |
| *Downey's, 2% Fat,* | | | |
| 1 Tbsp, 0.5 oz | 60 | 1 | 11 |
| **Garlic Butter,** (80% Fat): | | | |
| 1 Tbsp, 0.5 oz | 100 | 11 | 0 |
| **Sweet Cream Butter:** | | | |
| *Land O Lakes:* Regular, 1 Tbsp | 100 | 11 | 0 |
| Honey Butter Spread, 1 Tbsp | 70 | 6 | 4 |

### Butter & Butter Blends

*Per 1 Tablespoon*

| | C | F | Cb |
|---|---|---|---|
| **Challenge:** Stick, 0.5 oz | 100 | 11 | 0 |
| Tub, Whipped, 0.3 oz | 70 | 7 | 0 |
| **Brummel & Brown,** | | | |
| Spread Made with Yogurt, 0.5oz | 45 | 5 | 0 |
| **Land O'Lakes:** | | | |
| **Sticks,** Original, 0.5oz | 100 | 11 | 0 |
| **Tubs,** Butter With Olive Oil, 0.5 oz | 90 | 10 | 0 |
| **Smart Balance:** | | | |
| Original Buttery Spread, 0.5 oz | 90 | 10 | 0 |
| Omega-3, 0.5 oz | 80 | 9 | 0 |

### Ghee (Clarified Butter)  C F Cb

(Example ~ *Purity Farms*)
Note: Ghee is 100% fat compared to regular butter (80% fat + 20% water)

| | C | F | Cb |
|---|---|---|---|
| 1 tsp, 0.2 oz | 45 | 5 | 0 |
| 1 Tbsp, 0.5 oz | 120 | 14 | 0 |

### Light & Reduced Fat Spreads

*Per Tablespoon*

| | C | F | Cb |
|---|---|---|---|
| **bestlife,** Buttery Spread, 0.5 oz | 60 | 6 | 0 |
| **Benecol:** Regular, 0.5 oz | 70 | 8 | 0 |
| Light, 0.5 oz | 50 | 5 | 0 |
| **Blue Bonnet:** | | | |
| Stick, Light Spread, 0.5 oz | 50 | 5 | 0.5 |
| Tub, Original Soft Spread, 0.5 oz | 60 | 6 | 0.5 |
| **Country Crock** *(Shedd's)* | | | |
| **Tubs:** Original Spread, 0.5 oz | 50 | 6 | 0 |
| Light Spread, 0.5 oz | 35 | 4 | 0 |
| Churn Style, 0.5 oz | 100 | 11 | 0 |
| **Fleischmann's:** | | | |
| **Original:** Soft Spread, 0.4 oz | 60 | 7 | 0 |
| Spread, 0.5 oz | 80 | 9 | 0 |
| Light Spread, 0.5 oz | 40 | 4.5 | 0 |
| **I Can't Believe It's Not Butter!:** | | | |
| **Tubs:** Original Spread, 0.5 oz | 60 | 6 | 0 |
| Light, 0.5 oz | 40 | 4 | 0 |
| Olive Oil Spread, 1 Tbsp | 60 | 6 | 0 |
| **Parkay:** | | | |
| Original Spread, 0.4 oz | 70 | 7 | 0 |
| Spray, 5 sprays | 0 | 0 | 0 |
| Squeeze Bottle, 0.5 oz | 70 | 8 | 0 |
| **Promise:** | | | |
| Activ, Spread, 0.5 oz | 45 | 5 | 0 |
| Buttery Spread, 0.5 oz | 80 | 8 | 0 |
| Light Spread, 0.5 oz | 45 | 5 | 0 |
| **Smart Balance:** | | | |
| **Tubs,** Buttery Spread: | | | |
| Original, 0.5 oz | 90 | 10 | 0 |
| HeartRight, Light, 0.5 oz | 50 | 5 | 0 |
| Light with Flaxseed Oil. 0.5 oz | 50 | 5 | 0 |
| Omega 3: Reg., 0.5 oz | 80 | 9 | 0 |
| Light, 0.5 oz | 50 | 5 | 0 |

### Butter Substitutes

| | C | F | Cb |
|---|---|---|---|
| **Butter Buds:** | | | |
| **Butter Flavored:** Mix, 1 tsp | 5 | 0 | 2 |
| Sprinkles, 1 tsp | 5 | 0 | 2 |
| **Earth Balance,** | | | |
| Original, 1 Tbsp | 100 | 11 | 0 |
| **Molly McButter,** 1 tsp | 5 | 0 | 1 |
| **Sunsweet,** (Butter/Oil Replacement), | | | |
| Lighter Bake, 1 Tbsp, 0.7 oz | 35 | 0 | 9 |

## Animal Fats/Lards **C** **F** **Cb**

*Average All Types*
**Beef Tallow/Drippings, Lard (Pork),**
**Chicken, Duck, Goose, Turkey:**

| | | |
|---|---|---|
| 1 Tbsp, 0.5 oz | **115** 13 | 0 |
| 2.25 Tbsp, 1 oz | **255** 28 | 0 |
| 1 cup, 7.3 oz | **1850** 205 | 0 |
| ½ pound, 8 oz | **2040** 227 | 0 |

**Ghee/Butter/ Oil** ~ *See Page 93*

## Vegetable Shortening

*Average All Types*

| | | |
|---|---|---|
| 1 Tbsp, 0.5 oz | **115** 13 | 0 |
| 2.25 Tbsp, 1 oz | **250** 28 | 0 |
| 1 cup, 7.3 oz | **1810** 205 | 0 |

## Vegetable Oils

Includes almond, avocado, canola, corn, coconut, flaxseed, grapeseed, linseed, mustard, olive, palm, peanut, rice bran, safflower, sesame, sunflower, soybean, wheat germ. Note: Oil is 100% fat.

| | | |
|---|---|---|
| 1 tsp, 0.2 oz | **45** 5 | 0 |
| 1 Tbsp, 0.5 oz | **120** 14 | 0 |
| 2 Tbsp, 1 oz | **240** 28 | 0 |
| 1 cup, 7.3 oz | **1930** 205 | 0 |

## Fish Oils

*Average All Types*
(Includes Cod Liver, Herring, Salmon, Sardines): 1 Tbsp, 0.5 oz    **125**   14   0

## Cooking Sprays/Squeezes

Cooking Sprays: (PAM, Mazola, I Can't Believe It's Not Butter, Weight Watchers, Wesson):

| | | | |
|---|---|---|---|
| *Pam:* ¼ second spray | **2** | 0 | 0 |
| 1-3 second spray | **6** | 1 | 0 |
| *I Can't Believe It's Not Butter,* | | | |
| Original Spray | **0** | 0 | 0 |
| *Parkay,* Buttery Spray | **0** | 0 | 0 |

## Olestra (Olean) **C** **F** **Cb**

**Olestra** *(Olean)*    0    0    0
Note: Olean is Proctor & Gamble's brand name for Olestra – a no-calorie cooking oil that gives snacks (like potato chips, tortilla chips and crackers) taste and texture without adding fat or calories.
**Examples:**
• *Frito-Lay,* Light Products
  *(Lays, Ruffles, Tostitos, Doritos)*
• *Pringles,* Fat-Free Potato Crisps

## Quick Guide

### Mayonnaise: **C** **F** **Cb**

**Regular:** *Per 1 Tbsp, 0.5 oz Unless Indicated*

| | C | F | Cb |
|---|---|---|---|
| Average All Brands | 90 | 10 | 0 |
| ***Best Foods; Hellman's; Kraft:*** | | | |
| Original/Real | 90 | 10 | 0 |
| ½ cup, 4 oz | 720 | 80 | 0 |
| ***Hain,*** Safflower Mayonnaise | 100 | 11 | 0 |
| ***Spectrum,*** Canola Mayo | 100 | 11 | 0 |

**Light/Reduced Fat:** *Per 1 Tbsp, 0.5 oz*

| | C | F | Cb |
|---|---|---|---|
| ***Best Foods/Hellman's*** | 35 | 3.5 | 1 |
| ***Kraft,*** Light/Olive Oil | 35 | 3 | 1 |
| ***Smart Balance,*** Omega | 50 | 5 | 0 |
| ***Spectrum,*** Light Canola Mayo, | | | |
| Eggless | 35 | 3.5 | 0.5 |

**Fat Free:**

| | C | F | Cb |
|---|---|---|---|
| ***Kraft:*** Original, 1 Tbsp | 10 | 0 | 2 |
| ½ cup, 4 oz | 80 | 0 | 16 |

**Sugar Free:**

| | C | F | Cb |
|---|---|---|---|
| ***Dukes Mayo,*** 1 Tbsp | 100 | 12 | 0 |

### Mayonnaise Style Dressing:
*Per 1 Tbsp, 0.5 oz*

| | C | F | Cb |
|---|---|---|---|
| ***Best Foods,*** Sandwich Spread | 60 | 5 | 2 |
| ***Kraft:*** | | | |
| Miracle Whip Dressing: | | | |
| Original | 40 | 3.5 | 1 |
| Light | 20 | 1.5 | 1 |
| Fat Free | 15 | 0 | 3 |
| Mayo: | | | |
| Chipotle | 35 | 3 | 1 |
| Horseradish-Dijon | 35 | 3 | 1 |
| Sandwich Shop, Hot & Spicy | 100 | 11 | 0 |
| ***Nasoya,*** Egg & Dairy Free: | | | |
| Nayonaise: Regular/Whipped | 40 | 3.5 | 1 |
| Light | 20 | 1.5 | 1 |
| ***Sir Kensington's,*** Egg/Dairy Free | | | |
| Fabanaise (Vegan Mayo) | 90 | 10 | 0 |

## Quick Guide

**C** **F** **Cb**

### Fresh Fish

**Low Oil:** *Less than 2.5% fat*
**White/Lightly-colored flesh. Examples:**
Cod, Flounder, Haddock, Halibut, Mahi Mahi, Perch, Pike, Pollock, Snapper, Sole, Whiting.

| | C | F | Cb |
|---|---|---|---|
| **Raw,** without bones, 4 oz | 100 | 1 | 0 |
| **Steamed,** Broiled, Baked, 4 oz | 140 | 1.5 | 0 |
| **Fried:** Lightly Floured, 4 oz | 210 | 8 | 3.5 |
| Breaded, 4 oz | 260 | 12 | 8 |
| In Batter, 4 oz 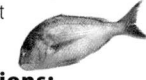 | 320 | 16 | 27 |

**Medium Oil:** *2.5-5% fat*
**Lightly-colored flesh. Examples:**
Bluefin Tuna, Catfish, Kingfish, Orange Roughy, Salmon (Pink), Swordfish, Rainbow Trout, Yellowtail.

| | C | F | Cb |
|---|---|---|---|
| **Raw,** without bones, 4 oz | 145 | 7 | 0 |
| **Baked/Broiled,** 4 oz | 195 | 8 | 0 |
| **Fried,** 4 oz | 230 | 11 | 8 |

**High Oil:** *Over 5% fat*
**Darker-colored flesh. Examples:**
Albacore Tuna, Mackerel, Salmon (Atlantic/Chinook/Sockeye), Sardines, Trout.

| | C | F | Cb |
|---|---|---|---|
| **Raw,** without bones, 4 oz | 220 | 14 | 0 |
| **Baked,** Broiled, 4 oz | 275 | 17 | 0 |
| **Fried,** 4 oz | 340 | 23 | 12 |

### Cooking Yields (Fin Fish):
4 oz Raw wt. = 3.5 oz Cooked weight
4 oz Cooked wt. = 5 oz Raw weight

### Calorie & Fat Variations:
The amount of fat/oil in fish varies with the species, season and locality. Within the same fish, fat/oil content is generally higher towards the head.

## Fish & Shellfish

*Edible Weights: (no bones/shell)*

| | C | F | Cb |
|---|---|---|---|
| **Abalone:** Raw, 3 oz | 90 | 0.5 | 5 |
| Fried, 3 oz | 160 | 6 | 9.5 |
| **Ahi Tuna,** grilled, 6 oz fillet (w/o fat) | 235 | 2 | 0 |
| **Anchovy:** Paste, 1 Tbsp, 0.5 oz | 45 | 3 | 0 |
| Canned in oil, drained, (5 ), 0.7 oz | 40 | 2 | 0 |
| **Barracuda (Pacific),** raw, 4 oz | 130 | 3 | 0 |
| **Basa/Swai,** raw, 4 oz fillet | 70 | 2 | 0 |
| **Bass:** | | | |
| Sea: Raw, 4.6 oz fillet | 125 | 2.5 | 0 |
| Baked, 3 oz | 105 | 2 | 0 |
| Striped: Raw, 1 fillet, 5.5 oz | 150 | 3.5 | 0 |
| Baked, 3 oz | 105 | 3 | 0 |
| Freshwater: Raw, 3 oz | 95 | 3 | 0 |
| Baked, 3 oz | 125 | 4 | 0 |

## Fish & Shellfish (Cont)

**C** **F** **Cb**

*Edible Weights: (no bones/shell)*

| | C | F | Cb |
|---|---|---|---|
| **Calamari/Squid:** | | | |
| Raw, 4 oz | 100 | 1.5 | 3.5 |
| Baked, 1 cup | 190 | 6.5 | 5.5 |
| Fried, 3 oz | 150 | 6 | 7 |
| **Catfish:** | | | |
| Farmed: Raw, 1 fillet 5.6 oz | 190 | 9.5 | 0 |
| Baked, 1 fillet 5 oz | 205 | 10 | 0 |
| Wild: Raw, 1 fillet, 5.6 oz | 150 | 4.5 | 0 |
| Baked, 1 fillet, 5 oz | 150 | 4 | 0 |
| Breaded, fried, 1 fillet, 3 oz | 200 | 12 | 0 |
| **Caviar,** black/red, 1 Tbsp, 16g | 40 | 3 | 0.5 |
| **Clams:** Raw (4 large/9 small), 3 oz | 70 | 1 | 3 |
| Breaded, Fried (20 small), 6.6 oz | 380 | 21 | 20 |
| Canned, drained, ½ cup, 2.8 oz | 115 | 1 | 0 |
| Steamed (10 small), 3.3 oz | 140 | 2 | 5 |
| **Clam Juice** *(Snow's)*, 1 Tbsp | 0 | 0 | 0 |
| **Cod:** | | | |
| Atlantic: Raw, 4 oz | 95 | 1 | 0 |
| Baked, 3 oz | 90 | 1 | 0 |
| Canned, solids & liquid | 90 | 0.5 | 0 |
| Pacific: Raw, 4 oz | 80 | 0.5 | 0 |
| Baked, 3 oz | 70 | 0.5 | 0 |
| **Crab:** | | | |
| Alaska King, 1 leg, cooked, 4.7 oz | 130 | 2 | 0 |
| Blue: Raw, 1 crab, 6 oz | 150 | 1 | 0 |
| Steamed, 3 oz | 70 | 0.5 | 0 |
| Canned, drained, 6.5 oz can | 105 | 0.5 | 0 |
| Dungeness: Raw, 1 crab, 5.8 oz | 140 | 1.5 | 0 |
| Steamed, 4.45 oz | 140 | 1.5 | 0 |
| **Crab Cakes** *(Capt. D's)*, (1), 2.8 oz | 250 | 16 | 16 |
| **Crayfish:** | | | |
| Farmed: Raw, 3 oz | 60 | 1 | 0 |
| Steamed, 3 oz | 75 | 1 | 0 |
| Wild: Raw 3 oz | 65 | 1 | 0 |
| Steamed, 3 oz | 70 | 1 | 0 |
| **Cuttlefish,** raw, 3 oz | 70 | 1 | 1 |
| **Dolphinfish** ~ *See Mahi-Mahi* | | | |
| **Eel:** Raw, 3 oz | 155 | 10 | 0 |
| Baked, 3 oz | 200 | 13 | 0 |
| **Fish & Chips** *(Red Lobster)*, battered, without condiments | 630 | 26 | 54 |
| **Fish Sandwich** *(Burger King)*, without Tartar Sauce | 410 | 12 | 53 |
| **Fish Oil,** 1 Tbsp, 0.5 oz | 125 | 14 | 0 |
| **Flounder/Sole:** | | | |
| Raw, 4 oz | 80 | 2 | 0 |
| Baked, 3 oz | 75 | 2 | 0 |
| **Frozen Fish** ~ *See Pages 114-122* | | | |

| Fish & Shellfish (Cont) | **C** | **F** | **Cb** |
|---|---|---|---|

*Edible Weights: Without Bones or Shell*

| | **C** | **F** | **Cb** |
|---|---|---|---|
| **Haddock:** Raw, 4 oz | 85 | 0.5 | 0 |
| Baked, 3 oz | 75 | 0.5 | 0 |
| Smoked, 3 oz | 100 | 1 | 0 |
| **Halibut:** | | | |
| Atlantic: Raw, 4 oz | 105 | 1.5 | 0 |
| Baked, ½ fillet, 5.6 oz | 175 | 2.5 | 0 |
| **Herring:** | | | |
| Atlantic, raw, 4 oz | 180 | 10 | 0 |
| Canned: Plain, drained, 3 oz | 130 | 8 | 0 |
| In Tomato Sauce, 3.5 oz | 140 | 8 | 2 |
| Pickled, 2 pieces, 1 oz | 75 | 5 | 3 |
| Smoked, kippered, 4 oz | 245 | 14 | 0 |
| **Jellyfish:** Raw, 4 oz | 30 | 0 | 0 |
| Dried, Salted, 1 cup, 2 oz | 20 | 1 | 0 |
| **Ling,** raw, 4 oz | 100 | 0.5 | 0 |
| **Lobster,** Northern: | | | |
| 1.5 lb Whole Lobster, edible portion: | | | |
| Raw, 6.3 oz | 140 | 1.5 | 0 |
| Boiled, 5 oz | 140 | 1 | 0 |
| Lobster Salads, average, ½ cup | 220 | 13 | 5 |
| Lobster Newberg, average, ¾ cup | 360 | 20 | 9 |
| Lobster Thermidor, av., 1 serving | 370 | 22 | 15 |
| **Lobster Tail,** | | | |
| *Red Lobster,* grilled/roasted | 170 | 1 | 1 |
| **Lox,** Regular/Nova, 2 oz | 65 | 2.5 | 0 |
| **Mackerel,** Atlantic: Raw, 4 oz | 230 | 16 | 0 |
| Baked, 3 oz fillet | 225 | 15 | 0 |
| Pacific/Jack: Raw, 4 oz | 180 | 9 | 0 |
| Baked, 3 oz | 170 | 9 | 0 |
| Spanish: Raw, 4 oz | 160 | 7 | 0 |
| Baked, 3 oz | 135 | 5.5 | 0 |
| **Mahi-Mahi/Dolphinfish:** | | | |
| Raw, 4 oz | 95 | 1 | 0 |
| Baked, 4 oz | 125 | 1 | 0 |
| **Monkfish:** Raw, 4 oz | 85 | 1.5 | 0 |
| Baked, 3 oz | 80 | 2 | 0 |
| **Mullet, Striped:** Raw, 4 oz | 135 | 4.5 | 0 |
| Baked, 3 oz | 130 | 4 | 0 |
| **Mussels:** | | | |
| Raw: 4 oz (edible wt) | 100 | 2.5 | 4 |
| 1 cup, 5.3 oz (edible weight) | 130 | 3.5 | 5 |
| Cooked, moist heat, 3 oz | 150 | 4 | 6 |
| **Ocean Perch:** | | | |
| Atlantic: Raw, 4 oz | 90 | 2 | 0 |
| Baked, 3 oz | 80 | 1.5 | 0 |
| **Octopus:** | | | |
| Common: Raw, 4 oz | 95 | 1 | 2.5 |
| Boiled, 3 oz | 140 | 2 | 4 |
| **Orange Roughy:** | | | |
| Raw, 4 oz | 85 | 1 | 0 |
| Baked, 3 oz | 90 | 1 | 0 |

| Fish & Shellfish (Cont) | **C** | **F** | **Cb** |
|---|---|---|---|

*Edible Weights: Without Bones or Shell*

| | **C** | **F** | **Cb** |
|---|---|---|---|
| **Oysters,** Common, Raw, 3 oz | 70 | 2 | 4 |
| Eastern: | | | |
| Farmed: Raw, 6 medium, 3 oz | 50 | 1.5 | 4.5 |
| Cooked, dry heat, 6 med., 2 oz | 45 | 1.5 | 4.5 |
| Wild: Raw, 6 medium, 3 oz | 45 | 1.5 | 2.5 |
| Cooked, dry heat, 6 med., 2 oz | 45 | 1.5 | 2.5 |
| Breaded & Fried, 6 med., 3 oz | 175 | 11 | 10 |
| Pacific: Raw, 1 medium, 1.8 oz | 40 | 1 | 2.5 |
| Steamed, 1 medium, 0.8 oz | 40 | 1 | 2.5 |
| **Perch ~** *See Ocean Perch* | | | |
| **Pike:** Northern: Raw, 4 oz | 100 | 1 | 0 |
| Baked, 3 oz | 95 | 1 | 0 |
| Walleye: Raw, 4 oz | 105 | 1.5 | 0 |
| Baked, 3 oz | 100 | 1.5 | 0 |
| **Pollock,** Atlantic: Raw, 4 oz | 105 | 1 | 0 |
| Baked, 3 oz | 100 | 1 | 0 |
| **Pompano,** Florida, raw, 4 oz | 185 | 11 | 0 |
| **Red Snapper ~** *See Snapper* | | | |
| Roe, raw, 2 Tbsp, 1 oz | 40 | 2 | 0.5 |
| **Sablefish:** Raw, 4 oz | 220 | 17 | 0 |
| Smoked, 3 oz | 220 | 17 | 0 |
| **Salmon:** | | | |
| Atlantic, Farmed: Raw, 4 oz | 235 | 15 | 0 |
| Baked, 3 oz | 175 | 10 | 0 |
| Steaks: Raw, 7 oz | 410 | 27 | 0 |
| Baked, 6 oz | 365 | 22 | 0 |
| Atlantic, Wild: Raw, 4 oz | 160 | 7 | 0 |
| Baked, 3 oz | 155 | 7 | 0 |
| Steaks: Raw, 7 oz | 280 | 13 | 0 |
| Baked, 6 oz | 310 | 14 | 0 |
| Chinook: Raw, 4 oz | 205 | 12 | 0 |
| Baked, 3 oz | 195 | 11 | 0 |
| Smoked, 3 oz | 100 | 3.5 | 0 |
| King: Raw, 3.5 oz | 185 | 12 | 0 |
| Kippered, 3.5 oz piece | 265 | 16 | 0 |
| Smoked & canned, 3.5 oz | 150 | 6 | 0 |
| Coho: | | | |
| Farmed: Raw, 4 oz | 180 | 8.5 | 0 |
| Baked, 3 oz | 150 | 7 | 0 |
| Wild: Raw, 4 oz | 165 | 6.5 | 0 |
| Steamed, 3 oz | 155 | 6.5 | 0 |
| Pink/Chum: Raw, 4 oz | 145 | 5 | 0 |
| Baked, 3.5 oz | 155 | 5.5 | 0 |
| Canned: Drained solids, 11 oz | 435 | 16 | 0 |
| Without skin & bones, 8.5 oz | 330 | 10 | 0 |
| Sockeye: Raw, 4 oz | 160 | 6.5 | 0 |
| Baked, 3 oz | 145 | 5.5 | 0 |
| Canned, Drained solids, 3 oz | 140 | 6.5 | 0 |
| Smoked, 3.5 oz | 205 | 7.5 | 0 |
| Salmon Cake (1), 3 oz | 240 | 15 | 6 |

## Fish & Shellfish (Cont)

| | C | F | Cb |
|---|---|---|---|
| **Sardines:** *Canned, Average all Brands* | | | |
| Drained of Oil: | | | |
| ¼ cup drained, 2.2 oz | 130 | 9 | 0 |
| 3.75 oz can, drained, 3.3 oz | 190 | 11 | 0 |
| 1 large/2 medium, ⅜", 0.8 oz | 50 | 3 | 0 |
| In Tomato Sauce, 3.8 oz | 150 | 8 | 3 |
| **Sashimi** ~ *See Japanese Foods, Page 171* | | | |
| **Scallops:** Raw, 6 lge/15 small, 3 oz | 65 | 0.5 | 3 |
| Breaded, Fried (6), 5 oz | 385 | 20 | 39 |
| Steamed, 3 oz | 95 | 0.5 | 0 |
| **Sea Bass** ~ *See Bass* | | | |
| **Seafood Salad,** Deli Style, | | | |
| ½ cup, 3.5 oz | 250 | 21 | 11 |
| **Shark:** Raw, 4 oz | 145 | 5 | 0 |
| Baked, 4 oz | 185 | 7 | 0 |
| Batter-dipped, fried, 4 oz | 260 | 16 | 7 |
| **Shrimp:** | | | |
| Raw: Small/Medium (4), 0.8 oz | 15 | 0 | 0 |
| Large (4), 1 oz | 20 | 0 | 0 |
| Breaded & Fried, 4.8 oz | 395 | 24 | 27 |
| Steamed, in shell, 3 oz | 100 | 1.5 | 0 |
| Canned, 1 can, 4.5 oz | 130 | 2 | 0 |
| **Snapper:** Raw, 4 oz | 115 | 1.5 | 0 |
| Baked: 3 oz | 110 | 1.5 | 0 |
| 6 oz fillet | 220 | 3 | 0 |
| **Sole:** Raw, 4 oz | 80 | 2 | 0 |
| Baked, 3 oz | 75 | 2 | 0 |
| **Squid** ~ *see Calamari* | | | |
| **Surimi,** (Imitation Crab), 4 oz | 110 | 0.5 | 17 |
| **Swai/Basa,** raw, 4 oz | 70 | 2 | 0 |
| **Swordfish:** Raw, 4 oz | 165 | 7.5 | 0 |
| Medium Steak, 6 oz | 250 | 11 | 0 |
| Baked: Small Steak, 4 oz | 205 | 7 | 0 |
| Medium Steak, 6 oz | 290 | 13 | 0 |
| **Tilapia:** Raw, 4 oz | 110 | 2 | 0 |
| Baked: 3 oz | 110 | 2.5 | 0 |
| **Trout,** Rainbow: | | | |
| Farmed: Raw, 4 oz | 160 | 7 | 0 |
| Baked, 3 oz | 145 | 6.5 | 0 |
| Wild: Raw, 4 oz | 135 | 4 | 0 |
| Baked, 3 oz | 130 | 5 | 0 |
| **Tuna:** | | | |
| **Raw:** Bluefin, 4 oz | 165 | 5.5 | 0 |
| Skipjack, Yellowfin, av., 4 oz | 120 | 1 | 0 |
| **Baked:** Bluefin, 3 oz | 155 | 5.5 | 0 |
| Skipjack, Yellowfin, av., 3 oz | 110 | 1 | 0 |
| **Canned:** *In Water, drained* | | | |
| Chunk Light: 2 oz | 50 | 1 | 0 |
| 3 oz can | 75 | 1.5 | 1 |
| 5 oz can | 125 | 2.5 | 1.5 |

| | C | F | Cb |
|---|---|---|---|
| **Tuna (Cont):** *In Water, drained (Cont)* | | | |
| Solid White: 2 oz | 60 | 0.5 | 0 |
| 5 oz can | 150 | 1.5 | 0 |
| 7 oz can | 210 | 2 | 0 |
| In Oil, drained: | | | |
| Chunk Light: 2 oz can | 80 | 4 | 0 |
| 5 oz can | 200 | 10 | 0 |
| Solid White: 2 oz can | 90 | 4 | 0 |
| 6 oz can | 270 | 12 | 0 |
| **Whitefish:** Raw, 4 oz | 150 | 6.5 | 0 |
| Baked, 3 oz | 145 | 6.5 | 1 |
| Smoked, 3 oz | 90 | 1 | 0 |
| **Whiting:** Raw, 4 oz | 100 | 1.5 | 0 |
| Baked, 3 oz | 100 | 1.5 | 0 |
| **Yellowtail:** Raw, 4 oz | 165 | 6 | 0 |
| Grilled, 3 oz | 160 | 6 | 0 |

## Other Canned/Packaged Fish

| | C | F | Cb |
|---|---|---|---|
| **Bumble Bee:** *Drained* | | | |
| **Mackerel,** in oil, skinless & boneless, | | | |
| drained, 1.9 oz | 160 | 15 | 0 |
| **Pink Salmon,** Skinless & Boneless, | | | |
| drained, 2 oz | 60 | 1.5 | 0 |
| **Red Salmon,** 2.2 oz | 100 | 5 | 0 |
| **Sardines,** in Olive Oil, drained, 3 oz | 210 | 15 | 0 |
| **Tuna Ready-To-Eat Kits:** *With Crackers:* | | | |
| Sensations, Tuna Medley: | | | |
| Tom. & Basil, 3 oz can & 3oz Crackers | 150 | 2.5 | 16 |
| Thai Chili, 3 oz can & 3Oz Crackers | 180 | 2.5 | 23 |
| **Tuna, Snack on the Run!:** *With Crackers Kit* | | | |
| Tuna Salad, 2.9 oz can, w/- Crackers | 300 | 23 | 18 |
| Tuna, Fat Free w/ Wheat Crackers, | | | |
| 2.9 oz | 130 | 2.5 | 20 |
| **Tuna, White Albacore:** | | | |
| Pouch, in water, 2 oz | 70 | 1.5 | 0 |
| Solid, in Oil, drained, 2 oz | 80 | 2.5 | 0 |
| **Chicken of the Sea:** | | | |
| Pink Salmon, skinless/boneless, | | | |
| 2.5 oz pouch | 70 | 2 | 0 |
| Sardines, in Oil, Smoked, 3.75 oz can | 150 | 10 | 0 |
| Tuna: Lunch Solutions, | | | |
| Tuna Salad Cup & Crackers, 3.4 oz | 80 | 0.5 | 7 |
| To-Go-Cups, Tuna Salad, 2.8 oz | 80 | 0.5 | 7 |
| **Starkist:** | | | |
| **Pouch:** *Per 2.6 oz Pouch* | | | |
| Albacore White Tuna in water | 80 | 1.5 | 0 |
| Chunk, Light, Tuna in water | 70 | 0.5 | 0 |
| **Lunch-To-Go Kit,** Chunk Light Tuna | | | |
| With Light Mayo & Crackers, 4 oz | 230 | 9 | 20 |
| **Tuna Creations:** *Per 2.6 oz* | | | |
| Herb & Garlic | 110 | 4 | 2 |
| Lemon Pepper | 80 | 0.5 | 1 |

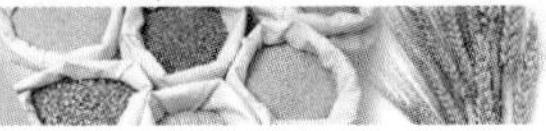

| Flours & Grains | C | F | Cb |
|---|---|---|---|
| **Amaranth Flour**, ½ cup, 3.5 oz | 365 | 6.5 | 65 |
| **Arrowroot Flour**, ½ cup, 2.3 oz | 230 | 0 | 56 |
| **Barley:** Grain, regular, ½ cup, 2.6 oz | 255 | 1 | 55 |
| Pearled, raw, 3.5 oz | 350 | 1 | 78 |
| **Buckwheat:** Grain, ½ cup, 3 oz | 290 | 3 | 61 |
| Flour, whole-groat, ½ cup, 2 oz | 200 | 2 | 42 |
| Groats: Rstd, dry, ½ cup, 3 oz | 285 | 2 | 62 |
| Roasted, cooked, 3.5 oz | 80 | 0.5 | 17 |
| **Bulgur:** Dry, ½ cup, 2.5 oz | 240 | 1 | 53 |
| Cooked, ½ cup, 3.2 oz | 75 | 0.5 | 17 |
| **Carob Flour**, ½ cup, 1.8 oz | 115 | 0.5 | 46 |
| **Corn Kernels**, cooked, av., ½ cup | 80 | 0.5 | 18 |
| **Corn Bran**, ½ cup, 1.3 oz | 85 | 0.5 | 33 |
| **Corn Flour/Masa**, ½ cup, 2 oz | 215 | 2.5 | 43 |
| **Corn Grits:** | | | |
| Dry, ½ cup, 2.8oz | 290 | 1 | 62 |
| Cooked, ½ cup, 4.3 oz | 70 | 0.5 | 15 |
| **Corn Germ**, toasted, ½ cup, 4 oz | 100 | 1.5 | 22 |
| **Cornmeal**, average all varieties: | | | |
| 3 Tbsp, 1 oz | 105 | 0.5 | 22 |
| ½ cup, 2.5 oz | 255 | 1 | 54 |
| Mixes, same as above | 230 | 1 | 48 |
| **Cornstarch:** 1 Tbsp, 0.3 oz | 30 | 0 | 8 |
| ½ cup, 2.3oz | 245 | 0 | 58 |
| **Couscous:** Dry, 1 oz | 110 | 0 | 22 |
| 1 cup cooked, 5.5 oz | 175 | 0.5 | 37 |
| **Farina:** Dry, ½ cup, 3 oz | 325 | 0.5 | 69 |
| Cooked, ½ cup, 4 oz | 55 | 0 | 12 |
| **Flaxseed:** Whole, 1 T., 0.3 oz | 45 | 3.5 | 2 |
| Ground, 2 Tbsp, 0.3 oz | 60 | 4.5 | 4 |
| **Garbanzo**, (Chick Pea), ½ cup, 1.6 oz | 180 | 3 | 27 |
| **Gluten Free Flour**, 3 Tbsp | 100 | 0 | 24 |
| **Matzo Meal**, ½ cup, 2.2 oz | 230 | 0.5 | 48 |
| **Millet:** Raw, ½ cup, 3.5 oz | 380 | 4 | 73 |
| Cooked, ½ cup, 3 oz | 105 | 1 | 21 |
| **Oat Bran:** Raw, ⅓ cup, 1 oz | 75 | 2 | 21 |
| Cooked, ½ cup, 3.8 oz | 45 | 1 | 13 |
| **Oats**, Rolled/Oatmeal: | | | |
| Dry/Groats, ½ cup, 1.5 oz | 160 | 3 | 28 |
| Cooked, ½ cup, 4.2 oz | 75 | 1 | 13 |
| **Polenta** ~ *See Cornmeal* | | | |
| **Potato Flour**, ½ cup, 2.8 oz | 285 | 0.5 | 66 |
| **Psyllium Husks**, 1 Tbsp, 0.2 oz | 10 | 0 | 4 |
| **Quinoa:** Dry ½ cup, 3 oz | 320 | 5 | 59 |
| Cooked, ½ cup, 3.8 oz | 130 | 2 | 24 |
| **Rice Bran**, ½ cup, 2 oz | 180 | 12 | 28 |
| **Rice Flour**, ½ cup, 2.8 oz | 290 | 1 | 63 |

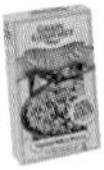

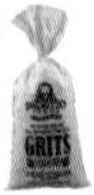

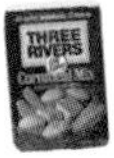

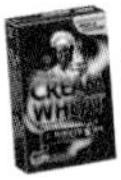

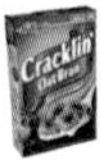

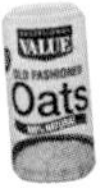

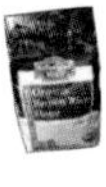

| Flours & Grains (Cont) | C | F | Cb |
|---|---|---|---|
| **Rice Polish**, ½ cup, 3.5 oz | 360 | 0.5 | 80 |
| **Rye Flour:** | | | |
| Dark, ½ cup, 2.3 oz | 210 | 2 | 44 |
| Light, ½ cup, 1.8 oz | 190 | 1 | 41 |
| Medium, ½ cup, 1.8 oz | 180 | 1 | 40 |
| **Rye Grain:** ½ cup, 3 oz | 280 | 2 | 59 |
| Flakes, ¼ cup, 1 oz | 100 | 0.5 | 21 |
| **Semolina Flour**, ½ cup, 3 oz | 300 | 1 | 61 |
| **Sorghum**, ½ cup, 3.4 oz | 325 | 3 | 72 |
| **Soy Flour:** | | | |
| Defatted, 1 cup, 3.5 oz | 330 | 1 | 38 |
| Low-Fat, 1 cup, 3 oz | 325 | 6 | 33 |
| Full-Fat, 1 cup, 3 oz | 365 | 17 | 29 |
| **Soy Meal**, defatted, 1 cup, 4.3 oz | 415 | 3 | 49 |
| **Spelt Flour**, ½ cup, 2 oz | 190 | 1 | 41 |
| **Tapioca Pearl:** | | | |
| Dry, ½ cup, 2.7 oz | 270 | 0 | 67 |
| 3 Tbsp, 1 oz | 100 | 0 | 25 |
| **Teff Seed Flour**, 2 oz | 215 | 2 | 42 |
| **Tortilla Flour Mix**, | | | |
| ½ cup, 2 oz | 220 | 6 | 37 |
| **Triticale:** | | | |
| ½ cup, 3.4 oz | 325 | 2 | 70 |
| Flour, wholegrain, ½ cup, 2.3 oz | 220 | 1 | 48 |
| **Wheat Bran**, unprocessed, ½ cup, 1 oz | 65 | 1 | 19 |
| **Wheat Flakes**, ½ cup, 1.5 oz | 160 | 1 | 35 |
| **Wheat Germ:** | | | |
| Raw, ¼ cup, 1 oz | 105 | 3 | 15 |
| Toasted, ¼ cup, 1 oz | 110 | 3 | 14 |
| **Wheat Flour:** | | | |
| White, All Purpose/Self-Rising: | | | |
| 1 level Tbsp, 0.3 oz | 30 | 0 | 6 |
| ½ cup, 2.2 oz | 230 | 0.5 | 48 |
| 1 cup, 4.4 oz | 455 | 1.5 | 95 |
| Whole Wheat, 1 cup, 4.2 oz | 405 | 2 | 87 |

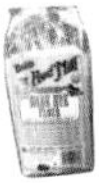

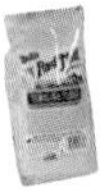

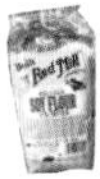

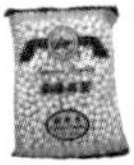

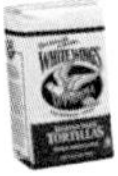

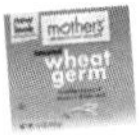

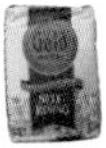

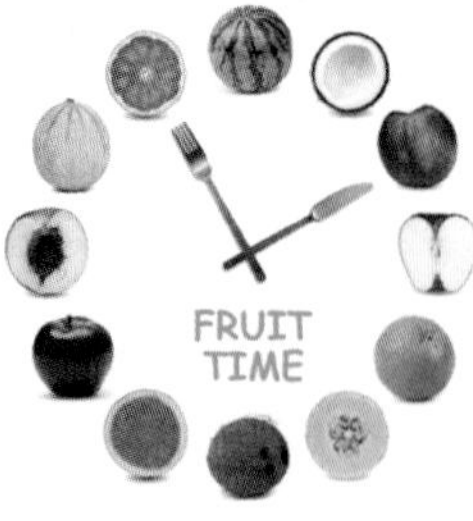

FRUIT TIME

## Fruit ~ Fresh

| | C | F | Cb |
|---|---|---|---|
| *Weights As Purchased* | | | |
| **Apples**, all varieties, average: | | | |
| Whole, with skin: 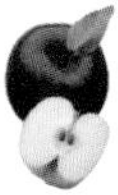 | | | |
| 1 small, 4 oz | 55 | 0 | 14 |
| 1 medium, 5.5 oz | 75 | 0 | 19 |
| 1 large, 8 oz | 110 | 0 | 28 |
| 1 extra large, 11 oz | 145 | 0 | 36 |
| Flesh only, no skin or core: 1 oz | 15 | 0 | 3.5 |
| Slices, 1 cup, 4 oz | 55 | 0 | 14 |
| Candy/Caramel Apple, 1 med., 6.5 oz | 245 | 4 | 54 |
| *Chiquita*, Apple Bites, 14 slices, 5 oz | 80 | 0 | 20 |
| **Apricots:** 1 small, 1.5oz 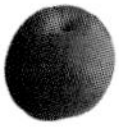 | 20 | 0 | 4 |
| 1 medium, 2 oz | 25 | 0 | 6 |
| 1 large, 3 oz | 40 | 0 | 10 |
| 1 extra large, 4 oz | 50 | 0 | 12 |
| **Asian Pear**, (Nashi Fruit), 1 med., 7 oz | 85 | 0 | 21 |
| **Avocado:** | | | |
| Fuerte (Florida) variety: 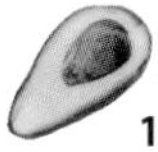 | | | |
| ¼ medium, 2.7 oz pulp | 90 | 7.5 | 6 |
| ½ medium, 5.4 oz pulp | 180 | 15 | 12 |
| Mashed, 2 Tbsp, 1 oz | 35 | 3 | 2 |
| Hass variety (Californian/Mexican): 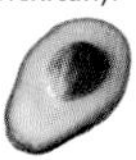 | | | |
| Cubes, ½ cup, 2.5 oz | 120 | 11 | 6 |
| Mashed: 2 Tbsp, 1 oz | 50 | 4 | 2 |
| ¼ cup, 2 oz | 95 | 8 | 5 |
| Pulp: ¼ medium, 1.5 oz | 70 | 6.5 | 3 |
| ½ medium, 3 oz | 140 | 13 | 7 |
| 1 medium (8.5 oz whole), 6 oz | 280 | 26 | 14 |
| Salad slices (3), 1 oz | 50 | 4 | 2 |

Note: The fat of avocados is heart-healthy. Avocados are very low in carbs ~ most is fiber. This benefits blood sugar and cholesterol levels. Use in place of butter and other high-fat spreads.

| | C | F | Cb |
|---|---|---|---|
| **Banana:** | | | |
| Weight with skin: 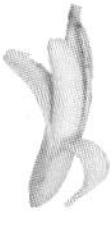 | | | |
| 1 baby, 3 oz | 50 | 0 | 12 |
| 1 small (5"), 4 oz | 65 | 0 | 16 |
| 1 medium (7"), 5 oz | 80 | 0 | 20 |
| 1 large (8"), 8 oz | 120 | 0 | 30 |
| 1 extra large (9"), 9 oz | 135 | 0 | 34 |
| Flesh only, weight without skin: 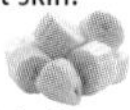 | | | |
| Mashed, ½ cup, 4 oz | 100 | 0 | 25 |
| Slices, ½ cup, 2.5 oz | 65 | 0 | 16 |
| Green Bananas, weight with skin: 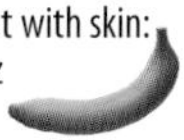 | | | |
| 1 medium (7"), 5 oz | 75 | 0 | 18 |
| 1 large (8"), 7 oz | 110 | 0 | 27 |
| **Blackberries**, 1 cup, 5 oz 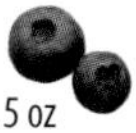 | 60 | 0.5 | 14 |
| **Blueberries:** ¼ cup, 1 oz | 15 | 0 | 4 |
| 1 cup or ½ pint container, 5 oz | 80 | 0 | 20 |
| 1 pint container, 10 oz | 160 | 0 | 40 |

| *Weights As Purchased* | C | F | Cb |
|---|---|---|---|
| **Boysenberries**, 1 cup, 4.5 oz | 60 | 4.5 | 14 |
| **Breadfruit**, ½ cup, 4 oz | 115 | 0 | 30 |
| **Cactus Fruit:** 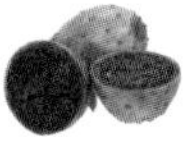 | | | |
| 1 small, 2 oz | 15 | 0 | 4 |
| 1 medium, 5 oz | 40 | 0 | 9 |
| 1 large, 7 oz | 55 | 0 | 13 |
| Pulp, no skin, 1 cup, 5.3 oz | 60 | 0 | 14 |
| **Cantaloupe:** Flesh, without skin, 1 oz | 10 | 0 | 2 |
| Pieces/Balls, 1 cup, 5.5 oz | 55 | 0 | 13 |
| Slices, ½ circle, without rind: 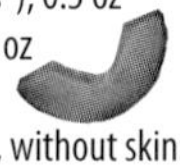 | | | |
| 1 thin (buffet), (⅛"), 0.5 oz | 5 | 0 | 1 |
| 1 medium (¼"), 1 oz | 10 | 0 | 2 |
| 1 thick (½"), 2 oz | 20 | 0 | 5 |
| Wedges, length cut, without skin: | | | |
| 1 thin, 1/16 medium, 2 oz | 20 | 0 | 5 |
| 1 thick, ⅛ medium, 4 oz | 40 | 0 | 9 |
| Whole, weight with seeds and skin: 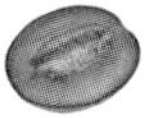 | | | |
| ½ small, 20 oz | 195 | 1 | 46 |
| ½ medium, 28 oz | 270 | 1.5 | 65 |
| ½ large, 2.5 lb | 370 | 2 | 90 |
| **Cape Gooseberries**, 1 cup, 5 oz | 70 | 1 | 15 |
| **Cherimoya:** Pulp, ½ cup, 3 oz | 60 | 0 | 14 |
| 1 Fruit (11 oz), 8 oz edible | 170 | 1 | 40 |
| **Cherries**, (Red/White), sweet, raw: 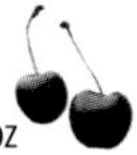 | | | |
| 6 medium or 4 large, 2 oz | 30 | 0 | 7 |
| 1 cup, 4.5 oz | 75 | 0 | 18 |
| ½ lb quantity | 130 | 0 | 32 |
| Sour, red, raw, 1 cup, 4 oz | 50 | 0 | 12 |
| **Clementine**, 1 medium, 2.6 oz | 35 | 0 | 9 |
| **Coconut:** raw: 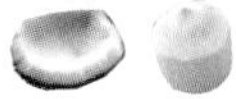 | | | |
| Young, sweet, | | | |
| Pieces: 1 piece (2"x 2"), 1.5 oz | 35 | 2 | 4 |
| ½ cup, 3.5 oz | 80 | 5 | 9 |
| Mature, hard, 1 piece (2"x 2"), 1.5 oz | 160 | 15 | 6 |
| **Crabapples**, slices, ½ cup, 2 oz | 40 | 0 | 11 |
| **Cranberries**, fresh, ¼ cup, 1 oz | 25 | 0 | 6.5 |
| **Custard Apple** ~ *See Cherimoya* | | | |
| **Dates:** Medium (1), 0.3 oz 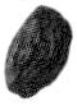 | 20 | 0 | 5 |
| Large Medjool (1), 0.5 oz | 40 | 0 | 10 |
| Extra Large Medjool (1), 0.9 oz | 65 | 0 | 16 |
| Chopped, ½ cup, 3 oz | 240 | 0 | 58 |
| **Dragon Fruit**, (Pitahaya): 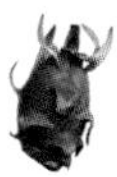 | | | |
| 1 medium, 4"long, 12 oz | 60 | 0 | 12 |
| 1 large, 5"long, 16 oz | 80 | 0 | 18 |
| **Durian**, pulp, 4 oz | 165 | 6 | 31 |
| **Elderberries**, ½ cup, 2.5 oz | 55 | 0.5 | 13 |

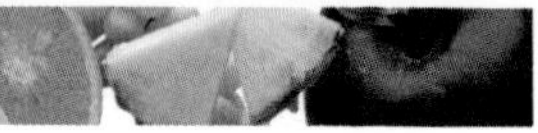

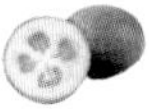

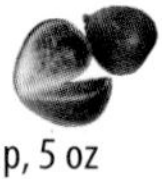

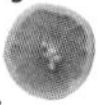

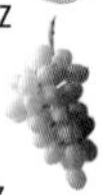

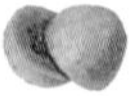

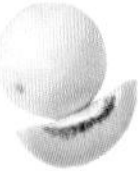

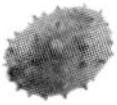

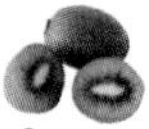

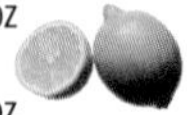

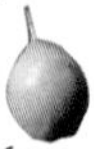

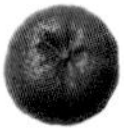

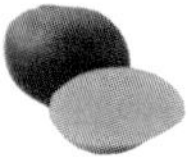

| Weights As Purchased | C | F | Cb |
|---|---|---|---|
| **Feijoa**, (Pineapple Guava), | | | |
| 1 medium, 2 oz | 30 | 0.5 | 5.5 |
| **Figs**, green/black: | | | |
| 1 medium, 2 oz | 40 | 0 | 10 |
| 1 large, 3 oz | 60 | 0 | 15 |
| **Gooseberries**, raw, 1 cup, 5 oz | 65 | 1 | 15 |
| **Grapefruit**, all varieties, average: | | | |
| ½ fruit, 10 oz (6 oz flesh) | 55 | 0 | 13 |
| 1 cup sections w/ juice, 8 oz | 75 | 0 | 18 |
| **Grapes**: Average, 1 cup, 5.5 oz | 105 | 0 | 28 |
| 1 small bunch, 4 oz | 80 | 0 | 20 |
| 1 medium bunch, 7 oz | 140 | 0 | 36 |
| 1 large bunch, 16 oz | 315 | 0 | 82 |
| **Granadilla**, pulp, ½ cup, 4 oz | 110 | 0 | 27 |
| **Guanabana**, pulp, ½ cup, 4 oz | 75 | 0 | 19 |
| **Guava**, 1 medium, 4 oz | 80 | 1 | 16 |
| **Honeydew**: | | | |
| 1 slice, ¾" thick, 3 oz | 30 | 0 | 7 |
| 1 wedge, (⅛ of 7" diameter), | | | |
| 12 oz (with rind) | 80 | 0 | 20 |
| Cubes/Balls, 1 cup, 6 oz | 60 | 0 | 14 |
| ½ small (4½ lb whole) | 180 | 0.5 | 42 |
| ½ medium (6lb whole) | 230 | 1 | 56 |
| **Honey Murcots**, 1 only, 5 oz | 45 | 0 | 11 |
| **Jaboticaba**, 1 cup, 5.5 oz | 55 | 0 | 14 |
| **Jackfruit**, flesh, ⅛, 4 oz | 105 | 0 | 27 |
| **Kiwano**, ½ medium, 5 oz | 35 | 0 | 8 |
| **Kiwifruit**: | | | |
| 1 Medium, 2.7 oz | 45 | 0 | 11 |
| 1 Large, 3.2 oz | 55 | 0 | 13 |
| **Langsat**, Duku, 1 medium, 2 oz | 25 | 0 | 5 |
| **Lemons**: 1 medium, 5oz | 20 | 0 | 4 |
| 1 wedge, 1 oz | 5 | 0 | 1 |
| **Limes**, 1 medium, 2.4 oz | 20 | 0 | 7 |
| **Loganberries**, frozen, ½ cup, 2.5 oz | 40 | 0 | 9 |
| **Longans**, 5 fruit, 0.5oz | 10 | 0 | 2.5 |
| **Loquats**, 4 fruit, 2.3 oz | 30 | 0 | 8 |
| **Lychees**, 4 fruit, 2.3 oz | 30 | 0 | 7 |
| **Mamey Apple**, Cubes, 1 cup, 6 oz | 85 | 1 | 20 |
| **Mandarin Orange:** | | | |
| 1 small, 3 oz | 35 | 0 | 9 |
| 1 medium, 4 oz | 45 | 0 | 11 |
| 1 large, 6 oz | 50 | 0 | 13 |
| **Mango:** | | | |
| Slices, ½ cup, 3 oz | 55 | 0 | 14 |
| 1 small mango, 7 oz | 90 | 0.5 | 24 |
| 1 medium, 10 oz | 130 | 0.5 | 34 |
| Side cheek, 4 oz | 60 | 0 | 14 |
| 1 large, 17 oz | 220 | 1 | 58 |
| 1 extra large, 24 oz | 310 | 1.5 | 82 |
| **Marionberries**, 1 cup, 5 oz | 75 | 1 | 15 |

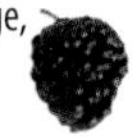

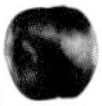

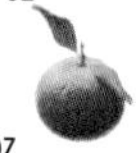

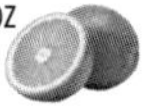

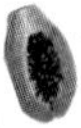

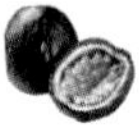

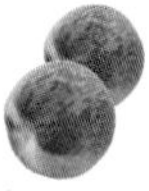

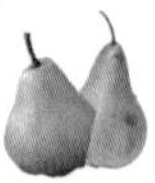

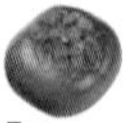

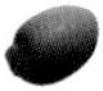

| Weights As Purchased | C | F | Cb |
|---|---|---|---|
| **Melons**, all varieties, average, | | | |
| cubes/balls, 1 cup, 6 oz | 60 | 0 | 14 |
| **Mulberries**, 20 fruit, 1 oz | 15 | 0 | 3 |
| **Nashi Fruit/Asian Pear**, 1 med. 7 oz | 85 | 0 | 21 |
| **Nectarines**: 1 medium, 5oz | 60 | 0 | 14 |
| 1 large, 7 oz | 80 | 0 | 18 |
| **Oheloberries**, ½ cup, 2.5 oz | 20 | 0 | 5 |
| **Olives**, Pickled: Green, 10 lge, 1.5 oz | 60 | 6.5 | 1.5 |
| Ripe, Greek Style, 10 medium, 1 oz | 70 | 6 | 4 |
| Ripe (Black) Californian: | | | |
| 1 small/medium | 5 | 0 | 0.2 |
| 1 large/extra large | 6 | 0.5 | 0.5 |
| 1 jumbo | 7 | 0.5 | 0.5 |
| 1 colossal | 11 | 1 | 0.5 |
| **Oranges**, all varieties, average, weights with skin: | | | |
| 1 small, (2.5" diam.), 5 oz | 45 | 0 | 11 |
| 1 medium (3"), 7 oz | 75 | 0 | 18 |
| 1 large, (3.5") 10 oz | 105 | 0 | 25 |
| 1 extra large, (4"), 14 oz | 130 | 0 | 30 |
| Flesh/Pulp only, 1 cup, 6 oz | 85 | 0 | 21 |
| Peel, 1 Tbsp | 0 | 0 | 0 |
| California Navel (3"), 7 oz | 70 | 0 | 17 |
| Californian Valencia, | | | |
| 1 medium (2¾" diam.) 6 oz | 60 | 0 | 14 |
| Florida Orange, 1 med., 7 oz | 70 | 0 | 17 |
| Sunkist Navel, large, 14 oz | 130 | 0 | 30 |
| **Papaya:** | | | |
| 1" pieces, 1 cup, 5 oz | 60 | 0 | 15 |
| 1 medium, 16 oz | 120 | 0 | 30 |
| Green (unripe), ½ cup, 3.5 oz | 20 | 0 | 5 |
| **Passionfruit:** | | | |
| 1 small, 1.5 oz | 15 | 0 | 3 |
| 1 large, 2.7 oz | 30 | 0 | 6 |
| Pulp, ½ cup, 4 oz | 110 | 0 | 27 |
| **Peaches**: 1 baby/donut, 3 oz | 30 | 0 | 7 |
| 1 small, 5 oz | 50 | 0 | 12 |
| 1 medium, 6 oz | 60 | 0 | 14 |
| 1 large, 7 oz | 70 | 0 | 16 |
| 1 extra large, 9 oz | 90 | 0 | 21 |
| **Pears**, all varieties, average: | | | |
| 1 mini, 2.5 oz | 35 | 0 | 8 |
| 1 small, 5 oz | 75 | 0 | 18 |
| 1 medium, 7 oz | 100 | 0 | 25 |
| 1 large, 9 oz | 130 | 0 | 33 |
| 1 extra large, 12 oz | 170 | 0 | 42 |
| **Pepino**, ½ medium, 4 oz | 20 | 0 | 4 |
| **Persimmons**: Native, 1 oz | 35 | 0 | 9 |
| Japanese (2½"d. x 2½"h), 7 oz | 120 | 0 | 30 |
| Seedless (Maui), 1 medium, 5 oz | 100 | 0 | 25 |

| Weights As Purchased | C | F | Cb |
|---|---|---|---|
| **Pineapple,** average all varieties: | | | |
| Weights without skin: 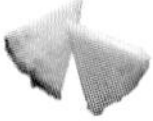 | | | |
| 1 thin slice (½"), 2 oz | 30 | 0 | 7 |
| 1 thick slice (¾"), 3 oz | 40 | 0 | 10 |
| 1 cup, chunks, 6 oz | 80 | 0 | 20 |
| Whole fruit, wt with skin: 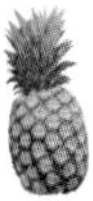 | | | |
| Baby/Mini, 16 oz | 150 | 0 | 39 |
| Medium size, 3 lbs | 450 | 1 | 118 |
| **Canned ~** See Page 102 | | | |
| **Pitanga,** (Surinam-Cherry) (5), 1.2 oz | 10 | 0 | 2 |
| **Plaintain:** | | | |
| Fresh/Raw, weight with skin: 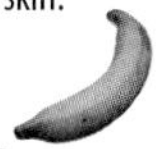 | | | |
| 1 medium, 10 oz | 220 | 0 | 55 |
| Slices, 1 cup, 5 oz | 180 | 0 | 44 |
| Cooked: | | | |
| Mashed, ½ cup, 3.5 oz | 115 | 0 | 30 |
| Slices, 1 cup, 5.5 oz | 180 | 0 | 47 |
| Fried in oil: 10 slices (¼"), 2 oz | 160 | 6 | 26 |
| 1 cup, 4.2 oz | 360 | 14 | 58 |
| **Plums,** all varieties, average: | | | |
| 1 mini/Damson, (1" diam), 0.5 oz | 10 | 0 | 1.5 |
| 1 small (2"), 2.3 oz | 30 | 0 | 7 |
| 1 medium (2½"), 3.5 oz | 45 | 0 | 10 |
| 1 large (3"), 5 oz | 60 | 0 | 14 |
| **Plumcot,** 1 medium, 6 oz | 75 | 0 | 18 |
| **Pomegranate:** 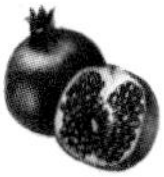 | | | |
| 1 small (3"), 5.5 oz | 70 | 1 | 15 |
| 1 medium (3½"), 10 oz | 125 | 2 | 27 |
| 1 large (4"), 16 oz | 230 | 3 | 50 |
| Seeds/Arils, ¼ cup, 2 oz | 40 | 1 | 10 |
| **Pomelo,** flesh, ½ cup, 3.5 oz | 35 | 0 | 9 |
| **Prickly Pear ~** See Cactus Fruit | | | |
| **Quince,** 1 medium, 3.5 oz 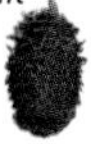 | 55 | 0 | 14 |
| **Rambutan/Rambotang,** | | | |
| Red/Yellow, 1 medium, 2 oz | 15 | 0 | 4 |
| **Raspberries:** ½ cup, 2 oz 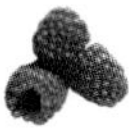 | 30 | 0 | 7 |
| 10 Raspberries, 0.8 oz | 10 | 0 | 2 |
| 1 Cup, 4.3 oz | 65 | 1 | 15 |
| 1 Pint, 11 oz | 160 | 2 | 37 |
| **Sapodilla:** 1 medium, 6 oz | 140 | 2 | 34 |
| Pulp, 1 cup, 8.5 oz | 200 | 2.5 | 45 |
| **Sapote:** 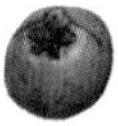 | | | |
| Black: 1 medium, 4.5 oz | 60 | 0 | 14 |
| Pulp only, ½ cup, 4 oz | 100 | 1 | 22 |
| Mamey, piece, 1 cup, 6 oz | 220 | 1 | 50 |
| **Satsuma Tangerine,** 1 medium, 3 oz | 45 | 0 | 11 |
| **Soursop,** pulp, 1 cup, 8 oz | 150 | 0.5 | 38 |
| **Starfruit,** (Carambola): 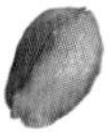 | | | |
| 1 medium, (3½" long), 3 oz | 30 | 0 | 6 |
| 1 large (4½"), 4.5 oz | 40 | 0 | 8 |
| **Strawberries:** 1 cup, 5.5 oz 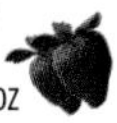 | 50 | 0.5 | 12 |
| 6 medium/3 large, 2 oz | 20 | 0 | 4 |
| 1 pint container, heaping, 16 oz | 130 | 0 | 32 |
| Chocolate Dipped, 1 large | 45 | 2.5 | 6 |

| Weights As Purchased | C | F | Cb |
|---|---|---|---|
| **Sugar-Apple (Sweetsop),** 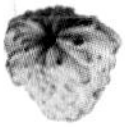 | | | |
| pulp, ½ cup, 4 oz | 120 | 0 | 28 |
| **Sugar Cane:** | | | |
| Unpeeled, 1 baton (7" long), 4 oz | 30 | 0 | 7 |
| Peeled, 1 small stick (3"), 2 oz | 35 | 0 | 8 |
| **Tamarillo,** 1 medium, 3 oz 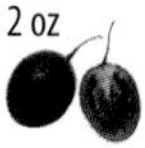 | 20 | 0 | 3 |
| **Tamarind:** 1 fruit (3"x1") | 5 | 0 | 1.5 |
| Pulp, ½ cup, 2 oz 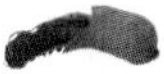 | 140 | 0.5 | 37 |
| **Tangelo:** 1 small, 4 oz 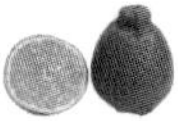 | 55 | 0 | 13 |
| 1 medium, 5 oz | 70 | 0 | 17 |
| 1 large, 7 oz | 95 | 0 | 23 |
| **Tangerine,** 1 med., (2½" diam.), 4 oz | 50 | 0 | 13 |
| **Tangor,** 1 medium, 4 oz | 35 | 0 | 7 |
| **Tomatillos:** 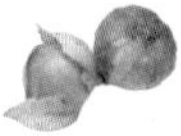 | | | |
| 3 medium, 3.5 oz | 35 | 0.5 | 6 |
| 1lb (16 oz) quantity | 160 | 2 | 27 |
| **Tomatoes:** 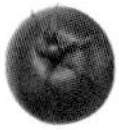 | | | |
| 1 small (2¼" diameter), 3 oz | 15 | 0 | 3 |
| 1 medium (2¾"), 5 oz | 25 | 0 | 5 |
| Sliced: 2 thin slices, 1 oz | 5 | 0 | 1 |
| 2 thick (⅜"), 2 oz 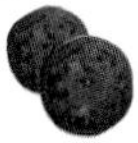 | 10 | 0 | 2 |
| Wedge, ¼, 1.3 oz | 6 | 0 | 1 |
| 1 large (3½"), 8 oz | 40 | 0.5 | 9 |
| 1 extra large (4"), 12 oz | 60 | 0.5 | 14 |
| Cherry: 4 medium, 2 oz | 10 | 0 | 2 |
| 1 cup, 5 oz 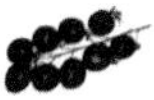 | 25 | 0 | 6 |
| Grape, 5 medium, 2 oz | 10 | 0 | 2 |
| Yellow Tear Drop, 3 medium, 1 oz | 5 | 0 | 2 |
| **Canned Tomatoes/Products ~** See Page 144 | | | |
| **Tree Tomato/Tamarillo,** 3 oz | 20 | 0 | 5 |
| **Ugli Fruit,** Tangelo type, 5 oz | 40 | 0 | 8 |
| **Watermelon:** | | | |
| Flesh only, weights without skin: | | | |
| 1 thin slice (½"), ¼ circle, 3 oz | 25 | 0 | 6 |
| 1 thick slice (1"): ¼ circle, 6 oz | 50 | 0 | 12 |
| ½ circle, 12 oz 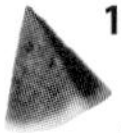 | 100 | 1 | 24 |
| Buffet Slice, small, thin, 1 oz | 8 | 0 | 2 |
| Cubes or Balls, 1 cup, 5.5 oz | 45 | 0 | 11 |
| Round Seedless Melon, weight with skin: | | | |
| Medium size, 13 lb, (8" diam.): | | | |
| Whole melon, 13 lb | 1160 | 5 | 280 |
| Wedge, ⅛ whole, 26 oz | 145 | 1 | 35 |
| Mini size, 6 lb, (6.5" diam.): 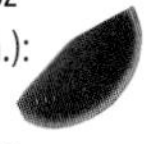 | | | |
| Whole melon, 6 lb | 480 | 2.5 | 110 |
| Wedge, ⅛ whole, 12 oz | 60 | 0 | 14 |

## Dried Fruit

| | C | F | Cb |
|---|---|---|---|
| **Apples**, 5 rings, 1 oz | 80 | 0 | 19 |
| **Apricots**, 8 halves, 1 oz | 65 | 0 | 16 |
| **Banana Chips**, ⅓ cup, 1 oz | 180 | 9 | 16 |
| **Banana Flakes**, 4 Tbsp, 1 oz | 80 | 0 | 20 |
| **Cranberries** (Craisins): | | | |
|   Original, ¼ cup | 130 | 0 | 33 |
|   Reduced Sugar, ¼ cup | 100 | 0 | 31 |
|   Chocolate Covered, ¼ cup, 2 oz | 180 | 8 | 28 |
| **Dates ~** See Dates in Fresh Fruit | | | |
| **Figs**, 3 medium figs, 1 oz | 90 | 0 | 23 |
| **Goji Berries**, 3 Tbsp, 1 oz | 100 | 0 | 21 |
| **Mango Slices**, 5 pieces, 1.4 oz | 25 | 0 | 6 |
| **Papaya Spears**, 2 pieces, 1.4 oz | 120 | 0 | 30 |
| **Peaches**, 2 halves, 1 oz | 60 | 0 | 15 |
| **Pears**, 3 halves, 2 oz | 140 | 0.5 | 34 |
| **Plums** (Sunsweet), (5), 1.4 oz | 100 | 0 | 24 |
| **Prunes/Dried Plums:** | | | |
|   With pits, 3 medium, 1 oz | 70 | 0 | 17 |
|   Without pits, 4 medium, 1 oz | 70 | 0 | 17 |
|   Cooked: With sugar, ½ cup, 5 oz | 155 | 0 | 38 |
|   Without sugar, ½ cup, 4.5 oz | 135 | 0 | 33 |
| **Raisins:** 2 Tbsp, 1 oz pack | 85 | 0 | 20 |
|   ½ cup, 2.8 oz | 220 | 0.5 | 56 |
| **White Mulberries**, 1 oz | 90 | 0.5 | 22 |

## Candied/Glazed Fruit

| | C | F | Cb |
|---|---|---|---|
| **Apricot**, 1 medium, 1 oz | 70 | 0 | 17 |
| **Cherry**, Maraschino (1) | 8 | 0 | 2 |
| **Citron/Fruit Peel**, 1 oz | 85 | 0 | 20 |
| **Ginger**, 1 oz | 90 | 0 | 21 |
| **Pineapple**, 1 slice, 1.3 oz | 120 | 0 | 29 |
| **Tamarind**, dried, sweetened, 1 oz | 70 | 0 | 17 |

## Fruit Leather Rolls

| | C | F | Cb |
|---|---|---|---|
| *Betty Crocker:* Fruit By The Foot, | | | |
|   1 roll, 0.8 oz | 80 | 0 | 17 |
|   Fruit Gushers, 1 oz | 90 | 1 | 20 |
|   Fruit Roll-Ups, 1 roll | 50 | 1 | 12 |
| *Stretch Island*, Leathers, 1 pouch, 0.5 oz | 45 | 0 | 12 |

## Canned/Bottled Fruit

**Solids & Liquids:**
*Per ½ Cup, 4½ oz Unless indicated*

| | C | F | Cb |
|---|---|---|---|
| **Apricots/Peaches/Pears:** | | | |
|   In juice, light | 60 | 0 | 15 |
|   In heavy syrup | 105 | 0 | 28 |
|   In water/diet | 35 | 0 | 8 |
| **Black/Blueberries:** | | | |
|   In heavy syrup | 120 | 0 | 30 |
|   In light syrup | 110 | 0 | 26 |

## Canned/Bottled Fruit (Cont)

| | C | F | Cb |
|---|---|---|---|
| **Cherries**, pitted: | | | |
|   In heavy syrup | 105 | 0 | 27 |
|   In light syrup | 85 | 0 | 22 |
|   In water | 55 | 0 | 15 |
|   Maraschino, 1 oz | 50 | 0 | 12 |
| **Fruit Cocktail/Salad:** | | | |
|   In heavy syrup | 95 | 0 | 25 |
|   In juice, light | 60 | 0 | 16 |
|   In water/diet | 35 | 0 | 10 |
| **Gooseberries**, light syrup | 90 | 0 | 24 |
| **Grapefruit**, in light syrup | 75 | 0 | 20 |
| **Lychees**, ½ cup, 4.5 oz | 105 | 0 | 26 |
| **Mixed Fruit:** In fruit juices/light syrup | 70 | 0 | 18 |
|   In heavy syrup | 90 | 0 | 24 |
|   In water/diet | 40 | 0 | 10 |
| **Pineapple**, all varieties: | | | |
|   In heavy syrup, 4.3 oz | 110 | 0 | 26 |
|   In own juice, 4 oz | 60 | 0 | 15 |
| **Prunes:** With syrup, 3 oz | 90 | 0 | 23 |
|   Stewed in water, ½ cup | 135 | 0 | 35 |

## Fruit Snack Cups

| | C | F | Cb |
|---|---|---|---|
| **Deli/Take-Out:** Small, 6 oz | 70 | 0 | 16 |
|   Large, 12 oz | 140 | 0 | 32 |
|   Yogurt and Fruit Cup, 15 oz | 380 | 4.5 | 75 |
| **Del Monte:** | | | |
| **Fruit & Veggie Fusions**, all flav., 4 oz | 70 | 0 | 17 |
| **Fruit Burst Squeezers**, av., 3.2 oz | 80 | 0 | 20 |
| **Fruit Refreshes**, average, 7 oz | 95 | 0 | 24 |
| **Fruit Snack Cups In Gel**, av., 4.5 oz | 80 | 0 | 20 |
| **Dole:** | | | |
| **Fruit Bowls:** *Per 4 oz Container* | | | |
|   Cherry Mixed Fruit; Tropical Fruit, av. | 80 | 0 | 17 |
|   Diced Pears | 90 | 0 | 22 |
| **Fruit in Gel:** *Per 4.3 oz Container* | | | |
|   Mixed Fruit, in Black Cherry Gel | 90 | 0 | 24 |
|   Average other fruits, in various Gels | 95 | 0 | 24 |

## Apple & Fruit Sauces

| | C | F | Cb |
|---|---|---|---|
| **Apple Sauce:** | | | |
| Regular/sweetened, 2 Tbsp, 1 oz | 20 | 0 | 6 |
|   4 oz package | 90 | 0 | 22 |
| **Cranberry**, Jellied, ¼ cup | 110 | 0 | 25 |
| **Fruit Sauces & Purees:** | | | |
| All fruit types, average: 2 Tbsp, 1 oz | 25 | 0 | 6 |
|   ½ cup, 4 oz | 100 | 0 | 24 |
| **Mott's:** | | | |
| Apple Sauce: Original, 4 oz | 90 | 0 | 24 |
|   Fruit Flavored, 4 oz | 90 | 0 | 23 |
|   Healthy Harvest, all flavors, 3.9 oz | 50 | 0 | 13 |
| **Ocean Spray,** | | | |
|   Jellied Cranberry, ¼ cup | 110 | 0 | 28 |

## Quick Guide  Ⓒ Ⓕ Ⓒⓑ

### Ice Cream
*Average all Flavors:*
**Regular (10% fat):**
*Examples: Dreyer's Grand, Hood, Friendly's*

| | C | F | Cb |
|---|---|---|---|
| ½ cup, 4 fl.oz | 140 | 7 | 16 |
| 1 cup, 8 fl.oz | 280 | 14 | 32 |
| 1 pint, 16 fl.oz | 560 | 28 | 64 |

**Rich/Premium (16-17% fat):**
*Examples: Baskin Robbins, Ben & Jerry's, Haagen-Dazs*

| | | | |
|---|---|---|---|
| ½ cup, 4 fl.oz | 250 | 16 | 24 |
| 1 cup, 8 fl.oz | 500 | 32 | 48 |
| 1 pint, 16 fl.oz | 1000 | 64 | 96 |

**Reduced-Fat/Light (5% fat):**
*Examples: Breyers ½ The Fat, Friendly's Light, Hood Light*

| | | | |
|---|---|---|---|
| ½ cup, 4 fl.oz | 140 | 5 | 21 |
| 1 cup, 8 fl.oz | 280 | 10 | 42 |
| 1 pint, 16 fl.oz | 560 | 20 | 84 |

**Fat-Free:**
*Example: Breyers*

| | | | |
|---|---|---|---|
| ½ cup, 4 fl.oz | 90 | 0 | 21 |
| 1 cup, 8 fl.oz | 180 | 0 | 42 |
| 1 pint, 16 fl.oz | 360 | 0 | 84 |

### Scoop Shops:
*Average all Brands*
Add extra for cone (see next column)

| | | | |
|---|---|---|---|
| **Kids,** 3 fl.oz | 125 | 8 | 12 |
| **Regular,** 6 fl.oz | 250 | 16 | 24 |
| **Large,** 9 fl.oz | 375 | 24 | 36 |

### Soft Serve:
*Average all Brands*

| | | | |
|---|---|---|---|
| **Regular:** ½ cup, 4 fl.oz | 255 | 15 | 25 |
| 1 cup, 8 fl.oz | 510 | 30 | 50 |
| **Light:** ½ cup, 4 fl.oz | 145 | 3 | 25 |
| 1 cup, 8 fl.oz | 290 | 6 | 50 |

## Quick Guide

### Frozen Yogurt
*Average all Brands*

| | | | |
|---|---|---|---|
| **Hard:** Low-Fat, ½ cup | 110 | 3 | 19 |
| Non-Fat, ½ cup | 110 | 0 | 24 |
| **Soft:** Low-Fat, ½ cup | 120 | 4 | 17 |
| Non-Fat, ½ cup | 100 | 0 | 30 |

**Brands** ~ *See Ice Cream & Novelties Section*

## Quick Guide  Ⓒ Ⓕ Ⓒⓑ

### Gelato/Ices/Frozen Custard
**Gelato:** *Per ½ Cup*

| | | | |
|---|---|---|---|
| Milk base: Vanilla | 160 | 6 | 25 |
| Chocolate Hazelnut | 230 | 15 | 21 |
| Water base, ½ cup | 100 | 0 | 26 |

**Frozen Custard**, Choc./Vanilla, av:

| | | | |
|---|---|---|---|
| ½ cup | 210 | 11 | 23 |
| Single Scoop, 5 oz wt | 300 | 15 | 38 |
| Double Scoop, 10 oz wt | 600 | 30 | 76 |

**Ice (Milk base):** *Average all flavors*

| | | | |
|---|---|---|---|
| Hard (4% fat),½ cup | 100 | 3 | 15 |
| Soft Serve (3% fat), ½ cup | 110 | 2 | 19 |
| **Shaved Ice**, average, 12 fl.oz | 160 | 0 | 40 |
| **Sherbet**, average, ½ cup | 110 | 1.5 | 22 |
| **Sorbet**, Fruit, fat free, ½ cup | 70 | 0 | 19 |
| **Fruit Ice Pops** | 80 | 0 | 20 |

### Sundaes

**Baskin Robbins:**

| | | | |
|---|---|---|---|
| **Classic:** Banana Royale | 680 | 33 | 90 |
| Banana Split | 970 | 39 | 146 |
| Brownie | 800 | 43 | 95 |

**Denny's,**

| | | | |
|---|---|---|---|
| Banana Split, 15 oz | 810 | 31 | 125 |

**Toppings** ~ *See Page 195*
**McDonald's:**
**Sundaes:**

| | | | |
|---|---|---|---|
| Hot Caramel, 6.4 oz | 340 | 8 | 60 |
| Hot Fudge, 6.3 oz | 340 | 10 | 52 |
| **Toppings,** Peanuts, 0.3 oz | 40 | 3.5 | 1 |

### Ice Cream Cones & Cups

*Average all Brands*

| | | | |
|---|---|---|---|
| **Wafer Cone/Cup**, average | 20 | 0 | 4 |
| **Sugar Cone**, average | 50 | 0 | 14 |
| **Waffle Cone:** | | | |
| Small | 50 | 1 | 10 |
| Large | 90 | 0.5 | 19 |
| **Brands:** | | | |
| *Comet,* Sugar Cone | 50 | 0 | 11 |
| *Keebler,* Sugar Cone | 50 | 0 | 10 |
| *Oreo,* Chocolate Cone | 50 | 1 | 10 |

## Ice Cream ~ Brands    **C** **F** **Cb**

### Amy's:
**Non Dairy Frozen Dessert:** *Per ½ Cup*

| | C | F | Cb |
|---|---|---|---|
| Chocolate; Vanilla, average, 3.3 oz | **175** | **12** | **15** |
| Mint /Mocha Choc. Chip, av., 3.5 oz | **230** | **16** | **20** |

**Baskin-Robbins** ~ *See Fast-Foods Section*

### Ben & Jerry's:
**Scoop Shop Ice Cream:** *Hand Scooped, per ½ Cup*

| | C | F | Cb |
|---|---|---|---|
| Americone Dream | **280** | **16** | **31** |
| Bourbon Brown Butter | **240** | **13** | **27** |
| Butter Pecan | **250** | **19** | **17** |
| Choc. Chip Cookie Dough | **280** | **15** | **32** |
| Chocolate Fudge Brownie | **260** | **13** | **20** |
| Chunky Monkey | **260** | **16** | **26** |
| Coconut Seven Layer Bar | **270** | **17** | **27** |
| Cookie Core | **260** | **17** | **23** |
| Mint Chocolate Chunk | **240** | **15** | **24** |
| Strawberry Cheesecake | **220** | **13** | **24** |
| Sweet Cream & Cookies | **230** | **13** | **25** |
| Vanilla Toffee Bar Crunch | **280** | **19** | **24** |

**Ice Cream, 1 Pint Tubs:** *Per ½ Cup*

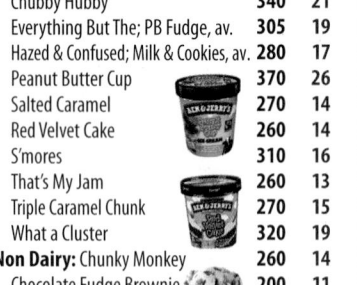

| | C | F | Cb |
|---|---|---|---|
| Banana Split; Bstn Cr. Pie, av. | **255** | **14** | **29** |
| Cake Batter; Cherry Garcia, av. | **265** | **16** | **27** |
| Chubby Hubby | **340** | **21** | **33** |
| Everything But The; PB Fudge, av. | **305** | **19** | **29** |
| Hazed & Confused; Milk & Cookies, av. | **280** | **17** | **29** |
| Peanut Butter Cup | **370** | **26** | **29** |
| Salted Caramel | **270** | **14** | **31** |
| Red Velvet Cake | **260** | **14** | **29** |
| S'mores | **310** | **16** | **36** |
| That's My Jam | **260** | **13** | **31** |
| Triple Caramel Chunk | **270** | **15** | **32** |
| What a Cluster | **320** | **19** | **31** |
| **Non Dairy:** Chunky Monkey | **260** | **14** | **31** |
| Chocolate Fudge Brownie | **200** | **11** | **23** |
| Coffee Caramel Fudge | **240** | **12** | **31** |
| PB & Cookies | **290** | **17** | **31** |

**Frozen Yogurt:** *Per ½ Cup*

| | C | F | Cb |
|---|---|---|---|
| **Fro Yo:** Cherry Garcia | **170** | **3** | **32** |
| Chocolate Fudge Brownie | **180** | **2.5** | **35** |
| Half Baked | **180** | **3** | **35** |
| Pfish Food, 3.6 oz | **250** | **7** | **42** |
| **Greek:** Peach Melba | **150** | **5** | **23** |
| Raspberry Fudge Chunk | **190** | **7** | **26** |
| Strawberry Shortcake | **170** | **5** | **26** |
| **Sorbet**, average all flavors | **95** | **0** | **23** |

### Blue Bunny:    **C** **F** **Cb**
**Premium Ice Cream (Pint Ctn):** *Per ½ Cup*

| | C | F | Cb |
|---|---|---|---|
| Banana Split | **160** | **7** | **23** |
| Bunny Tracks | **190** | **11** | **21** |
| Chocolate | **130** | **7** | **17** |
| Cookies 'n Cream | **150** | **7** | **20** |

**Fat Free, No Sugar Added:** *Per ½ Cup*

| | C | F | Cb |
|---|---|---|---|
| Brownie Sundae | **90** | **0** | **23** |
| Caramel Toffee Crunch | **90** | **0** | **23** |
| Vanilla | **80** | **0** | **20** |
| *Note: Carb figures include 4-8 g sugar alcohols* | | | |

**Frozen Yogurt:** *Per ½ Cup*

| | C | F | Cb |
|---|---|---|---|
| Caramel Praline Crunch | **120** | **4** | **20** |
| Strawberry Banana | **100** | **2** | **19** |
| White Mint Choc. Chunk | **130** | **4** | **21** |

**Bars/Pops** ~ *See Page 108*

### Breyers:
**Original Ice Cream:** *Per ½ Cup*

| | C | F | Cb |
|---|---|---|---|
| Butter Pecan | **140** | **6** | **18** |
| Cherry Vanilla; Cookies & Cream | **130** | **4** | **22** |
| Chocolate Truffle | **170** | **9** | **21** |
| Mint Chocolate Chip | **150** | **8** | **18** |
| Natural Strawberry | **110** | **5** | **14** |
| Salted Caramel | **130** | **3.5** | **23** |
| Vanilla, Chocolate | **130** | **7** | **16** |
| **Fat Free**, av. all flavors | **90** | **0** | **21** |

**Half The Fat:** *Per ½ Cup*

| | C | F | Cb |
|---|---|---|---|
| Cookies & Cream | **120** | **4** | **20** |
| Creamy, Chocolate or Vanilla, av. | **100** | **3** | **16** |

**No Added Sugar Dairy Dessert:**

| | C | F | Cb |
|---|---|---|---|
| Butter Pecan | **100** | **5** | **14** |
| Salted Cararmel Swirl | **90** | **4** | **16** |
| Vanilla; Vanilla, Choc., Strawberry | **80** | **3** | **13** |
| *Note: Carb figures include 1-6g sugar alcohol and 0-2g fiber* | | | |

**Blasts!:** *Per ½ Cup*

| | C | F | Cb |
|---|---|---|---|
| Girl Scout Cookies Thin Mint | **140** | **4.5** | **23** |
| Mrs Field's Choc Fudge Brownie | **140** | **4** | **25** |
| Oreo Cookies and Cream Mint | **120** | **4** | **20** |
| Strawberry Waffle Cone | **130** | **4** | **22** |
| **CarbSmart**, average all flav., ½ cup | **115** | **6** | **14** |
| *Carb figure includes 5g sugar alcohol and 4g fiber* | | | |

### Bruster's:

| | C | F | Cb |
|---|---|---|---|
| **Ice Cream**, Choc./Vanilla, av., ½ cup | **210** | **12** | **24** |

**Fat Free, No Added Sugar:** *Per ½ Cup*

| | C | F | Cb |
|---|---|---|---|
| Chocolate | **100** | **0** | **26** |
| Choc. Caramel/Fudge Swirl | **120** | **0** | **31** |
| Cinnamon; Coffee; Van., av. | **100** | **0** | **23** |

**Frozen Yogurt,**

| | C | F | Cb |
|---|---|---|---|
| Chocolate; Vanilla, average, ½ cup | **150** | **4.5** | **24** |

## Ice Cream ~ Brands (Cont)

| | **C** | **F** | **Cb** |
|---|---|---|---|
| **Clemmy's:** *Per ½ Cup* | | | |
| Chocolate | 160 | 11 | 20 |
| Coffee; Vanilla Bean, av. | 160 | 11 | 21 |
| Orange Cream | 120 | 6 | 23 |
| Toasted Almond | 220 | 16 | 20 |
| *Note: Carb figures include 12-15g sugar alcohol* | | | |
| **Carvel Ice Cream** ~ *See Fast-Foods Section* | | | |
| **Coldstone Creamery** ~ *See Fast-Foods Section* | | | |
| **Dairy Queen/Brazier** ~ *See Fast-Foods Section* | | | |
| **Dannon:** | | | |
| **Oikos Greek Frozen Yogurt:** *Per ½ Cup* | | | |
| Cookies & Cream; Strawberry, av. | 145 | 3 | 24 |
| Salted Caramel | 160 | 3 | 28 |
| Average other flavors | 150 | 3 | 26 |
| **Dippin' Dots:** | | | |
| **Original Dots:** *Per ½ Cup* | | | |
| Banana Split | 160 | 8 | 20 |
| Caramel Brownie Sundae | 190 | 9 | 23 |
| Cookies 'n Cream | 200 | 11 | 22 |
| Cotton Candy | 160 | 8 | 18 |
| Mint Chocolate | 170 | 8 | 21 |
| Strawberry | 160 | 8 | 18 |
| Vanilla | 160 | 8 | 18 |
| **Dove:** | | | |
| **Ice Cream:** *Per ½ Cup* | | | |
| Mint/Vanilla Choc. Chunk | 180 | 11 | 17 |
| Unconditional Chocolate | 200 | 12 | 23 |
| **Dreyer's/Edy's:** | | | |
| **Ice Cream:** *Per ½ Cup* | | | |
| **Grand:** Chocolate | 140 | 7 | 17 |
| Mint Chocolate Chip | 150 | 8 | 18 |
| Neapolitan | 130 | 6 | 16 |
| Strawberry | 120 | 5 | 16 |
| Vanilla | 140 | 7 | 16 |
| **Slow Churned, ½ The Fat:** *Per ½ Cup* | | | |
| Chocolate | 100 | 3.5 | 15 |
| Double Fudge Brownie | 120 | 3 | 19 |
| Fudge Tracks | 120 | 3.5 | 19 |
| Mint Chocolate Chip | 120 | 4.5 | 17 |
| Peanut Butter Cup | 130 | 5 | 18 |
| **Friendly's:** | | | |
| **Rich & Creamy Ice Cream:** *Per ½ Cup* | | | |
| Butter Crunch; Classic Chocolate, av. | 150 | 7 | 18 |
| Chocolate Almond Chip | 160 | 9 | 17 |
| Coffee | 130 | 7 | 15 |
| Strawberry; Vanilla, av. | 140 | 7 | 16 |
| Vienna Mocha Chunk | 170 | 9 | 19 |

| | **C** | **F** | **Cb** |
|---|---|---|---|
| **Friendly's (Cont):** *Per ½ Cup* | | | |
| **Light:** Chocolate Peanut Butter Swirl | 150 | 7 | 20 |
| Pistachio Almond | 120 | 4.5 | 17 |
| **Smooth Churned Ice Cream:** *Per ½ Cup* | | | |
| **Light:** Mint Chocolate Chip | 120 | 4.5 | 19 |
| Vanilla | 110 | 3.5 | 17 |
| **SundaeXtreme:** *Per ½ Cup* | | | |
| Chocolate Fudge | 150 | 5 | 25 |
| Choc. Chip Cookie Dough | 170 | 6 | 26 |
| Chocolate P'nut Butter | 190 | 9 | 22 |
| **Sherbet**, Rasp Orange Lemon, ½ cup | 130 | 1.5 | 28 |
| **Yogurt Frozen,** | | | |
| Regular, average all flavors, ½ cup | 140 | 4.5 | 23 |
| **Gelati-da:** | | | |
| **Gelato:** *Per ½ Cup* | | | |
| Amaretto Chocolate | 150 | 4.5 | 23 |
| Choc Mint Milano | 120 | 2.5 | 22 |
| Coffee Fudge Latte | 130 | 2 | 22 |
| Limoncello; Vanilla Marsala, average | 120 | 3 | 21 |
| Red Raspberry | 130 | 1.5 | 25 |
| **Great Value** *(Walmart):* | | | |
| **Ice Cream:** *Per ½ cup* | | | |
| Chocolate Chip Cookie Dough | 150 | 8 | 19 |
| Coffee | 130 | 7 | 15 |
| Decadent Fudge Tracks | 180 | 10 | 20 |
| Homestyle Vanilla | 140 | 7 | 17 |
| Peanut Butter Cup | 160 | 9 | 17 |
| **Sherbet**, average all flav. | 110 | 0 | 26 |
| **Haagen-Dazs:** | | | |
| **Tubs, Regular:** *Per ½ Cup* | | | |
| Butter Pecan | 300 | 22 | 20 |
| Chocolate Peanut Butter | 340 | 23 | 26 |
| Dulce de Leche | 270 | 16 | 27 |
| White Chocolate Raspberry Truffle | 280 | 16 | 31 |
| **Gelato:** *Per ½ Cup* | | | |
| Black Cherry Amaretto | 240 | 9 | 35 |
| Sea Salt Caramel | 270 | 11 | 38 |
| **Healthy Choice,** | | | |
| **Greek Frozen Yogurt,** | | | |
| average all varieties, | 105 | 2 | 19 |
| **Bars ~** *See Page 109* | | | |

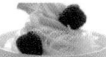 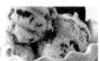

## Ice Cream ~ Brands (Cont)

### Hood:

| | C | F | Cb |
|---|---|---|---|
| **Ice Cream:** *Per ½ Cup* | | | |
| Chocolate | 140 | 6 | 18 |
| Classic Trio | 140 | 7 | 17 |
| Cookie Dough | 170 | 8 | 21 |
| Cookies 'N Cream | 150 | 8 | 19 |
| Creamy Coffee | 140 | 7 | 16 |
| Fudge Twister | 140 | 6 | 20 |
| Golden/Natural Vanilla; Patchwork | 140 | 7 | 17 |
| Maple Walnut | 150 | 9 | 17 |
| **Churned, Light:** *Per ½ Cup* | | | |
| Chocolate Chip | 120 | 4.5 | 18 |
| Coffee | 100 | 3 | 16 |
| Moosehead Lake Fudge | 160 | 7 | 21 |
| Under The Stars | 160 | 8 | 18 |
| Vanilla | 110 | 3 | 16 |
| **Frozen Fat-Free Yogurt:** *Per ½ Cup* | | | |
| Chocolate; Strawberry, av. | 85 | 0 | 19 |
| Chocolate Chip | 110 | 1.5 | 20 |
| Mocha Fudge | 100 | 0 | 22 |

### New England Creamery ~ www.CalorieKing.com
### Jerseymaid *(Vons): Per ½ Cup*

| **Ice Cream:** | | | |
|---|---|---|---|
| Cookies & Cream | 160 | 8 | 18 |
| Choc Chip; Mint Choc Chip | 150 | 9 | 16 |
| Heavenly Hash | 165 | 9 | 19 |
| Mocha Almond Fudge; Chocolate | 150 | 9 | 16 |
| Neapolitan; Real Vanilla | 140 | 8 | 15 |
| Strawberry | 130 | 6 | 17 |

### Oberweis:

| **Super Premium Ice Cream:** *Per 6 oz Scoop* | | | |
|---|---|---|---|
| Chocolate | 480 | 31 | 43 |
| Chocolate Peanut Butter | 550 | 39 | 42 |
| Cookie Dough | 500 | 28 | 56 |
| Vanilla | 460 | 31 | 40 |

### Oikos ~ *see Dannon*
### Pinkberry:

| **Frozen Yogurt:** *Without Toppings* | | | |
|---|---|---|---|
| Original: Mini, 3.2 oz wt | 90 | 0 | 19 |
| Small, 5 oz wt | 140 | 0 | 29 |
| Medium, 8 oz wt | 230 | 0 | 48 |
| Large, 13 oz wt | 370 | 0 | 78 |
| Chocolate Hazelnut, 13 oz | 560 | 15 | 96 |
| Cookies & Cream, 13 oz | 520 | 7.5 | 96 |
| Mango, 13 oz | 405 | 0 | 89 |

### Red Mango:

| **Frozen Yogurt:** *No Toppings Included* | C | F | Cb |
|---|---|---|---|
| **Original:** 3.3 oz wt | 80 | 0 | 19 |
| Small, 4.7 oz wt | 120 | 0 | 27 |
| Regular, 7.5 oz wt | 190 | 0 | 43 |
| Large, 11.4 oz wt | 290 | 0 | 65 |
| **Blueberry:** 3.3 oz wt | 100 | 0 | 23 |
| Small, 4.7 oz wt | 150 | 0 | 33 |
| Regular, 7.5 oz wt | 230 | 0 | 53 |
| Large, 11.4 oz wt | 350 | 0 | 81 |
| **Dulce de Leche:** 3.3 oz wt | 80 | 0 | 18 |
| Small, 4.7 oz wt | 120 | 0 | 27 |
| Regular, 7.5 oz wt | 190 | 0 | 43 |
| Large, 11.4 oz wt | 290 | 0 | 65 |
| **Pomegranate:** 3.3 oz wt | 90 | 0 | 21 |
| Small, 4.6 oz wt | 130 | 0 | 30 |
| Regular, 7.5 oz wt | 210 | 0 | 48 |
| Large, 11.4 oz wt | 320 | 0 | 73 |

### Rice Dream:

| **Frozen Dessert:** *Per ½ Cup* | | | |
|---|---|---|---|
| Cocoa Marble Fudge | 170 | 6 | 31 |
| Mint Carob Chip | 180 | 7 | 28 |
| Strawberry | 170 | 6 | 30 |
| Vanilla | 160 | 6 | 26 |

### Bars ~ *See Page 110*
### Skinny Cow:
**Bars/Sandwiches/Cones ~** *See Page 110*

### So Delicious:

| **Coconut Based:** *Per ½ Cup* | | | |
|---|---|---|---|
| Cherry Amaretto | 130 | 5 | 23 |
| Chocolate | 140 | 7 | 21 |
| Choc. P'Nut Butter Swirl | 200 | 14 | 22 |
| Coconut | 140 | 8 | 20 |
| **Soy Based:** *Per ½ Cup* | | | |
| Chocolate Velvet | 130 | 3.5 | 23 |
| Cookie Dough | 170 | 7 | 29 |
| Creamy Vanilla | 120 | 3 | 24 |
| Neapolitan | 120 | 3.5 | 24 |
| Peanut Butter Zig Zag | 210 | 11 | 28 |

### Soy Dream:

| **Frozen Dessert:** *Per ½ Cup* | | | |
|---|---|---|---|
| Butter Pecan | 190 | 11 | 23 |
| French Vanilla | 170 | 9 | 21 |
| Vanilla Fudge Swil | 170 | 9 | 23 |

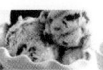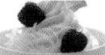

# Ice Cream & Frozen Yogurt  Ⓘ

## Ice Cream ~ Brands (Cont)

| | C | F | Cb |
|---|---|---|---|
| **Stonyfield Farm:** | | | |
| **Frozen Yogurt:** *Per ½ Cup* | | | |
| After Dark Chocolate | 100 | 0 | 21 |
| Creme Caramel | 130 | 1.5 | 26 |
| Gotta Have Vanilla | 100 | 0 | 20 |
| **Stop & Shop:** | | | |
| **Ice Cream:** *Per ½ Cup* | | | |
| Chocolate | 150 | 8 | 18 |
| Neapolitan; Vanilla, average | 140 | 7.5 | 17 |
| Vanilla Fudge Swirl | 140 | 7 | 18 |
| Light: Moose Tracks | 130 | 5 | 18 |
| Vanilla | 100 | 3 | 17 |
| **Premium:** | | | |
| Cookies & Cream | 170 | 9 | 21 |
| Mint Chocolate Chip | 160 | 9 | 18 |
| **Simply Enjoy:** | | | |
| Chocolate | 210 | 12 | 22 |
| Strawberry; Vanilla, average | 225 | 13 | 25 |
| **Tasti D-Lite:** | | | |
| **Soft Serve:** *Per 4 fl.oz* | | | |
| Banana, 2.5 oz | 70 | 1 | 13 |
| Blueberry Cheesecake, 2.6 oz | 80 | 1.5 | 15 |
| Brownie Batter, 2.6 oz | 70 | 1.5 | 13 |
| Buttercrunch Mania, 2.5 oz | 90 | 3.5 | 13 |
| Coffee 'n Cream, 2.5 oz | 70 | 1.5 | 12 |
| Marshmallow, 2.6 oz | 80 | 1 | 14 |
| **Tofutti:** | | | |
| **Premium Pints:** *Per ½ Cup* | | | |
| Better Pecan | 250 | 15 | 27 |
| Chocolate | 210 | 13 | 20 |
| Vanilla | 210 | 13 | 21 |
| Vanilla Almond Bark | 240 | 15 | 24 |
| Van. Fudge; Wild Berry Supreme, av. | 190 | 9 | 25 |
| **TCBY** ~ *See Page 250* | | | |
| **Turkey Hill:** | | | |
| **All Natural:** *Per ½ Cup* | | | |
| Chocolate Chip | 170 | 10 | 18 |
| Mint Chocolate Chip | 180 | 10 | 18 |
| **Light:** *Per ½ Cup* | | | |
| Moose Tracks | 140 | 6 | 20 |
| Vanilla Bean | 100 | 2 | 17 |

| | C | F | Cb |
|---|---|---|---|
| **Turkey Hill (Cont)** | | | |
| **No Sugar Added:** *Per ½ Cup* | | | |
| Dutch Chocolate; Vanilla Bean, av. | 70 | 0 | 20 |
| Moose Tracks | 120 | 5 | 22 |
| **Premium Ice Cream:** *Per ½ Cup* | | | |
| Black Cherry | 130 | 6 | 18 |
| Butter Pecan; Choco Mint Chip, av. | 160 | 10 | 16 |
| Chocolate Peanut Butter Cup | 180 | 11 | 18 |
| Cookies 'n Cream; Tin Roof Sundae | 150 | 8 | 19 |
| Rocky Road | 170 | 8 | 23 |
| Vanilla Bean | 130 | 7 | 16 |
| **Frozen Yogurt:** *Per ½ Cup* | | | |
| Mint Cookies 'n Cream | 110 | 1.5 | 22 |
| Fat-Free: Chocolate Marshmallow | 110 | 0 | 24 |
| Other flavors | 90 | 0 | 19 |
| **Gelato:** *Per ½ Cup, 3.1 oz* | | | |
| Chocolate Chocolate Chip | 220 | 12 | 26 |
| Chocolate Peanut Butter | 230 | 15 | 21 |
| Hazelnut | 240 | 14 | 24 |
| Sea Salted Caramel | 220 | 11 | 27 |
| **Sherbet,** Fruit Rainbow | 120 | 1 | 26 |
| **Wawa:** | | | |
| **Premium Ice Cream:** *Per ½ Cup* | | | |
| Butter Pecan; Mint Choc. Chip, av. | 180 | 10 | 20 |
| Chocolate; Vanilla Bean, average | 160 | 8 | 20 |
| Cookies & Cream | 180 | 9 | 21 |
| Strawberry Shortcake | 160 | 7 | 22 |
| **Wegmans:** *Per ½ Cup* | | | |
| **Regular:** Chocolate | 130 | 7 | 15 |
| French Van./ Vanilla, average | 145 | 7 | 19 |
| **Light Extra Churned:** Cookie Dough | 130 | 3 | 23 |
| French Vanilla | 120 | 3.5 | 19 |
| **Yoplait:** | | | |
| **Go-Gurt!,** average all flavors, 2.3 oz | 60 | 0.5 | 12 |
| **Frozen Yogurt:** *Per ½ Cup* | | | |
| Original Fruit flavors, average | 115 | 2 | 21 |
| Vanilla | 110 | 2.5 | 19 |
| Greek: | | | |
| Fruit Flavors, average | 130 | 2 | 21 |
| Honey Caramel | 140 | 2.5 | 22 |
| Vanilla | 120 | 2.5 | 17 |

# Ice Cream Bars & Pops

## Ice Cream Bars & Pops ~ Brands

*Per Bar/Serving Unless Indicated*

| | **C** | **F** | **Cb** |
|---|---|---|---|
| **Ben & Jerry's:** | | | |
| **Bars:** Cherry Garcia | 270 | 17 | 26 |
| Half Baked | 340 | 20 | 34 |
| **Big Bear** ~ *See Klondike* | | | |
| **Blue Bunny:** | | | |
| **Single Bars:** | | | |
| Chocolate Eclair, 2.8 oz | 210 | 9 | 29 |
| Chocolate Raspberry Bar, 2.8 oz | 260 | 16 | 26 |
| Cookies 'n Cream, 3 oz | 240 | 11 | 33 |
| Heath Bar, 3 oz | 290 | 20 | 26 |
| Hot Fudge Bar, 3.6 oz | 360 | 24 | 33 |
| Strawberry Shortcake, 2.8 oz | 200 | 10 | 27 |
| Turtle Bar, 3.5 oz | 350 | 23 | 33 |
| Vanilla Choc Chip, 3.2 oz | 310 | 18 | 34 |
| **12 Pack:** Caramel Crunch, 1.4 oz | 120 | 7 | 12 |
| English Toffee, 1.4 oz | 120 | 8 | 13 |
| **Cones, 6 Pack:** | | | |
| Caramel Lovers, 3.4 oz | 310 | 16 | 38 |
| Chocolate Lovers, 3.2 oz | 270 | 13 | 36 |
| Cookies 'n Cream, 3.2 oz | 270 | 13 | 37 |
| King Size: | | | |
| Brownie Sundae, 5.6 oz | 450 | 23 | 57 |
| Bunny Tracks, 5.7 oz | 470 | 26 | 54 |
| Big Swirls, Choc., Van., 3 oz | 250 | 12 | 32 |
| **Ice Cream Sandwiches:** | | | |
| Singles: Chips Galore, 3.4 oz | 310 | 14 | 43 |
| Cookies 'N Cream, 3 oz | 240 | 10 | 37 |
| 8 Packs: Birthday Party, 2.5 oz | 180 | 5 | 30 |
| Chocolate Lovers, 2.7 oz | 190 | 6 | 32 |
| Simply Vanilla, 2.5 oz | 160 | 5 | 27 |
| **Big:** Alaska Bar, 3.3 oz | 250 | 15 | 27 |
| Bopper, 5 oz | 450 | 20 | 63 |
| Double Strawberry, 3.9 oz | 250 | 7 | 42 |
| Mississippi Mud, 4 oz | 280 | 8 | 47 |
| **Breyers:** | | | |
| **Carb Smart, 6 Pack:** | | | |
| Fudge Bar, 1.7 oz | 70 | 3 | 11 |
| *Note: Carb figure includes 5g sugar alcohol* | | | |
| Vanilla Ice Cream Bar, 2 oz | 150 | 11 | 13 |
| *Note: Carb figure includes 4g sugar alcohol* | | | |
| Vanilla Almond Ice Cream Bar, 2 oz | 160 | 12 | 13 |
| *Note: Note: Carb figures include 4g sugar alcohol* | | | |

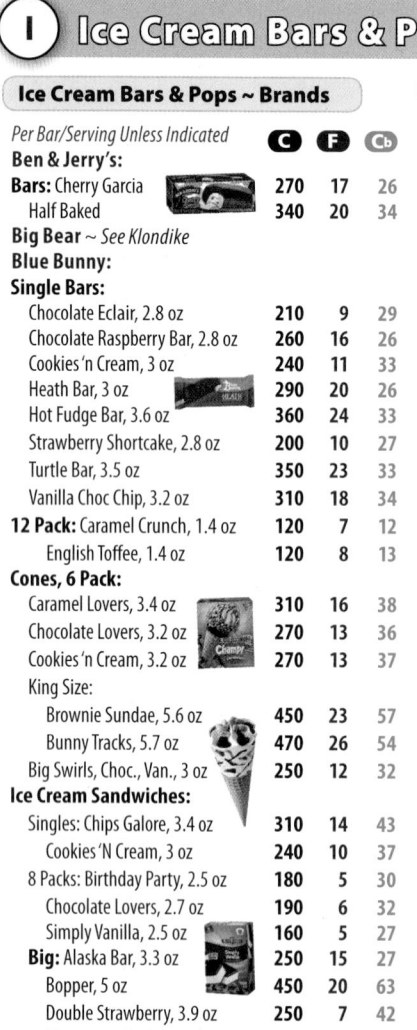

*Per Bar/Serving Unless Indicated*

| | **C** | **F** | **Cb** |
|---|---|---|---|
| **Butterfinger** *(Nestle),* | | | |
| **Loaded Ice Cream Bar** | 280 | 18 | 27 |
| **Clemmy's,** | | | |
| **Bars,** average all flavors, 2 oz | 70 | 3 | 16 |
| **Cool Classics:** | | | |
| **Arctic Blasters:** | | | |
| Crispy Bar | 160 | 11 | 15 |
| Fudge Bar | 100 | 1 | 21 |
| Ice Cream Bar | 150 | 10 | 13 |
| Orange Cream | 100 | 2.5 | 18 |
| Strawberry Shortcake | 150 | 8 | 20 |
| Toffee Bar | 160 | 11 | 14 |
| **Icepix:** Grape; Cherry; Orange | 35 | 0 | 8 |
| Honeydew; Watermelon; Cantelope | 35 | 0 | 9 |
| **Swirl Pops**, Mango-Cherry | 80 | 0 | 20 |
| **Creamsicles:** *Per Bar* | | | |
| **Box of 12**, 100 Cal. Orange Crm Pops | 100 | 1.5 | 19 |
| **Box of 18**, Sugar-Free Cream Pops | 30 | 0 | 6 |
| *Note: Sugar-Free carb figure includes 5g Sucralose sweetener* | | | |
| **Diana's Bananas:** | | | |
| **Banana Babies:** | | | |
| Milk/Dark Chocolate (1) | 130 | 6 | 18 |
| Milk Choc. & Peanuts (1) | 215 | 13 | 21 |
| **Banana Bites**, (5), 2 oz | 130 | 8 | 16 |
| **Dove:** | | | |
| **Bars:** *Per 2.6 oz Bar* | | | |
| Vanilla: | | | |
| With Milk Chocolate | 250 | 16 | 24 |
| And Almonds | 250 | 17 | 21 |
| Caramel Swirl & Cashews | 250 | 16 | 23 |
| Vanilla, | | | |
| with Dark Chocolate | 250 | 17 | 24 |
| **Miniatures**, Variety Pack, | | | |
| w/ Milk/Dark Choc., 5 pcs, 3.2 oz, av. | 330 | 21 | 32 |
| **Dreyer's/Edy's** *(Nestle)* : | | | |
| **Outshine Fruit Bars:** | | | |
| Creamy Coconut | 120 | 3 | 20 |
| Grape; Strawberry; Tangerine | 60 | 0 | 15 |
| Lemon; Lime | 70 | 0 | 18 |
| Mango; Pineapple | 75 | 0 | 18 |
| Peach | 90 | 0 | 23 |
| Pomegranate | 60 | 0 | 16 |
| Raspberry | 70 | 0 | 18 |

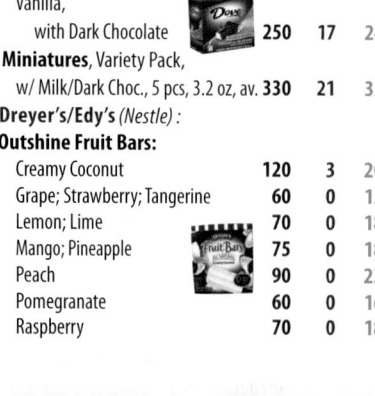

## Ice Cream Bars/Pops ~ Brands (Cont)

*Per Bar/Serving* — **C** **F** **Cb**

**Drumstick** *(Nestlé)*:

| | C | F | Cb |
|---|---|---|---|
| **Classic Cones:** Vanilla | 290 | 15 | 34 |
| Vanilla Caramel | 300 | 15 | 38 |
| Super Nugget: Van. Fudge | 320 | 17 | 37 |
| Strawberry | 310 | 17 | 34 |
| **S'mores,** Toasted Marshmallow | 270 | 12 | 39 |
| **Strawberry,** with Fudge | 300 | 15 | 37 |
| **King Size:** Triple Chocolate | 350 | 14 | 51 |
| Vanilla with Chocolate Layers | 360 | 16 | 49 |
| **Lil' Drums:** Choc with Choc Swirls | 130 | 6 | 16 |
| Average other flavors | 110 | 6 | 18 |
| **Simply Dipped:** Mint | 260 | 12 | 37 |
| Vanilla | 260 | 12 | 37 |
| **Edy's** ~ See Dreyer's | | | |
| **Eskimo Pie** *(Nestle)*: | | | |
| **Milk Chocolate,** Vanilla | 150 | 10 | 14 |
| **Dark Chocolate,** No Sugar Added | 150 | 10 | 13 |
| **Fat Boy:** | | | |
| **Sundae On A Stick:** | | | |
| Nut Sundae | 270 | 20 | 23 |
| Toffee Crunch | 280 | 20 | 26 |
| Vanilla Dipped | 260 | 19 | 22 |
| **Sandwiches:** Chocolate, 3 oz | 210 | 9 | 31 |
| Cookies n' Cream, 3 oz | 220 | 8 | 34 |
| Mint Chocolate Chip, 3 oz | 220 | 9 | 33 |
| Prem. Van.; Lime, 3 oz | 210 | 8 | 31 |
| Rasp. Cheesecake, 3 oz | 210 | 7 | 35 |
| Strawberry, 3 oz | 210 | 7 | 35 |
| **Fresh & Easy,** Vanilla Sundae Cone | 260 | 15 | 29 |
| **Fudge Bar** *(Nestle)*, Regular, 2.8 oz | 110 | 2 | 21 |
| **Fudgesicle:** | | | |
| **100 Calorie:** Fudge Bar | 100 | 2 | 17 |
| Low Fat Fudge Bar | 60 | 1.5 | 12 |
| **Good Humor:** | | | |
| **Dessert Bars, Singles:** | | | |
| Original Vanilla, 2.8 oz | 240 | 14 | 27 |
| Birthday Cake, 2.6 oz | 200 | 10 | 25 |
| Chocolate Eclair, 2.6 oz | 190 | 9 | 27 |
| Oreo 2.6 oz | 210 | 11 | 26 |
| Toasted Almond, 2.6 oz | 200 | 11 | 24 |
| **Cones, Singles:** | | | |
| Giant King Cone, | | | |
| Vanilla Chocolate, 5 oz | 390 | 22 | 44 |
| King Cone, Vanilla, 2.7 oz | 230 | 14 | 25 |
| Multi-Packs, | | | |
| King Cones, Vanilla, 3 oz | 240 | 12 | 31 |
| **Sandwiches:** | | | |
| Chocolate Chip Cookie, 2.7 oz | 250 | 10 | 40 |
| Giant, Neapolitan; Vanilla, av. | 220 | 5 | 40 |
| **Stickless:** Reese's PB Dessert Cup Bar | 260 | 17 | 25 |
| Girl Scout's Thin Mint Bar | 190 | 11 | 22 |

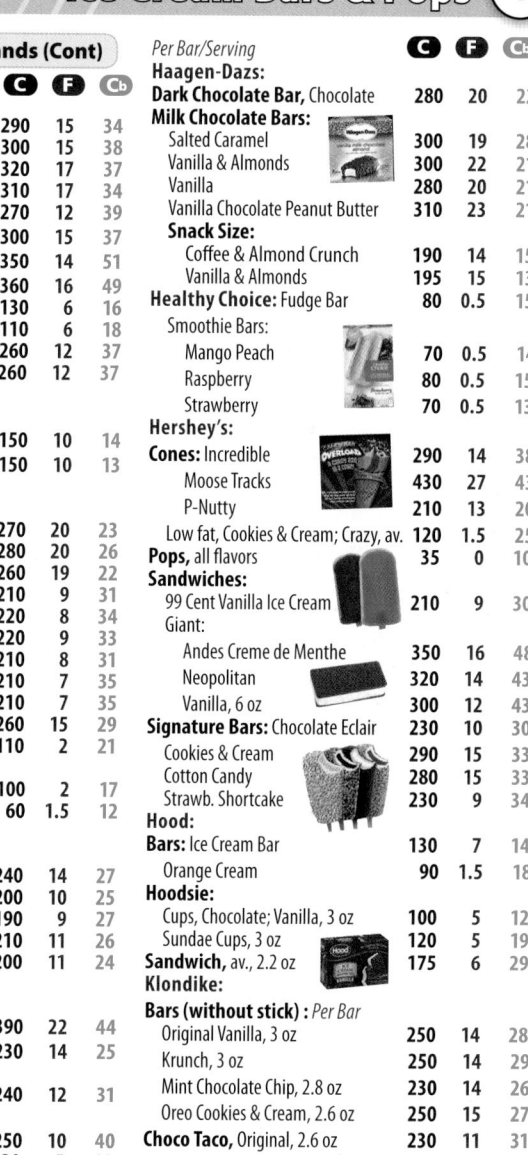

*Per Bar/Serving* — **C** **F** **Cb**

**Haagen-Dazs:**

| | C | F | Cb |
|---|---|---|---|
| **Dark Chocolate Bar,** Chocolate | 280 | 20 | 22 |
| **Milk Chocolate Bars:** | | | |
| Salted Caramel | 300 | 19 | 28 |
| Vanilla & Almonds | 300 | 22 | 21 |
| Vanilla | 280 | 20 | 21 |
| Vanilla Chocolate Peanut Butter | 310 | 23 | 21 |
| **Snack Size:** | | | |
| Coffee & Almond Crunch | 190 | 14 | 15 |
| Vanilla & Almonds | 195 | 15 | 13 |
| **Healthy Choice:** Fudge Bar | 80 | 0.5 | 15 |
| Smoothie Bars: | | | |
| Mango Peach | 70 | 0.5 | 14 |
| Raspberry | 80 | 0.5 | 15 |
| Strawberry | 70 | 0.5 | 13 |
| **Hershey's:** | | | |
| **Cones:** Incredible | 290 | 14 | 38 |
| Moose Tracks | 430 | 27 | 43 |
| P-Nutty | 210 | 13 | 20 |
| Low fat, Cookies & Cream; Crazy, av. | 120 | 1.5 | 25 |
| **Pops,** all flavors | 35 | 0 | 10 |
| **Sandwiches:** | | | |
| 99 Cent Vanilla Ice Cream | 210 | 9 | 30 |
| Giant: | | | |
| Andes Creme de Menthe | 350 | 16 | 48 |
| Neopolitan | 320 | 14 | 43 |
| Vanilla, 6 oz | 300 | 12 | 43 |
| **Signature Bars:** Chocolate Eclair | 230 | 10 | 30 |
| Cookies & Cream | 290 | 15 | 33 |
| Cotton Candy | 280 | 15 | 33 |
| Strawb. Shortcake | 230 | 9 | 34 |
| **Hood:** | | | |
| **Bars:** Ice Cream Bar | 130 | 7 | 14 |
| Orange Cream | 90 | 1.5 | 18 |
| **Hoodsie:** | | | |
| Cups, Chocolate; Vanilla, 3 oz | 100 | 5 | 12 |
| Sundae Cups, 3 oz | 120 | 5 | 19 |
| **Sandwich,** av., 2.2 oz | 175 | 6 | 29 |
| **Klondike:** | | | |
| **Bars (without stick)** : *Per Bar* | | | |
| Original Vanilla, 3 oz | 250 | 14 | 28 |
| Krunch, 3 oz | 250 | 14 | 29 |
| Mint Chocolate Chip, 2.8 oz | 230 | 14 | 26 |
| Oreo Cookies & Cream, 2.6 oz | 250 | 15 | 27 |
| **Choco Taco,** Original, 2.6 oz | 230 | 11 | 31 |
| **Sandwiches:** *Each* | | | |
| Mrs Fields, 2.3 oz | 210 | 8 | 34 |
| Vanilla, 2.7 oz | 180 | 5 | 31 |

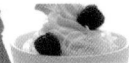
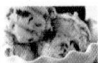

## Ice Cream Bars/Pops ~ Brands (Cont)

*Per Bar/Serving*

| | C | F | Cb |
|---|---|---|---|
| **Luigi's:** | | | |
| **Real Italian Ice:** Cherry | 100 | 0 | 26 |
| Chocolate Fudge | 150 | 0 | 36 |
| Mango | 100 | 0 | 26 |
| Watermelon; Blue Raspberry | 160 | 0 | 39 |
| **M&M's:** | | | |
| Cone, Single, 2.6 oz | 240 | 11 | 32 |
| Cookie Ice Cream Sandwich, 2.9 oz | 250 | 13 | 34 |
| **Magnum:** Almond, 2.8 oz | 270 | 18 | 24 |
| Dark, 3.2 oz | 240 | 17 | 20 |
| Double Caramel, 3.6 oz | 320 | 20 | 32 |
| Gold, 3 oz | 290 | 20 | 25 |
| White, 2.7 oz | 250 | 16 | 23 |
| Minis: Almond (2), 3.7 oz | 320 | 22 | 28 |
| Double Caramel (2), 3.8 oz | 380 | 22 | 38 |
| **Minute Maid,** Juice Bars, 2.25 fl.oz | 40 | 0 | 10 |
| **Nestlé:** | | | |
| **Bars:** Crunch Bar | 180 | 11 | 19 |
| Orange & Cream | 80 | 1.5 | 17 |
| Strawberry Shortcake | 210 | 9 | 31 |
| **Dibs,** Crunch, 4 oz container | 340 | 24 | 30 |
| **Drumsticks ~ See Page 109** | | | |
| **Ice Pop,** Wildberry & Zesty Lemon | 90 | 0 | 22 |
| **Sandwiches:** Neapolitan | 240 | 7 | 40 |
| Vanilla | 160 | 4 | 29 |
| **Toll House,** | | | |
| Choc. Chip Cookie Sandwich | 380 | 16 | 54 |
| **Popsicle:** | | | |
| Firecracker, all flavors (1) | 35 | 0 | 9 |
| Hello Kitty; Scribbles (2) | 60 | 0 | 14 |
| Marvel Avengers Assemble (1) | 40 | 0 | 10 |
| SpongeBob Pop-Ups (1) | 80 | 1 | 11 |
| Slow Melts, Mighty Minis, 5 pieces | 60 | 0 | 11 |
| **Reese's** *(Good Humor),* | | | |
| P'nut Butter Ice Cream Cup, 2.4 oz | 260 | 17 | 25 |
| **Skinny Cow:** | | | |
| **Bars:** Fudge | 110 | 1 | 22 |
| Chocolate Truffle | 100 | 2.5 | 19 |
| Vanilla Almond Crunch | 190 | 11 | 19 |
| **Candy Bars,** av. all flavors | 155 | 9 | 17 |
| **Cones,** average all flavors | 155 | 3 | 28 |
| **Sandwiches,** all flavors | 180 | 9 | 22 |
| **Snickers:** | | | |
| **Bars:** Regular, 1.8 oz | 180 | 11 | 18 |
| Mini Bar, 1 piece, 0.9 oz | 90 | 6 | 9 |
| **Cone,** 2.9 oz | 250 | 13 | 29 |
| **Ice Cream Brownie,** 3.3 oz | 300 | 13 | 41 |

*Per Bar/Serving*

| | C | F | Cb |
|---|---|---|---|
| **Snow Cone** *(Wonder)*, av. all, 7 fl.oz | 60 | 0 | 15 |
| **So Delicious** *(Turtle Mountain):* | | | |
| **Almond Based Minis:** | | | |
| Bars, Mocha ALm. Fudge (1), 1.8 oz | 150 | 10 | 14 |
| Sandwich, Vanilla, 1.3 oz | 90 | 3.5 | 13 |
| **Coconut Based Minis:** | | | |
| Bars: Almond, 1.8 oz | 180 | 13 | 17 |
| Simply Strawberry, 2 oz | 80 | 3.5 | 14 |
| **Soy Based Minis:** | | | |
| Sandwiches, av. all varieties, 1.4 oz | 90 | 2 | 18 |
| **Soy Dream:** Almond Bar (1), 3 oz | 140 | 16 | 24 |
| Bites, Choc/Vanilla/Coconut, 15 pcs | 140 | 16 | 22 |
| Lil' Dreamers, Vanilla | 100 | 4 | 15 |
| **Tampico,** Freezer Pops, all var., 1.4 oz | 30 | 0 | 7 |
| **Tofutti:** | | | |
| **Bars:** | | | |
| Chocolate Fudge/Coffee Break Treats | 30 | 0 | 6 |
| Hooray Hooray Bar | 120 | 8 | 8 |
| Marry Me Bar | 170 | 8 | 22 |
| Totally Fudge Pops | 95 | 1.5 | 19 |
| *Note: Carb figures include 0-7g sugar alcohols* | | | |
| **Cones,** (1), all flavors | 220 | 13 | 24 |
| **Cuties,** average all flavors | 130 | 6 | 18 |
| **Turkey Hill:** | | | |
| **Bar,** Vanilla Ice Cream, 3.3 oz | 320 | 23 | 26 |
| **Sandwiches:** Double Decker, 2.5 oz | 190 | 7 | 30 |
| Vanilla Bean, 2.5 oz | 190 | 7 | 29 |
| **Sundae Cone,** Van. Fudge | 320 | 18 | 33 |
| **Twix Bar,** 2.4 oz | 250 | 14 | 28 |
| **Wegmans:** | | | |
| **Bars:** Fudge, low fat | 100 | 1 | 20 |
| Peanut Butter Sundae Crunch | 200 | 11 | 22 |
| Vanilla, Choc Coated, 2 oz | 160 | 11 | 14 |
| **Cones:** Nutty Sundae, 2.5 oz | 210 | 11 | 25 |
| Sundae Nut, 3 oz | 260 | 15 | 29 |
| **Weight Watchers:** | | | |
| **Bars:** | | | |
| Dark Chocolate: | | | |
| Dulce de Leche | 120 | 4.5 | 19 |
| Raspberry | 120 | 5 | 18 |
| Giant, Fudge Bar | 90 | 1 | 21 |
| **Cones,** Double Caramel Swirl, snack | 90 | 2 | 17 |
| **Cups,** Chocolate Chip Cookie Dough | 140 | 3 | 26 |
| **Sandwiches:** Giant Vanilla | 140 | 2 | 31 |
| Mint | 140 | 1.5 | 31 |
| Red Velvet, snack size | 100 | 1.5 | 20 |
| **Sundae,** Peanut Butter Cup | 130 | 3 | 23 |
| **Yoplait** ~ *See Frozen Yogurt* | | | |
| **Yosicle,** Swirlz, average all flavors, (1) | 45 | 1 | 7 |

## Canned & Packaged Meals ~ Brands

**Amy's:** *Per Serve*

**Frozen:**

| | **C** | **F** | **Cb** |
|---|---|---|---|
| **Asian Meals:** | | | |
| Stir-Fry: Asian Noodle, 10 oz | 300 | 7 | 50 |
| Thai, 9.5 oz | 310 | 11 | 45 |
| **Bowls:** Baked Ziti, 9.5 oz | 390 | 12 | 62 |
| Broccoli & Cheddar Bake, 9.5 oz | 430 | 20 | 44 |
| Pesto Tortellini, 9.5 oz | 440 | 20 | 50 |
| **Burritos:** Bean & Cheese, 6 oz | 310 | 9 | 46 |
| Bean & Rice, 6 oz | 320 | 8 | 52 |
| Breakfast Burrito, 6 oz | 270 | 8 | 38 |
| **Entrees:** Cheese Enchilada, 4.5 oz | 240 | 14 | 18 |
| Cheese Lasagna, 10.3 oz | 410 | 16 | 46 |
| Macaroni & Soy Cheese, 9 oz | 370 | 15 | 42 |
| Roasted Vegetable Tamale, 10.3 oz | 280 | 7 | 44 |
| **Light & Lean:** *Per 8 oz Serve* | | | |
| Black Bean & Cheese Enchilada | 250 | 5 | 44 |
| Mattar Paner | 260 | 6 | 42 |
| Soft Taco Fiesta | 220 | 4.5 | 40 |
| **Pot Pies:** | | | |
| Broccoli, 7.5 oz | 460 | 24 | 50 |
| Mex. Tamale; Shephd's Pie, av., 8 oz | 165 | 4 | 27 |
| Vegetable, 7.5 oz | 430 | 20 | 54 |
| **Snacks:** Cheese Pizza, 5-6 pieces | 210 | 9 | 25 |
| Nacho, Cheese & Bean, 5-6 pcs | 220 | 9 | 25 |
| Swirls: Artichoke & Parmesan (2) | 210 | 11 | 20 |
| Cheddar Jalepeno (2) | 220 | 9 | 25 |
| Mushroom & Cheese; Pesto (2) | 180 | 9 | 19 |
| **Whole Meals:** | | | |
| Black Bean Enchil., 10 oz | 330 | 8 | 53 |
| Veggie Loaf, 10 oz | 340 | 10 | 47 |
| Veggie, Steak & Gravy, 11 oz | 380 | 16 | 50 |
| **Wraps:** | | | |
| Indian Samosa, 5 oz | 250 | 9 | 35 |
| Teriyaki, gluten free, 5.5 oz | 250 | 6 | 38 |
| Tofu Scramble, gluten free, 5.5 oz | 300 | 13 | 35 |
| **Atkins:** *Per 9 oz Tray/Bowl* | | | |
| **Frozen:** | | | |
| Beef Merlot | 310 | 21 | 9 |
| Chicken & Broccoli Alfredo | 330 | 20 | 9 |
| Chili Con Carne | 320 | 21 | 8 |
| Crustless Chicken Pot Pie | 330 | 22 | 8 |
| Italian Style Pasta Bake | 320 | 15 | 17 |
| Meatloaf w/ Portobello Mshrm Gravy | 340 | 23 | 11 |
| **Bagel Bites:** | | | |
| **Frozen:** | | | |
| Cheese, Sausage & Pepperoni, 4 pcs | 200 | 6 | 28 |
| Supreme; Three Cheese, av., 4 pcs, 3 oz | 195 | 5 | 31 |

| **B&M:** | **C** | **F** | **Cb** |
|---|---|---|---|
| **Baked Beans:** *Per 16 oz Can, ½ cup, 4.6 oz* | | | |
| Original | 170 | 2 | 31 |
| Boston's Best | 170 | 1.5 | 32 |
| Maple Flavor | 150 | 1 | 28 |
| Vegetarian | 160 | 1 | 25 |
| **Brown Bread,** Raisin, ½ slice, 2 oz | 130 | 0.5 | 29 |
| **Banquet:** | | | |
| **Homestyle Bakes:** *1 Cup, Prepared* | | | |
| Cheeseburger Mac | 240 | 6 | 36 |
| Chicken Taco Bake | 280 | 7 | 41 |
| Creamy Turkey & Stuffing | 240 | 10 | 29 |
| Pitza Pasta Bake | 280 | 6 | 46 |
| **Frozen:** | | | |
| **Meals:** Boneless Pork Rib, 10.5 oz | 370 | 14 | 45 |
| Cheesy & Macaroni & Beef, 7 oz | 230 | 9 | 27 |
| **Chicken:** Fingers, 6.5 oz | 310 | 12 | 33 |
| Fried Chicken, 10 oz | 330 | 14 | 40 |
| Nuggets, 6.2 oz | 300 | 13 | 32 |
| Parmesan, 8.5 oz | 320 | 11 | 41 |
| Fettuccine Alfredo, 8 oz | 300 | 12 | 36 |
| Fish Sticks, w/ Mac & Cheese, 7.5 oz | 260 | 9 | 33 |
| Homestyle Grilled Patty, 10 oz | 340 | 17 | 32 |
| Lasagna, w/ Meat Sce | 250 | 9 | 31 |
| Meat Loaf, 9.5 oz | 330 | 11 | 43 |
| Pepper Steak, 10 oz | 320 | 13 | 39 |
| Rigatoni & Italian Sausage, 8 oz | 300 | 12 | 35 |
| Salisbury Steak, 9.5 oz | 350 | 14 | 44 |
| Spaghetti & Meatballs, 10 oz | 320 | 14 | 34 |
| Spaghetti & Chicken Nuggets, 7 oz | 230 | 7 | 32 |
| Sweet & Sour Chicken, 8 oz | 420 | 10 | 70 |
| Turkey, 10 oz | 280 | 11 | 29 |
| **Family:** | | | |
| Broccoli Chicken & Cheese, with Rice & Sce, 7.7 oz | 210 | 7 | 26 |
| Chicken Alfredo, with Broccoli & Noodles, 8 oz | 210 | 6 | 29 |
| Salisbury Steak & Gravy, 4.5 oz | 180 | 12 | 11 |
| **Pies:** *Per 7 oz* | | | |
| **Deep Dish:** | | | |
| Breakfast Cheesy Ham & Potato | 440 | 25 | 46 |
| Breakfast Sausage & Gravy | 450 | 33 | 44 |
| **Pot Pie:** Chicken; Turkey, average | 335 | 19 | 32 |
| Chicken & Broccoli | 330 | 18 | 31 |

| Barilla: | C | F | Cb |
|---|---|---|---|
| **Microwaveables:** *Per 9 oz Container* | | | |
| Ital. Ssg; Meat Sauce Gemelli, av | 350 | 7 | 60 |
| Marinara/Tomato & Basil Penne, av. | 310 | 4 | 60 |

**Betty Crocker:**
**Bowl Appetit:**

| | C | F | Cb |
|---|---|---|---|
| Herb Chicken Flavored Veggie Rice | 250 | 3 | 51 |
| Pasta Alfredo | 350 | 9 | 55 |
| Three-Cheese Rotini | 340 | 7 | 59 |

**Hamburger Helper:** *Per 1 Cup, Prep'd*

| | | | |
|---|---|---|---|
| Bacon Cheeseburger | 320 | 14 | 27 |
| Beef Pasta | 280 | 12 | 24 |
| Cheeseburger Macaroni | 310 | 13 | 57 |
| Cheesy Baked Potatoes | 310 | 12 | 30 |
| Cheesy Italian Shells | 310 | 12 | 27 |
| Salisbury | 280 | 11 | 27 |
| Strogaoff | 310 | 12 | 30 |
| Three Cheese | 320 | 13 | 30 |

**Potatoes:** *Per Serving, Prepared*

| | | | |
|---|---|---|---|
| Casserole: Au Gratin, ½ cup | 150 | 6 | 24 |
| Cheddar & Bacon, ½ c. | 150 | 6 | 24 |
| Roasted Garlic, ½ cup | 130 | 4 | 21 |
| Scalloped, ⅔ cup | 130 | 3 | 24 |
| Sour Cream and Chives, ⅔ cup | 150 | 6.5 | 17 |

**Seasoned Skillet:**

| | | | |
|---|---|---|---|
| Hash Brown, ½ cup | 120 | 3 | 20 |
| Rstd Garlic & Herb Potatoes, ⅔ c. | 170 | 10 | 21 |
| Trad'nl Recipe Potatoes, ½ cup | 180 | 9 | 22 |

**Tuna Helper:** *Per 1 Cup, Prepared*

| | | | |
|---|---|---|---|
| Creamy Pasta | 250 | 10 | 27 |
| Average other varieties | 265 | 10 | 30 |

**Ultimate Helper:** *1 Cup Prepared*

| | | | |
|---|---|---|---|
| Cheddar Broccoli | 310 | 10 | 27 |
| Creamy Parmesan Alfedo | 340 | 10 | 30 |
| Sweet & Spicy Teriyaki | 300 | 9 | 33 |

**Biggest Loser:**
**Refrigerated:**
**Simply Sensible:** *Per ½ Package*

| | | | |
|---|---|---|---|
| Beef Pot Roast & Gravy | 220 | 5 | 16 |
| Beef Tips & Gravy | 200 | 3.5 | 21 |
| Lasagna | 200 | 5 | 28 |
| Mediterranean-Style Chicken | 250 | 6 | 36 |
| Zing Chicken | 230 | 1.5 | 38 |

| Birds Eye: | C | F | Cb |
|---|---|---|---|
| **Frozen:** | | | |
| **Voila!:** *Per 1 Cup Prepared Unless Indicated* | | | |
| Alfredo Chicken, 1½ cups | 280 | 12 | 37 |
| Beef & Broccoli Stir Fry | 160 | 6 | 13 |
| Chicken Florentine | 230 | 6 | 27 |
| Chicken Parmesan | 360 | 11 | 50 |
| Garlic Shrimp | 230 | 9 | 30 |
| Shrimp Scampi | 190 | 2.5 | 31 |
| Sweet & Sour Chicken | 200 | 1 | 38 |

**Boca:**
**Frozen:**
**Burger:**

| | | | |
|---|---|---|---|
| All American Flame Grilled, 2.5 oz | 120 | 5 | 6 |
| Cheeseburger, 2.5 oz | 100 | 4.5 | 6 |
| Grilled Vegetables, 2.5 oz | 80 | 1 | 7 |
| Original Vegan, 2.5 oz | 70 | 0.5 | 6 |

| **Chik'n:** Orig. Nuggets, 3 oz | 180 | 7 | 17 |
|---|---|---|---|
| Patties (1), 2.5 oz | 160 | 6 | 15 |
| Spicy Patties (1), 2.5 oz | 160 | 6 | 15 |

**Boston Market:**
**Frozen:**

| **Dinners:** Beef Steak & Pasta, 14 oz | 470 | 14 | 52 |
|---|---|---|---|
| Chicken Parmesan, 13 oz | 500 | 13 | 70 |
| Oven Roasted Chicken, 13 oz | 280 | 7 | 32 |
| Salisbury Steak, 14.5 oz | 530 | 32 | 38 |
| Swedish M'balls, 13 oz | 660 | 30 | 67 |

**Buitoni:**
**Refrigerated:**

| **Ravioli:** Four Cheese, 3.7 oz | 330 | 12 | 42 |
|---|---|---|---|
| Spinach & Artichoke, 3.8 oz | 310 | 11 | 42 |
| **Tortelloni:** Mixed Cheese, 3.7 oz | 320 | 8 | 47 |
| Chicken & Proscuitto, 3.8 oz | 330 | 9 | 46 |

**Other Pasta Dishes ~ See Page 133**
**Bush's Best:** *Per ½ Cup, 4.6 oz*

| **Baked Beans:** Original | 140 | 1 | 29 |
|---|---|---|---|
| Vegetarian | 130 | 0 | 29 |
| Average other varieties | 150 | 1 | 32 |
| Black Beans | 100 | 0 | 18 |
| Black Eyed Peas | 80 | 0 | 15 |
| **Chili Beans,** Pinto, medium | 110 | 1 | 20 |
| Dark Red Kidney Beans | 120 | 0 | 22 |
| Garbanzo Beans | 120 | 2 | 20 |

**Grillin' Beans:**

| Bourbon & Brown Sugar | 170 | 0.5 | 35 |
|---|---|---|---|
| Smokehouse Tradition | 160 | 1 | 33 |
| Southern Pit | 170 | 0.5 | 35 |
| Steakhouse | 180 | 0.5 | 39 |

| **Refried Beans:** Cocina Latina | 150 | 3 | 23 |
|---|---|---|---|
| Cocina Latina, Fat Free | 130 | 0 | 24 |

## Campbell's:

| | C | F | Cb |
|---|---|---|---|
| **Pork & Beans,** 11 oz can, | | | |
| 4.6 oz serving | 140 | 1.5 | 25 |
| **Chunky Microwaveable Bowls:** | | | |
| Firehouse; Roadhouse, | | | |
| Chunky Beef & Beans Chili, 1 cup | 220 | 6 | 28 |
| **Spaghetti O's:** *Per 1 Cup* | | | |
| Original | 170 | 1 | 34 |
| With Meatballs | 210 | 6 | 30 |
| With Sliced Franks | 160 | 4 | 25 |
| **Chef Boyardee:** | | | |
| **Big Bowl:** *Per 1 Cup* | | | |
| Creamy Tomato Chicken, 8.7 oz | 150 | 1.5 | 26 |
| Italian Sausage Marinara, 8.6 oz | 200 | 6 | 28 |
| **Canned:** *Per ½ Can, 7.5 oz* | | | |
| Beefaroni | 215 | 9 | 26 |
| Lasagna | 215 | 8 | 27 |
| **Ravioli:** *Per 1 Cup* | | | |
| Beef, in Tomato & Meat Sauce: | | | |
| Regular, 8.7 oz | 220 | 7 | 31 |
| 99% Fat Free, 8.6 oz | 170 | 2 | 31 |
| Overstuffed, 9.2 oz | 230 | 5 | 37 |
| Chicken Ravioli, 8.7 oz | 170 | 1.5 | 33 |
| in Meat & Tomato Sce, 8.7 oz | 230 | 6 | 34 |
| Mac & Cheese, 8.2 oz | 210 | 8 | 28 |
| Mini Bites, Beef Ravioli & M'balls, | | | |
| 1 cup, 8.6 oz | 220 | 7 | 32 |
| **Microwaveable:** *Per 7.5 oz Cup* | | | |
| Beefaroni | 220 | 8 | 28 |
| Beef Ravioli | 200 | 7 | 28 |
| Cheeze Ravioli | 190 | 5 | 28 |
| Mini Beef Ravioli | 160 | 4 | 25 |
| With Meatballs | 250 | 10 | 32 |
| **Boxed Pizza Maker Kits:** *Single Kits* | | | |
| Cheese, ¼ package, 4 oz | 260 | 4.5 | 47 |
| Pepperoni, ¼ package, 4 oz | 280 | 8 | 42 |
| Pizza Sauce, w/ Chse, ¼ c., 2 oz | 35 | 1.5 | 4 |
| **Dennison's Chili:** *Per Cup* | | | |
| **Chili Con Carne:** | | | |
| Original: w/ Beans, 9 oz | 350 | 15 | 31 |
| without Beans, 8.8 oz | 310 | 16 | 20 |
| **Chili:** | | | |
| Original, with Beans, 9 oz | 360 | 14 | 38 |
| Chunky, w/ Beans, 8.8 oz | 300 | 10 | 32 |
| Hot, with Beans, 9 oz | 350 | 14 | 36 |
| Vegetarian, 99% fat free, 9 oz | 190 | 1.5 | 34 |

## Dinty Moore *(Hormel)*:

| | C | F | Cb |
|---|---|---|---|
| **Big Bowl (Microwave):** *Approx. ½ of 15 oz Bowl* | | | |
| Beef Stew, 8.3 oz | 200 | 10 | 17 |
| Chicken & Dumplings, 8.5 oz | 220 | 7 | 29 |
| Scalloped Potatoes & Ham, 8.7 oz | 280 | 16 | 23 |
| **Dr. McDougall's:** *Per 2 oz Package* | | | |
| **Asian Noodle Entree Cups,** | | | |
| average all varieties | 200 | 1.5 | 41 |
| **Quinoa Cups:** Black Bean | 320 | 4 | 57 |
| Curry Almond and Br. Rice | 260 | 3 | 51 |
| Sweet Potato Kale | 260 | 3.5 | 48 |
| **Eden Organics:** *Per ½ Cup* | | | |
| **Baked Beans,** w/ Sorghum, 4.6 oz | 150 | 0 | 27 |
| **Chili Black Beans & Quinoa,** 4.4 oz | 100 | 1 | 18 |
| **Lentils,** w/ Onions & Bay Leaf, 4.6 oz | 90 | 0 | 13 |
| **Refried Beans:** | | | |
| Black Beans, 4.6 oz | 110 | 1.5 | 18 |
| Pinto; Kidney, av., 4.6 oz | 85 | 1 | 17 |
| **Farmhouse:** | | | |
| **Rice:** *Per 1 Cup, Prepared* | | | |
| Long Grain & Wild Herb | | | |
| & Butter | 250 | 7 | 44 |
| Mexican | 230 | 5 | 42 |
| Roasted Chicken Flavor | 230 | 5 | 44 |
| **French's:** | | | |
| **French Crispy Fried Onions:** | | | |
| Original; Cheddar: | | | |
| 2 Tbsp, 0.3 oz | 45 | 3.5 | 3 |
| ¼ cup, 0.5 oz | 90 | 7 | 6 |
| 1 cup, 2 oz | 360 | 28 | 24 |
| **GardenBurger:** | | | |
| **Veggie Burger:** *Per Burger* | | | |
| Original | 110 | 3 | 16 |
| Black Bean Chipotle | 90 | 3 | 16 |
| Portabella | 100 | 2.5 | 16 |
| **Garden Lites:** | | | |
| **Entrees:** *Per 7 oz Serving* | | | |
| Cheddar Broccoli | 210 | 6 | 29 |
| Kale & Quinoa Souffle | 200 | 6 | 23 |
| Mac & Cheese | 240 | 10 | 26 |
| Roasted Vegetable Souffle | 170 | 3 | 28 |
| **Bites:** | | | |
| Broccoli & Brown Rice (4) | 130 | 5 | 16 |
| Corn Bread (4) | 170 | 2.5 | 31 |
| Italian (4) | 130 | 5 | 16 |
| Kale & Brown Rice (4) | 130 | 5 | 17 |

| Gorton's: | C | F | Cb |
|---|---|---|---|
| **Battered Pollock Fillets,** | | | |
| Beer/Crispy (2), 3.6 oz | 255 | 14 | 24 |
| **Breaded Pollock Fillets:** | | | |
| Crunchy (2), 3.8 oz | 230 | 9 | 26 |
| Lemon Herb Crunchy (2), 3.7 oz | 220 | 9 | 25 |
| **Gourmet,** Signat. S'snd Salmon, 3.5 oz | 90 | 2 | 2 |
| **Grilled Fillets:** *Per Fillet* | | | |
| Garlic Butter Pollock, 3.5 oz | 80 | 3 | 0 |
| Lemon Butter Pollock, 3.5 oz | 90 | 3 | 0 |
| Signature Tilapia, 3.2 oz | 80 | 2 | 2 |
| **Shrimp:** | | | |
| Crispy Beer Batter (9), 3.5 oz | 240 | 12 | 25 |
| Crunchy Butterfly Shrimp (5), 3.5 oz | 220 | 8 | 27 |
| Garl. Butter Shrimp Scampi (6), 4 oz | 120 | 5 | 8 |
| **Simple Bake:** Salmon, 4.4 oz | 140 | 2.5 | 8 |
| Hadddock Garlic Herb Butter, 4.9 oz | 130 | 2.5 | 8 |
| Tilapia, Signature Seasoning, 5.2 oz | 120 | 3 | 3 |
| **Skillet Crisp,** Tilapia, av., 3.5 oz | 195 | 9 | 16 |
| **Smart & Crunch,** Fish Sticks (5), 3 oz | 180 | 5 | 24 |
| **Great Value** (Walmart): | | | |
| **Breakfast Bowls:** Bacon, 7 oz | 430 | 27 | 19 |
| Sausage, 7 oz | 390 | 25 | 22 |
| Sausage & Gravy, 7 oz | 360 | 24 | 21 |
| **Complete Skillet Meals,** | | | |
| Shrimp Scampi & Linguini, 12 oz | 550 | 23 | 58 |
| **Packaged Meals:** *Per 10 oz Pkg* | | | |
| Chicken Parmesan & Penne | 400 | 16 | 45 |
| Meatloaf & Mashed Potatoes | 370 | 21 | 29 |
| Rstd Turkey Breast w/ Mshd Potatoes | 260 | 11 | 23 |
| Salisbury Steak with Potatoes | 340 | 19 | 26 |
| Health Valley: | | | |
| **Vegetarian Chili:** *Per 8.7 oz Cup* | | | |
| 3 Bean Chipotle | 200 | 3 | 37 |
| Spicy Chili | 190 | 3 | 36 |
| Tame Tomato | 210 | 2.5 | 41 |
| Healthy Choice: | | | |
| **Asian Cafe Steamer:** | | | |
| Beef Teriyaki, 9.5 oz | 270 | 5 | 39 |
| General Tso's Spicy Chicken, 10.3 oz | 290 | 3.5 | 47 |
| Sweet Sesame Chicken, 9.7 oz | 280 | 7 | 31 |
| **Cafe Steamers:** Chkn & Noodles, 10 oz | 270 | 8 | 29 |
| Spaghetti & Meatballs, 9.5 oz | 300 | 7 | 40 |
| Sweet & Sour Chicken, 10 oz | 350 | 3.5 | 68 |
| **Complete Meals:** | | | |
| Beef Pot Roast, 11 oz | 260 | 7 | 32 |
| Chicken Parmig., 11.6 oz | 330 | 10 | 43 |
| Lem. Pepp. Fish, 10.7 oz | 340 | 4 | 59 |
| **Simply Cafe Steamers:** | | | |
| Chicken & Vegetable Stir Fry, 9.2 oz | 190 | 4 | 15 |
| Gr. Chicken & Broccoli Alfredo, 9.1 oz | 190 | 6 | 8 |
| Gr. Chicken Pesto & Veggies, 9.1 oz | 200 | 6 | 11 |

| Healthy Choice (Cont): | C | F | Cb |
|---|---|---|---|
| **Vegetarian Cafe Steamers:** | | | |
| Asian Potstickers | 330 | 3.5 | 67 |
| Portabella Spinach Parm. | 230 | 5 | 38 |
| Pumpkin Squash Ravioli | 260 | 6 | 44 |
| **Whole Grain Steamers:** | | | |
| Grilled Basil Chkn, 9.9 oz | 240 | 5 | 30 |
| Kung Pao Chicken, 9.5 oz | 280 | 4.5 | 41 |
| Pineapple Chicken, 9.9 oz | 310 | 5 | 49 |
| **Extra Product Listings ~** *www.CalorieKing.com* | | | |
| **Heinz,** Vegetarian Beans, ½ cup, 4 oz | 140 | 0.5 | 27 |
| Hormel: | | | |
| **Chili w/ Beans:** *Per 8.7 oz* | | | |
| Regular; Hot; Chunky, av. | 260 | 7 | 31 |
| Turkey | 210 | 3 | 28 |
| Vegetarian | 190 | 1 | 35 |
| **Chili w/out Beans:** *Per 8.3 oz* | | | |
| Chunky/Hot Chili, average | 215 | 9 | 19 |
| Turkey | 190 | 3 | 16 |
| **Compleats, Comfort Classics:** *Per 7.5 oz* | | | |
| Beefy Mac & Cheese | 220 | 4 | 35 |
| Chicken & Noodles | 180 | 6 | 20 |
| Dumplings & CHicken | 170 | 4 | 25 |
| Noodles & Beef | 150 | 2 | 26 |
| Spaghetti & Meat Sauce | 230 | 7 | 32 |
| **Compleats, Homesyle:** | | | |
| Beef Pot Roast, 9 oz | 230 | 6 | 22 |
| Chicken Alfredo, 10 oz | 340 | 18 | 28 |
| Chkn Breast & Msh'd Pot., 10 oz | 210 | 4.5 | 26 |
| Meatloaf & Mashed Pot., 9 oz | 280 | 12 | 27 |
| Salisbury Steak, 9 oz | 300 | 17 | 23 |
| Swedish Mtballs, 9 oz | 270 | 12 | 27 |
| **Refrigerated Meals:** | | | |
| H'style Meat Loaf & Tom. Sce, 5 oz | 220 | 9 | 14 |
| Sliced Rst Tukey Brst & Gravy, 5 oz | 110 | 2 | 3 |
| Slow Simmered Beef Tips, 4.3 oz | 170 | 10 | 4 |
| **Side Dishes:** | | | |
| Garlic Mashed Potatoes, 5 oz | 120 | 4 | 24 |
| HomeStyle Mashed Potatoes, 5 oz | 140 | 7 | 18 |
| Loaded Mashed Potatoes, 5 oz | 190 | 11 | 18 |
| Mashed Sweet Potato, 5 oz | 170 | 6 | 27 |
| Horizon Organic: | | | |
| **Mac & Cheese:** *Per 1 Cup Prepared* | | | |
| **Cheesy Mac:** 2.5 oz dry | 260 | 1.5 | 53 |
| Microwaveable, 2.1 oz dry | 220 | 2 | 44 |
| **Org. Cheesy Deluxe,** av., | | | |
| ⅓ box, 3.3 oz dry | 320 | 10 | 46 |
| **Organic Mac,** av., 2.5 oz dry | 260 | 2.5 | 50 |
| **Protein Mac,** 2.5 oz dry | 270 | 2.5 | 47 |

| Hot Pockets: | C | F | Cb |
|---|---|---|---|
| **Sandwiches:** *Per Sandwich* | | | |
| Crispy Buttery Crust: BBQ Rcpe Beef | 320 | 13 | 44 |
| Cheddar Cheeseburger | 290 | 11 | 39 |
| Hickory Ham & Chse | 280 | 11 | 38 |
| Crispy Crust: | | | |
| Five Cheese Pizza | 350 | 18 | 37 |
| Pepperoni Pizza | 340 | 19 | 35 |
| Croissant Crust: | | | |
| Hickory Ham & Cheddar | 310 | 15 | 35 |
| Philly Steak | 320 | 16 | 35 |
| Ssausage, Egg & Cheese | 320 | 17 | 35 |
| Flaky Crust, Chicken Pot Pie | 240 | 10 | 30 |
| Garlic Buttery Seasoned Crust | | | |
| Four Cheese Pizza | 320 | 13 | 39 |
| Four Meat & Four Cheese | 310 | 14 | 37 |
| Meatballs & Mozzarella | 310 | 13 | 38 |
| Pepperoni & Sausage Pizza | 310 | 14 | 38 |
| Pretzel Bread, | | | |
| Appwd Bacon Chedd. Chse Melt | 310 | 13 | 36 |
| Seasoned Crust, | | | |
| Philly Steak & Cheese | 300 | 12 | 38 |
| **Hungry Jack:** | | | |
| **Casserole Potatoes,** | | | |
| av. all varieties, ½ cup prepared | 165 | 7 | 21 |
| **Hashbrowns:** | | | |
| Original, ⅓ cup prepared | 100 | 4.5 | 14 |
| Cheesy, ½ cup prepared | 140 | 7 | 17 |
| **Mashed Potatoes,** average, | | | |
| Dry Mix only, ⅓ cup unprepared | 80 | 0 | 19 |
| **Hungry Man:** | | | |
| **Dinners:** | | | |
| Boneless Fried Chicken | 790 | 37 | 88 |
| Boneless Pork Rib Shaped Patties | 730 | 33 | 85 |
| Country Fried Chicken | 580 | 26 | 56 |
| Grilled Beef Patty | 450 | 22 | 39 |
| Home-Style Meatloaf | 530 | 22 | 64 |
| Roasted Carved White Meat Turkey | 430 | 11 | 62 |
| Salisbury Steak | 540 | 28 | 49 |
| **Pub Favorites:** | | | |
| Beer Battered Chkn | 760 | 38 | 75 |
| Honey Bourbon Chicken Strips | 600 | 25 | 69 |

| Hungry Man (Cont): | C | F | Cb |
|---|---|---|---|
| **Selects:** *Per Package* | | | |
| Classic Fried Chicken | 840 | 41 | 77 |
| Spicy Classic Fried Chicken | 700 | 34 | 61 |
| **XXL Sandwiches:** *Per Package* | | | |
| Angus Beef Charbroil | 740 | 47 | 52 |
| BBQ Pork Ribs | 690 | 39 | 62 |
| Buffalo Fried Chicken | 650 | 27 | 73 |
| Chicken Parmesan | 610 | 29 | 63 |
| Crispy Fried Chicken | 670 | 32 | 64 |
| **José Olé:** | | | |
| **Breakfast Burritos:** | | | |
| Egg & Bacon, 4 oz | 260 | 10 | 30 |
| Egg & Sausage, 4 oz | 240 | 10 | 28 |
| **Premium Burritos:** | | | |
| Chicken Monterey (1) | 270 | 6 | 41 |
| Steak & Cheese (1) | 300 | 10 | 40 |
| **Premium Chimichangas:** | | | |
| Chicken & Cheese (1), 5 oz | 330 | 11 | 45 |
| Steak & Cheese (1), 5 oz | 350 | 14 | 41 |
| **Snacks:** | | | |
| Mini: Chimichangas, | | | |
| Steak & Cheddar (3) | 370 | 20 | 37 |
| Quesadillas, | | | |
| Grilled Chicken & 3 Cheese (4) | 210 | 8 | 25 |
| Tacos, Beef & Cheese (4) | 230 | 12 | 23 |
| **Taquitos:** Chicken, Corn Tortillas, (3) | 200 | 8 | 26 |
| Steak & Cheese, Flour Tortillas, (2) | 250 | 12 | 26 |
| **Kashi:** | | | |
| **Entrees:** *Per 10 oz Package* | | | |
| Black Bean Mango | 340 | 8 | 58 |
| Chicken Enchilada | 280 | 9 | 38 |
| Chicken Florentine | 290 | 9 | 31 |
| Chicken Pasta Pomodoro | 280 | 6 | 38 |
| Mayan Harvest Bake | 340 | 9 | 58 |
| Pesto Pasta Primavera | 290 | 11 | 37 |
| Southwest Style Chicken | 310 | 5 | 49 |
| **Kid Cuisine:** *Per Meal* | | | |
| Cheese Stuffed Crust Pizza | 330 | 7 | 54 |
| Chicken Breast Nuggets, 8 oz | 400 | 13 | 55 |
| Fish Sticks, 7.6 oz | 320 | 11 | 45 |
| Fried Chicken, 10 oz | 530 | 22 | 53 |
| Hot Dog, 7.2 oz | 320 | 5 | 55 |
| Mac. & Cheese, 10.6 oz | 420 | 11 | 69 |
| Pancakes, 7.2 oz | 400 | 15 | 59 |
| Popcorn Chicken, 8.6 oz | 370 | 12 | 53 |
| Spaghetti w/ Mini Meatballs, 10.2 oz | 290 | 6 | 45 |

# Meals ◆ Entrees ◆ Sides ~ Canned/Packaged

| Knorr: Sides, Prepared as Directed | C | F | Cb |
|---|---|---|---|
| **Asian:** Chicken Fried Rice | 290 | 7 | 48 |
| Teriyaki Noodles | 280 | 9 | 45 |
| Teriyaki Rice | 280 | 7 | 48 |
| **Cajun,** Garlic Butter Rice | 260 | 4 | 48 |
| **Fiesta:** Mexican Rice/Spanish | 280 | 6 | 48 |
| Taco Rice | 270 | 6 | 46 |
| **Pasta:** Alfredo; Parmesan | 290 | 10 | 39 |
| Alfredo Broccoli | 300 | 10 | 39 |
| Butter; Butter & Herb;Stroganoff | 260 | 8 | 39 |
| Cheesy Cheddar | 270 | 7 | 39 |
| **Rice:** Cheddar Broccoli | 280 | 6 | 48 |
| Chicken Flavor Broccoli | 270 | 5 | 48 |
| Chicken Flavor | 280 | 6 | 48 |

**Kraft:**

**Macaroni & Cheese Dinner:** *Prepared*

| | C | F | Cb |
|---|---|---|---|
| Blue Box: Original flavor, 2.5 oz dry | 350 | 13 | 47 |
| Cheddar Explosion, 2.5 oz dry | 300 | 6 | 51 |
| Thick 'N Creamy, 2.5 oz dry | 370 | 12 | 50 |
| Three Cheese, 2.5 oz dry | 360 | 12 | 51 |
| Deluxe: Original, 3.5 oz dry | 310 | 10 | 42 |
| White Chedd. & Bacon, 3.5 oz | 320 | 11 | 41 |
| Microwaveable: Orig., 2 oz dry | 220 | 3.5 | 41 |
| White Cheddar, 2 oz dry | 220 | 3.5 | 41 |

**Velveeta Cheesy Potatoes:** *Dry Ingredients*

| | C | F | Cb |
|---|---|---|---|
| Au Gratin, 2 oz dry | 180 | 5 | 24 |
| Bacon Scalloped, 2.1 oz dry | 190 | 5 | 24 |
| Sthwest Diced, 1.9 oz dry | 170 | 5 | 24 |

**Velveeta Shells & Cheese,**

| | C | F | Cb |
|---|---|---|---|
| Original, 2.4 oz dry | 220 | 8 | 29 |

**Kroger:**

**Kitchen Creation Skillet Dinners:** *Per Cup, Prepared*

| | C | F | Cb |
|---|---|---|---|
| Creamy Broccoli | 300 | 12 | 33 |
| Creamy Pasta | 300 | 13 | 33 |
| Double Cheeseburger | 320 | 13 | 30 |
| Lasagna | 280 | 12 | 26 |
| Stroganoff | 320 | 14 | 27 |

**Frozen:**

**Healthy Meals Made Simple:** *Refrigerated, Per Cup*

| | C | F | Cb |
|---|---|---|---|
| Braised Beef Pot Roast & Gravy | 220 | 5 | 15 |
| Lean Beef Tips & Gravy | 210 | 4 | 20 |
| Lem. Herb Chkn w/ Rice | 170 | 1.5 | 23 |
| Sweet & Spicy Chicken | 270 | 1.5 | 48 |

| Kroger (Cont): | C | F | Cb |
|---|---|---|---|
| **Frozen (Cont):** | | | |
| **Meals Made Simple:** | | | |
| Beef Stir Fry, 1¾ cups | 180 | 4 | 26 |
| Chicken Florentine, 2¼ cups, 6.9 oz | 320 | 18 | 22 |
| Chicken Stir Fry, 1½ cups | 180 | 2 | 25 |
| Shrimp Fried Rice, 1¼ cups, 8 oz | 240 | 0 | 44 |
| **Oven Ready:** | | | |
| Breaded Calamari Rings (10), 3 oz | 200 | 10 | 21 |
| Coconut Shrimp (5), with 1 oz sweet chili sauce | 350 | 20 | 34 |

**La Choy:**

**Family Meals, Canned:** *Per 1 Cup*

| | C | F | Cb |
|---|---|---|---|
| Beef Pepper Oriental, 8.9 oz | 80 | 1 | 11 |
| Beef Chow Mein, 8.7 oz | 80 | 0 | 11 |
| Chicken Chow Mein, 8.8 oz | 100 | 4 | 11 |
| Sweet & Sour Chicken, 8.9 oz | 180 | 1.5 | 35 |

**Lean Cuisine:**

**Culinary Collection:** *Per Complete Meal*

| | C | F | Cb |
|---|---|---|---|
| Asparagus &Cheese Ravioli | 260 | 7 | 40 |
| Beef Chow Fun | 320 | 5 | 54 |
| Broccoli Cheddar Dip with Pita Bread | 200 | 6 | 29 |
| Chicken Pecan | 320 | 7 | 49 |
| Chkn in Peanut Sauce | 280 | 6 | 35 |
| Chicken with Almonds | 270 | 4 | 44 |
| Chicken with Basil Cream Sauce | 230 | 5 | 28 |
| Chili Lime Chicken | 240 | 2 | 38 |
| Fiesta Grilled Chicken | 260 | 6 | 33 |
| Lemon Pepper Fish | 300 | 8 | 40 |
| Mushroom Mezzaluna Ravioli | 290 | 9 | 39 |
| Orange Chicken | 310 | 8 | 46 |
| Parmesan Crusted Fish | 300 | 8 | 43 |
| Ranchero Braised Beef | 240 | 5 | 32 |
| Roasted Chicken & Garden Veggies | 230 | 3 | 35 |
| Sesame Chicken | 330 | 9 | 47 |
| Spinach Artichoke Ravioli | 280 | 7 | 41 |
| Sweet & Sour Chicken | 300 | 3 | 51 |
| Spring Rolls: | | | |
| Fajita Style Chicken (2) | 220 | 8 | 22 |
| Garlic/Thai Chicken (2), average | 200 | 7 | 24 |

*continued next page...*

| Lean Cuisine (Cont): | C | F | Cb |
|---|---|---|---|
| **Market Collections:** | | | |
| Chicken Pot Stickers | 280 | 7 | 43 |
| Garlic Chicken | 290 | 5 | 38 |
| Roasted Turkey Breast | 290 | 7 | 38 |
| Salisbury Steak | 260 | 6 | 38 |
| Shanghai Style Shrimp | 250 | 3 | 41 |
| Shrimp Scampi | 250 | 7 | 32 |
| Sweet & Spicy Ginger Chicken | 290 | 2 | 45 |
| **Simple Favorites:** | | | |
| BBQ Chicken Quesadilla | 280 | 6 | 37 |
| Chicken Chow Mein | 200 | 2 | 34 |
| French Bread Cheese Pizza | 340 | 6 | 53 |
| Spaghetti with Meat Sauce | 310 | 4 | 53 |
| **Spa Collection:** | | | |
| Butternut Squash Ravioli | 260 | 7 | 40 |
| Lemongrass Chicken | 240 | 4 | 38 |
| Salmon with Basil | 250 | 2 | 38 |
| **Pizzas ~** *See Page 136* | | | |
| **Extra Product Listings ~** *www.CalorieKing.com* | | | |
| **Lean Pockets:** | | | |
| **Sandwiches:** *Per Single Pocket* | | | |
| Garlic Buttery Crust, Pepp. Pizza | 320 | 15 | 35 |
| Pretzel Bread: BBQ Recipe Chicken | 250 | 5 | 41 |
|    Chicken Japalpeno Cheddar | 260 | 8 | 35 |
|    Three Cheese & Spinach | 250 | 7 | 37 |
| Seasoned Crust, | | | |
|    Four Cheese Pizza | 260 | 6 | 42 |
| Whole Grain Crust: | | | |
|    Bacon, Egg & Cheese | 260 | 8 | 35 |
|    Garlic Chicken White Pizza | 260 | 8 | 37 |
|    Hickory Ham & Cheddar | 270 | 8 | 39 |
|    Supreme Pizza | 220 | 7 | 33 |
|    Three Cheese & Broccoli | 250 | 6 | 40 |
| **Lightlife (Meatless):** | | | |
| **Beef:** | | | |
| Gimme Lean Beef, 2 oz | 60 | 0 | 7 |
| Smart Grounds: | | | |
|    Mexican Crumbles, 2 oz | 60 | 0 | 6 |
|    Original Crumbles, 2 oz | 70 | 0 | 6 |
| **Burgers:** | | | |
| Orig., with Quinoa (1) | 100 | 2.5 | 10 |
| Black Bean (1) | 100 | 2.5 | 11 |
| **Chick'n:** | | | |
| Smart Cutlets/Tenders, 3 oz | 110 | 1 | 7 |
| Smart Strips, 3 oz | 80 | 0 | 5 |
| Smart Wings, 4 wings, 3 oz | 110 | 0 | 6 |
| **Tempeh:** | | | |
| Fakin' Bacon Strips, 4 slices | 140 | 5 | 10 |
| Flax, 3 oz | 160 | 7 | 9 |

| Lunchables: | C | F | Cb |
|---|---|---|---|
| **Crackers Stackers:** *Without Drink* | | | |
| Ham & Swiss, 3.4 oz | 320 | 10 | 42 |
| Light Bologna & Am. Cheese, 2.8 oz | 310 | 16 | 34 |
| Turkey & Cheddar, 2.9 oz | 340 | 14 | 42 |
| Extra Cheesy Pizza | 270 | 9 | 30 |
| Ham & Cheddar, | | | |
|    with Crackers, 3.2 oz | 260 | 13 | 22 |
| Nachos, Cheese Dip & Salsa, 4.7 oz | 500 | 23 | 65 |
| Pizza, with Pepperoni | 300 | 13 | 32 |
| Turkey & Cheddar, w/ Crackers, 3.2 oz | 260 | 13 | 22 |
| **Lunchmakers** *(Armour): Per Package* | | | |
| Bologna Cracker Crunchers | 350 | 14 | 46 |
| Cheese Pizza | 340 | 12 | 51 |
| Nachos | 480 | 17 | 77 |
| Pepperoni Pizza | 330 | 10 | 55 |
| Turkey Cracker Crunchers | 350 | 14 | 45 |
| **Marie Callender's:** | | | |
| **Beef:** *Per Container* | | | |
| Beef & Broccoli | 370 | 9 | 50 |
| Beef Pot Roast | 320 | 11 | 35 |
| Country Fried Beef Steak & Gravy | 660 | 31 | 75 |
| **Chicken:** *Per Container* | | | |
| Chicken Parmigiana | 530 | 27 | 47 |
| Country Fried Chicken & Gravy | 560 | 27 | 61 |
| Fettuccini with Chicken & Broccoli | 500 | 24 | 41 |
| Sweet & Sour Chicken | 560 | 13 | 93 |
| **Pasta:** *Per Container* | | | |
| Fettuccini Alfredo & Garlic Bread | 610 | 31 | 59 |
| Grilled Chicken Alfredo Bake | 480 | 21 | 45 |
| **Pot Pies:** *Per 1 Cup, 7 oz* | | | |
| Beef | 410 | 23 | 39 |
| Cheesy Chicken & Bacon | 520 | 31 | 43 |
| Chicken | 380 | 21 | 38 |
| Chicken Corn Chowder | 470 | 27 | 44 |
| Creamy: | | | |
|    Mushroom Chicken | 450 | 27 | 41 |
|    Parmesan Chicken | 420 | 24 | 35 |
| Turkey | 480 | 28 | 46 |
| **Under 500 Calories:** | | | |
| Country Fried Pork Chop & Gravy | 460 | 19 | 55 |
| Golden Battered Fish Filet | 410 | 11 | 58 |
| Herb Roasted Chicken | 470 | 17 | 46 |
| Meat Loaf & Gravy | 450 | 17 | 43 |
| Spaghetti & Meatballs | 420 | 13 | 52 |
| Steak & Roasted Potatoes | 350 | 11 | 40 |
| **Family size:** *Per 1 Cup* | | | |
| Cheesy Chicken Lasagna, 8 oz | 320 | 14 | 33 |
| Vermont White Cheddar | | | |
|    Mac & Cheese, 6.3 oz | 350 | 20 | 31 |

| Maruchan: | C | F | Cb |
|---|---|---|---|
| **Bowls,** all varieties, 3.3 oz | 380 | 16 | 50 |
| **Ramen,** Noodle Soup, average all, 3 oz pkg | 380 | 16 | 52 |
| **Instant Lunch,** average, 1 package | 290 | 11 | 39 |
| **Yakisoba:** *Per 4 oz Pkg* | | | |
| Chicken/Teriyaki Beef Flavor, av. | 520 | 21 | 72 |
| Sweet & Sour Chicken | 560 | 22 | 78 |
| **Michael Angelo's:** | | | |
| **Organic:** Chicken Parmesan, 10 oz | 350 | 6 | 47 |
| Four Cheese Lasagna, 10 oz | 380 | 11 | 46 |
| Lasagna with Meat Sauce, 10 oz | 390 | 16 | 38 |
| Manicotti, with Sauce, 10 oz | 410 | 18 | 35 |
| **Signature:** Chicken Alfredo, 11 oz | 410 | 12 | 47 |
| Meat Lasagna, 11 oz | 420 | 13 | 51 |
| Shrimp Scampi, 10 oz | 540 | 28 | 46 |
| **Minute Rice:** | | | |
| **Ready To Serve:** *Per 4.4 oz Container, Prepared* | | | |
| Brown/Chicken Rice Mix, average | 230 | 5 | 42 |
| Fried/Yellow Rice Mix, average | 225 | 2.5 | 46 |
| **Morningstar Farms (Meatless):** | | | |
| **Breakfast,** Hot & Spicy Ssg Patty (1) | 70 | 3 | 3 |
| **Burgers:** *Per Patty* | | | |
| Grillers Original (1) | 130 | 6 | 5 |
| Mushroom Lovers (1) | 110 | 5 | 6 |
| Spicy Black Bean (1) | 110 | 4 | 13 |
| **Chik'n:** | | | |
| Buffalo Wings (5) | 200 | 9 | 19 |
| Chik'n Nuggets (4) | 180 | 8 | 18 |
| Patties: | | | |
| Chik, Original (1) | 160 | 6 | 19 |
| Grillers Chik'n Veggie (1) | 80 | 3 | 7 |
| Hot & Spicy Sausage (1) | 70 | 3 | 3 |
| **Entree:** Baja Black Bean Pizza (1) | 380 | 11 | 59 |
| Mediterranean Chickpea Pizza (1) | 380 | 12 | 59 |
| **Newman's Own:** | | | |
| **Comp[lete Skillets:** *Per ½ Package, 11-12 oz* | | | |
| Chicken: Fettuccini Alfredo | 410 | 12 | 49 |
| Florentine & Farfalle | 370 | 10 | 42 |
| Parmigiana & Penne | 490 | 25 | 47 |
| Garlic Chicken Lo Mein Noodles | 320 | 7 | 42 |
| Italian Ssge & Rigatoni | 510 | 28 | 48 |
| Steak Fajita | 290 | 6 | 47 |
| Sweet & Sour Chicken | 330 | 10 | 46 |

| Nissin: | C | F | Cb |
|---|---|---|---|
| **Chow Mein:** *Per 4 oz Package* | | | |
| Chicken Flavor | 480 | 18 | 70 |
| Spicy Chicken Flavor | 560 | 28 | 66 |
| Teriyaki Beef | 520 | 20 | 68 |
| With Shrimp | 540 | 24 | 68 |
| **Cup Noodles,** | | | |
| Beef/Chicken/Shrimp Flav., 1 cup | 280 | 11 | 40 |
| **Top Ramen,** average, 3 oz package | 380 | 14 | 52 |
| **Old El Paso:** | | | |
| **Dinner Kits:** *Per Serving, Prepared with Chicken* | | | |
| Chicken Soft Taco | 300 | 10 | 30 |
| Enchilada | 390 | 16 | 27 |
| **Frozen Meals:** *Per ½ Pkg* | | | |
| Chicken Burritos (1) | 480 | 17 | 59 |
| Chicken Quesadillas (1) | 620 | 30 | 57 |
| Shredded Beef Burritos (1) | 490 | 16 | 63 |
| **Pasta Roni:** *Per Cup, Prepared* | | | |
| Angel Hair Pasta varieties, average | 310 | 14 | 40 |
| Butter & Herb Italiano | 300 | 11 | 41 |
| Chicken & Broccoli | 360 | 15 | 49 |
| Chicken Flavor | 300 | 12 | 40 |
| Fettuccine Alfredo | 450 | 24 | 44 |
| Four Cheese Corkscrew | 370 | 15 | 49 |
| Stroganoff | 350 | 13 | 48 |
| Tomato Parmesan | 270 | 9 | 40 |
| White Cheddar & Broccoli | 300 | 13 | 39 |
| **P.F. Chang's:** *Per ½ Package, 11 oz* | | | |
| **Meals:** Beef with Broccoli | 360 | 17 | 30 |
| General Chang's Chicken | 350 | 14 | 35 |
| King Pao Chicken | 360 | 17 | 27 |
| Mongolian Style Beef | 340 | 11 | 41 |
| Mongolian Style Chicken | 310 | 9 | 40 |
| Orange Chicken | 430 | 18 | 44 |
| Sweet & Sour Chicken | 335 | 12 | 40 |
| Shrimp Lo Mein | 390 | 12 | 52 |

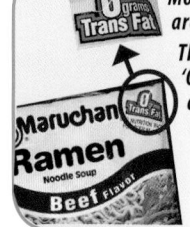

*Most packaged noodle soups are high in calories and fat.*

*Their promotion of 'O Grams Trans Fat' does not make them heart-healthy.*

*They are still high in saturated fat as well as salt/sodium.*

| | C | F | Cb |
|---|---|---|---|
| **Rice-A-Roni:** | | | |
| **Classic Favorites:** *Per Cup, Prepared* | | | |
| Beef; Herb & Butter; Rice Pilaf, av. | 310 | 9 | 52 |
| Broccoli Au Gratin | 350 | 16 | 46 |
| Chicken Flavor | 300 | 9 | 50 |
| Chicken & Broccoli | 220 | 5 | 40 |
| Spanish Rice | 260 | 8 | 44 |
| **Whole Grain Blends:** | | | |
| Roasted Garlic Italiano | 270 | 9 | 41 |
| Spanish | 250 | 8 | 42 |
| **Rosarita:** | | | |
| Kidney Beans, 4.5 oz | 110 | 0 | 20 |
| Chili Beans, 4.5 oz | 130 | 0.5 | 24 |
| **Refried Beans:** | | | |
| Traditional, 4.5 oz | 120 | 2 | 18 |
| No Fat, 14.5 oz | 100 | 0 | 18 |
| **Safeway Select:** | | | |
| **Frozen:** | | | |
| Beef Salisbury Steak, 9.4 oz | 410 | 28 | 23 |
| Chicken Cacciatore, 8.8 oz | 290 | 10 | 34 |
| Fettucini Alfredo, 11.5 oz | 380 | 12 | 55 |
| Five Vegetable Lasagna, 10.6 oz | 330 | 8 | 48 |
| Homestyle Baked Chicken, 9 oz | 260 | 11 | 31 |
| Orange Chicken, 9 oz | 360 | 7 | 61 |
| Penne Pasta, 8 oz | 300 | 11 | 42 |
| Pot Roast, 9 oz | 270 | 11 | 23 |
| Spaghetti with Meat Sauce, 12 oz | 450 | 16 | 61 |
| Swedish Meat Balls, 11.5 oz | 470 | 24 | 43 |
| Three Cheese Tortellini, 7.5 oz | 350 | 16 | 38 |
| **S & W:** *Per ½ Cup* | | | |
| Black Beans, 4.5 oz | 110 | 0.5 | 22 |
| Chili Beans, in Zesty Tomato Sauce, 4.6 oz | 130 | 1.5 | 23 |
| Kidney Beans, 4.7 oz | 110 | 0 | 22 |
| White Beans, 4.5 oz | 110 | 0.5 | 21 |
| **Seapak** ~ *See www.calorieking.com* | | | |
| **Simply Asia:** | | | |
| **Noodle Bowls:** *Per 8.5oz Bowl* | | | |
| Roasted Peanut | 460 | 12 | 75 |
| Sesame Teriyaki | 390 | 13 | 82 |
| Soy Ginger | 420 | 6 | 84 |
| Spicy Mongolian | 430 | 6 | 86 |

| | C | F | Cb |
|---|---|---|---|
| **Simply Asia:** | | | |
| **Noodle Bowls:** *Per 8.5oz Bowl* | | | |
| Roasted Peanut | 460 | 12 | 75 |
| Sesame Teriyaki | 390 | 13 | 82 |
| Soy Ginger | 420 | 6 | 84 |
| Spicy Mongolian | 430 | 6 | 86 |
| **Noodles & Sauce:** *Per ⅓ Package* | | | |
| Sesame Teriyaki | 300 | 3 | 60 |
| Soy Ginger | 320 | 4.5 | 60 |
| Spicy Kung Pao | 350 | 7 | 63 |
| **Quick Noodles:** *Per 8.8 oz Tray* | | | |
| Honey Teriyaki | 430 | 3.5 | 85 |
| Pad Thai | 460 | 3 | 93 |
| Szechwan Garl. Chow Mein | 460 | 7 | 83 |
| **Smart Ones** *(Weight Watchers):* | | | |
| **Classic Favorites:** *Per Meal* | | | |
| Angel Hair Marinara | 180 | 2 | 34 |
| Chkn Enchiladas Suiza | 290 | 6 | 46 |
| Lasagna Bake with Meat Sauce | 250 | 5 | 39 |
| Lasagna Florentine | 320 | 10 | 43 |
| Lemon Herb Chicken Piccata | 210 | 2.5 | 32 |
| Macaroni & Cheese | 260 | 2 | 51 |
| Pasta Primavera | 200 | 2.5 | 35 |
| Pasta with Ricotta & Spinach | 290 | 5 | 44 |
| Ravioli Florentine | 210 | 3.5 | 37 |
| Spaghetti with Meat Sauce | 280 | 3.5 | 50 |
| Swedish Meatballs | 290 | 7 | 38 |
| Three Cheese Macaroni | 300 | 6 | 48 |
| Traditional Lasagna w/ Meat Sauce | 310 | 8 | 45 |
| Tuna Noodle Gratin | 250 | 3 | 44 |
| **Smart Beginnings:** *Per Meal* | | | |
| Breakfast Quesadilla | 230 | 7 | 29 |
| Canadian Bacon English Muffin | 210 | 6 | 27 |
| English Muffin S'wich, Egg White & Cheese | 210 | 5 | 28 |
| Three Cheese Omelet | 200 | 7 | 20 |
| **Smart Creations:** *Per Meal* | | | |
| Chicken Fettucini | 300 | 4 | 45 |
| Chicken Parmesan | 280 | 5 | 37 |
| Homestyle Turkey Breast, with Stuffing | 280 | 6 | 36 |
| Meatloaf | 270 | 9 | 25 |
| Teriyaki Chicken & Vegetables | 250 | 2.5 | 41 |

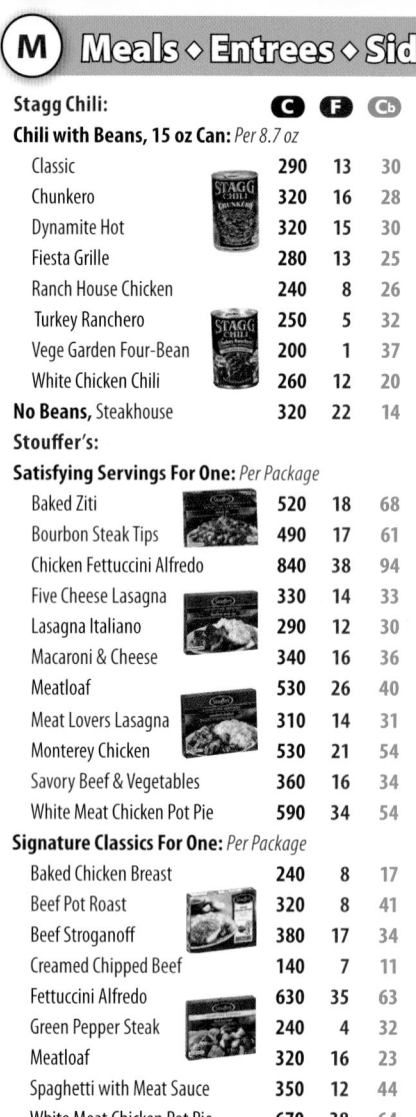

| Stagg Chili: | C | F | Cb |
|---|---|---|---|
| **Chili with Beans, 15 oz Can:** *Per 8.7 oz* | | | |
| Classic | 290 | 13 | 30 |
| Chunkero | 320 | 16 | 28 |
| Dynamite Hot | 320 | 15 | 30 |
| Fiesta Grille | 280 | 13 | 25 |
| Ranch House Chicken | 240 | 8 | 26 |
| Turkey Ranchero | 250 | 5 | 32 |
| Vege Garden Four-Bean | 200 | 1 | 37 |
| White Chicken Chili | 260 | 12 | 20 |
| **No Beans,** Steakhouse | 320 | 22 | 14 |

| Stouffer's: | | | |
|---|---|---|---|
| **Satisfying Servings For One:** *Per Package* | | | |
| Baked Ziti | 520 | 18 | 68 |
| Bourbon Steak Tips | 490 | 17 | 61 |
| Chicken Fettuccini Alfredo | 840 | 38 | 94 |
| Five Cheese Lasagna | 330 | 14 | 33 |
| Lasagna Italiano | 290 | 12 | 30 |
| Macaroni & Cheese | 340 | 16 | 36 |
| Meatloaf | 530 | 26 | 40 |
| Meat Lovers Lasagna | 310 | 14 | 31 |
| Monterey Chicken | 530 | 21 | 54 |
| Savory Beef & Vegetables | 360 | 16 | 34 |
| White Meat Chicken Pot Pie | 590 | 34 | 54 |
| **Signature Classics For One:** *Per Package* | | | |
| Baked Chicken Breast | 240 | 8 | 17 |
| Beef Pot Roast | 320 | 8 | 41 |
| Beef Stroganoff | 380 | 17 | 34 |
| Creamed Chipped Beef | 140 | 7 | 11 |
| Fettuccini Alfredo | 630 | 35 | 63 |
| Green Pepper Steak | 240 | 4 | 32 |
| Meatloaf | 320 | 16 | 23 |
| Spaghetti with Meat Sauce | 350 | 12 | 44 |
| White Meat Chicken Pot Pie | 670 | 38 | 64 |
| **Simple Dishes For One:** *Per ½ Package* | | | |
| Cheddar Potato Bake | 270 | 17 | 21 |
| Garlic Parmesan Mac & Cheese | 340 | 15 | 36 |
| Macaroni & Cheese | 340 | 16 | 33 |
| Spinach Souffle | 150 | 10 | 9 |

| Stouffer's (Cont): | C | F | Cb |
|---|---|---|---|
| **Family Size Meals:** *Per Serving* | | | |
| Cheese Manicotti | 340 | 16 | 33 |
| Cheesy Chicken & Broccoli Rice Bake | 330 | 15 | 30 |
| Chicken & Broccoli Pasta Bake | 300 | 14 | 24 |
| Chicken & Vegetable Rice | 360 | 15 | 37 |
| Chicken Cordon Bleu | 330 | 15 | 28 |
| Chicken Enchiladas | 290 | 9 | 38 |
| Lasagna Italiano | 250 | 9 | 30 |
| Lasagna with Meat Sauce | 320 | 12 | 32 |
| Macaroni & Cheese | 350 | 17 | 34 |
| Meatloaf in Gravy | 190 | 10 | 9 |
| Meat Lovers Lasagna | 330 | 16 | 31 |
| Rigatoni with Chicken & Pesto | 270 | 12 | 25 |
| Salisbury Steak | 220 | 15 | 7 |
| Stuffed Green Peppers | 190 | 8 | 20 |

| Swanson: | | | |
|---|---|---|---|
| **Dinners:** *Per Package* | | | |
| Chicken Nuggets | 590 | 25 | 71 |
| Rib Style Bnless Pork | 540 | 23 | 71 |
| Salisbury Steak | 450 | 22 | 44 |
| **Skillets:** *For Two* | | | |
| Alfredo Chicken | 370 | 12 | 42 |
| Beef Lo Mein | 360 | 6 | 55 |
| Chicken Parmesan | 430 | 14 | 60 |
| Garlic Chicken | 420 | 15 | 51 |
| Teriyaki Chicken | 290 | 2.5 | 51 |

| Tasty Bite: | | | |
|---|---|---|---|
| **Vegetarian Entrees:** *Per ½ Package, 5 oz* | | | |
| Bengal Lentils | 160 | 6 | 20 |
| Bombay Potatoes | 130 | 4 | 19 |
| Jaipur Vegetables | 180 | 11 | 12 |
| Jodhpur Lentils | 110 | 2.5 | 16 |
| Madras Lentils | 150 | 6 | 18 |
| Punjab Eggplant | 150 | 9 | 13 |

| TGI Friday's: | | | |
|---|---|---|---|
| Cheese & Bacon Loaded Fries, 3 oz | 220 | 14 | 14 |
| Chicken Parmesan Sliders, 3 oz | 260 | 13 | 27 |
| Chicken Wings, Buffalo Style Sce, 3.4 oz | 180 | 13 | 4 |
| Cream Cheese Stuffed Jalap., 2.7 oz | 200 | 11 | 20 |
| Crispy Green Bean Fries & Sce, 3 oz | 190 | 9 | 26 |
| Dill Pickle Chips, w/ Horseradish Sce | 200 | 11 | 22 |
| Mozzarella Sticks (1), with Marinara Sauce | 100 | 4.5 | 10 |
| Potato Skins, Cheddar & Bacon (3) | 200 | 10 | 21 |

| Thai Kitchen: | C | F | Cb |
|---|---|---|---|
| **Take-Out Meals:** *Per ½ Package* | | | |
| Original Pad Thai | 250 | 2 | 54 |
| Thai Basil & Chili | 250 | 3 | 50 |
| Thai Peanut | 270 | 5 | 51 |
| **Noodle Carts:** *Per 9 oz Tray* | | | |
| Pad Thai | 460 | 2 | 104 |
| Thai Peanut | 510 | 9 | 96 |
| **Rice Noodle Soup Bowls,** | | | |
| average all varieties, 2.5 oz | 240 | 2 | 50 |
| **Stir-Fry Rice Noodles:** *Per ½ Package* | | | |
| Original Pad Thai | 390 | 3.5 | 84 |
| Thai Peanut | 390 | 2 | 87 |
| **Tofurky:** | | | |
| **Chick'n:** | | | |
| BBQ Style, 3.2 oz | 200 | 5 | 14 |
| Sesame, 3.2 oz | 210 | 9 | 10 |
| Tandoori, 3.2 oz | 180 | 6 | 9 |
| **Pies:** | | | |
| Chick'N Pot Pie (1), 8 oz | 520 | 33 | 45 |
| Sausage & Veggie Quiche (1), 7.5 oz | 520 | 28 | 43 |
| **Pockets:** BBQ Chick'N (1), 4.5 oz | 290 | 4 | 50 |
| Broccoli Cheddar (1), 4.5 oz | 240 | 5 | 40 |
| Pepp. Pizza (1), 4.5 oz | 300 | 5 | 43 |
| **Trader Joe's:** | | | |
| **Baked Beans,** Organic, | | | |
| average all varieties, ½ cup | 140 | 0 | 29 |
| **Black Beans:** | | | |
| Regular, ½ cup | 110 | 0 | 19 |
| Cuban Style, ½ cup | 100 | 0.5 | 19 |
| Chicken Chili with Beans, 1 cup | 290 | 9 | 32 |
| Pasta, Shells & White Cheddar, 1 cup | 280 | 6 | 47 |
| **Potatoes:** Garlic Mashed, ½ cup | 150 | 7 | 19 |
| Cheddar Cheese Au Gratin, ½ cup | 140 | 5 | 21 |
| Turkey Chili w/ Beans, 1 cup | 240 | 4.5 | 30 |
| **Frozen:** | | | |
| Butter Chicken w/ Basmati Rice, 1 cup | 270 | 8 | 33 |
| Chicken Chow Mein, ⅓ package, 6.7 oz | 210 | 2 | 35 |
| Chicken Quesadilla (1), 6 oz | 320 | 16 | 26 |
| Citrus Glazed Chicken with Rice, 8 oz | 270 | 5 | 40 |
| Mac & Cheese: Regular, 1 cup, 7 oz | 360 | 15 | 42 |
| Reduced Guilt, 7 oz | 270 | 6 | 40 |
| Shrimp Stir Fry, 6.4 oz | 70 | 0.5 | 6 |
| Spag. & Beef Meatballs, | | | |
| 1 cup, 9 oz | 380 | 13 | 48 |
| Spicy Beef & Broccoli, | | | |
| 1¾ cups | 430 | 13 | 64 |
| Thai Vegetable Kao Soi, 12.6 oz | 430 | 20 | 55 |
| Vegetable Pad Thai, 10.5 oz tray | 520 | 21 | 74 |
| **Pies:** Chicken Pot Pie, ½ pie, 8 oz | 360 | 22 | 28 |
| Shepherd's Pie, 1 cup, 8 oz | 170 | 3 | 22 |

| Tyson: | C | F | Cb |
|---|---|---|---|
| **Any'tizers Snacks:** | | | |
| H'style Chicken Fries (7), 3.2 oz | 230 | 13 | 14 |
| Stuffed Chicken Cordon Bleu, | | | |
| Minis, 3 pieces, 3 oz | 200 | 12 | 11 |
| Chicken Wings: Buffalo Style Hot Wings | | | |
| bone-in, 3 oz | 190 | 13 | 3 |
| Honey BBQ, 3 oz | 190 | 12 | 8 |
| Hot & Spicy, 3 oz | 190 | 13 | 1 |
| Chicken Wyngz, Boneless: | | | |
| Buffalo Style, 3 pcs | 150 | 7 | 8 |
| Honey BBQ, 3 oz | 200 | 8 | 20 |
| **Better For You:** *Per 3 oz Serving* | | | |
| Grilled & Ready Chicken Breast Strips: | | | |
| 100% Natural | 100 | 2.5 | 1 |
| Fajita | 110 | 4 | 1 |
| Southwestern | 120 | 3 | 5 |
| **Breaded Chicken:** | | | |
| 100% All Natural: | | | |
| Breast Patties (1), 2.7 oz | 200 | 13 | 10 |
| Chicken Nuggets (5), 3.2 oz | 270 | 17 | 15 |
| Crispy Chicken Strips, 3 oz | 190 | 9 | 12 |
| Breast Nuggets (5), 3.1 oz | 220 | 13 | 15 |
| Buffalo Chicken Strips, 3 oz | 190 | 9 | 17 |
| **Fully Cooked Beef:** | | | |
| Country Fried Steak, 1 pattie, 2.6 oz | 250 | 17 | 13 |
| Steak Fingers, 2 pieces, 2.5 oz | 250 | 18 | 14 |
| **To Go Products:** | | | |
| Mini Chicken Sandwich: | | | |
| Original, breaded | 390 | 16 | 46 |
| With Cheese | 440 | 20 | 47 |
| **Uncle Ben's:** | | | |
| **Country Inn:** *Per Cup, Prepared with Water Only* | | | |
| Broccoli Rice Au Gratin | 200 | 2 | 41 |
| Chicken & Vegetable Rice | 200 | 1 | 43 |
| Chicken Flavored Rice | 200 | 1 | 42 |
| Rice Pilaf | 200 | 1 | 43 |
| **Flavored Grains:** *1 Cup cooked As Directed* | | | |
| 5 Grain Medley Quinoa Pilaf | 200 | 1.5 | 41 |
| Basmati Medley Savory Herb | 200 | 0.5 | 43 |
| Brown Rice Medley, | | | |
| Roasted Garlic & Herbs, 2 oz | 200 | 2 | 40 |
| **Ready Rice:** *Per Package, Heat & Serve* | | | |
| Butter & Garlic Flavored | 220 | 4 | 41 |
| Garden Vegetable | 200 | 2.5 | 41 |
| Roasted Chicken Flavored | 210 | 3 | 42 |
| Teriyaki Style | 220 | 3 | 42 |
| **Ready Whole Grain Medley,** | | | |
| average all varieties, 1 pkt | 210 | 3 | 41 |

| Van Camp's: | C | F | Cb |
|---|---|---|---|
| Baked Beans, Original, ½ cup, 4.8 oz | 160 | 1 | 30 |
| Hickory Baked Beans, ½ cup, 4.8 oz | 170 | 1 | 32 |
| Pork & Beans, 28 oz can, ½ cup, 4.6 oz | 110 | 1 | 23 |
| **Van De Kamp's:** | | | |
| Beer Battrd Fillets, 3.8 oz | 210 | 10 | 21 |
| Crispy Fish Tenders, 3.6 oz | 230 | 2.5 | 21 |
| Cracked Blk Pepper & Sea Salt Salmon, 4.3 oz | 230 | 8 | 20 |
| Crunchy Fish Fillets, 1.8 oz | 90 | 4 | 13 |
| Garlic Herb Cod, 5 oz | 260 | 10 | 26 |
| Parmesan & Rsted Garlic Tilapia, 5 oz | 280 | 10 | 26 |
| **Whole Foods (365):** | | | |
| Chickenless Nuggets, breaded (4), 2.8 oz | 180 | 7 | 16 |
| Meatless Meatballs (4), 2 oz | 110 | 4 | 9 |
| Meatless Burgers (1), 2.5 oz | 120 | 4.5 | 7 |
| Pasta Rings in Tomato Sauce, 1 cup | 150 | 1 | 31 |
| Vegetarian Chili, 1 cup | 130 | 2 | 25 |
| **Worthington/Loma Linda:** | | | |
| Big Franks: 1 link, 1.8 oz | 110 | 6 | 3 |
| Low-fat, 1 link, 1.8 oz | 80 | 2.5 | 3 |
| Chili, 1 cup, 8.10 oz | 280 | 10 | 25 |
| Choplets, 2 slices, 3.2 oz | 90 | 1 | 4 |
| Diced Chik, 2 oz | 50 | 0 | 2 |
| FriChik, Original, low fat, 2 pieces, 3 oz | 80 | 2.5 | 4 |
| Linketts (1), 1.3 oz | 70 | 4 | 1 |
| Little Links (2), 1.6 oz | 90 | 5 | 3 |
| Redi-Burger, ⅝" slice, 3 oz | 120 | 2.5 | 7 |
| Super Links (1), 1.5 oz | 110 | 8 | 2 |
| Tender Rounds (6), 2.8 oz | 120 | 4.5 | 6 |
| Vegetable Skallops, ½ cup, 3 oz | 90 | 1 | 4 |
| Vegetarian Burger, ¼ cup, 1.9 oz | 70 | 1.5 | 3 |
| Veja-Links (1), 1 oz | 50 | 3 | 1 |
| **Frozen:** | | | |
| Chic-ketts, 2 slices | 110 | 5 | 3 |
| Dinner Roast, ¾" slice | 180 | 11 | 6 |
| FriPats, 1 pattie, 2.3 oz | 130 | 6 | 5 |
| Leanies, 1 link, 1.4 oz | 100 | 7 | 2 |
| **Meatless:** | | | |
| Chicken Style Roll, ⅜" slice | 90 | 4.5 | 2 |
| Smoked Turkey Roll, ⅜" slice | 130 | 8 | 4 |
| Prosage Links (2), 1.6 oz | 80 | 3 | 3 |
| Stakelets, 2.5 oz piece | 150 | 7 | 7 |
| Stripples, 2 strips, 0.6 oz | 60 | 4.5 | 2 |

| Yves Veggie Cuisine: | C | F | Cb |
|---|---|---|---|
| **Brats:** *Per Brat* | | | |
| Veggie Classic, 3.5 oz | 160 | 5 | 9 |
| Zesty Italian, 3.5 oz | 150 | 5 | 9 |
| **Burgers:** Meatless Beef Burger (1) | 110 | 4 | 8 |
| Meatless Chicken (1) | 100 | 3 | 5 |
| **Deli Slices:** | 80 | 2.5 | 2 |
| Meatless: Bologna, 4 slices | 80 | 2.5 | 2 |
| Ham, 4 slices | 100 | 2 | 5 |
| Pepperoni, 6 slices | 80 | 1 | 4 |
| Roast without the Beef, 4 slices | 110 | 2.5 | 4 |
| Salami, 4 slices | 80 | 0 | 4 |
| Smoked Chicken, 4 slices | 100 | 1.5 | 5 |
| Turkey, 4 slices | 100 | 1.5 | 5 |
| **Ground Rounds:** | | | |
| Meatless: Taco Stuffers, ⅓ cup, 2 oz | 90 | 2.5 | 5 |
| Turkey, ⅓ cup, 2 oz | 60 | 1 | 4 |
| **Hot Dog:** | | | |
| Good Dog (1), 2 oz | 70 | 3.5 | 1 |
| Hot Dog (1), 1.5 oz | 50 | 0.5 | 2 |
| Jumbo Hot Dog (1), 2.8 oz | 110 | 3 | 5 |
| Tofu Dog (1), 1.5 oz | 45 | 1 | 2 |
| **Skewers & Strips:** | | | |
| Chicken Skewers (1) | 100 | 1 | 7 |
| Meatless Beef/Chicken Strips, average, 2.8 oz | 115 | 1 | 4 |
| **Veggie Seafood:** | | | |
| Shrimp, 3 oz | 50 | 1.5 | 8 |
| Shrimp Scampi, 3.5 oz | 100 | 7 | 8 |
| Tuna Steak, with Sesame Ginger Sce, 3.5 oz | 250 | 20 | 8 |
| **Zatarain's:** | | | |
| **New Orleans Style:** *Per Dry Mix Only* | | | |
| Black Beans & Rice, Original, 2.3 oz | 230 | 1 | 47 |
| Caribbean Rice Mix, 2.5 oz | 250 | 2 | 52 |
| Chicken Creole Rice Mix, 1.5 oz | 140 | 1 | 29 |
| Chicken Flavor Rice, 2 oz | 210 | 0.5 | 45 |
| Garlic & Herb & Rice Mix, 1.5 oz | 130 | 0.5 | 29 |
| Rice Pilaf, 2 oz | 210 | 0.5 | 45 |
| Smothered Chicken Rice Mix, 1.6 oz | 160 | 0.5 | 34 |
| Yellow Rice, 2 oz | 200 | 0.5 | 43 |
| **Frozen:** | | | |
| **Meals:** *Per Meal* | | | |
| Blackened Chicken Alfredo, 10.5 oz | 500 | 21 | 56 |
| Dirty Rice with Beef & Pork, 10 oz | 430 | 13 | 64 |
| Jambalaya Flavored w/ Ssg, 12 oz | 490 | 10 | 86 |
| Red Beans & Rice w/ Sausage, 12 oz | 540 | 17 | 79 |
| Shrimp Scampi with Pasta, 10.5 oz | 350 | 10 | 49 |

Note: Cooking reduces weight of meat by 20-45% due to water and fat losses. Average weight loss is 30%. Actual loss depends on cooking method and cooking time.

Examples:

4 oz raw weight = approx. 3 oz cooked weight

4 oz cooked weight = approx. 5½ oz raw weight

### What 3 oz Cooked Meat Looks Like:
- Rectangular piece (4" x 2½" x ½" thick)
- Deck of cards (3½" x 2½" x ⅝" thick)

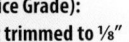

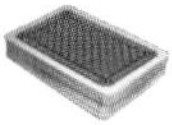

### Quick Guide   **C  F  Cb**

**Sirloin (Choice Grade):**
**External fat trimmed to ⅛"**
*Broiled, Edible Portion (no bone)*

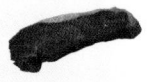

#### Small/Regular Serving, 3 oz, cooked weight:
(from 4-4½ oz raw)

| | | | |
|---|---|---|---|
| Lean + external fat (⅛"), 3 oz | 220 | 13 | 0 |
| Lean + marbling, 3 oz | 185 | 9 | 0 |
| Lean only, 3 oz | 160 | 6 | 0 |

(No external fat or marbling)

#### Medium Serving, 5 oz, cooked weight:
(from approximately 7 oz raw)

| | | | |
|---|---|---|---|
| Lean + external fat (⅛"), 5 oz | 365 | 22 | 0 |
| Lean + marbling, 5 oz | 310 | 15 | 0 |
| Lean only, 5 oz | 265 | 10 | 0 |

#### Large Serving, 8 oz, cooked weight:
(from approximately11-12 oz raw)

| | | | |
|---|---|---|---|
| Lean + external fat (⅛"), 8 oz | 585 | 36 | 0 |
| Lean + marbling, 8 oz | 500 | 24 | 0 |
| Lean only, 8 oz | 425 | 15 | 0 |

#### Extra Large Serving, 12 oz, cooked weight:
(from approximately 16-17 oz raw)

| | | | |
|---|---|---|---|
| Lean + external fat (⅛"), 12 oz | 875 | 54 | 0 |
| Lean + marbling, 12 oz | 745 | 36 | 0 |
| Lean only, 12 oz | 640 | 22 | 0 |

#### Pan Fried:
Sirloin (Choice), medium serving,

| | | | |
|---|---|---|---|
| Lean + external fat (⅛"), 5 oz | 445 | 30 | 0 |

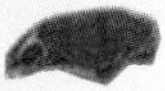

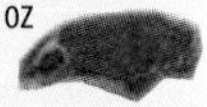

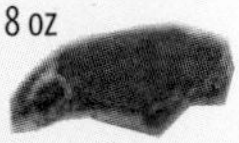

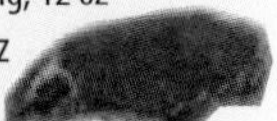

### Other Steaks   **C  F  Cb**

**Filet Mignon (Tenderloin):**
1 Medium steak, 6 oz raw weight:
Broiled, with ¼" fat trim:

| | | | |
|---|---|---|---|
| Lean + fat (¼"), 4 oz | 360 | 27 | 0 |
| Lean only, 3.5 oz | 230 | 12 | 0 |

**New York/Club Steak:**
Top Loin/Short Loin:
1 steak, regular (9.25 oz raw, ¼" fat):
Broiled: Lean + fat (¼"), 6.3 oz

| | | | |
|---|---|---|---|
| Broiled: Lean + fat (¼"), 6.3 oz | 580 | 43 | 0 |
| Lean + marbling, 5.5 oz | 400 | 25 | 0 |
| Lean only, 5.25 oz | 360 | 20 | 0 |

**Porterhouse Steak:**
1 Medium, 6 oz raw weight, without bone, broiled:

| | | | |
|---|---|---|---|
| Lean + fat (¼"), 4.3 oz | 410 | 33 | 0 |
| Lean only, 3.5 oz | 210 | 11 | 0 |

1 Large ,12 oz raw weight, without bone, broiled:

| | | | |
|---|---|---|---|
| Lean + fat (¼") 8.5 oz cooked | 820 | 66 | 0 |
| Lean only, 7 oz cooked | 420 | 22 | 0 |

**T-Bone Steak:** *Broiled or Grilled*
**Medium Size:** *8 oz raw weight, without bone*
Approximately 6 oz cooked:

| | | | |
|---|---|---|---|
| Lean + Fat (¼"), 5 oz | 400 | 28 | 0 |
| Lean only, 4 oz | 265 | 12 | 0 |

**Large Size:** *12 oz raw weight*
Approximately 9 oz cooked:

| | | | |
|---|---|---|---|
| Lean + fat (¼"), 7 oz, without bone | 560 | 39 | 0 |
| Lean only, 6 oz, without bone | 400 | 18 | 0 |

**Extra Large Size:** *20 oz raw weight*
Approximately 16 oz cooked:

| | | | |
|---|---|---|---|
| Lean + Fat (¼"), 12 oz, without bone | 960 | 66 | 0 |
| Lean Only, 10 oz, without bone | 660 | 30 | 0 |

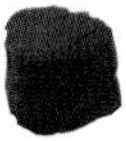

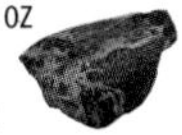

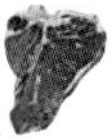

### Also See Fast-Foods & Restaurants Section ~
*Lone Star Steakhouse; Outback Steakhouse*

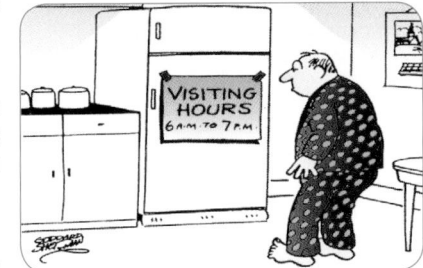

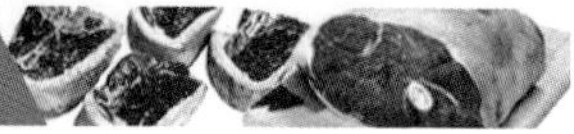

## Beef – Individual Cuts   C  F  Cb

*Average All Grades*
Edible Weight, Without Bone

| | C | F | Cb |
|---|---|---|---|
| **Brisket, whole, braised:** | | | |
| Lean + fat (¼" trim), 3 oz | 330 | 27 | 0 |
| Lean + marbling, 3 oz | 250 | 17 | 0 |
| Lean only, 3 oz | 185 | 9 | 0 |
| **Chuck blade, braised:** | | | |
| Lean + fat (¼"), 3 oz | 310 | 24 | 0 |
| Lean + marbling, 3 oz | 295 | 22 | 0 |
| Lean only, 3 oz | 245 | 13 | 0 |
| **Flank:** Raw, 4 oz | 175 | 8 | 0 |
| Braised, 3 oz | 225 | 14 | 0 |
| Broiled, 3 oz | 155 | 6 | 0 |
| **Round, bottom, braised:** | | | |
| Lean + marbling, 3 oz | 190 | 7.5 | 0 |
| Lean only, 3 oz | 185 | 6.5 | 0 |
| **Round, eye/tip, rstd:** | | | |
| Lean + fat (¼"), 3 oz | 205 | 11 | 0 |
| Lean, w/ marbling, 3 oz | 150 | 5 | 0 |
| **Round, top:** *Per 3 oz, Cooked Weight* | | | |
| Braised, Lean + fat | 210 | 10 | 0 |
| Lean only | 170 | 4 | 0 |
| Broiled, Lean + fat | 180 | 8 | 0 |
| Lean only | 160 | 5 | 0 |
| Pan-fried, Lean + fat | 235 | 13 | 0 |
| Lean only | 195 | 7 | 0 |

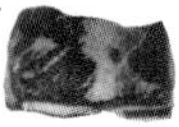

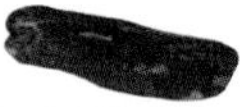

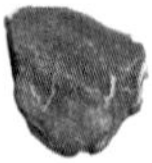

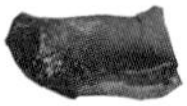

## Beef Ribs

**Back Ribs:** *7" long, visible fat trimmed to ¼"*
10.3 oz raw w/ bone or 3.5 oz cooked, braised, w/o bone

| | C | F | Cb |
|---|---|---|---|
| 1 average rib | 410 | 34 | 0 |
| 3 ribs | 1230 | 102 | 0 |

**Short Ribs:** *2½" long, visible fat trimmed to ¼"*
6 oz raw with bone or 2.52 oz cooked, braised, w/o bone

| | C | F | Cb |
|---|---|---|---|
| 1 average rib | 320 | 28 | 0 |
| 3 ribs | 960 | 85 | 0 |

## Ground Beef

**Ground Beef, Raw:** *Per 4 oz*

| | C | F | Cb |
|---|---|---|---|
| 70% lean (30% fat) | 380 | 34 | 0 |
| 75% lean (25% fat) | 335 | 29 | 0 |
| 80% lean (20% fat) | 290 | 23 | 0 |
| 85% lean (15% fat) | 245 | 17 | 0 |
| 90% lean (10% fat) | 200 | 12 | 0 |
| 95% lean (5% fat) | 155 | 6 | 0 |
| **Baked/Broiled:** Regular (70%), 3 oz | 230 | 16 | 0 |
| Lean (80%), 3 oz | 215 | 14 | 0 |
| Extra lean (90%), 3 oz | 185 | 10 | 0 |
| **Pan-Broiled:** | | | |
| Regular (70%), 3 oz | 230 | 15 | 0 |
| Lean (80%), 3 oz | 210 | 14 | 0 |
| Extra lean (90%), 3 oz | 195 | 10 | 0 |
| **Ground Beef Patties:** *Average, 23% Fat* | | | |
| Raw, 4 oz | 330 | 25 | 0 |
| Broiled, 3 oz (from 4 oz raw) | 250 | 19 | 0 |

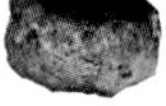

## Quick Guide   C  F  Cb

### Roast Beef

**Round (Eye/Tip, average):** *Average All Cuts*
**Small/Regular Serving:** *3 oz*
(2 thin slices/1 thick slice)

| | C | F | Cb |
|---|---|---|---|
| Lean + fat (⅛" fat trim) | 180 | 9 | 0 |
| Lean only | 145 | 4 | 0 |
| **Medium Serving:** *5 oz* | | | |
| (3-4 thin slices) | | | |
| Lean + fat (⅛" fat trim) | 300 | 15 | 0 |
| Lean only | 245 | 6.5 | 0 |
| **Large Serving, 8 oz:** *3 thick slices* | | | |
| Lean + fat (⅛" fat trim) | 480 | 24 | 0 |
| Lean only | 385 | 11 | 0 |

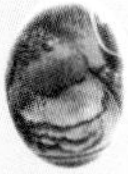

### Roast Dinner Extras

| | C | F | Cb |
|---|---|---|---|
| **Gravy:** Thin, 2 Tbsp | 20 | 0.5 | 3.5 |
| Thick, 2 Tbsp | 50 | 2 | 0.5 |
| 1 Ladle/4 Tbsp | 100 | 4 | 1 |
| **Veggies:** Beans, green, ½ cup | 20 | 0 | 5 |
| Cauliflower with cheese sauce, 4 oz | 135 | 9 | 15 |
| Corn, kernels, ¼ cup | 35 | 0 | 9 |
| Carrots, ¼ cup | 20 | 0 | 3 |
| Peas, ¼ cup | 35 | 0 | 6 |
| **Potato:** | | | |
| Baked in jacket: Plain, 1 large | 280 | 0 | 63 |
| With sour cream, 2 Tbsp | 270 | 5 | 64 |
| With whipped butter, 1 Tbsp | 350 | 8 | 63 |
| Roasted with fat, 1 small | 155 | 8 | 30 |
| **Sweet Potato/Yam,** 1 medium | 105 | 1 | 24 |
| **Yorkshire Pudding,** 1 oz | 90 | 3.5 | 11 |

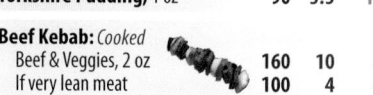

| **Beef Kebab:** *Cooked* | C | F | Cb |
|---|---|---|---|
| Beef & Veggies, 2 oz | 160 | 10 | 4 |
| If very lean meat | 100 | 4 | 4 |

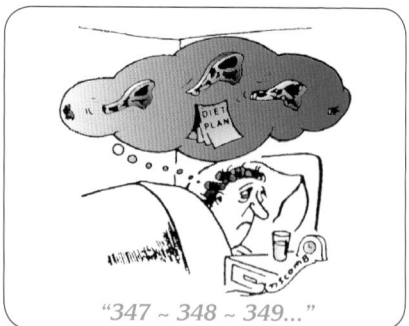

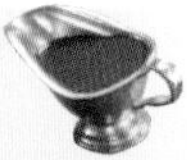

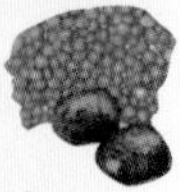

*"347 ~ 348 ~ 349..."*

## Lamb  C  F  Cb

**Choice Grade:**

**Leg (Whole), roasted:**
| | C | F | Cb |
|---|---|---|---|
| Lean + fat, 3 oz | 220 | 14 | 0 |
| Lean only, 3 oz | 160 | 7 | 0 |

**Leg (Sirloin Half), roasted:**
| | | | |
|---|---|---|---|
| Lean + fat, 3 oz | 250 | 18 | 0 |
| Lean only, 3 oz | 175 | 8 | 0 |

**Leg (Shank Half), roasted:**
| | | | |
|---|---|---|---|
| Lean + fat, 3 oz | 190 | 11 | 0 |
| Lean only, 3 oz | 155 | 6 | 0 |

**Loin Chop, broiled:**
1 chop (raw weight, 4.25 oz):
| | | | |
|---|---|---|---|
| Lean + fat (2.25 oz edible) | 180 | 12 | 0 |
| Lean only (1.6 oz edible) | 85 | 3.5 | 0 |

**Rib Chop, broiled:**
1 chop (raw wt., 3.5 oz):
| | | | |
|---|---|---|---|
| Lean + fat (2.5 oz edible) | 255 | 21 | 0 |
| Lean only (1.75 oz edible) | 105 | 6 | 0 |

**Shoulder (Arm/Blade):**
| | | | |
|---|---|---|---|
| Braised: Lean + fat, 3 oz | 295 | 21 | 0 |
| Lean only, 3 oz | 240 | 12 | 0 |
| Broiled: Lean + fat, 3 oz | 240 | 17 | 0 |
| Lean only, 3 oz | 170 | 8 | 0 |
| Roasted: Similar to Broiled | | | |

**Cubed Lamb (Leg/Shoulder):**
For stew or kebab:
| | | | |
|---|---|---|---|
| Braised, lean only, 3 oz | 190 | 8 | 0 |
| Broiled, lean only, 3 oz | 160 | 6 | 0 |

## Veal

**Edible Weights:**

**Leg (Top Round):**
| | | | |
|---|---|---|---|
| Braised: Lean + fat, 3 oz | 180 | 6 | 0 |
| Lean only, 3 oz | 175 | 5 | 0 |

Pan-fried, breaded:
| | | | |
|---|---|---|---|
| Lean + fat, 3 oz | 195 | 8 | 9 |
| Lean only, 3 oz | 185 | 6 | 9 |

Pan-fried, not breaded:
| | | | |
|---|---|---|---|
| Lean + fat, 3 oz | 180 | 7 | 0 |
| Lean only, 3 oz | 155 | 4 | 0 |
| Roasted: Lean + fat, 3 oz | 135 | 4 | 0 |
| Lean only, 3 oz | 130 | 3 | 0 |

## Veal (Cont)  C  F  Cb

**Loin Chop:** *1 chop, 7 oz raw weight*
| | C | F | Cb |
|---|---|---|---|
| Braised: Lean + fat, 3 oz | 240 | 15 | 0 |
| Lean only, 3 oz | 190 | 8 | 0 |
| Roasted: Lean + fat, 3 oz | 185 | 11 | 0 |
| Lean only, 3 oz | 150 | 6 | 0 |

**Rib, roasted:** *Lean + fat, 3 oz*
| | | | |
|---|---|---|---|
| | 195 | 12 | 0 |
| Lean only, 3 oz | 150 | 7 | 0 |

**Shoulder, Arm/Blade, roasted:**
| | | | |
|---|---|---|---|
| Lean + fat, 3 oz | 155 | 7 | 0 |
| Lean only, 3 oz | 140 | 5 | 0 |

**Sirloin, roasted:**
| | | | |
|---|---|---|---|
| Lean + fat, 3 oz | 170 | 9 | 0 |
| Lean only, 3 oz | 145 | 6 | 0 |

**Cubed for Stew, braised:**
| | | | |
|---|---|---|---|
| Leg/Shoulder, lean only, 3 oz | 160 | 4 | 0 |

(1 lb raw yields approximately 9.25 oz cooked)

## Pork

**Fresh Pork:** *Cooked Weight, without bone):*
*4 oz raw weight = approx. 3 oz cooked weight*

**BBQ, Pulled:**
| | | | |
|---|---|---|---|
| 2 oz | 90 | 2.5 | 10 |
| 4 oz | 180 | 5 | 20 |
| 8 oz | 360 | 10 | 40 |

**Blade Steak, broiled:**
| | | | |
|---|---|---|---|
| Lean + fat, 3 oz | 220 | 15 | 0 |
| Lean only, 3 oz | 190 | 11 | 0 |

**Country Style Ribs, broiled/roasted:**
| | | | |
|---|---|---|---|
| Lean + fat, 3 oz | 280 | 22 | 0 |
| Lean only, 3 oz | 210 | 13 | 0 |

**Spareribs, braised:** *Lean & fat, 6 oz*
(from 1 lb raw weight)  675  52  0

**Leg (Ham), whole, roasted:**
| | | | |
|---|---|---|---|
| Lean + fat, 3 oz | 230 | 15 | 0 |
| Lean only, 3 oz | 180 | 8 | 0 |

**Loin Chops, broiled:** *Average*
(From 1 chop: 5 oz raw weight with bone or 4 oz raw weight, without bone)
| | | | |
|---|---|---|---|
| Lean + fat, 3 oz | 200 | 11 | 0 |
| Lean only, 3 oz | 165 | 7 | 0 |

**Loin Roast, roasted:**
| | | | |
|---|---|---|---|
| Lean + fat, 3 oz | 210 | 13 | 0 |
| Lean only, 3 oz | 180 | 8 | 0 |

**Rib Chops, (Boneless), broiled:**
| | | | |
|---|---|---|---|
| Lean + fat, 3 oz | 220 | 14 | 0 |
| Lean only, 3 oz | 185 | 9 | 0 |

**Rib Roast:**
| | | | |
|---|---|---|---|
| Lean + fat, 3 oz | 215 | 13 | 0 |
| Lean only, 3 oz | 180 | 9 | 0 |

| Pork (Cont) | C | F | Cb |
|---|---|---|---|
| **Sirloin Chop, broiled:** | | | |
| Lean + fat, 3 oz | 180 | 8 | 0 |
| Lean only, 3 oz | 165 | 6 | 0 |
| **Sirloin Roast, roasted:** | | | |
| Lean + fat, 3 oz | 175 | 8 | 0 |
| Lean only, 3 oz | 170 | 7 | 0 |
| **Tenderloin (Boneless), roasted:** | | | |
| Lean + fat, 3 oz | 125 | 4 | 0 |
| Lean only, 3 oz | 120 | 3 | 0 |
| **Ground Pork:** | | | |
| Raw, average, ¼ lb, 4 oz | 300 | 24 | 0 |
| Broiled, 3 oz | 250 | 18 | 0 |
| Pan-fried, drained, 3 oz | 260 | 19 | 0 |

| Bacon | C | F | Cb |
|---|---|---|---|
| **Raw:** 1 med. slice, 0.75 oz | 95 | 9 | 0 |
| 1 thick slice, 1.3 oz | 175 | 17 | 0 |
| (1 lb raw yields approximately 5 oz cooked) | | | |
| **Broiled/Pan-Fried:** | | | |
| 1 medium slice, 0.3 oz | 40 | 3 | 0 |
| 3 medium slices, 0.8 | 125 | 10 | 0 |
| 2 thin slices, 0.5 oz | 75 | 6 | 0 |
| 1 thick slice, 0.9 oz | 65 | 5 | 0 |
| **Canadian Bacon:** | | | |
| Cooked: 1 slice, 1 oz | 45 | 2 | 0.5 |
| 2 slices, 2 oz | 90 | 4 | 1 |
| **Bacon Bits,** 1 Tbsp, 0.3 oz | 35 | 2 | 0 |
| **Breakfast Strips,** Broiled, 1 sl., 0.4 oz | 50 | 4 | 0 |

| Ham | C | F | Cb |
|---|---|---|---|
| **Boneless Ham,** cooked: | | | |
| Regular, (approximately 13% fat): | | | |
| Roasted, 3 oz | 150 | 8 | 0 |
| Extra Lean (5% fat), | | | |
| Roasted, 3 oz | 125 | 5 | 0 |
| **Whole Ham,** cooked: | | | |
| Lean + fat (as purchased) | | | |
| Roasted, 3 oz | 210 | 15 | 0 |
| Lean only, Roasted, 3 oz | 135 | 5 | 0 |
| **Canned Ham:** *Similar to boneless ham* | | | |
| Chopped, canned, 3 oz | 200 | 16 | 0 |
| **Ham Patties,** cooked, (1), 2.3 oz | 220 | 20 | 1 |
| **Ham Steak,** extra lean, 2 oz | 70 | 2.5 | 0 |
| **Lunch Slices** ~ *See Deli Meats, Page 128* | | | |

| Game & Other Meats | C | F | Cb |
|---|---|---|---|
| **Bison Steak,** | | | |
| lean, 6 oz (raw) | 205 | 4 | 0 |
| **Boar (wild),** roasted, 3 oz | 140 | 4 | 0 |
| **Buffalo Steak,** | | | |
| *New West Foods,* 4 oz | 70 | 3 | 0 |
| **Caribou,** roasted, 3 oz | 140 | 4 | 0 |
| **Deer/Venison,** roasted 3 oz | 135 | 3 | 0 |
| **Goat (Capretto):** | | | |
| Raw, 3 oz | 95 | 2 | 0 |
| Roasted, 3 oz | 120 | 2.5 | 0 |
| **Ostrich:** | | | |
| *Blackwing Ostrich Meats:* | | | |
| Sausage Patties (2) 2 oz | 60 | 0.5 | 0 |
| Sport Jerky, 0.5 oz piece | 25 | 0 | 0 |
| *New West Foods:* | | | |
| Ground Ostrich, 4 oz | 165 | 7 | 0 |
| Ostrich Steak, 4 oz steak | 130 | 2.5 | 0 |
| **Rabbit:** Roasted, 3 oz | 165 | 7 | 0 |
| Stewed, 1 cup, diced, 5 oz | 290 | 12 | 0 |

| Variety & Organ Meats | C | F | Cb |
|---|---|---|---|
| **Brain (Lamb):** Braised, 3 oz | 125 | 9 | 0 |
| Pan-fried, 3 oz | 230 | 19 | 0 |
| **Chitterlings,** pork, simmered, 3 oz | 260 | 25 | 0 |
| **Ears,** pork, simmered, 1 ear, 4 oz | 185 | 12 | 0 |
| **Feet,** Pork: Simmered, 3 oz | 200 | 14 | 0 |
| Cured, pickled, 3 oz | 170 | 14 | 0 |
| *Hormel,* 2 oz | 80 | 6 | 0 |
| **Head Cheese (Pork Snouts/Ears/Vinegar/Spices),** | | | |
| 1 oz slice | 50 | 4 | 0 |
| **Heart,** Beef, braised, 3 oz | 140 | 4 | 0 |
| **Jowl,** pork, raw, 4 oz | 750 | 80 | 0 |
| **Kidneys,** braised, 3 oz | 140 | 5 | 0 |
| **Liver (beef):** Raw, 4 oz | 150 | 4 | 4 |
| Braised, 3 oz | 140 | 4 | 3 |
| Pan-fried, 3 oz | 185 | 7 | 7 |
| **Pancreas,** pork, braised, 3 oz | 185 | 8 | 0 |
| **Pork Cracklins,** 0.5 oz | 80 | 6 | 0 |
| **Pork Hocks,** 1 piece, 6 oz | 340 | 23 | 0 |
| **Scrapple,** pork, 2 oz | 120 | 8 | 8 |
| **Spleen,** pork, braised, 3 oz | 130 | 3 | 0 |
| **Stomach,** pork, raw, 4 oz | 185 | 12 | 0 |
| **Sweetbreads:** | | | |
| Beef,/Lamb, cooked, 3 oz | 125 | 9 | 0 |
| **Tail,** pork, simmered, 3 oz | 340 | 31 | 0 |
| **Tongue:** Raised Veal, 3 oz | 170 | 9 | 0 |
| Beef/Lamb/Pork, av., 3 oz | 235 | 17 | 0 |
| **Tripe,** beef, raw, 3 oz | 85 | 3.5 | 0 |

### Quick Guide | C | F | Cb

#### Franks & Weiners
*Average All Brands*

**Regular (Pork Mix):** *Per Frank*

| | C | F | Cb |
|---|---|---|---|
| Regular, 1.5 oz | 140 | 13 | 1 |
| Bun Length/Jumbo, 2 oz | 185 | 17 | 2 |
| Extra Long, 2.75 oz | 255 | 24 | 2 |
| Small/Cocktail, each | 30 | 3 | 0.5 |

**Beef Franks:** *Per Frank*

| | C | F | Cb |
|---|---|---|---|
| Regular, 1.5 oz | 140 | 13 | 2 |
| Bun Length/Jumbo, 2 oz | 175 | 17 | 2.5 |
| ¼ lb Dog, 4 oz | 375 | 33 | 5 |

#### Franks & Weiners

**Ball Park:** *Per 2 oz Frank Unless Indicated*
**Angus Beef:**

| | C | F | Cb |
|---|---|---|---|
| Original; Bun Size, 2 oz | 170 | 15 | 3 |
| Lean, 1.8 oz | 70 | 5 | 2 |
| **Beef:** Original, Bun Size, 2 oz | 190 | 16 | 4 |
| Deli Style: Regular, 1.8 oz | 150 | 12 | 2 |
| BunSize, 1.8 oz | 150 | 12 | 2 |
| Park's Finest, Chili Beef, 2 oz | 180 | 15 | 4 |
| **Better For You,** Turkey, 2 oz | 110 | 7 | 6 |
| **Foster Farms,** Chicken; Turkey, 2 oz | 140 | 12 | 1 |

**Hebrew National:** *Per Frank*
**Beef:** Regular, 1.7 oz

| | C | F | Cb |
|---|---|---|---|
| Beef: Regular, 1.7 oz | 150 | 14 | 1 |
| ¼ Pounder, 4 oz | 360 | 33 | 3 |
| Jumbo, 3 oz | 270 | 25 | 2 |
| 97% Fat-Free, 1.6 oz | 40 | 1 | 3 |
| Beef Frank in a Blanket, 5 pcs, 3 oz | 300 | 24 | 12 |

**Jennie-O:** *Per Frank*

| | C | F | Cb |
|---|---|---|---|
| **Turkey Franks:** 1.2 oz | 70 | 6 | 1 |
| Jumbo, 2 oz | 120 | 10 | 2 |

**Oscar Mayer:** *Per Frank*
**Beef:** Classic, 1.6 oz

| | C | F | Cb |
|---|---|---|---|
| Beef: Classic, 1.6 oz | 140 | 13 | 0 |
| Lean, 1.8 oz | 60 | 3.5 | 1 |
| **Turkey:** Classic, 1.6 oz | 100 | 8 | 2 |
| Classic Bun Length, 2 oz | 120 | 10 | 3 |

**Shelton's:** *Per Frank*

| | C | F | Cb |
|---|---|---|---|
| **Chicken,** uncured, 1.2 oz | 80 | 7 | 1 |
| **Turkey,** Regular, 1.2 oz | 60 | 4.5 | 1 |
| **Zacky Farms,** Chkn; Turkey, av, 2 oz | 115 | 10 | 4 |

### Quick Guide | C | F | Cb

#### Fresh Sausages
**Pork/Beef:** *Average All Types*

| | C | F | Cb |
|---|---|---|---|
| **Small:** Raw, 4" link, 1 oz | 85 | 7.5 | 0 |
| Broiled/Pan-fried | 80 | 7 | 0 |
| **Medium:** Raw, 2 oz | 170 | 15 | 0 |
| Broiled/Pan-fried | 165 | 14 | 0 |
| **Large:** Raw, 3 oz | 255 | 22 | 0 |
| Broiled/Pan-fried | 245 | 21 | 0 |
| **Italian:** Raw, 3.2 oz | 315 | 28 | 1 |
| Cooked, 2.4 oz | 230 | 18 | 3 |
| **Chorizo:** Beef Chorizo, 2.5 oz piece | 250 | 23 | 5 |
| Pork Chorizo, 2 oz piece | 250 | 23 | 5 |

**Note:** Fat is lost in broiling/pan frying.
Cooked weight = approx. 60-70% raw weight

#### Smoked Sausages

*Per Link:*

| | C | F | Cb |
|---|---|---|---|
| **Butterball,** Turkey, 2 oz | 100 | 6 | 4 |
| **Eckrich:** | | | |
| **Grillers:** Original, 2 oz | 180 | 15 | 4 |
| Cheese | 190 | 17 | 1 |
| **Hillshire Farm:** | | | |
| Angus Beef, 2 oz | 170 | 15 | 3 |
| Cheddar Wurst, 2 oz | 180 | 16 | 2 |
| Chicken Hardwood, 2 oz | 100 | 7 | 3 |

**Johnsonville** ~ *See CalorieKing.Com*

#### Breakfast Sausages/Patties

**Butterball:** *Fully Cooked*
Turkey:

| | C | F | Cb |
|---|---|---|---|
| B'fast Sausage Links (3), 2.5 oz | 110 | 6 | 2 |
| Sausage Patties (2), 2.5 oz | 110 | 6 | 2 |

**Jimmy Dean:** *Fully Cooked*
**Heat 'N Serve Sausage Links:**

| | C | F | Cb |
|---|---|---|---|
| Pork, Regular (3), 1.9 oz | 210 | 19 | 2 |
| Turkey (3), 2 oz | 130 | 8 | 2 |
| **Maple Pork Sausages,**(3), 2.4 oz | 260 | 22 | 3 |

**Heat 'N Serve Sausage Patties:**

| | C | F | Cb |
|---|---|---|---|
| Pork, Original (2), 1.8 oz | 200 | 17 | 2 |
| Turkey (2), 1.8 oz | 120 | 8 | 1 |
| **Maple Pork Patties,** (2), 2.4 oz | 260 | 22 | 3 |

**Breakfast Sandwiches** ~ *See Page 92*
**Jones Dairy Farm:**
**All Natural Golden Brown Sausages:** *Fully Cooked*

| | C | F | Cb |
|---|---|---|---|
| Mild Pork Sausages (3), 2 oz | 250 | 24 | 1 |
| Pork Sausage Patty (1),1.2 oz | 120 | 12 | 0 |

#### Vegetarian Patties:

**Boca** ~ *See Page 117*
**GardenBurer** ~ *See Page 114*

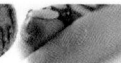

## Bagel, Corn & Hot Dogs  C  F  Cb

### Hot Dogs, Ready-To-Go:
*Includes Ketchup/Relish*

| | C | F | Cb |
|---|---|---|---|
| **Regular,** 1.5 oz frank, 1.5 oz bun | 260 | 15 | 22 |
| **Bun Length,** 2 oz frank, 1.5 oz bun | 290 | 18 | 21 |
| **Jumbo Dog,** 2 oz frank, 2 oz bun | 360 | 20 | 36 |
| **¼ lb Beef Dog,** 2 oz bun | 480 | 15 | 36 |
| **Mile Long Dog,** 2.6 oz dog, 1.5 oz bun | 360 | 24 | 23 |

### Corn Dogs:
| | | | |
|---|---|---|---|
| Beef/Pork Frank, average, 2.6 oz | 170 | 10 | 16 |

**Foster Farms:**

### Corn Dogs:
| | | | |
|---|---|---|---|
| Chili Cheese: (1), 2.7 oz | 180 | 9 | 19 |
| Honey Crunchy: | | | |
| Regular (1), 2.7 oz | 180 | 9 | 19 |
| Jumbo (1), 4 oz | 280 | 15 | 27 |
| Mini (4), 2.7 oz | 210 | 12 | 18 |

**State Fair:**
| | | | |
|---|---|---|---|
| Beef Corn Dog (1), 2.7 oz | 230 | 11 | 26 |
| Classic Corn Dog (1), 2.7 oz | 190 | 8 | 23 |
| Fiesta (1), 2.7 oz | 180 | 9 | 19 |

### Bagel Dogs:
**Einstein Bros/Noah's:**
| | | | |
|---|---|---|---|
| **N.Y. Bagels:** Asiago | 620 | 33 | 58 |
| Original | 610 | 32 | 57 |

**Vienna Beef:**
| | | | |
|---|---|---|---|
| **Bageldog:** 5.5 oz | 400 | 1 | 64 |
| 6.5 oz | 470 | 18 | 56 |
| Mini (4), 3 oz | 220 | 13 | 16 |

## Hot Dog Toppings/Extras:
| | | | |
|---|---|---|---|
| **American Cheese,** 1 slice, 1 oz | 110 | 9 | 1 |
| **Chili Con Carne,** ¼ cup | 50 | 2 | 5.5 |
| **Ketchup,** 1 Tbsp | 15 | 0 | 4 |
| **Mustard,** 1 Tbsp | 20 | 0 | 1 |
| **Onions,** chopped, 1 Tbsp | 5 | 0 | 1 |
| **Pickle Relish,** 1 Tbsp | 20 | 0 | 5 |
| **Sauerkraut,** ½ cup | 20 | 0 | 5 |

## Deli/Lunch Meats & Sausage

| | C | F | Cb |
|---|---|---|---|
| **Beef Jerky/Meat Snacks,** | | | |
| Berliner (pork/beef), 1 oz | 65 | 5 | 1 |
| **Beerwurst (Beef):** | | | |
| Small (2¾"diam), 1/16" slice | 20 | 2 | 0 |
| Large (4" diam), 1/8" slice | 75 | 7 | 0.5 |
| **Beerwurst (Pork):** | | | |
| Small (2.75"diameter), 1/16" slice | 15 | 1 | 0 |
| Large (4"diameter), 1/8" Slice | 55 | 4 | 0.5 |
| **Blood Sausage,** 1 oz | 100 | 9 | 0.5 |

## Deli/Lunch Meats & Sausages (Cont)

| | C | F | Cb |
|---|---|---|---|
| **Bologna:** | | | |
| Beef Bologna: 1 slice, 1 oz | 90 | 8 | 1 |
| Light, 1 slice, 1 oz | 60 | 4 | 2 |
| *Oscar Mayer:* Regular, 1 oz | 90 | 8 | 1 |
| 98% Fat Free, 1 oz | 25 | 0.5 | 3 |
| Light, 1 slice, 1 oz | 60 | 4 | 2 |
| *Boar's Head,* Ring, 2 oz | 150 | 13 | 1 |
| Pork Bologna: 1 Slice, 1 oz | 65 | 6 | 1 |
| Fat-Free, 1 slice, 1 oz | 20 | 0 | 2 |
| Turkey Bologna, average, 1 oz | 60 | 5 | 0.5 |
| **Bratwurst:** Average, 1 oz | 80 | 7 | 1 |
| *Bob Evan's,* Beer B'wurst, 2.2 oz link | 170 | 14 | 0 |
| **Braunschweiger,** (Pork/Liver/Sausage), | | | |
| *Oscar Mayer,* 2 oz slice | 190 | 17 | 1 |
| **Chicken,** average: | | | |
| 1 thick or 2 thin slices, 1 oz | 30 | 1 | 1 |
| 2 oz slice | 60 | 2 | 2 |
| *Hillshire Farm,* | | | |
| Rotiss. Seas'nd Chicken Breast, 2 oz | 50 | 0.5 | 2 |
| **Corned Beef,** average, full fat, 1 oz | 60 | 5 | 0.5 |
| **Ham, Sliced:** | | | |
| Baked/Broiled, 1 oz slice | 35 | 1 | 1 |
| *Oscar Mayer,* Baked, Lean, | | | |
| 3 slices, 2.3 oz | 80 | 2.5 | 1 |
| Honey/Brown Sugar, av., 1 oz | 35 | 1 | 1 |
| Prosciutto, average, 1 oz | 70 | 5 | 0 |
| **Ham & Cheese Loaf,** average, 1 oz | 70 | 5 | 1 |
| **Italian Sausage,** 2.6 oz | 250 | 20 | 3 |
| **Kielbasa:** Polish Sausage, 2 oz | 65 | 5 | 1 |
| Beef, 2 oz link | 190 | 17 | 1 |
| *Hillshire Farm,* | | | |
| Polska Kielbasa, 2 oz | 180 | 16 | 3 |
| **Knockwurst,** av., 1 oz | 90 | 8 | 0.5 |
| **Linguica** *(Gaspar's),* 2 oz | 130 | 9 | 1 |
| **Liverwurst,** 1 oz | 65 | 5 | 2 |
| **Liver Pate,** fresh, average, 1 oz | 90 | 8 | 1 |
| **Mortadella,** 1 oz | 105 | 9 | 0 |
| **Olive Loaf:** Average, 1 oz | 70 | 5 | 3 |
| *Oscar Mayer,* 1 oz | 80 | 6 | 3 |
| **Pancetta,** *Boars Head, 1 slice* | 50 | 4.5 | 0 |

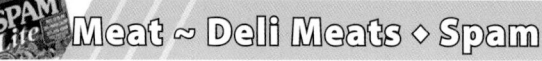

## Deli/Lunch Meats & Sausages (Cont)

| | **C** | **F** | **Cb** |
|---|---|---|---|
| **Pastrami (Beef):** | | | |
| *Boar's Head:* | | | |
|   1st cut Brisket, 2 oz | 90 | 4 | 2 |
|   Cap-Off Top Round, 2 oz | 80 | 3 | 1 |
| *Hillshire,* Deli Select, | | | |
|   Ultra Thin, 7 slices., 2 oz | 60 | 1.5 | 1 |
| **Peppered Beef,** 1 oz slice | 40 | 2 | 1 |
| **Pepperoni,** 5 slices, 1 oz | 140 | 13 | 0 |
| **Pickle Loaf,** average, 1 oz | 70 | 5 | 5 |
| **Pickle & Pepper Loaf,** | | | |
| *Boars Head,* 2 oz | 150 | 13 | 2 |
| **Proscuitto/Proscuitti,** av., 1 oz | 70 | 5 | 1 |
| **Roast Beef,** Lean, 1 oz | 40 | 2 | 0 |
| **Salami:** Beef, av., 1 oz | 80 | 7 | 1 |
| *Oscar Mayer,* Hard, 1 slice, 1.8 oz | 100 | 8 | 1 |
|   Beer Salami, average, 1 oz | 50 | 4 | 0.5 |
| *Oscar Mayer,* Cotto, 1 slice, 1 oz | 70 | 6 | 1 |
|   Dry, Hard, average, 4 slices, 1 oz | 100 | 8 | 1 |
|   Genoa: Average, 1 oz | 100 | 8 | 1 |
|     Stick, 1.8 oz | 175 | 14 | 2 |
| *Bridgford,* Italian, 1 oz | 120 | 11 | 0 |
| **SPAM (Hormel):** *Per 2 oz* | | | |
|   Classic: 2 oz serving | 180 | 16 | 1 |
|     7 oz can | 630 | 56 | 3.5 |
|     12 oz can | 1080 | 96 | 6 |
|   Spam Lite: 2 oz | 110 | 8 | 1 |
|     12 oz can | 660 | 48 | 6 |
| **Other Spam Products:** *Per 2 oz* | | | |
|   Hickory Smoked | 170 | 16 | 2 |
|   Hot & Spicy | 180 | 16 | 2 |
|   Oven Roasted Turkey | 80 | 4 | 2 |
|   Spam Spresd | 140 | 12 | 0 |
|   Spam with Bacon | 180 | 16 | 1 |
|   Spam with Cheese | 170 | 15 | 2 |
|   25% Less Sodium | 180 | 16 | 1 |
| **Spam Singles:** *Per 3 oz* | | | |
|   Classic, 3 oz package | 210 | 16 | 0 |
|   Lite, 3 oz package | 160 | 11 | 2 |

## Deli/Lunch Meats & Sausages (Cont)

| | **C** | **F** | **Cb** |
|---|---|---|---|
| **Summer Sausage:** | | | |
| *Armour,* 2 oz | 190 | 17 | 2 |
| *Hillshire Farm,* 2 oz | 190 | 16 | 1 |
| **Treet** *(Armour),* Luncheon Loaf, | | | |
|   Original, 2 oz | 140 | 11 | 4 |
| **Turkey**, average: 1 oz slice | 30 | 1 | 0.5 |
|   0.8 oz slice | 22 | 0.5 | 0.5 |
| **Turkey Breast:** | | | |
| *Butterball,* Oven Roasted: | | | |
|   Thick Slice, 1 slice 1 oz | 30 | 0.5 | 2 |
|   Deli Inspirations, | | | |
|     Extra Thin Slices, 4 slices, 2 oz | 50 | 1 | 3 |
| *Hillshire,* Deli Select, | | | |
|   Oven Roasted, 6 slices, 2 oz | 50 | 0.5 | 2 |
| **Turkey Ham,** 1 slice, 1 oz | 35 | 1.5 | 0.5 |
| **Turkey Loaf,** 1 oz | 30 | 1 | 0.5 |
| **Turkey Pastrami,** 1 oz | 35 | 1.5 | 1 |
| **Turkey Roll,** 1 oz | 40 | 2 | 0.5 |
| **Vegetarian Deli** ~ *See Page 118* | | | |

### Meat Spreads

| | **C** | **F** | **Cb** |
|---|---|---|---|
| **Average All Brands:** *Per 2 oz* | | | |
| Chicken, white meat | 130 | 10 | 2 |
| Ham, Deviled | 140 | 11 | 0 |
| Liverwurst | 190 | 16 | 2 |
| Roast Beef | 130 | 10 | 2 |
| Sandwich Spread | 140 | 10 | 9 |
| Turkey | 110 | 7 | 2 |
| **Underwood:** *Per 2 oz* | | | |
| Chicken, White Meat | 140 | 11 | 2 |
| Deviled Ham | 180 | 15 | 1 |
| Liverwurst | 160 | 13 | 4 |
| Roast Beef | 130 | 10 | 2 |

### Paté

| | **C** | **F** | **Cb** |
|---|---|---|---|
| **Les Trois Petit Cochons:** *Per 2 oz* | | | |
| **Pate:** de Campagne 2 oz | 240 | 22 | 2 |
|   de Canard a l'Orange; Forestier, 2 oz | 210 | 18 | 3 |
|   Paysan, 2 oz | 150 | 12 | 2 |
|   Rustique, 2 oz | 240 | 22 | 2 |
|   Venison, 2 oz | 200 | 16 | 4 |
|   Wild Boar, 2 oz | 180 | 15 | 4 |
| **Old Wisconsin Pate,** | | | |
|   Braunschweiger, 2 oz | 210 | 18 | 3 |

## Nuts

| | **C** | **F** | **Cb** |
|---|---|---|---|
| *Per 1 oz Unless Indicated* | | | |
| **Acorns,** raw 1 oz 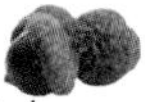 | 110 | 7 | 12 |
| **Almonds:** Dried/Dry Roasted: | | | |
| Whole: 12 medium size, 0.5 oz | 85 | 7.5 | 3 |
| 23-25 medium size, 1 oz | 170 | 15 | 6 |
| ½ cup, 2.5 oz 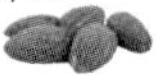 | 420 | 37 | 13 |
| Ground, 1 cup, 3.4 oz | 545 | 47 | 20 |
| Sliced, ½ cup, 1.6 oz 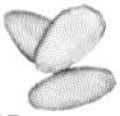 | 260 | 22 | 10 |
| Slivered, ½ cup, 2 oz | 310 | 27 | 12 |
| Chocolate Coated (5-6), 1 oz | 150 | 10 | 15 |
| Honey Roasted, 1 oz 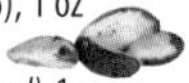 | 170 | 14 | 8 |
| Oil Roasted (*Blue Diamond*), 1 oz | 170 | 16 | 5 |
| **Brazil Nuts,** 8 medium, 1 oz | 185 | 19 | 3.5 |
| **Cashews,** dry or oil roasted: | | | |
| 14 large/18 med./26 small: 1 oz | 165 | 14 | 9 |
| ½ cup, 2.4 oz | 375 | 31 | 20 |
| Honey Roasted, 1 oz 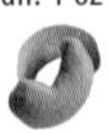 | 165 | 13 | 10 |
| **Chestnuts:** | | | |
| Average, dried, 1 oz | 105 | 1 | 22 |
| Raw/Fresh, 5-6 nuts, 1 oz 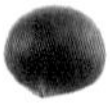 | 60 | 0 | 13 |
| Canned, water chestnuts, | | | |
| sliced/whole/drained, 1 oz | 30 | 0 | 7 |
| **Coconut, Fresh:** | | | |
| 1 piece, 2"x2"x ½", 1 oz 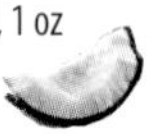 | 185 | 18 | 7 |
| Shredded, fresh, ½ cup, 1.4 oz | 140 | 13 | 6 |
| Dried (Desiccated): | | | |
| Sweetened: Shredded, 1 oz | 145 | 10 | 14 |
| Grated, ½ cup, 1.3 oz | 185 | 13 | 18 |
| Unsweetened, 1 oz | 185 | 18 | 7 |
| Cream (canned), ½ cup, 5.2 oz 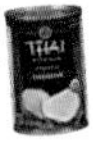 | 285 | 26 | 12 |
| Milk (canned), unsweetened, | | | |
| ¼ cup, 2 fl.oz | 100 | 10 | 3 |
| Water (center liquid), ½ cup, 4.3 oz | 25 | 0 | 4.5 |
| **Filberts or Hazelnuts:** | | | |
| Shelled, 18-20 nuts 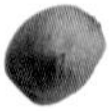 | 180 | 17 | 4.5 |
| Chopped, ¼ cup, 1 oz | 180 | 18 | 5 |
| Ground, ¼ cup, 0.6 oz | 120 | 12 | 3 |
| **Ginkgo Nuts,** canned, 14 med., 1 oz | 32 | 0.5 | 6.5 |
| **Hickory,** | | | |
| 30 small nuts, 1 oz | 200 | 18 | 5 |
| **Macadamia Nuts,** Shelled: | | | |
| Raw or Dry Roasted, avg: | | | |
| 12 small or 8 med., 1 oz 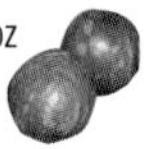 | 200 | 21 | 4 |
| 6-7 large, 1 oz | 200 | 21 | 4 |
| ½ cup, 2.3 oz | 480 | 51 | 10 |
| **Mixed Nuts:** Raw, 18-22 nuts, 1 oz | 170 | 15 | 7 |
| Oil Roasted, all types 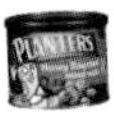 | 170 | 16 | 6 |
| Sweet Roasts, 26 pieces, 1 oz | 160 | 12 | 10 |
| *Planters*, Dry Roasted/Honey | 160 | 12 | 9 |
| **Nut Toppings,** chopped, 1 Tbsp, 0.3 oz | 40 | 4 | 1.5 |

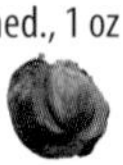

| | **C** | **F** | **Cb** |
|---|---|---|---|
| *Per 1 oz Unless Indicated* | | | |
| **Peanuts,** dry or oil roasted, average: | | | |
| Small handful, 0.5 oz 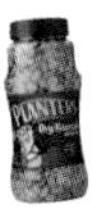 | 85 | 7 | 3 |
| ⅕ cup, 1 oz | 165 | 14 | 6 |
| ½ cup, 2.5 oz | 415 | 35 | 15 |
| 3 oz bag | 500 | 42 | 18 |
| 7 oz bag | 1160 | 98 | 42 |
| *Planters:* | | | |
| Cocktail, all varieties 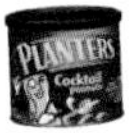 | 170 | 14 | 5 |
| Honey Roasted | 160 | 13 | 7 |
| Spanish Redskins 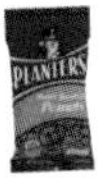 | 170 | 15 | 4 |
| Sweet N' Crunchy | 140 | 8 | 15 |
| Japanese Style Peanuts, | | | |
| Coated in Crunchy Shell | 150 | 8 | 13 |
| Raw: Shelled, 1 oz 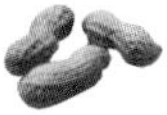 | 160 | 14 | 4.5 |
| In shell, 1 oz | 115 | 110 | 3 |
| **Pecans,** roasted: | | | |
| 10 halves, 0.5 oz 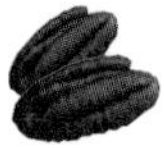 | 95 | 10 | 2 |
| 20 Halves, 1 oz | 195 | 20 | 4 |
| 1 cup, halves, 3.5 oz | 680 | 71 | 14 |
| **Pilinuts,** dried, 1 oz | 215 | 24 | 1 |
| **Pine Nuts,** | | | |
| dried, 1 Tbsp, 0.3 oz | 70 | 7 | 1.5 |
| **Pistachios,** raw: | | | |
| Shelled, 45 nuts, 1 oz | 160 | 13 | 8 |
| Unshelled, 2 oz | 165 | 14 | 7 |
| *Lance,* Roasted, 1.5 oz 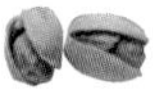 | 120 | 9 | 6 |
| **Sesame Nut Mix,** 1 oz | 160 | 13 | 9 |
| **Soy Nuts:** Dry Roasted 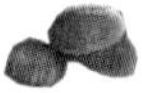 | 130 | 6 | 9 |
| ½ cup, 3 oz | 390 | 18 | 28 |
| *Dr Soy*, Chocolate coated, 1 oz pkg | 140 | 7 | 13 |
| **Trail Mix** (*Planters*): | | | |
| Daybreak, Berry Almond, 1.5 oz | 180 | 7 | 27 |
| Energy Mix, 1.5 oz 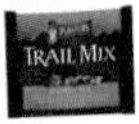 | 250 | 20 | 14 |
| Fruit & Nut | 140 | 9 | 14 |
| Nut & Chocolate, 1.3oz | 150 | 9 | 14 |
| Nuts, Seeds & Raisins, 1 oz 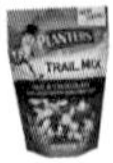 | 160 | 11 | 11 |
| Spicy Nuts & Cajun Sticks | 150 | 11 | 10 |
| Sweet & Nutty, 1 oz | 150 | 9 | 13 |
| **Walnuts,** average all types: | | | |
| 7-10 halves, 0.5 oz 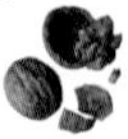 | 90 | 9 | 2 |
| 15-20 halves, 1 oz | 175 | 17 | 3 |
| Chopped, ½ cup, 2.2 oz | 380 | 36 | 6 |
| Ground, ¼ cup, 0.7 oz | 130 | 13 | 3 |

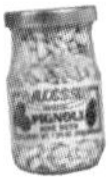

### Quick Guide | C F Cb

**Peanut Butter:** *Average All Brands*

| | C | F | Cb |
|---|---|---|---|
| 1 level tsp, 0.2 oz | 35 | 3 | 1 |
| 1 level Tbsp, 0.6 oz | 100 | 8.5 | 3.5 |
| 1 oz Quantity | 165 | 14 | 6 |
| ½ cup, 5 oz | 835 | 72 | 29 |

### Peanut Butter ~ Brands

| | C | F | Cb |
|---|---|---|---|
| Jif: Regular, all varieties, 2 Tbsp | 190 | 16 | 8 |
| Natural, average all varieties, 2 Tbsp | 190 | 16 | 9 |
| Reduced Fat, all varieties, 2 Tbsp | 190 | 12 | 15 |
| To Go: Crmy/Crunch, 1.5 oz cup | 250 | 22 | 11 |
| Reduced Fat, 1.7 oz cup | 250 | 16 | 20 |
| Whipped: Creamy, 2 Tbsp | 140 | 12 | 6 |
| Chocolate flavored, 2 Tbsp | 150 | 11 | 11 |
| Laura Scudder's, Natural, Smooth; Nutty, 2 Tbsp | 200 | 16 | 6 |
| Peanut Wonder, Original, 2 Tbsp | 100 | 2 | 13 |
| Peter Pan: Natural, Creamy/Crunchy, 2 Tbsp | 210 | 17 | 6 |
| Creamy/Crunchy, Red.-Fat, 2 Tbsp | 200 | 13 | 14 |
| Creamy, Whipped, 2 Tbsp | 150 | 12 | 5 |
| Planters, Creamy/Crunchy, 2 Tbsp | 180 | 15 | 8 |
| Smucker's, Goober, Grape/Srawberry, 3 Tbsp. 2 oz | 240 | 13 | 24 |
| Skippy: Natural, Creamy/Chunky, 2 T. | 190 | 16 | 6 |
| Reduced Fat, all varieties, 2 Tbsp | 180 | 12 | 15 |
| Dark Chocolate Spread, 2 Tbsp | 200 | 14 | 12 |
| PB Bites, average all, 15 pcs, 1 oz | 160 | 10 | 14 |

### Peanut Butter & Jelly Sandwich

| 1 sandwich: *With 2 oz Bread* | C | F | Cb |
|---|---|---|---|
| Thin Spread, 1 Tbsp Peanut Butter + 1 Tbsp Jelly | 310 | 10 | 48 |
| Thick Spread, 2 Tbsp Peanut Butter + 2 Tbsp Jelly | 480 | 19 | 67 |

### Nut & Chocolate Spread

| Nutella: | C | F | Cb |
|---|---|---|---|
| 1 Tbsp, 0.7 oz | 110 | 6 | 11 |
| 2 Tbsp, 1.3 oz | 200 | 11 | 22 |

Note: Nutella contains approx. 50% sugar & 13% hazelnuts

### Other Nut & Seed Butters

*Per 1 Tbsp, 0.5 oz*

| | C | F | Cb |
|---|---|---|---|
| Almond Butter | 100 | 10 | 3.5 |
| Cashew Butter | 95 | 8 | 4.5 |
| Hazelnut Butter; Pecan Butter | 110 | 10 | 2 |
| Pistachio Butter | 90 | 6.5 | 4.5 |
| Sesame Butter (Tahini) | 90 | 8 | 3 |
| Soy Nut Butter | 75 | 5 | 4 |

### Seeds | C F Cb

| | C | F | Cb |
|---|---|---|---|
| Alfalfa Seeds, sprouted, ½ cup, 0.5 oz | 5 | 0 | 1 |
| Caraway/Fennel, 1 tsp | 7 | 0.5 | 1 |
| Chia Seeds: 1 Tbsp, 0.4 oz | 45 | 3 | 4 |
| 3 Tbsp, 1 oz | 140 | 8.5 | 12 |
| Cottonseed Kernels, roasted, 1 Tbsp | 50 | 3.5 | 2 |
| Flax Seeds, 3 Tbsp, 1 oz | 140 | 9 | 9 |
| Lotus Seeds, dried, ½ cup, 0.5 oz | 55 | 0.5 | 10 |
| Poppy Seeds, 1 tsp | 15 | 1 | 1 |
| Pumpkin/Pepita Seeds, whole: Roasted/Tamari: 1 oz | 150 | 12 | 4 |
| ½ cup, 4 oz | 590 | 48 | 15 |
| Dried (hulled), ¼ cup, 1 oz | 155 | 13 | 5 |
| Safflower Kernels, dried, 1 oz | 150 | 11 | 10 |
| Sesame Seeds: Dried, 1 Tbsp, 0.3 oz | 50 | 4.5 | 2 |
| Roasted/Toasted, 1 oz | 160 | 14 | 7.5 |
| Sunflower Kernels/Seeds: Dried, ¼ cup w/out hulls, 0.3 oz | 200 | 18 | 7 |
| Dry Roasted: 1 Tbsp, 0.3 oz | 45 | 4 | 2 |
| ¼ cup, 1 oz | 165 | 14 | 7 |
| Oil Roasted, ⅓ cup, 1 oz | 170 | 14 | 6.5 |
| Watermelon Seeds, dried, ¼ cup, 1 oz | 150 | 13 | 4 |

*N*ut eaters are healthier and live longer, say scientists.

Nuts are a nutritious source of protein, vitamins, minerals, fiber, healthy fats, and antioxidants.

The fat and fiber of nuts can help reduce blood cholesterol. Their protein and fiber also promotes meal satiety (fullness) and reduces hunger levels – of benefit in weight control.

Eat nuts instead of high-sugar snacks, candy and soft drinks. Add chopped nuts to breakfast cereals.

## Quick Guide    C   F   Cb

### Pancakes:

**Plain:** *Average All Types*

| | C | F | Cb |
|---|---|---|---|
| Small (3" diameter), 0.8 oz | 50 | 2 | 6 |
| Medium (4" diameter), 1.3 oz | 85 | 3.5 | 11 |
| Large (6" diameter), 2.5 oz | 175 | 7.5 | 22 |

*Add Extra for Syrups/Butter*

**Pancake Syrup:** Regular, 1 Tbsp

| | | | |
|---|---|---|---|
| Regular, 1 Tbsp | 50 | 0 | 12 |
| ¼ cup, 4 Tbsp | 185 | 0 | 49 |
| Lite, 1 Tbsp | 25 | 0 | 6.5 |
| ¼ cup, 4 Tbsp | 100 | 0 | 27 |

**Butter/Margarine:**

| | | | |
|---|---|---|---|
| Regular, 1 Tbsp | 100 | 11 | 0 |
| Whipped, 1 Tbsp | 65 | 7.5 | 0 |

### Waffles:

| | | | |
|---|---|---|---|
| **Homemade,** 7" waffle, 2.5 oz | 220 | 11 | 25 |
| **Frozen + Toasted,** (4" diam.), 1 oz | 105 | 3 | 16 |

## Pancake Brands

*Prepared As Directed*

**Aunt Jemima:** *Prepared*

**Mixes:** *Per 4" Pancake*

| | | | |
|---|---|---|---|
| Original (4) | 250 | 8 | 36 |
| Original Complete (2) | 160 | 1.5 | 32 |
| Buttermilk (4) | 160 | 3 | 27 |
| Whole Wheat Blend (3) | 200 | 6.5 | 30 |

**Bisquick:** *Prepared*

**Pancake/Waffle Mix:**

| | | | |
|---|---|---|---|
| Complete, Simply Buttermilk, with Whole Grain (3) | 210 | 4 | 39 |
| Shake 'n Pour, Buttermilk (3) | 220 | 3 | 43 |

**Hungry Jack:**

**Pancake & Waffle Mixes:** *Per 4" Pancake*

Complete Mixes: Just Add Water

| | | | |
|---|---|---|---|
| Blueberry Wheat, 1.9 oz | 190 | 2 | 39 |
| Chocolate Chip, 1.9 oz | 190 | 2.5 | 39 |
| Cinnamon spice, 1.9 oz | 190 | 1 | 41 |

**Easy Packs:** *Dry Mix Only*

| | | | |
|---|---|---|---|
| Blueberry Wheat, 1.9 oz | 190 | 2 | 39 |
| Buttermilk, 1.6 oz | 150 | 1.5 | 31 |

**Traditional:** *Dry Mix Only*

| | | | |
|---|---|---|---|
| Original, 1.7 oz | 160 | 1 | 34 |
| Buttermilk, 1.7 oz | 160 | 1 | 34 |
| Extra Light & Fluffy, 1.6 oz | 150 | 1 | 32 |

**Northern Pines,**

| | | | |
|---|---|---|---|
| Premium Mix (3), 4", 3.5 oz, prep'd | 200 | 3.5 | 38 |

## Frozen Breakfasts    C   F   Cb

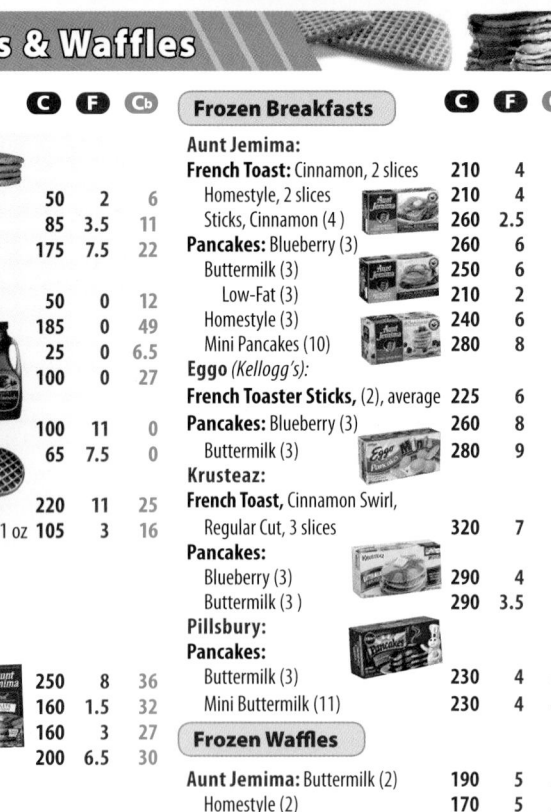

**Aunt Jemima:**

| | C | F | Cb |
|---|---|---|---|
| **French Toast:** Cinnamon, 2 slices | 210 | 4 | 35 |
| Homestyle, 2 slices | 210 | 4 | 34 |
| Sticks, Cinnamon (4) | 260 | 2.5 | 39 |
| **Pancakes:** Blueberry (3) | 260 | 6 | 45 |
| Buttermilk (3) | 250 | 6 | 41 |
| Low-Fat (3) | 210 | 2 | 42 |
| Homestyle (3) | 240 | 6 | 41 |
| Mini Pancakes (10) | 280 | 8 | 45 |

**Eggo** *(Kellogg's):*

| | | | |
|---|---|---|---|
| **French Toaster Sticks,** (2), average | 225 | 6 | 37 |
| **Pancakes:** Blueberry (3) | 260 | 8 | 42 |
| Buttermilk (3) | 280 | 9 | 45 |

**Krusteaz:**

| | | | |
|---|---|---|---|
| **French Toast,** Cinnamon Swirl, Regular Cut, 3 slices | 320 | 7 | 53 |

**Pancakes:**

| | | | |
|---|---|---|---|
| Blueberry (3) | 290 | 4 | 55 |
| Buttermilk (3) | 290 | 3.5 | 57 |

**Pillsbury:**

**Pancakes:**

| | | | |
|---|---|---|---|
| Buttermilk (3) | 230 | 4 | 45 |
| Mini Buttermilk (11) | 230 | 4 | 45 |

## Frozen Waffles

| | | | |
|---|---|---|---|
| **Aunt Jemima:** Buttermilk (2) | 190 | 5 | 29 |
| Homestyle (2) | 170 | 5 | 28 |

**Eggo** *(Kellogg's):*

| | | | |
|---|---|---|---|
| Blueberry (2) | 180 | 6 | 29 |
| Chocolatey Chip (2) | 200 | 7 | 31 |
| Homestyle (2) | 190 | 7 | 27 |

Nutri-Grain:

| | | | |
|---|---|---|---|
| Blueberry (2) | 180 | 6 | 30 |
| Whole Wheat (2) | 170 | 6 | 27 |
| **Kashi,** all varieties (2) | 150 | 5 | 25 |

**Nature's Path:**

| | | | |
|---|---|---|---|
| Ancient Grains; Maple Cinn., av, (2) | 180 | 6 | 29 |
| Buckwheat Wildberry (2) | 190 | 7 | 33 |
| Chia Plus; Homestyle, (2) | 210 | 7 | 34 |
| Flax Plus (2) | 200 | 8 | 30 |
| **Van's:** 8 Whole Grains, Berry (2) | 170 | 6 | 27 |
| Belgian, Homestyle (2) | 250 | 10 | 37 |
| **Wheat Gluten Free,** Apple Cinnamon (2) | 200 | 6 | 35 |
| **Mini,** Chocolate Chip (8) | 160 | 5 | 29 |

### Spaghetti/Pasta   **C** **F** **Cb**

- Pasta includes all shapes and sizes; (e.g. spaghetti, fettuccini, elbows, shells, twists, sheets, cannelloni, linguini, tubes, ziti).
- All regular pasta products have the same cals/fat/carbs on a weight basis.
- 1 oz Dry = approximately 2.5 -3 oz cooked.

### Dry Spaghetti/Pasta

| | C | F | Cb |
|---|---|---|---|
| 1 oz quantity | 105 | 0.5 | 21 |
| 1lb box/pkg, 16 oz | 1685 | 7 | 339 |
| Elbows, 1 cup, 4 oz | 380 | 2 | 80 |
| Shells, small, 1 cup, 3.3 oz | 330 | 1.5 | 69 |
| Spirals, 1 cup, 3 oz | 305 | 1.5 | 64 |

### Cooked Spaghetti/Pasta

| | C | F | Cb |
|---|---|---|---|
| **Plain, All Types (no added fat):** | | | |
| Firm/Al Dente (8-10 minutes), 1 oz | 42 | 0.5 | 8.5 |
| Medium (11-13 minutes), 1 oz | 37 | 0.5 | 7.5 |
| Tender (14-20 minutes), 1 oz | 32 | 0.5 | 7 |
| Longer cooking increases water absorbed | | | |
| **Spaghetti:** ½ cup, 2.5 oz | 90 | 0.5 | 18 |
| Medium serving, 1 cup, 5 oz | 225 | 1.5 | 44 |
| Large serving, 2 cups, 10 oz | 450 | 3 | 88 |
| Extra large, 3 cups, 15 oz | 675 | 5 | 132 |
| **Elbows/Spirals,** 1 cup, 5 oz | 220 | 1.5 | 43 |
| **Small Shells,** 1 cup, 4 oz | 180 | 1 | 36 |
| **Protein-fortified:** Dry, 1 c., 3.4 oz | 350 | 2 | 63 |
| Cooked, 1 cup, 5 oz | 230 | 0.5 | 46 |
| **Spinach/Vegetable:** Dry, 1 cup, 3 oz | 310 | 1 | 61 |
| Cooked, 1 cup, 5 oz | 180 | 0.5 | 38 |
| **Whole-wheat:** Dry, 1 cup, 3.8 oz | 365 | 1.5 | 79 |
| Cooked, 1 cup, 5 oz | 175 | 1 | 37 |

### Fresh Pasta (Refrigerated)

| | C | F | Cb |
|---|---|---|---|
| *Average All Brands:* | | | |
| **Plain/Spinach/Tomato:** | | | |
| As purchased, 4.5 oz | 370 | 3 | 70 |
| Cooked, 1 cup, 5 oz | 185 | 1.5 | 35 |
| Home-made, w/o egg, cooked, 1 c. 5 oz | 175 | 1 | 35 |
| **Buitoni:** | | | |
| **Cut Pasta:** | | | |
| Angel Hair, 3 oz | 230 | 2 | 43 |
| Fettuccine/Linguine, 3 oz | 240 | 2 | 45 |
| **House Foods:** | | | |
| **Tofu Shirataki Noodles:** | | | |
| Traditional, 1.6 oz | 0 | 0 | 1 |
| Angel Hair/Fettuccini, Macaroni/Spaghetti, 4 oz | 15 | 0.5 | 3 |
| **Nasoya,** | | | |
| Shirataki Spaghetti, Pasta Zero, ⅔ cup, 4 oz | 20 | 0 | 4 |

### Buitoni: *Per 1 Cup Unless Indicated*   **C** **F** **Cb**

| | C | F | Cb |
|---|---|---|---|
| **Agnolotti:** Butternut Squash, 3.7 oz | 300 | 12 | 37 |
| Wild Mushroom, 3.8 oz | 280 | 10 | 34 |
| **Ravioli:** Beef & Sausage, 3.8 oz | 260 | 8 | 33 |
| Chicken Marsala, 3.9 oz | 280 | 8 | 36 |
| Light 4-Cheese, 1¼ cups, 3.3 oz | 260 | 6 | 39 |
| **Tortellini:** Herb Chicken, 3.9 oz | 330 | 8 | 52 |
| Mixed Cheese, 3.7 oz | 320 | 8 | 48 |
| **Tortelloni:** Italian Sausage, 4 oz | 350 | 10 | 51 |
| Spinach & Ricotta, 3.7 oz | 270 | 7 | 39 |
| **Other Varieties ~** See Page 112 | | | |
| **Pasta Sauces ~** See Page 144 | | | |

### Macaroni & Cheese

| | C | F | Cb |
|---|---|---|---|
| **Packaged (Kraft) ~** See Page 116 | | | |
| **Restaurant:** *Average* | | | |
| Side Serve, 6 oz | 265 | 13 | 26 |
| Medium serve, 1 cup, 9 oz | 350 | 17 | 34 |
| Large serve, 2 cups, 18 oz | 700 | 34 | 68 |

### Noodles

| | C | F | Cb |
|---|---|---|---|
| **Plain/Egg:** Dry, 1 oz | 110 | 1.5 | 20 |
| 1 cup, 1.4 oz | 145 | 1.5 | 27 |
| **Cooked:** 1 oz | 40 | 0.5 | 7 |
| ½ cup, 2.8 oz | 110 | 1.5 | 20 |
| 1 cup, 5.5 oz | 220 | 3.5 | 40 |
| **Stir-Fried:** 1 cup, 5.5 oz | 270 | 9 | 40 |
| 2 cup serving, 11 oz | 540 | 18 | 80 |
| **Low Carb Noodles,** | | | |
| Quest Pasta, 4 oz | 10 | 0 | 3 |
| *Note: Carbs are from glucomannan fiber* | | | |
| **Yolk Free (Cooked):** | | | |
| Manischewitz, Yolk Free, 2 oz | 200 | 1 | 41 |
| **Chinese:** Cellophane/Rice, dry, 1 oz | 100 | 0 | 25 |
| Chow Mein/hard, dry, 1 oz | 150 | 9 | 16 |
| **Japanese:** Soba: Dry, 1 oz | 95 | 0.5 | 21 |
| Cooked, 1 cup, 4 oz | 115 | 0.5 | 24 |
| Somen: Dry, 1 oz | 100 | 0.5 | 21 |
| Cooked, 1 cup, 6 oz | 230 | 0.5 | 49 |
| **Japanese Style Pan Fried,** | | | |
| Yaki-Soba (*Maruchan's*), av., 5.6 oz | 260 | 3 | 50 |
| **Ramen Noodles ~** See Page 118 | | | |
| **Rice Noodles:** Dry, 3.5 oz | 365 | 0.5 | 83 |
| Cooked, 1 cup, 6.2 oz | 190 | 0.5 | 44 |
| *Yakisoba,* Stir Fry, 3.5 oz | 430 | 6 | 52 |
| *House Foods,* Tofu Shirataki, 4 oz | 20 | 0.5 | 3 |
| *Chikara,* Udon, average, 7.5 oz pkt | 250 | 1 | 52 |
| *Simply Asia/Thai Kitchen ~* See Pages 119 & 121 | | | |

### Egg Roll/Won Ton Wrappers

| | C | F | Cb |
|---|---|---|---|
| Egg/Spring Roll (1), 0.8 oz | 65 | 0 | 15 |
| Won Ton Wrapper (1), 0.3 oz | 20 | 0 | 4 |

## Quick Guide  C  F  Cb

**Fruit Pies:** *Average All Brands, 9" Pie*
**Apple; Blueberry; Cherry:**

| | C | F | Cb |
|---|---|---|---|
| Small Serving, | | | |
| 1/8 pie, 4.8 oz | 350 | 16 | 49 |
| Medium Serving, | | | |
| 1/6 pie, 6.5 oz | 465 | 22 | 65 |
| Large Serving | | | |
| 1/4, 9.5 oz | 700 | 33 | 98 |
| Whole Pie (9"), 38 oz | 2800 | 131 | 392 |

**Other Pies:** *Per Serving, 1/6 of 9" Pie*

| | | | |
|---|---|---|---|
| Chocolate Cream Pie | 345 | 22 | 38 |
| Custard: Egg Pie | 220 | 12 | 22 |
| Coconut Pie | 330 | 18 | 35 |
| Lemon Meringue Pie | 305 | 10 | 53 |
| Peach Pie | 260 | 12 | 39 |
| Pecan Pie | 440 | 23 | 57 |
| Pumpkin Pie | 315 | 14 | 41 |
| Shoo-Fly Pie | 400 | 13 | 70 |

## Dessert/Fruit Pies ~ Brands

**Hostess:**

| | | | |
|---|---|---|---|
| Cherry Pie, 4.5 oz | 480 | 20 | 69 |
| Lemon Pie, 4.5 oz | 490 | 22 | 69 |

**Marie Callender's:**

| | | | |
|---|---|---|---|
| Almond Glazed Cherry, 1/10 pie, 4.3 oz | 370 | 17 | 53 |
| Banana Cream, 1/9 pie, 4.2 oz | 310 | 17 | 37 |
| Peach, w/- Crmy Glaze, 1/10 pie, 4.2 oz | 360 | 16 | 50 |

**Mrs Smith's:**
**Original Flaky Crust:** *Per 1/8 Pie, 4.6 oz*

| | | | |
|---|---|---|---|
| Apple | 340 | 17 | 45 |
| Cherry | 350 | 17 | 47 |
| Peach | 340 | 19 | 41 |
| Pumpkin | 300 | 13 | 42 |
| Sweet Potato | 330 | 13 | 48 |
| Very Berry | 340 | 17 | 44 |

**Sara Lee:**
**Creme Pies:**

| | | | |
|---|---|---|---|
| Chocolate, 1/5 pie, 3.9 oz | 450 | 27 | 50 |
| Coconut, 1/6 pie, 4.5 oz | 370 | 20 | 44 |
| Key Lime, 1/5 pie | 410 | 17 | 60 |
| Lemon Meringue, 1/5 pie, 4.6 oz | 390 | 13 | 64 |

**Oven Fresh Pies:** *Per 9" Pie, 4.6 oz Slice*

| | | | |
|---|---|---|---|
| Apple | 340 | 16 | 43 |
| Cherry | 340 | 17 | 44 |
| Peach | 320 | 14 | 42 |
| Seasonal: Pumpkin, 4.6 oz | 270 | 10 | 41 |
| Sthrn Sweet Potato, 4.6 oz | 280 | 9 | 46 |

**Tastykake:** Apple | 270 | 11 | 41
| Lemon | 300 | 14 | 44 |

## Croissants  C  F  Cb

**Average all Brands**
**Plain/Butter/Cheese:**

| | C | F | Cb |
|---|---|---|---|
| Mini, 1 oz | 115 | 6 | 13 |
| Small, 1.5 oz | 170 | 9 | 19 |
| Medium, 2 oz | 230 | 12 | 26 |
| Large, 2.5 oz | 290 | 15 | 32 |

**Sweet Croissants:**

| | | | |
|---|---|---|---|
| Almond Filled, 3 oz | 330 | 18 | 39 |
| Chocolate Filled, 3 oz | 360 | 19 | 43 |
| **Dunkin' Donuts,** Plain Croissant | 330 | 17 | 37 |

**Sara Lee:**

| | | | |
|---|---|---|---|
| French Style: Original, 1.8 oz | 185 | 9 | 21 |
| Mini, 1 oz | 230 | 11 | 26 |

**Croissant Sandwiches** ~ *See Page 165*

## Pastry & Pie Crust

**Pie Crust,** Baked, 9" diameter shell:

| | | | |
|---|---|---|---|
| 1 Pie Shell, 6.5 oz | 970 | 64 | 87 |
| 2-crust Pie, 9", 11.3 oz | 1660 | 109 | 150 |
| **Filo Pastry:** 4 sheets, 2.5 oz | 210 | 2.5 | 40 |
| *Athens,* Filo Dough, 5 sheets, 2 oz | 170 | 1 | 36 |

**Puff:**

| | | | |
|---|---|---|---|
| *Pepperidge Farm:* 1/2 sheet | 480 | 30 | 48 |
| Bake & Fill Shell (1) | 180 | 11 | 18 |

**Arrowhead Mills,**

| | | | |
|---|---|---|---|
| Graham Cracker Pie Crust, 1/8 of 9" | 110 | 5 | 14 |

**Keebler:**
**Ready Crust:** *Per 1/8 of 9" Crust*

| | | | |
|---|---|---|---|
| Chocolate | 100 | 4.5 | 14 |
| Graham: Regular | 100 | 5 | 14 |
| Reduced Fat | 100 | 3.5 | 15 |
| Shortbread Crust | 100 | 5 | 14 |

**Marie Callenders,**

| | | | |
|---|---|---|---|
| Deep Dish Pie Crust, 1/8 pie, 1 oz | 140 | 10 | 11 |

**Mrs Smith's,**

| | | | |
|---|---|---|---|
| Deep Dish, 1/8 pie, 1 oz | 130 | 7 | 14 |

**Nabisco:**
**Honey Maid,**

| | | | |
|---|---|---|---|
| Graham Cacker, 1/8 pie, 0.75 oz | 110 | 5 | 14 |

**Nilla,** Pie Crust,

| | | | |
|---|---|---|---|
| 1/6 of 9", 1 oz | 140 | 8 | 18 |

**Pillsbury,**

| | | | |
|---|---|---|---|
| Rolled, 1/8, 0.9 oz | 100 | 6 | 12 |
| **Trader Joe's,** Pie Crust, 1/8 pie, 1.2 oz | 190 | 13 | 17 |

## Pie Fillings ~ Canned

**Apple/Blueb./Cherry/Strawb.,** average:

| | | | |
|---|---|---|---|
| Sweetened: 1/3 cup, 3.2oz | 90 | 0 | 22 |
| 1 cup, 9.5 oz | 270 | 0 | 66 |
| 1 can, 21 oz | 600 | 0 | 150 |
| Light/Lite, 1/3 cup, 3.2 oz | 60 | 0 | 15 |
| Unsweetened, 1/3 cup, 3.2 oz | 35 | 0 | 8 |
| **Lemon Crm/Creme,** 1/3 cup, 3.2 oz | 130 | 1.5 | 28 |

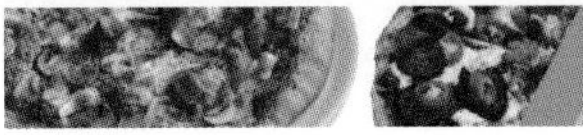

## Pizzas ~ Ready to Eat  **C** **F** **Cb**

*Figures Based On Pizza Hut Unless Indicated*

### Cheese

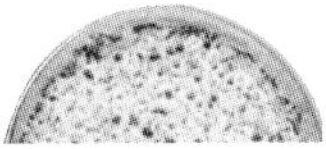

| Medium Size (12"): | C | F | Cb |
|---|---|---|---|
| **Hand Tossed/Classic Crust:** | | | |
| ⅛ Pizza (1 slice) | 210 | 8 | 26 |
| ½ Pizza (4 slices) | 840 | 32 | 104 |
| Whole Pizza (8 slices) | 1680 | 64 | 208 |
| **Original Pan:** ⅛ Pizza (1 slice) | 240 | 10 | 26 |
| ½ Pizza (4 slices) | 960 | 40 | 104 |
| Whole Pizza (8 slices) | 1920 | 80 | 208 |
| **Thin 'N Crispy Crust:** | | | |
| ⅛ Pizza (1 slice) | 190 | 8 | 22 |
| ½ Pizza (4 slices) | 760 | 32 | 88 |
| Whole Pizza (8 slices) | 1520 | 64 | 176 |

### Ham & Pineapple

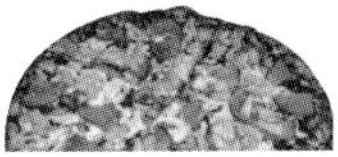

*Figures Based On Domino's*

| Medium Size (12"): | C | F | Cb |
|---|---|---|---|
| **Hand Tossed/Classic Crust:** | | | |
| ⅛ Pizza (1 slice) | 200 | 7 | 26 |
| ½ Pizza (4 slices) | 800 | 26 | 104 |
| Whole Pizza (8 slices) | 1600 | 52 | 208 |
| **Pan Crust:** ⅛ Pizza (1 slice) | 300 | 13 | 30 |
| ½ Pizza (4 slices) | 1180 | 52 | 120 |
| Whole Pizza (8 slices) | 2360 | 104 | 240 |
| **Thin Crust:** | | | |
| ⅛ Pizza (1 slice) | 155 | 7.5 | 16 |
| ½ Pizza (4 slices) | 620 | 30 | 64 |
| Whole Pizza (8 slices) | 1240 | 60 | 128 |

### Meat Lovers

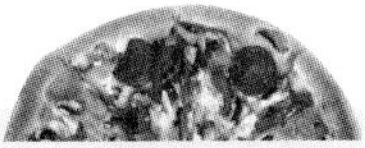

| Medium Size (12"): | C | F | Cb |
|---|---|---|---|
| **Hand Tossed/Classic Crust:** | | | |
| ⅛ Pizza (1 slice) | 280 | 15 | 25 |
| ½ Pizza (4 slices) | 1120 | 60 | 100 |
| Whole Pizza (8 slices) | 2240 | 120 | 200 |
| **Original Pan:** ⅛ Pizza (1 slice) | 310 | 17 | 27 |
| ½ Pizza (4 slices) | 1240 | 68 | 108 |
| Whole Pizza (8 slices) | 2480 | 136 | 216 |
| **Thin Crust:** ⅛ Pizza (1 slice) | 260 | 14 | 22 |
| ½ Pizza (4 slices) | 1040 | 56 | 88 |
| Whole Pizza (8 slices) | 2080 | 112 | 176 |

### Pepperoni    **C** **F** **Cb**

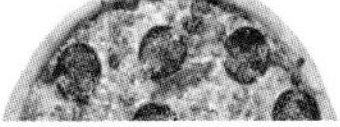

| Medium Size (12"): | C | F | Cb |
|---|---|---|---|
| **Hand Tossed/Classic Crust:** | | | |
| ⅛ Pizza (1 slice) | 220 | 9 | 25 |
| ½ Pizza (4 slices) | 880 | 36 | 100 |
| Whole Pizza (8 slices) | 1760 | 72 | 200 |
| **Original Pan:** ⅛ Pizza (1 slice) | 260 | 12 | 27 |
| ½ Pizza (4 slices) | 1040 | 48 | 108 |
| Whole Pizza (8 slices) | 2080 | 96 | 216 |
| **Thin Crust:** ⅛ Pizza (1 slice) | 200 | 9 | 21 |
| ½ Pizza (4 slices) | 800 | 36 | 84 |
| Whole Pizza (8 slices) | 1600 | 72 | 168 |

### Large Pizzas

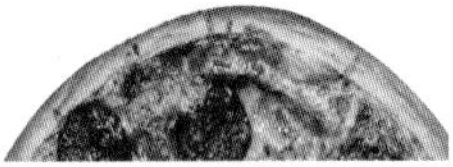

| Large (14") | C | F | Cb |
|---|---|---|---|
| **Hand Tossed:** | | | |
| **Cheese:** ⅛ Pizza (1 slice) | 290 | 11 | 33 |
| ½ Pizza (4 slices) | 1150 | 45 | 134 |
| **Meat Lovers:** ⅛ Pizza (1 slice) | 390 | 21 | 33 |
| ½ Pizza (4 slices) | 1560 | 84 | 133 |
| **Pepperoni:** ⅛ Pizza (1 slice) | 310 | 13 | 35 |
| ½ Pizza (4 slices) | 1240 | 52 | 140 |

### Extra Large, Single Slice

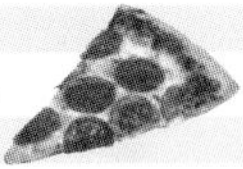

*Figures Based On Sbarro*

| | C | F | Cb |
|---|---|---|---|
| Cheese | 430 | 15 | 51 |
| Ham & Pineapple | 490 | 16 | 60 |
| Pepperoni | 650 | 31 | 69 |
| Sausage-Pepperoni | 850 | 44 | 76 |

### Individual Personal Pizzas

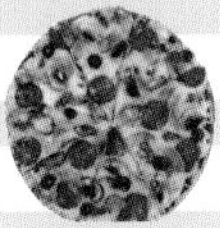

*Pan (6"): Figures Based On Pizza Hut*

| | C | F | Cb |
|---|---|---|---|
| Buffalo Chicken | 630 | 25 | 72 |
| Cheese | 600 | 25 | 68 |
| Pepperoni | 630 | 29 | 67 |
| Supreme | 700 | 35 | 69 |
| Veggie Lovers | 560 | 22 | 70 |

*Chicago-Style Deep Dish: Individual*
*Figures Based On Uno Pizzeria*

| | C | F | Cb |
|---|---|---|---|
| Cheese & Tomato, 20 oz | 1750 | 119 | 117 |
| Pepperoni, 19 oz | 1750 | 121 | 114 |
| Sausage, Tomato & Cheese, 27 oz | 2300 | 164 | 119 |
| Sausage, Pepperoni & Cheese, 24 oz | 1850 | 128 | 120 |

### Frozen Pizzas

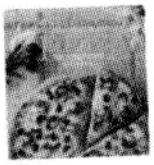

| | C | F | Cb |
|---|---|---|---|
| **Amy's:** *Per ⅓ Pizza* | | | |
| Cheese Pizza | 290 | 12 | 33 |
| Mushroom & Olive | 260 | 10 | 33 |
| Pesto | 310 | 12 | 39 |
| Roasted Vegetable | 280 | 9 | 42 |
| Vegan, Roasted Vegetables, no Cheese | 260 | 4.5 | 50 |
| **California Pizza Kitchen:** | | | |
| **Crispy Thin Crust:** *Per ⅓ Pizza* | | | |
| Margherita | 320 | 16 | 31 |
| Sicilian Recipe | 360 | 18 | 30 |
| Signature Pepperoni | 350 | 19 | 29 |
| White | 320 | 17 | 30 |
| **Small Crispy Thin Crust:** *Per Whole Pizza* | | | |
| BBQ Recipe Chicken; Margh., av | 390 | 15 | 43 |
| Four Cheese | 400 | 18 | 40 |
| Hawaiian | 350 | 12 | 43 |
| Sicilian | 420 | 20 | |
| **Hand Tossed Style:** *Per ⅓ Pizza* | | | |
| BBQ Recipe Chicken, with Bacon | 360 | 9 | 50 |
| Californian Style White | 310 | 7 | 49 |
| The Works | 350 | 11 | 48 |
| **Celeste:** | | | |
| **Pizza For One:** Original, 1 pizza | 320 | 14 | 42 |
| Deluxe | 340 | 15 | 41 |
| Four Cheese | 330 | 15 | 38 |
| Pepperoni | 340 | 13 | 43 |
| Sausage & Pepperoni | 380 | 19 | 41 |
| Zesty Four Cheese | 350 | 16 | 43 |
| **DiGiorno:** *Per Slice, Unless Indicated* | | | |
| **Cheese Stuffed Crust:** | | | |
| Bacon Cheeseburger, ⅙ pizza, 4.5 oz | 310 | 13 | 34 |
| Five Cheese, ⅕ Pizza, 5.3 oz | 380 | 16 | 40 |
| Pepperoni, ⅕ pizza, 5.3 oz | 380 | 16 | 40 |
| Three Meat, ⅙ pizza 4.8 oz | 340 | 16 | 34 |
| Supreme, ⅙ pizza, 5 oz | 350 | 16 | 34 |
| **Classic Thin Crust**, Supreme, ⅕ pizza, 5 oz | 310 | 14 | 32 |
| **Garlic Bread:** *Per ⅙ Pizza* | | | |
| Pepperoni, 5 oz | 380 | 17 | 40 |
| Supreme, 4.3 oz | 300 | 12 | 36 |

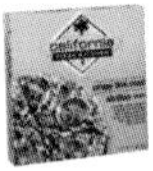

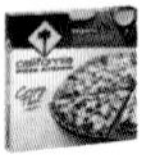

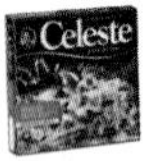

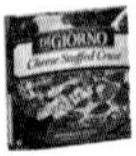

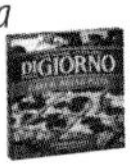

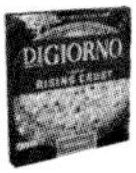

| | C | F | Cb |
|---|---|---|---|
| **DiGiorno (Cont):** | | | |
| **Original Rising Crust:** *Per ⅙ Pizza* | | | |
| Four Cheese, 4.7 oz | 310 | 10 | 39 |
| Italian Sausage, 5 oz | 350 | 14 | 39 |
| Spicy Chicken Supreme, 5.3 oz | 300 | 9 | 40 |
| **Small Pizzas:** *Per ½ Pizza* | | | |
| Cheese Stuffed Crust: | | | |
| Four Cheese, 4.2 oz | 320 | 15 | 34 |
| Pepperoni, 4.2 oz | 330 | 16 | 34 |
| Three Meat, 4.6 oz | 360 | 18 | 34 |
| Traditional Crust: | | | |
| Pepperoni, 4.6 oz | 380 | 18 | 42 |
| Three Meat, 4.7 oz | 360 | 16 | 40 |
| **Freschetta:** | | | |
| **Brick Oven:** *Per ⅕ Pizza Unless Indicated* | | | |
| 5 Italian Cheese, ¼ Pizza, 5.2 oz | 380 | 18 | 40 |
| Chicken Club, ¼ Pizza, 5.5 oz | 360 | 15 | 41 |
| Pepp. & Italian Style Cheese, 4.6 oz | 340 | 17 | 33 |
| Rstd Portab. M'shrms & Spin., 4.6 oz | 270 | 10 | 34 |
| Three Meat Medley, 4.6 oz | 350 | 18 | 33 |
| Zesty Italian Supreme, 4.6 oz | 310 | 15 | 33 |
| **Naturally Rising:** *Per ⅙ of Large Pizza Unless Indicated* | | | |
| 4 Cheese Medley, ⅕ Pizza, 5 oz | 380 | 14 | 47 |
| Canada Style Bacon P'apple, 4.5 oz | 290 | 9 | 40 |
| Classic Supreme, 5 oz | 360 | 15 | 41 |
| Ssg & Pepperoni, 4.9 oz | 370 | 16 | 40 |
| Signat. Pepperoni, 4.5 oz | 340 | 13 | 40 |
| **Jeno's:** *Per Pizza* | | | |
| **Crispy 'N Tasty:** | | | |
| Cheese, 5 oz | 320 | 14 | 37 |
| Pepperoni, 5 oz | 350 | 18 | 36 |
| **Kashi:** | | | |
| **Thin Crust:** *Per ⅓ Pizza* | | | |
| Margherita, 4 oz | 260 | 9 | 29 |
| Mediterranean, 4.2 oz | 290 | 9 | 37 |
| Mushroom Trio & Spinach, 4 oz | 250 | 9 | 28 |
| **Kroger:** | | | |
| **3 Minute Microwave:** *Per 8 oz Pizza* | | | |
| 3-Meat | 500 | 17 | 64 |
| Cheese | 490 | 16 | 66 |
| Combination | 520 | 20 | 64 |
| Pepperoni | 530 | 20 | 65 |
| Supreme | 490 | 18 | 63 |
| **French Bread,** Pepperoni, 5 oz | 380 | 17 | 42 |

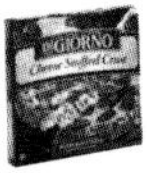

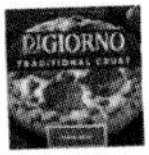

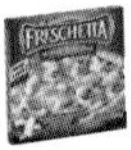

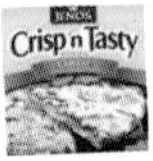

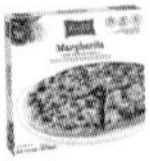

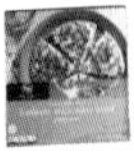

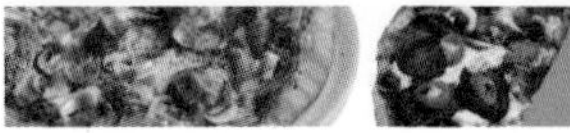

## Frozen Pizzas (Cont)

| | C | F | Cb |
|---|---|---|---|
| **Lean Cuisine:** | | | |
| **Craveables:** Four Cheese, 6 oz | 380 | 7 | 60 |
| Pepperoni, 6 oz | 390 | 9 | 58 |
| **Deep Dish:** | | | |
| Three Meat, 6 oz | 390 | 9 | 56 |
| Spinach & Mushroom, 6 oz | 350 | 7 | 54 |
| **Woodfired:** BBQ Recipe Chicken | 340 | 7 | 50 |
| Garlic Chicken | 380 | 8 | 55 |
| Margherita | 320 | 7 | 48 |
| **Snack:** Cheese & Tomato, (1), 3 oz | 160 | 4 | 23 |
| Pepperoni (1), 3 oz | 210 | 6 | 28 |
| **Red Baron:** | | | |
| **Brick Oven:** Per ¼ Pizza | | | |
| Cheese Trio, 4.4 oz | 320 | 14 | 36 |
| Meat Trio, Pepperoni, 4.6 oz | 340 | 16 | 36 |
| Sausage Supreme, 4.7 oz | 320 | 14 | 37 |
| **Classic Crust:** Per ¼ Pizza | | | |
| 4 Cheese, 5.2 oz | 370 | 16 | 41 |
| Sausage & Pepp., 5.3 oz | 390 | 18 | 42 |
| Supreme, 4.7 oz | 310 | 14 | 34 |
| **Deep Dish Minis:** | | | |
| Cheese, 4 pieces, 5.4 oz | 420 | 20 | 46 |
| Pepperoni, 4 pieces, 5.4oz | 470 | 25 | 46 |
| **Rising Crust:** | | | |
| Cheese; Pepperoni, average, 4.8 oz | 335 | 12 | 44 |
| Sausage & Pepperoni, 5 oz | 360 | 14 | 45 |
| **Thin & Crispy Crust:** Per ⅓ Pizza | | | |
| 5 Cheese, 5 oz | 360 | 16 | 40 |
| Pepperoni, 5.3 oz | 400 | 19 | 40 |
| **Singles:** Per Pizza | | | |
| **Deep Dish:** Hawaiian Style, 5.3 oz | 350 | 13 | 47 |
| Meat-Trio, 5.6 oz | 400 | 17 | 47 |
| Sausage, 5.8 oz | 420 | 19 | 48 |
| **French Bread:** | | | |
| 5 Cheese & Garlic (1) | 430 | 23 | 41 |
| Pepperoni (1) | 370 | 15 | 44 |
| **Safeway Select:** | | | |
| **Pizzeria Crust:** | | | |
| Cheese Trio, ¼ pizza | 340 | 15 | 34 |
| Fajita Chicken Ole, ⅕ pizza | 250 | 10 | 29 |
| Pepperoni & Sausage, ⅕ pizza | 320 | 17 | 30 |
| **Self Rising:** Per ⅙ Pizza | | | |
| Four Cheese | 300 | 9 | 41 |
| Pepperoni | 350 | 14 | 41 |
| Sausage & Pepperoni | 340 | 13 | 41 |

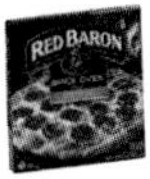

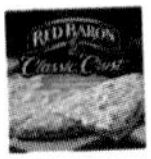

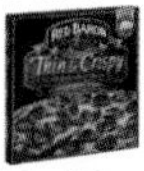

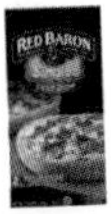

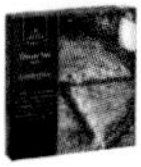

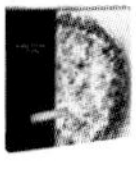

| | C | F | Cb |
|---|---|---|---|
| **Smart Ones** (Weight Watchers): | | | |
| **Classic Favorites,** Thin Crust, | | | |
| Cheese Pizza, 6 oz | 290 | 6 | 42 |
| **Smart Anytime,** Brick Oven Style, | | | |
| Pepperoni Pizza, 6 oz | 430 | 13 | 57 |
| **Stouffer's:** | | | |
| **French Bread Pizzas:** | | | |
| **Two Per Box:** | | | |
| Deluxe, 1 piece, 6.2 oz | 430 | 21 | 44 |
| Sausage & Pepperoni, | | | |
| 1 piece, 6.3 oz | 460 | 24 | 43 |
| **Nine Per Box:** | | | |
| Cheese, 1 piece, 5.9 oz | 380 | 16 | 43 |
| Pepperoni, 1 piece, 5.7 oz | 430 | 21 | 44 |
| **Tombstone:** | | | |
| **Original:** Per ¼ Pizza | | | |
| Canadian Style Bacon | 320 | 12 | 37 |
| Extra Cheese | 350 | 15 | 36 |
| Pepperoni | 390 | 20 | 37 |
| Pepperoni & Sausage | 360 | 17 | 37 |
| **Thin Crust:** Per ¼ Pizza | | | |
| Three Cheese | 310 | 15 | 28 |
| Pepperoni; Sausage, average | 315 | 16 | 28 |
| **Brick Oven Style:** Cheese, ⅓ pizza | 350 | 15 | 37 |
| Pepperoni; Supreme, av., ¼ pizza | 315 | 16 | 29 |
| **Tony's:** | | | |
| **Pizzeria Style Crust:** Per ¼ Pizza | | | |
| Bacon Cheeseburger, 4.8 oz | 360 | 16 | 39 |
| Cheese, 4.8 oz | 330 | 13 | 42 |
| Pepperoni, 4.7 oz | 330 | 14 | 41 |
| Supreme, 5.3 oz | 350 | 15 | 42 |
| **Singles:** | | | |
| Classic, 7 oz | 480 | 19 | 67 |
| Combination, 7.4 oz | 510 | 22 | 66 |
| Deluxe, 7.4 oz | 470 | 18 | 66 |
| Pepperoni, 7.1 oz | 490 | 20 | 66 |
| **Totino's:** | | | |
| **Crisp Crust Party Pizza:** Per ½ Pizza | | | |
| Cheese | 320 | 15 | 35 |
| Combination | 360 | 19 | 36 |
| Hamburger | 350 | 18 | 36 |
| Pepperoni | 360 | 19 | 35 |
| **Pizza Rolls:** | | | |
| Cheese (6), 3 oz | 210 | 8 | 28 |
| Pepperoni (6), 3 oz | 220 | 9 | 26 |
| **Trader Joe's:** | | | |
| 3 Cheese, ⅓ pizza | 310 | 9 | 42 |
| Parlanno, ¼ pizza | 340 | 16 | 34 |
| Pizza 4 Formaggi, ⅓ pizza | 310 | 9 | 42 |
| Spinach, ⅓ pizza | 300 | 12 | 38 |

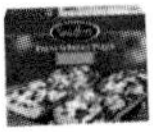

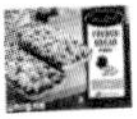

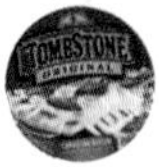

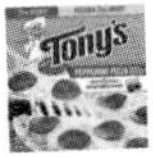

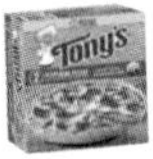

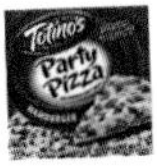

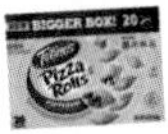

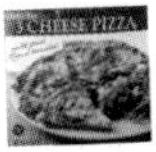

## Chicken

### Chicken
From 3lb ready-to-cook chicken

| | C | F | Cb |
|---|---|---|---|
| **Breast/Wing Quarter:** | | | |
| **Roasted:** with skin | 300 | 15 | 0 |
| without skin | 185 | 5 | 0 |
| **Fried,** batter dipped | 530 | 30 | 17 |
| **Leg Quarter:** | | | |
| **Thigh & Drumstick:** | | | |
| **Roasted:** with skin | 270 | 16 | 0 |
| without skin | 185 | 8 | 0 |
| **Fried,** batter dipped | 435 | 25 | 15 |

**KFC ~ See Fast-Foods Section**

### Per 4 oz Edible Portion

| | C | F | Cb |
|---|---|---|---|
| **Average of Light Meat:** *Per 4 oz without Bone* | | | |
| **Roasted:** with skin | 250 | 12 | 0 |
| without skin | 175 | 4.5 | 0 |
| **Stewed:** with skin | 230 | 12 | 0 |
| without skin | 180 | 4.5 | 0 |
| **Fried:** Batter-dipped, with skin, 4 oz | 315 | 17 | 11 |
| Flour-coated, with skin, 4 oz | 280 | 14 | 2 |
| **Average of Dark Meat:** *Per 4 oz without Bone* | | | |
| **Roasted:** with skin | 290 | 18 | 0 |
| without skin | 235 | 11 | 0 |
| **Stewed:** with skin | 265 | 17 | 0 |
| without skin | 220 | 10 | 0 |
| **Fried:** Batter-dipped, with skin, 4 oz | 340 | 21 | 11 |
| Flour-coated, with skin, 4 oz | 325 | 19 | 5 |

### Chicken Parts

| | C | F | Cb |
|---|---|---|---|
| **Broilers or Fryers:** *Edible Weights (no bone)* | | | |
| **Breast:** *Per ½ Breast* | | | |
| Raw: with skin, 5 oz | 250 | 14 | 0 |
| without skin, 4.25 oz | 140 | 3 | 0 |
| Roasted: with skin, 3.5 oz | 195 | 8 | 0 |
| without skin, 3 oz | 140 | 3 | 0 |
| Stewed: with skin, 4 oz | 200 | 8 | 0 |
| without skin, 3.3 oz | 145 | 3 | 0 |
| Fried: Batter-dipped, w/ skin, 5 oz | 365 | 19 | 13 |
| Flour-coated, with skin, 3.5 oz | 220 | 9 | 2 |
| **Drumstick:** *Per Drumstick* | | | |
| Roasted: with skin, 2 oz | 115 | 6 | 0 |
| without skin, 1.5 oz | 75 | 2.5 | 0 |
| Stewed: with skin, 2 oz | 115 | 6 | 0 |
| without skin, 1.5 oz | 80 | 3 | 0 |
| Fried: Batter-dipped, w/ skin, 2.5 oz | 195 | 11 | 6 |
| Flour-coated, with skin, 1.8 oz | 120 | 7 | 1 |

| | C | F | Cb |
|---|---|---|---|
| **Broilers or Fryers (Cont):** *Edible Weights (no bone)* | | | |
| **Thigh Portion:** | | | |
| Raw: with skin, 3.3 oz | | | |
| (4¼ oz with bone) | 200 | 14 | 0 |
| without skin, 2.4 oz | 80 | 3 | 0 |
| Roasted: with skin, 2.3 oz | 155 | 10 | 0 |
| without skin, 2 oz | 110 | 6 | 0 |
| Stewed: with skin, 2.5 oz | 160 | 10 | 0 |
| without skin, 2 oz | 105 | 5 | 0 |
| Fried: Batter-dipped, with skin 3 oz | 240 | 14 | 8 |
| Flour-coated, with skin, 2.3 oz | 165 | 9 | 2 |
| **Wing:** *Per Wing, Bone In* | | | |
| Raw Weight, 3.2 oz | | | |
| Raw: with skin | 110 | 8 | 0 |
| without skin | 35 | 1 | 0 |
| Roasted: with skin | 100 | 7 | 0 |
| without skin | 45 | 2 | 0 |
| Fried: Batter-dipped, with skin | 160 | 11 | 5 |
| Flour-coated, with skin | 105 | 7 | 1 |
| Stewed: with skin, 4 oz | 100 | 7 | 0 |
| **Buffalo Wings ~ See Fast-Foods Section** | | | |
| **Neck:** Simmered, with skin | 95 | 7 | 0 |
| without skin | 30 | 2 | 0 |
| **Skin Only:** *Skin from ½ Chicken* | | | |
| Raw skin, 3 oz | 275 | 26 | 0 |
| Roasted skin, 2 oz | 255 | 23 | 0 |
| Stewed skin, 2.5 oz | 260 | 24 | 0 |
| Fried, flour-coated, 2 oz | 280 | 24 | 5 |
| Fried, batter-dipped, 6.8 oz | 750 | 55 | 44 |
| **Roasters:** *Average of Light & Dark Meat* | | | |
| **Roasted:** with skin, 4 oz | 250 | 15 | 0 |
| without skin, 4 oz | 190 | 8 | 0 |
| Dark Meat, without skin | 200 | 10 | 0 |
| Light Meat, without skin | 175 | 5 | 0 |
| **Stewing Chicken:** *Per 4 oz, average of Light & Dark Meat* | | | |
| **Stewed:** with skin | 325 | 22 | 0 |
| without skin | 270 | 14 | 0 |
| Dark Meat, without skin | 290 | 17 | 0 |
| Light Meat, without skin | 240 | 9 | 0 |
| **Capon Chicken:** | | | |
| **Roasted:** with skin, 4 oz | 260 | 13 | 0 |
| ½ Chicken, with skin, 22.5 oz | 1460 | 74 | 0 |
| **Chicken Offal & Stuffing:** | | | |
| **Giblets:** Simmered, 1 cup | 230 | 7 | 0.5 |
| Fried, flour-coated, 1 cup | 400 | 20 | 6 |
| **Gizzard,** simmered, 1 cup | 210 | 4 | 0 |
| **Heart,** simmered, 1 cup | 270 | 12 | 0.2 |
| **Liver:** Raw, 4 oz | 130 | 5.5 | 0 |
| Simmered, 1 cup | 215 | 8.5 | 1 |
| **Liver Pate,** fresh, 1 Tbsp, 0.5 oz | 30 | 2 | 1 |
| **Stuffing,** average, ½ cup | 180 | 9 | 22 |

## Chicken Products    C   F   Cb

**Bumble Bee:**
**Chicken In Water:** *Per 2 oz Drained*

| | C | F | Cb |
|---|---|---|---|
| Premium White | 70 | 1.5 | 0 |
| Premium Breast | 70 | 1 | 1 |

**Foster Farms:**

| | | | |
|---|---|---|---|
| **Chicken Breast Strips**, grilled, 3 oz | 100 | 2 | 1 |
| **Wings:** Chipotle, 3 wings, 3 oz | 190 | 13 | 4 |
| Honey BBQ Glazed, 3 wings, 3 oz | 190 | 11 | 7 |
| Hot 'n' Spicy, 3 wings, 3 oz | 190 | 14 | 1 |

**Tyson:**
**Anytizers, Frozen:**
  **Wings:**

| | | | |
|---|---|---|---|
| Hot Wings, Buffalo Style (3) | 190 | 13 | 1 |
| Honey BBQ Seasoned (3) | 190 | 12 | 8 |

  **Wyngz, Boneless:**

| | | | |
|---|---|---|---|
| Buffalo Style, 3 pieces, 3 oz | 150 | 7 | 8 |
| Sweet Garlic Glazed, 3 pcs, 2.8 oz | 130 | 5 | 10 |

## Duck, Goose, Quail

**Duck, Roasted:**

| | | | |
|---|---|---|---|
| with skin, 3 oz | 290 | 24 | 0 |
| without skin, 3 oz | 170 | 10 | 0 |
| ½ duck, with skin, 13.5 oz | 1290 | 108 | 0 |
| **Goose:** Roasted with skin, 3 oz | 260 | 19 | 0 |
| without skin, 3 oz | 200 | 11 | 0 |
| **Pheasant,** cooked, 3 oz | 210 | 10 | 0 |
| **Quail,** cooked, 1 whole, 6 oz | 385 | 24 | 0 |

## Turkey

**Fryer-Roasters:** *Per 3 oz Serving*
**Roasted:**

| | | | |
|---|---|---|---|
| Light Meat: with skin | 140 | 4 | 0 |
| without skin | 120 | 1 | 0 |
| Dark Meat: with skin | 155 | 6 | 0 |
| without skin | 140 | 4 | 0 |

**½ of Whole Turkey:** (Approx. 3.3 lbs raw weight without neck and giblets; 1.8 lbs cooked weight)

| | | | |
|---|---|---|---|
| **Roasted:** with skin | 1650 | 74 | 0 |
| without skin | 1125 | 31 | 0 |

**Ground Turkey,** raw: (4 oz raw wt. = 3 oz ckd wt.)

| | | | |
|---|---|---|---|
| 85% lean, regular, 4 oz | 170 | 10 | 0 |
| 93% lean: Average, 4 oz | 160 | 8 | 0 |
| *Jennie-O,* 4 oz | 170 | 8 | 0 |
| *Trader Joe's,* 4 oz | 150 | 8 | 0 |
| 94% lean, | | | |
| *Foster Farms,* 4 oz | 150 | 7 | 0 |
| Breast, no skin, 4 oz | 115 | 1 | 0 |
| Patties: Small, 3 oz | 130 | 7 | 0 |
| Medium, 4 oz | 170 | 10 | 0 |

## Turkey Parts    C   F   Cb

**Roasted, Edible Weights, without bone:**
**Breast,** (½), (from 17.3 oz raw weight with bone):

| | C | F | Cb |
|---|---|---|---|
| with skin, 12 oz (no bone) | 525 | 11 | 0 |
| without skin, 10.8 oz | 415 | 2 | 0 |
| **Back (½):** with skin, 4.5 oz | 265 | 13 | 0 |
| without skin, 3.5 oz | 165 | 6 | 0 |

**Leg (Thigh & Drumstick):**
(from 1 lb raw weight with bone)

| | | | |
|---|---|---|---|
| with skin, 8.5 oz (without bone) | 410 | 13 | 0 |
| without skin, 7.8 oz (w/out bone) | 355 | 8.5 | 0 |

**Wing:** (From 7.3 oz raw weight)

| | | | |
|---|---|---|---|
| with skin, 3 oz (without bone) | 185 | 9 | 0 |
| without skin, 2 oz (w/out bone) | 100 | 2 | 0 |
| **Neck:** Simmered, 1 neck, 9 oz (with bone) | 275 | 11 | 0 |
| **Giblets,** simmered, 1 cup, 5 oz | 240 | 7 | 3 |

## Young Hens (Roasted)

**Light Meat:**

| | | | |
|---|---|---|---|
| with skin, 3 oz | 175 | 8 | 0 |
| without skin, 3 oz | 135 | 3 | 0 |
| **Dark Meat:** with skin, 3 oz | 200 | 11 | 0 |
| without skin, 3 oz | 165 | 7 | 0 |

**Young Toms ~** *Similar to Young Hens*

## Turkey Products

**Foster Farms:** *Cooked & Frozen*
Meatballs, cooked:

| | | | |
|---|---|---|---|
| Homestyle (3) | 160 | 9 | 3 |
| Italian Style (3) | 160 | 8 | 5 |
| **Hormel,** Canned Turkey Breast, in water, 2 oz | 50 | 1 | 0 |

**Jennie-O:**

| | | | |
|---|---|---|---|
| Bacon, 1 slice, 0.5 oz | 30 | 2.5 | 0 |
| Bratwurst, lean, 1 link, 3.85 oz | 170 | 10 | 2 |
| Burgers, uncooked, All Natural, White Meat, 5.3 oz | 200 | 10 | 0 |
| Meatballs, Fully Cooked: Italian, 3 oz | 180 | 13 | 2 |
| Home Style, 3 oz | 180 | 13 | 3 |
| **Spam,** Oven Roasted Turkey, 2 oz | 80 | 4 | 2 |

**Trader Joe's,**

| | | | |
|---|---|---|---|
| Italian Turkey Meatloaf, 3 oz | 140 | 8 | 5 |

**Valley Fresh,** 100% Natural,
Canned Prem. White Turkey Breast,

| | | | |
|---|---|---|---|
| in water, 2 oz | 45 | 1 | 0 |

## White Rice

| | C | F | Cb |
|---|---|---|---|
| **Raw:** | | | |
| Glutinous, 1 cup, 6.5 oz | 685 | 1 | 151 |
| Long Grain, 1 cup, 6.5 oz | 675 | 1 | 148 |
| Short Grain, 1 cup, 7 oz | 715 | 1 | 158 |
| Wild Rice, 1 cup, 5.5 oz | 570 | 2 | 120 |
| **Cooked Rice:** *Boiled/Steamed* | | | |
| **Short/Medium Grain:** | | | |
| ½ cup, 3.3 oz | 140 | 0 | 30 |
| 1 cup (½ Pint), 7.2 oz | 265 | 0.5 | 59 |
| 2 cups (1 Pint), 13 oz | 480 | 1 | 106 |
| **Long Grain:** ½ cup, 2.8 oz | 100 | 0 | 22 |
| 1 cup, 5.5 oz | 205 | 0.5 | 44 |
| **Glutinous/Sticky,** 1 cup, 6 oz | 170 | 0.5 | 37 |
| **Parboiled,** ½ cup, 3 oz | 105 | 0.5 | 22 |
| **Precooked/Instant:** | | | |
| Dry, ½ cup, 3.5 oz | 380 | 1 | 82 |
| Cooked, ½ cup, 3 oz | 95 | 0.5 | 21 |
| **Wild Rice,** | | | |
| Cooked, 1 cup, 5.8 oz | 165 | 0.5 | 35 |

## Brown Rice

*Average of Short or Long Grain*

| | C | F | Cb |
|---|---|---|---|
| **Raw/Dry:** ½ cup, 3.3 oz | 340 | 2.5 | 71 |
| 1 cup, 6.5 oz | 685 | 5.5 | 143 |
| **Cooked:** ½ cup, 3.5 oz | 110 | 1 | 22 |
| 1 cup, 7 oz | 220 | 2 | 46 |

## Rice Dishes

| | C | F | Cb |
|---|---|---|---|
| **Chinese Fried Rice:** | | | |
| ½ cup, 2.5 oz | 140 | 4.5 | 21 |
| 1 cup, (½ Pint), 5 oz | 280 | 9 | 42 |
| 2 cups, (1 Pint), 10 oz | 565 | 18 | 84 |
| **Mexican Style Rice:** | | | |
| *Taco John's,* Cilantro Lime, 6 oz | 220 | 3 | 39 |
| *Taco Time,* Mexi, 3.5 oz | 80 | 0.5 | 17 |
| **Rice-A-Roni** ~ *See Page 119* | | | |
| **Rice with Raisins/Pinenuts,** 1 cup | 400 | 11 | 60 |
| **Rice Pilaf:** Restaurant, 1 cup | 275 | 7.5 | 46 |
| *O'Charley's,* A La Carte, 1 order | 220 | 6 | 36 |
| **Rice Pudding,** | | | |
| *Kozy Shack,* Original, 1 pudding cup | 130 | 2.5 | 24 |
| **Risotto,** 1 cup | 420 | 12 | 70 |
| **Saffron Rice,** 4 oz | 175 | 7 | 25 |
| **Spanish Rice:** 1 cup, 5 oz | 390 | 9 | 72 |
| *El Pollo Loco,* Small, 4.5 oz | 170 | 2.5 | 33 |
| *Taco Cababa,* 3.6 oz | 120 | 0.5 | 25 |
| **Sticky Rice,** 1 cup, 5 oz | 155 | 0.5 | 34 |
| **Sushi Rice:** 1 Tbsp | 25 | 0 | 5 |
| 1 cup, 5.2 oz | 390 | 0 | 77 |
| **Other Packaged Rice Products:** | | | |
| **Uncle Ben's / Zatarain's** ~ *See Page 121* | | | |

---

## CalorieKing.com Recipes

*See the CalorieKing website for a salubrious selection of healthy recipes – all analyzed for calories, fat, protein, carbohydrate, fiber and sodium.*

**Choose from:**
- **Starters/Appetizers**
- **Salads**
- **Entrees: Meat, Fish and Chicken**
- **Vegetarian**
- **Desserts**
- **Cakes, Cookies**
- **Drinks**

*www.CalorieKing.com/recipes*

### HEALTHY RECIPE TIPS

- **Use non-fat milk** in place of whole or 2% milk
- **Use low-fat yogurt** in place of sour cream
- **Skim fat** from surface of soups and casseroles after cooling
- **Add extra vegetables** to soups and hot entreés
- **Cakes/cookies/muffins:** Replace most or all the fat/oil with applesauce and/or prune puree (Example, *Sunsweet Lighter Bake*)

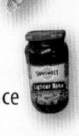

- **Drinks:** Replace sugar with no-calorie sweeteners such as *Equal, Stevia, Splenda and Sweet 'N Low*

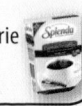

## Deli Salads

**C** **F** **Cb**

*Average All Outlets*

| | C | F | Cb |
|---|---|---|---|
| **Antipasto Salad,** ½ cup | 135 | 8 | 13 |
| **3-Bean Salad,** ½ cup | 90 | 4.5 | 12 |
| **Bulgur Salad,** ½ cup | 70 | 2 | 12 |
| **Caesar Salad,** Classic, 1 cup | 200 | 14 | 15 |
| **Side Salad,** without Dressing | 25 | 0 | 6 |
| **Carrot Raisin:** with Dressing, ½ cup | 135 | 12 | 6 |
| without Dressing, ½ cup | 20 | 0 | 5 |
| **Chef's Salad:** Regular, w/o Dressing | 620 | 37 | 8 |
| with 2 oz Thousand Island Drssng | 860 | 61 | 8 |
| **Chicken Salad,** ½ cup/scoop, 4 oz | 280 | 21 | 2 |
| **Coleslaw:** Traditional, ½ cup | 150 | 8 | 18 |
| w/ Low Cal Dressing, ½ c. | 50 | 2 | 8 |
| **Corn,** Mexican, ½ cup | 240 | 12 | 33 |
| **Cucumber:** Non-Oil Dressing, ½ cup | 60 | 0 | 14 |
| with Oil Dressing, ½ cup | 140 | 12 | 8 |
| **Eggplant Salad,** ½ cup | 75 | 5 | 7 |
| **Fettucini,** with veges, ½ cup | 135 | 6 | 16 |
| **Garden Salad,** without Dressing, 1 cup | 10 | 0 | 2 |
| **Greek Salad,** 1 cup | 105 | 8 | 7 |
| **Greek Vegetables,** 1 cup | 110 | 8 | 6 |
| **Lobster Salad,** ½ cup, 4 oz | 250 | 21 | 11 |
| **Macaroni Salad,** ½ cup, 5 oz | 360 | 26 | 26 |
| **Nicoise,** 1 cup | 450 | 32 | 18 |
| **Pasta Salad,** ½ cup | 200 | 11 | 19 |
| **Potato Salad:** Dijon, 3 oz | 120 | 7 | 13 |
| with Mayonnaise, ½ cup, 4 oz | 215 | 15 | 17 |
| Lowfat, ½ cup | 110 | 1.5 | 21 |
| **Rice Salad,** ½ cup | 150 | 10 | 13 |
| **Saffron Rice,** 4 oz | 175 | 7 | 25 |
| **Spinach Salad,** 1 cup | 180 | 13 | 13 |
| **Tabouli,** ½ cup | 125 | 7 | 13 |
| **Three Bean Salad,** ½ cup | 90 | 4.5 | 12 |
| **Tomato & Mozzarella,** ½ cup | 180 | 14 | 10 |
| **Tortellini,** with Basil Pesto, ½ cup | 150 | 9 | 15 |
| **Waldorf,** with Mayo, ½ cup | 110 | 7 | 12 |

**Signature Salads:** *Per 6 oz Serving*
(Supplied to Deli's and Institutions)

| | C | F | Cb |
|---|---|---|---|
| **Antipasto Salad** | 510 | 50 | 4 |
| **Artichoke Salad,** marinated | 400 | 41 | 8 |
| **California Medley** | 120 | 7 | 15 |
| **Cheese Agnolotti** | 250 | 8 | 23 |
| **Chicken Salad** | 420 | 33 | 11 |
| **Crabmeat Flavored** | 450 | 38 | 20 |
| **Egg Salad** | 300 | 23 | 14 |
| **Fresh Button Mushroom** | 190 | 16 | 6 |

**Signature Salads (Cont):** *Per 6 oz* **C** **F** **Cb**

| | C | F | Cb |
|---|---|---|---|
| **Fresh Button Mushroom** | 190 | 16 | 6 |
| **Ham Salad** | 400 | 32 | 14 |
| **Prima Pasta Salad** | 360 | 30 | 18 |
| **Seafood Pasta Del Mar** | 170 | 10 | 21 |
| **Seafood, Crab & Shrimp** | 420 | 34 | 20 |
| **Shrimp Salad** | 360 | 32 | 14 |
| **Tuna Salad** | 450 | 36 | 14 |

*~ Also See Fast-Foods & Restaurants Section*

## Fresh Salad Packs

*Pre-Packaged (Supermarkets):*
**Dole:**
**Kits:** *Per 3.5 oz, with Dressing*

| | C | F | Cb |
|---|---|---|---|
| Caesar | 150 | 12 | 8 |
| Chopped: Chipotle & Cheddar | 120 | 8 | 10 |
| Sesame Asian | 160 | 16 | 13 |
| Southwest | 140 | 10 | 10 |

**Salad Blends:** *without Dressing*

| | C | F | Cb |
|---|---|---|---|
| American; Mediterranean, 3 oz | 15 | 0 | 3 |
| Arugula; Baby Spinach, average, 3 oz | 20 | 0.5 | 3 |

**Fresh Express:**
**Complete Salad Kits:** *Per 3½ oz, Prepared*

| | C | F | Cb |
|---|---|---|---|
| Asian | 120 | 5 | 17 |
| Caesar: Regular | 150 | 12 | 7 |
| Lite | 90 | 6 | 7 |
| Supreme | 160 | 14 | 6 |
| Pear Gorganzola | 130 | 6 | 17 |

**Gourmet Cafe:** *Per Package*

| | C | F | Cb |
|---|---|---|---|
| Chopped Santa Fe | 290 | 19 | 18 |
| Tuscan | 330 | 28 | 9 |

**Ready Pac:**
**Bowl Salads:** *Per Container, with Dressing*

| | C | F | Cb |
|---|---|---|---|
| Apple Bleu Pecan, 4.5 oz | 230 | 17 | 15 |
| Asian Style Chkn, 6.2 oz | 210 | 11 | 14 |
| Cranb. Walnut, 4.5 oz | 220 | 9 | 26 |

**Dinner Solutions:** *with Dressing*

| | C | F | Cb |
|---|---|---|---|
| Chef, 3.5 oz | 160 | 11 | 7 |
| Southwestern, 3.5 oz | 130 | 9 | 7 |

**Gourmet:** *Per Container, with Dressing*

| | C | F | Cb |
|---|---|---|---|
| Baby Kale Apple Harvest, 8 oz | 390 | 23 | 42 |
| Turkey Cobb with Bacon, 11.5 oz | 460 | 32 | 24 |

## Salad Toppings

| | C | F | Cb |
|---|---|---|---|
| **Bac'n Pieces,** McCormick, 1Tbsp, 0.3 oz | 30 | 1 | 2 |
| **Bacon Bits** (Hormel), 1Tbsp | 25 | 1 | 0 |
| **Bac-Os, Bits** (Betty Crocker), 1 Tbsp | 30 | 1 | 2 |
| **Chow Mein Noodles,** dry, ½ cup | 120 | 7 | 13 |
| **Croutons,** 2 Tbsp, 0.3 oz | 40 | 1 | 7 |
| **Salad Toppins,** McCormick, 4 tsp | 35 | 1.5 | 3 |
| **Sunflower Seeds,** 1 Tbsp, 0.3 oz | 45 | 4 | 1.5 |
| **Toasted Sliced Almonds,** 2 T., 0.5 oz | 85 | 7 | 3 |

# S Salad Dressings

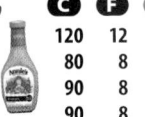

## Quick Guide

### Salad Dressings
**Average All Brands:** *Per 2 Tbsp, Approx 1 fl.oz*

| | C | F | Cb |
|---|---|---|---|
| **Balsamic Vinaigrette:** | | | |
| Regular | 90 | 9 | 3 |
| Light, 2 Tbsp | 45 | 4 | 2 |
| Fat Free, 2 Tbsp | 25 | 0 | 6 |
| **Blue Cheese:** Regular, 2 Tbsp | 145 | 15 | 1.5 |
| Regular, ¼ cup, 2 oz | 280 | 30 | 3 |
| Light, 2 Tbsp | 30 | 1 | 4 |
| **Caesar:** Regular, 2 Tbsp | 165 | 17 | 1 |
| Regular, ¼ cup, 2 oz | 310 | 34 | 2 |
| Light, 2 Tbsp | 35 | 1.5 | 5.5 |
| **Coleslaw:** Regular, 2 Tbsp | 125 | 11 | 8 |
| Regular, ¼ cup, 2 oz | 245 | 21 | 15 |
| Light, 2 Tbsp | 110 | 7 | 14 |
| **French:** Regular | 145 | 14 | 5 |
| Regular, ¼ cup, 2 oz | 260 | 25 | 9 |
| Light, 2 Tbsp | 65 | 4 | 9 |
| Fat/Oil-Free, 2 Tbsp | 40 | 0 | 10 |
| **Italian:** Regular, 2 Tbsp | 85 | 8.5 | 3 |
| Regular, ¼ cup, 2 oz | 165 | 16 | 6 |
| Light, 2 Tbsp | 55 | 5.5 | 2 |
| Fat/Oil-Free, 2 Tbas | 15 | 0 | 2.5 |
| **Ranch:** Regular, 2 Tbsp | 145 | 16 | 2 |
| Regular, ¼ cup, 2 oz | 290 | 30 | 4 |
| Light, 2 Tbsp | 60 | 4 | 6.5 |
| Fat-Free, 2 Tbsp | 35 | 0.5 | 8 |
| **Thousand Island:** Reg., 2 T. | 115 | 11 | 4.5 |
| Regular, ¼ cup, 2 oz | 210 | 20 | 9 |
| Light, 2 Tbsp | 60 | 3.5 | 7 |
| Fat-Free, 2 Tbsp | 40 | 0.5 | 10 |

**Enjoy a healthy salad but don't drown it in high-fat salad dressings.**

**Use 'light' dressings to halve the fat and calories.**

## Brands ~ Salad Dressings

| | C | F | Cb |
|---|---|---|---|
| **Annie's Naturals:** *Per 2 Tbsp* | | | |
| Organic: Goddess Dressing | 120 | 12 | 2 |
| Green Garlic | 80 | 8 | 2 |
| Papaya Poppy Seed | 90 | 8 | 5 |
| Thousand Island | 90 | 8 | 5 |
| Vinaigrettes: | | | |
| Red Wine & Olive Oil | 140 | 15 | 0 |
| Sesame Ginger | 90 | 8 | 4 |
| Shitake & Sesame | 120 | 13 | 1 |
| **Bernstein's:** *Per 2 Tbsp* | | | |
| Creamy Caesar | 120 | 13 | 1 |
| Herb Garden French | 130 | 12 | 6 |
| Italian | 110 | 12 | 1 |
| Restaurant Recipe Italian | 120 | 12 | 1 |
| Sweet Herb Italian | 130 | 11 | 8 |
| Fat-Free, Cheese & Garlic Italian | 10 | 0 | 2 |
| Light Fantastic: Cheese Fantastico | 25 | 1.5 | 3 |
| Roasted Garlic Balsamic | 45 | 3.5 | 3 |
| **Best Foods:** *Per 1 Tbsp Unless Indicated* | | | |
| Dijonnaise, 1 tsp | 5 | 0 | 1 |
| Mayonnaise: Real | 90 | 10 | 0 |
| Light | 35 | 3.5 | 1 |
| Low-Fat | 15 | 1 | 2 |
| Canola | 40 | 4 | 1 |
| Olive Oil | 60 | 6 | 1 |
| Mayonesa, Lemom-Lime | 90 | 10 | 0 |
| **Cardini's:** *Per 2 Tbsp* | | | |
| Aged Parmesan Ranch | 150 | 16 | 1 |
| **Caesar:** Original | 160 | 17 | 1 |
| Fat-Free Caesar | 40 | 0 | 9 |
| Light Caesar | 80 | 7 | 5 |
| Honey Mustard | 120 | 11 | 6 |
| Roasted Asian Sesame | 120 | 10 | 6 |
| Vinaigrette, Balsamic: | | | |
| Regular | 100 | 8 | 5 |
| Lite | 50 | 3 | 5 |
| **Great Value** (Walmart): *Per 2 Tbsp* | | | |
| Caesar | 120 | 12 | 2 |
| **Ranch:** Bacon | 140 | 14 | 1 |
| Buttermilk | 110 | 11 | 2 |
| Chipotle | 120 | 13 | 2 |
| Classic | 130 | 14 | 1 |
| Zesty Italian | 70 | 6 | 3 |
| **Hampton Creek** (Vegan): *Per 1 Tbsp* | | | |
| **Just Mayo:** | | | |
| Original | 90 | 10 | 0 |
| Chipotle; Sriracha | 90 | 10 | 1 |
| Garlic | 100 | 10 | 0 |

## Brands ~ Salad Dressings (Cont)

### Hidden Valley:

| | C | F | Cb |
|---|---|---|---|
| **Buttermilk** | 130 | 14 | 2 |
| **Farmhouse Originals**, | | | |
| Dijon Mustard Vinaigrette | 100 | 9 | 4 |
| Homestyle Italian | 100 | 10 | 3 |
| Southwest Chipotle | 100 | 10 | 2 |
| **Ranch Originals:** Regular | 140 | 14 | 2 |
| Light Original | 80 | 7 | 3 |
| Bacon; Spicy, average | 145 | 15 | 2 |

### Kraft: *Per 2 Tbsp*
**Regular Dressings:**

| | C | F | Cb |
|---|---|---|---|
| Caesar Vinaigrette, with Parmesan | 70 | 6 | 3 |
| Catalina | 90 | 6 | 9 |
| Classic Caesar | 120 | 12 | 2 |
| Creamy Ranch | 110 | 11 | 2 |
| Creamy Italian | 100 | 10 | 2 |
| Greek Vinaigrette | 110 | 11 | 2 |
| Roka Blue Cheese | 120 | 13 | 1 |
| Sweet Honey Catalina | 100 | 8 | 8 |
| Thousand Island | 130 | 12 | 4 |
| Tuscan House, Italian | 130 | 13 | 3 |
| **Fat Free:** Catalina; Classic Ranch | 50 | 0 | 11 |
| French Style | 45 | 0 | 11 |
| Italian | 15 | 0 | 3 |
| Thousand Island | 45 | 0 | 10 |
| **Lite:** Asian Toasted Sesame | 50 | 2.5 | 7 |
| Balsamic Vinaigrette | 30 | 1 | 4 |
| Creamy Caesar | 35 | 2 | 4 |
| Zesty Italian | 25 | 1.5 | 3 |

### Seven Seas:

| | C | F | Cb |
|---|---|---|---|
| Green Goddess | 130 | 13 | 2 |
| Viva Italian Anything | 50 | 4.5 | 1 |
| Reduced Fat: Viva Italian | 45 | 4 | 2 |
| Red Wine Vinaigrette | 45 | 4 | 3 |

### Marie's: *Per 2 Tbsp*

| | C | F | Cb |
|---|---|---|---|
| Blue Cheese, Premium Super | 160 | 17 | 1 |
| Caesar | 170 | 19 | 1 |
| Ranch: Buttermilk | 150 | 16 | 1 |
| Jalapeno Ranch | 160 | 17 | 1 |
| **Classics:** | | | |
| Chunky Blue Cheese | 160 | 17 | 0 |
| Coleslaw | 140 | 13 | 7 |
| Creamy Italian Garlic | 170 | 19 | 1 |
| Creamy Ranch | 170 | 19 | 1 |
| Thousand Island | 150 | 15 | 4 |
| **Specialty:** Honey Dijon | 130 | 12 | 5 |
| Poppy Seed | 150 | 13 | 8 |

### Marzetti's:

| | C | F | Cb |
|---|---|---|---|
| **Organic:** Blue Cheese | 130 | 14 | 1 |
| Caesar | 140 | 15 | 1 |
| Parmesan Ranch | 130 | 14 | 2 |
| Chunky Blue Cheese | 150 | 15 | 1 |
| Classic Ranch | 160 | 17 | 1 |
| Honey Dijon | 130 | 12 | 6 |

### Newman's Own: *Per 2 Tbsp*

| | C | F | Cb |
|---|---|---|---|
| **Regular:** Balsamic Vinaigrette | 90 | 9 | 3 |
| Creamy Caesar | 170 | 18 | 1 |
| Family Recipe Italian | 130 | 13 | 1 |
| Olive Oil & Vinegar | 150 | 16 | 1 |
| Parmesan & Rstd Garlic | 110 | 11 | 2 |
| Ranch | 150 | 16 | 2 |
| **Lite:** Italian | 60 | 6 | 1 |
| Raspberry & Walnut | 70 | 5 | 7 |
| **Organic:** | | | |
| Light Balsamic Vinaigrette | 45 | 4 | 4 |
| Tuscan Italian | 100 | 11 | 2 |

### Wish-Bone: *Per 2 Tbsp*

| | C | F | Cb |
|---|---|---|---|
| **Creamy:** Chunky Blue Cheese | 150 | 14 | 1 |
| Caesar | 180 | 18 | 1 |
| Deluxe French | 120 | 11 | 5 |
| Italian | 110 | 10 | 4 |
| Ranch | 130 | 13 | 2 |
| Russian | 110 | 6 | 14 |
| Sweet 'n Spicy French | 140 | 12 | 7 |
| Thousand Island | 130 | 12 | 5 |
| **Light:** Blue Cheese | 70 | 6 | 2 |
| Creamy Caesar | 70 | 6 | 2 |
| Honey Dijon | 70 | 5 | 6 |
| Italian | 35 | 2.5 | 3 |
| Parmesan Peppercorn Ranch | 60 | 5 | 2 |
| Ranch | 70 | 5 | 4 |
| Thousand Island | 60 | 5 | 4 |
| Vinaigrette: Balsamic & Basil | 50 | 4 | 3 |
| Asian with Sesame & Ginger | 70 | 5 | 5 |
| Raspberry Walnut | 70 | 4 | 7 |
| **Fat-Free:** | | | |
| Chunky Blue Cheese | 30 | 0 | 7 |
| Ranch | 30 | 0 | 6 |
| **Oil & Vinegar:** | | | |
| Balsamic Vinaigrette | 60 | 5 | 3 |
| House Italian | 110 | 10 | 3 |
| Red Wine Vinaigrette | 70 | 5 | 6 |
| Robusto Italian | 80 | 7 | 4 |

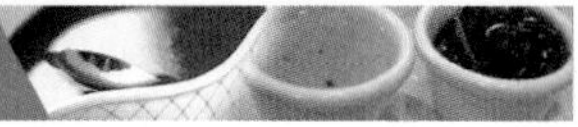

## Gravy

| | C | F | Cb |
|---|---|---|---|
| **Homemade Gravy,** average: | | | |
| Thin, little fat, 2 Tbsp, 1 oz | 20 | 1 | 3 |
| Thick: 2 Tbsp, 1.3 oz | 50 | 2 | 9 |
| ¼ cup, 2.5 oz | 100 | 4 | 18 |
| **McCormick:** | | | |
| Brown, 1 Tbsp | 25 | 0.5 | 3 |
| Turkey, 1 Tbsp | 20 | 0.5 | 4 |

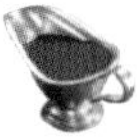

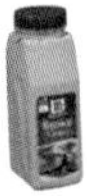

## Gravy-In-Jars

| | C | F | Cb |
|---|---|---|---|
| **Boston Market,** | | | |
| Classic Beef, ¼ cup, 2 oz | 30 | 1 | 4 |
| **Campbell's,** Slow Roast, | | | |
| Beef/Chicken/Turkey, ¼ cup, 2 oz | 25 | 1 | 3 |
| **Heinz:** *Per ¼ Cup, 2 oz* | | | |
| Homestyle: Classic Chicken | 30 | 2 | 3 |
| Savory Beef | 30 | 1 | 4 |
| Sausage | 45 | 1.5 | 6 |
| Other varieties, average | 20 | 0.5 | 3 |
| Fat-Free, all varieties | 20 | 0 | 4 |
| **Safeway,** all varieties, ¼ cup, 2 oz | 20 | 0.5 | 4 |

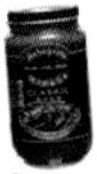

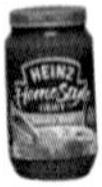

## Tomato Products

| | C | F | Cb |
|---|---|---|---|
| **Whole/Chopped/Crushed/Diced:** | | | |
| Regular: 1 cup, 8.5 oz | 50 | 0 | 10 |
| In Aspic, ½ cup | 50 | 0 | 12 |
| with Green Chili, 1 c., 8.5 oz | 60 | 0 | 16 |
| Stewed, ½ cup, 1.7 oz | 40 | 1.5 | 7 |
| Wedges in Tomato Juice, 1 cup | 70 | 0.5 | 18 |
| Salsa, average, 2 Tbsp, 1 oz | 25 | 0 | 6 |
| **Tomato Ketchup:** | | | |
| Regular: 1 Tbsp, 0.5 oz | 15 | 0 | 4 |
| Single Serve, 1 packet | 10 | 0 | 3 |
| *Heinz,* Simply Heinz 1 Tbsp, 0.5 oz | 15 | 0 | 4 |
| **Tomato Paste:** | | | |
| Regular: 2 Tbsp, 1 oz | 25 | 0 | 6 |
| ¾ cup, 6 oz | 140 | 1 | 32 |
| **Tomato Puree,** ½ cup, 4.5 oz | 50 | 0 | 10 |
| **Tomato Sauce:** | | | |
| Regular, ½ cup, 4.4 oz | 50 | 0 | 11 |
| Spanish Style, ½ cup, 4.3 oz | 40 | 0 | 9 |
| with Mushr., ½ cup, 4.3 oz | 45 | 0 | 10 |
| with Onions, ½ cup, 4.3 oz | 50 | 0 | 12 |
| **Tomato Seasoning,** 3 tsp | 20 | 0 | 4 |
| **Sundried Tomatoes:** | | | |
| Natural, 5-6 pieces, 0.4 oz | 20 | 0 | 5 |
| In Oil, drained, 6 pieces, 0.5 oz | 40 | 2.5 | 4 |

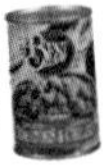

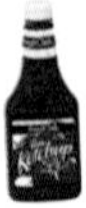

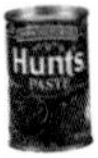

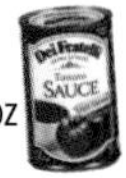

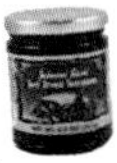

## Sauces ~ Brands

| | C | F | Cb |
|---|---|---|---|
| **A-1:** | | | |
| **Marinades:** *Per Tbspn, ½ oz* | | | |
| Chicago Steakhouse | 20 | 1 | 3 |
| Classic | 15 | 0 | 4 |
| New Orleans Cajun | 25 | 0 | 5 |
| New York Steakhouse | 20 | 0 | 5 |
| **Steak Sauce:** Original | 15 | 0 | 3 |
| Bold & Spicy | 20 | 0 | 4 |
| Cracked Peppercorn | 15 | 0 | 0 |
| Thick & Hearty | 25 | 0 | 6 |
| **Barilla:** | | | |
| **Pasta Sauces:** *Per ½ Cup* | | | |
| Marinara; Tom. & Basil, av. | 70 | 1 | 15 |
| Mushroom | 80 | 2.5 | 12 |
| Rstd Garlic; Traditional, av. | 70 | 1 | 14 |
| Spicy Marinara | 60 | 0.5 | 13 |
| Sweet Peppers; Three Cheese, av. | 70 | 1 | 13 |
| Tuscan Herb | 70 | 0.5 | 14 |
| **Bertolli:** | | | |
| **Alfredo Sauces:** *Per ¼ Cup* | | | |
| Alfredo; Four Cheese Rosa | 110 | 10 | 3 |
| Garlic | 100 | 10 | 2 |
| Mushroom | 80 | 7 | 2 |
| **Gold Label:** | | | |
| Asiago Cheese with Artichokes | 110 | 6 | 10 |
| Balsamic Vinegar w/ Caramel Onions | 90 | 2.5 | 11 |
| Porcini Mushrooms with Truffle Oil | 100 | 5 | 9 |
| **Traditional:** *Per ½ Cup* | | | |
| Five Cheese | 90 | 3.5 | 14 |
| Italian Sausage | 90 | 3 | 14 |
| Olive Oil & Garlic | 80 | 3 | 14 |
| **Vineyard,** Marinara; Portobello Mshrm | 80 | 25 | 13 |
| **Best Foods/Hellmann's,** | | | |
| Tartar Sauce, 2 Tbsp | 80 | 7 | 4 |
| **Buitoni:** | | | |
| **Pasta Sauces:** | | | |
| Alfredo: Regular, ¼ cup | 140 | 12 | 4 |
| Light, ¼ cup | 90 | 6 | 4 |
| Marinara: Regular ½ cup | 70 | 3 | 10 |
| with Roasted Garlic, ½ cup | 60 | 1 | 10 |
| Pesto: with Basil, ¼ cup | 270 | 26 | 4 |
| Reduced Fat, ¼ cup | 230 | 17 | 8 |
| **Bull's-Eye:** *Per 2 Tbsp* | | | |
| BBQ Sauce: Origianl | 50 | 0 | 12 |
| Hickory Smoke | 60 | 0 | 15 |
| Regional, average all varieties | 50 | 0 | 11 |
| **Catelli:** *Per ½ Cup* | | | |
| **Pasta,** Garden Select Six Vegetable: | | | |
| Country Mushroom | 70 | 1.5 | 11 |
| Diced Tomato & Basil | 70 | 1 | 12 |
| **Meat Sauce** | 80 | 2.5 | 11 |
| **Pizza Sauce,** Tomato & Basil | 60 | 1.5 | 11 |

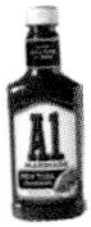

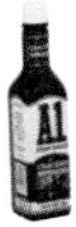

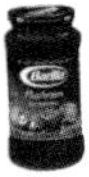

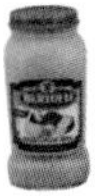

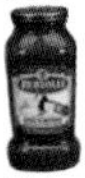

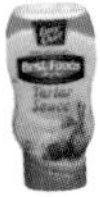

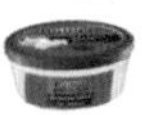

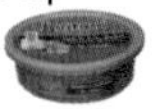

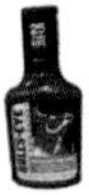

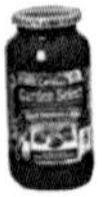

## Sauces ~ Brands (Cont)

| | **C** | **F** | **Cb** |
|---|---|---|---|
| **Cento:** *Per ½ Cup* | | | |
| **Clam,** Red, 4.3 oz | 60 | 2 | 6 |
| **San Marzano Pasta:** | | | |
| Arrabbiata, 4.3 oz | 70 | 3.5 | 6.5 |
| Marinara, 4.3 oz | 60 | 3.5 | 6 |
| Vodka, 4.3 oz | 75 | 3.5 | 6 |
| **Classico:** | | | |
| **Alfredo:** *Per ¼ Cup* | | | |
| Creamy | 60 | 4.5 | 3 |
| Roasted Red Pepper | 60 | 4 | 4 |
| **Pesto:** *Per ¼ Cup* | | | |
| Basil Pesto | 240 | 24 | 5 |
| Sun-Dried Tomato Pesto | 100 | 6 | 9 |
| **Red Sauces:** *Per ½ Cup* | | | |
| Family Favorites: Meat | 60 | 1 | 10 |
| Parmesan & Romano | 70 | 2 | 10 |
| Traditional | 80 | 2.5 | 13 |
| Seasonal Selection: Bolognese | 60 | 1.5 | 10 |
| Creamy Spinach & Parmesan | 80 | 4 | 8 |
| Signature Recipes: | | | |
| Cabernet Marinara with Herbs | 60 | 1.5 | 10 |
| Caramelized Onion & Rstd Garlic | 70 | 1.5 | 12 |
| Traditional Pizza Sauce | 40 | 1 | 7 |
| Tomato Cream Collection: | | | |
| Creamy Tomato & Roasted Garlic | 35 | 1.5 | 5 |
| Four Cheese Tomato | 40 | 2 | 5 |
| Spicy tomato & Parmesan | 40 | 2 | 5 |
| Traditional Favorites, Sweet Basil | 70 | 1 | 13 |
| **Colgin,** Liquid Smoke, 1 tsp | 0 | 0 | 0 |
| **Contadina:** | | | |
| **Pizza Sauce:** *Per 2.2 oz* | | | |
| Flavored with Pepperoni | 35 | 1 | 5 |
| Original; Four Cheese | 30 | 0.5 | 6 |
| **Tomato Sauce,** average | 20 | 0.5 | 4 |
| **Crosse & Blackwell:** | | | |
| **Meat:** Ham Glaze, 1 Tbsp | 25 | 0 | 7 |
| Mint Meat Sauce, 1 tsp | 5 | 0 | 2 |
| **Seafood:** | | | |
| Cocktail, ¼ cup, 2.5 oz | 80 | 0 | 20 |
| Shrimp, ¼ cup, 2.5 oz | 80 | 0 | 21 |
| **Dave's Gourmet:** *Per ½ Cup* | | | |
| **Pasta Sauce:** | | | |
| Butternut Squash | 100 | 4 | 17 |
| Organic: Red Heirloom | 45 | 1.5 | 7 |
| Rstd Garlic & Sweet Basil | 70 | 4.5 | 8 |
| **Del Monte:** | | | |
| **Pasta Sauces:** *Per ½ Cup* | | | |
| Four Cheese; Traditional, av. | 60 | 1 | 12 |
| Mushroom | 50 | 1 | 11 |
| Average other varieties | 70 | 1 | 13 |
| Sloppy Joe Sauce, Orig., ¼ cup | 50 | 0 | 13 |

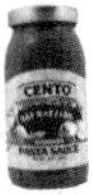

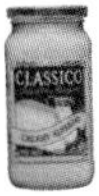

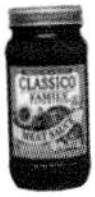

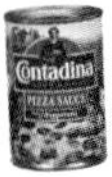

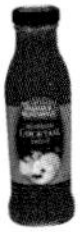

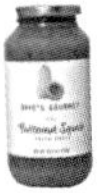

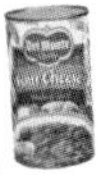

| | **C** | **F** | **Cb** |
|---|---|---|---|
| **Emeril's:** | | | |
| **Pasta Sauces:** *Per ½ Cup* | | | |
| Homestyle Marinara | 90 | 3 | 14 |
| Kicked Up Tomato | 80 | 3.5 | 11 |
| Roasted Gaaahlic | 80 | 3.5 | 12 |
| Roasted Red Pepper | 70 | 3.5 | 9 |
| Vodka Sauce | 110 | 7 | 12 |
| **Francesco Rinaldi:** *Per ½ Cup* | | | |
| **Hearty:** Super Mushroom | 110 | 4.5 | 17 |
| Three Cheese | 90 | 2 | 16 |
| **Traditional:** Original | 80 | 3 | 14 |
| Meat Flavored | 90 | 3.5 | 14 |
| Mushroom | 80 | 3 | 13 |
| **French's,** | | | |
| **Worcestershire Sce,** 1 Tbsp | 5 | 0 | 1 |
| **Heinz:** *Per 1 Tbsp* | | | |
| 57/Steak Sauce | 20 | 0 | 4 |
| Chili Sauce | 20 | 0 | 5 |
| Cocktail Sauce, Original, | | | |
| ¼ cup, 2.2 oz | 60 | 0 | 15 |
| Horseradish Sauce | 75 | 6 | 3 |
| Tomato Ketchup: Regular | 20 | 0 | 5 |
| Reduced Sugar | 5 | 0 | 1 |
| Worcestershire Sauce, 1 Tbsp | 5 | 0 | 1 |
| **House of Tsang:** *Per 1 Tbsp* | | | |
| Bangkok Peanut Sauce | 40 | 2 | 4 |
| Ginger Flavored Soy | 20 | 0 | 4 |
| General Tsao | 45 | 0.5 | 10 |
| Ginger Sriracha | 15 | 0 | 4 |
| Hibachi Grill, Sweet Ginger Sesame | 40 | 1 | 8 |
| Hoisin, 1 tsp | 15 | 0 | 4 |
| Oyster Flavored | 30 | 0 | 7 |
| Saigon Sizzle Stir-Fry | 45 | 2 | 7 |
| Sweet & Sour Stir-Fry | 35 | 0 | 9 |
| **Hunt's:** | | | |
| BBQ Sauce, Original, 2 Tbsp | 60 | 0 | 15 |
| Hickory & Brown Sugar BBQ Sce, 2 Tbsp | 70 | 0 | 18 |
| **Manwich,** Sloppy Joe Sauce, | | | |
| Original, ¼ cup, 2.3 oz | 35 | 0 | 7 |
| **Pasta Sauce:** *Per ½ Cup* | | | |
| Four Cheese | 60 | 1 | 10 |
| Garlic & Herb | 40 | 1 | 8 |
| Meat Flavor | 60 | 1 | 10 |
| Mushroom | 50 | 0.5 | 10 |
| Traditional | 60 | 1 | 11 |

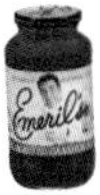

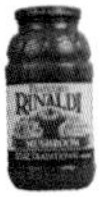

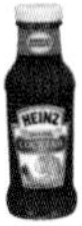

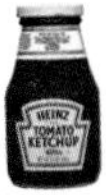

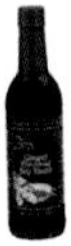

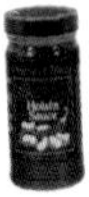

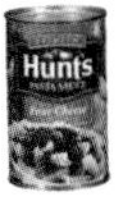

## Brands (Cont)

| | C | F | Cb |
|---|---|---|---|
| **Kikkoman:** | | | |
| **Asian Authentic:** | | | |
| Black Bean Sauce, w/ Garlic, 2 Tbsp | 50 | 1 | 6 |
| Hoisin Sauce, 2 Tbsp | 80 | 0 | 19 |
| **Marinades:** Gourmet Teriyaki | 30 | 0 | 7 |
| Honey Mustard, 1 Tbsp | 30 | 0 | 6 |
| Roasted Garlic & Herbs | 20 | 0 | 4 |
| **Knorr:** | | | |
| **Classic Sauce:** *Per Whole Package* | | | |
| Bernaise, dry mix only | 100 | 0 | 20 |
| Hollandaise, dry mix only | 100 | 0 | 20 |
| **Kraft:** | | | |
| Barbecue Sauces, av, 2 Tbsp | 65 | 0 | 15 |
| **Specialty Sauce:** Cocktail, 2 Tbsp | 60 | 0.5 | 11 |
| Coleslaw Dressing, 1.2 oz | 110 | 8 | 9 |
| Horseradish, 1 oz | 100 | 9 | 4 |
| Sandwich Spread, 1 Tbsp | 35 | 2.5 | 3 |
| Tartar, Original, 1 Tbsp | 60 | 5 | 4 |
| **Las Palmas:** | | | |
| Green Enchilada Sauce, all varieties, 2 oz | 25 | 1.5 | 3 |
| Red Chili Sauce, 2 oz | 15 | 0.5 | 3 |
| **La Victoria,** | | | |
| Red/Green Enchilada Sauce, av, 2 oz | 15 | 0.5 | 3 |
| **Lawry's:** | | | |
| **30 Minute Marinade:** *Per Tbsp* | | | |
| Caribbean Jerk | 30 | 0 | 7 |
| Herb & Garlic; Lemon Pepper | 10 | 0 | 2 |
| Mesquite, w/ Lime Juice | 10 | 0 | 2 |
| Steak & Chop, w/ Garl. Pepp. | 5 | 0 | 0.5 |
| Sesame Ginger, w/ Mandarin | 30 | 0 | 7 |
| **Packet Seasonings:** *Dry* | | | |
| Fajitas; Taco, average, 2 tsp | 15 | 0 | 3 |
| Other varieties, average, 2 tsp | 20 | 0 | 4 |
| **Lea & Perrins:** | | | |
| Marinade In-A-Bag, av. all var, 0.5 oz | 15 | 0 | 4 |
| Marinade for Chicken, 1 Tbsp | 15 | 0 | 1 |
| Steak Sauce, Bold, 1 Tbsp | 20 | 0 | 5 |
| Worcestershire Sauce, Original 1 tsp, 5 ml | 5 | 0 | 1 |
| **McCormicks:** | | | |
| **Seafood Sauces:** *Per 2 Tbsp* | | | |
| Asian | 50 | 1.5 | 7 |
| Cajun Style | 15 | 0 | 3 |
| Lemon Butter Dill | 100 | 9 | 4 |
| Lemon Herb | 140 | 15 | 0.5 |
| Mediterranean; Santa Fe Style | 20 | 0 | 4 |
| Scampi | 160 | 17 | 2 |

| | C | F | Cb |
|---|---|---|---|
| **Mrs. Dash:** | | | |
| **Marinades:** *Per 1 Tbsp* | | | |
| Garlic Herb | 15 | 0 | 3 |
| Lemon Pepper | 10 | 0 | 2 |
| Lime Garlic | 15 | 0 | 3 |
| Sweet Teriyaki | 35 | 0 | 9 |
| **Newman's Own:** *Per ½ Cup* | | | |
| Five Cheese | 80 | 2 | 11 |
| Fra Diavolo | 80 | 3 | 10 |
| Marinara; Sockarooni | 70 | 1 | 12 |
| Roasted Garlic & Peppers | 70 | 1.5 | 11 |
| Tomato & Basil Bombolina | 80 | 2 | 13 |
| Vodka | 120 | 5 | 13 |
| **O Organics** (Von's): *Per ½ Cup* | | | |
| Marinara; Roasted Garlic, av. | 60 | 1.5 | 9 |
| Mushroom; Tomato Basil | 50 | 1.5 | 8 |
| **Old El Paso:** | | | |
| **Enchilada Sauce:** | | | |
| Green Chile, ¼ cup | 25 | 1.5 | 4 |
| Other varieties, ¼ cup | 20 | 0 | 4 |
| **Salsa,** Thick & Chunky, all var, 2 Tbsp | 10 | 0 | 2 |
| **Taco Sauce,** all varieties, 1 Tbsp | 5 | 0 | 1 |
| **Pace:** *Per 2 Tbsp* | | | |
| Picante Sauce | 10 | 0 | 3 |
| **Salsa:** Thick & Chunky, av. | 10 | 0 | 2 |
| Fire, Mango & Habanero | 10 | 0 | 2 |
| Restaurant Style, Peach Mango | 15 | 0 | 4 |
| **Prego:** *Per ½ Cup* | | | |
| **Alfredo,** average all varieties | 150 | 14 | 6 |
| **Classic Italian:** | | | |
| Flavored with Meat | 90 | 3 | 13 |
| Fresh Mushroom; Traditional | 70 | 1.5 | 13 |
| Italian Sausage & Garlic | 90 | 3 | 13 |
| Marinara | 80 | 3 | 10 |
| Roasted Garlic & Herb | 80 | 2 | 13 |
| Three Cheese | 70 | 1.5 | 12 |
| Tomato, Basil & Garlic | 80 | 2.5 | 12 |
| **Chunky Garden:** | | | |
| Combo | 70 | 1.5 | 12 |
| Mushroom Supreme | 80 | 2.5 | 13 |
| **Heart Smart:** Ricotta Parmesan | 90 | 2.5 | 13 |
| Other varieties | 70 | 1.5 | 13 |
| **Pizza Sauce,** Pizzeria Style | 70 | 2 | 12 |
| **Premier Japan,** Hoisin; Teriyaki, 1 Tbsp | 15 | 0 | 3 |
| **Progresso:** *Per ½ Cup* | | | |
| **Recipe Starters:** | | | |
| Creamy Roasted Garlic | 70 | 5 | 4 |
| Fire Roasted Tomato | 60 | 2 | 10 |
| Average other varieties | 90 | 7 | 5 |

### Brands (Cont)

**C** **F** **Cb**

**Ragu:**
**Cheesy:** *Per ¼ Cup*

| | C | F | Cb |
|---|---|---|---|
| Classic Alfredo | 90 | 8 | 2 |
| Creamy Mozzarella | 80 | 7 | 2 |
| Creamy Tomato | 90 | 8 | 4 |
| Double Cheddar | 100 | 9 | 3 |
| Four Cheese | 80 | 8 | 2 |
| Light Parmesan Alfredo | 60 | 4 | 2 |
| Roasted Garlic Parmesan | 100 | 9 | 3 |
| Six Cheese | 90 | 3 | 13 |

**Chunky:** *Per ½ Cup*

| | C | F | Cb |
|---|---|---|---|
| Roasted Garlic | 80 | 2.5 | 14 |
| Average other varieties | 90 | 2.5 | 14 |

**Old World Style:** *Per ½ Cup*

| | C | F | Cb |
|---|---|---|---|
| Flavored with Meat | 70 | 2.5 | 10 |
| Marinara | 80 | 2.5 | 11 |
| Traditional | 80 | 2 | 11 |
| Light, Tomato & Basil | 50 | 0 | 10 |

**Pizza:** Homemade Style, ¼ cup — 30 | 1 | 5
Quick Sauce, Traditional, ¼ cup — 45 | 1.5 | 6

**Safeway Select:**
Salsa, all varieties, average, 2 Tbsp — 15 | 0 | 3

**Select Sauces:** *Per ½ Cup*

| | C | F | Cb |
|---|---|---|---|
| Arrabbiata | 110 | 8 | 10 |
| Artichoke Pesto | 60 | 2 | 9 |
| Four Cheese | 80 | 3.5 | 11 |
| Marinara | 60 | 2 | 10 |
| Spicy Red Bell Pepper | 50 | 1 | 9 |
| Sundried Tomato & Olive | 60 | 1.5 | 11 |
| Tomato Alfredo; Vodka | 130 | 10 | 9 |

**Taco Bell,** Creamy Jalapeno Sauce,
1 Tablespoon, 0.5 oz — 70 | 7 | 1

**Tony Roma's:**
Bold & Spicy BBQ Sauce, 2 Tbsp — 50 | 0 | 12
Carolina Honeys BBQ Sauce,
2 Tablespoons — 70 | 0 | 18

**Trader Joe's:**
BBQ Sauce,
Kansas City Style, 2 Tbsp — 60 | 0 | 15
Tomato Basil Marinara, ½ cup — 80 | 4.5 | 10

**Walnut Acres,**
Organic Pasta Sauces,
average all var., ½ cup, 4.5 oz — 50 | 1 | 9

### Seasonings & Flavorings

**C** **F** **Cb**

| | C | F | Cb |
|---|---|---|---|
| **Auromatic Bitters** (Angostua), 1 tsp | 15 | 0 | 4 |
| **Bacon Bits,** average, 1 Tbsp | 35 | 2 | 2 |
| **Bacon Chips** (Durkee), 1 Tbsp | 30 | 1 | 2 |
| **Bac-Os** (Betty Crocker), 1Tbsp | 30 | 1.5 | 2 |
| **Blends** (Mrs Dash), 1 tsp | 0 | 0 | 0 |
| **Butter Buds,** 1 tsp | 5 | 0 | 2 |
| **Flavor Enhancer** (Accent), 1 tsp | 0 | 0 | 0 |
| **Flavor Sprinkles** (Molly McButter), Natural/Cheese, 1 tsp | 5 | 0 | 1 |
| **Garlic Bread Sprinkle,** 1 tsp | 8 | 0.5 | 1 |
| **Garlic Salt,** 1 tsp | 2 | 0 | 0 |
| **Italian Seasoning,** 1 tsp | 4 | 0 | 1 |
| **Lemon Pepper Seasoning,** 1 tsp | 7 | 0 | 1 |
| **Meat Tenderizer,** av., 1 tsp | 7 | 0 | 1 |
| **Salad Crunchies** (McCormick), 1 tsp | 10 | 0.5 | 2 |
| **Salt,** Reg., Sea Salt, Lite Salt | 0 | 0 | 0 |
| **Seasoning** (Old Bay), ¼ tsp | 0 | 0 | 0 |
| **Seasoning Mix** (Vegit), ¼ tsp | 0 | 0 | 0 |
| **Seasoning Mixes,** av., ¼ pkg | 70 | 1 | 9 |
| **Taco Seasoning,** av., ¼ pkg | 30 | 0.5 | 4 |
| **Bragg's,** Liquid Aminos | 0 | 0 | 0 |
| **Old El Paso:** Chili Season. Mix, 1 Tbsp | 8 | 0.5 | 1.5 |
| Cheesy Taco Seasoning Mix, 1 Tbsp | 10 | 0.5 | 2 |
| Taco/Burrito Seasoning Mix, 2 tsp | 15 | 0 | 4 |
| Fajita Seasoning Mix, 1 tsp | 5 | 0 | 1.5 |

### Spices & Herbs

| | C | F | Cb |
|---|---|---|---|
| **Average all types,** 1 tsp | 5 | 0 | 1 |
| **All Purpose,** 1 tsp | 0 | 0 | 0 |
| **Allspice,** ground | 5 | 0 | 1 |
| **Chili Powder** | 8 | 0 | 1 |
| **Cinnamon,** ground | 6 | 0 | 2 |
| **Curry Powder** | 6 | 0 | 1 |
| **Garlic Powder** | 9 | 0 | 2 |
| **Nutmeg,** ground | 12 | 0 | 1 |
| **Onion Powder** | 7 | 0 | 2 |
| **Parsley,** dried | 4 | 0 | 1 |
| **Pepper,** average | 6 | 0 | 1 |
| **Saffron** | 2 | 0 | 0 |
| **Salt-Free Blends,** 1 tsp | 0 | 0 | 0 |
| **Tumeric,** ground | 8 | 0 | 1 |
| **Seeds:** Fenugreek | 12 | 1 | 2 |
| Mustard, Poppyseed | 15 | 1 | 1 |
| Other varieties, average | 7 | 0 | 1 |

## Home-Popped Popcorn | C | F | Cb |

| | C | F | Cb |
|---|---|---|---|
| **Popping Corn Kernels,** | | | |
| 2 Tbsp, 1 oz | 110 | 1 | 26 |
| (makes approximately 5 cups) | | | |
| **Air-popped,** without oil: Plain, 1 oz | 110 | 1 | 22 |
| 1 cup, 0.2 oz | 20 | 0 | 5 |
| **Oil-popped:** Plain, 1 oz | 145 | 8 | 16 |
| 1 cup, 0.4 oz | 55 | 3 | 6 |
| **Popcorn Oil,** 1 Tbsp | 120 | 14 | 0 |

## Microwave Popcorn

**Average all Brands:** *Per 1 Cup Popped, Unless Indicated*

| | C | F | Cb |
|---|---|---|---|
| Butter: Regular, 1 cup | 35 | 2 | 4 |
| Light, 1 cup | 25 | 1 | 4 |
| **Act II Popcorn:** | | | |
| **Butter:** 1 cup | 25 | 1 | 4 |
| 4½ cups, 1 oz | 120 | 5 | 19 |
| **94% Fat-Free Butter:** | | | |
| 1 cup | 20 | 0.5 | 4 |
| 6½ cups, 1 oz | 130 | 2 | 27 |
| **Butter Lovers:** 1 cup | 25 | 1 | 4 |
| 4½ cups, 1 oz | 120 | 4 | 19 |
| **Xreme Butter:** 1 cup | 25 | 1 | 4 |
| 4½ cups | 120 | 4 | 19 |
| **BodyKey** *(Amway),* Slim Popcorn, | | | |
| Sea Salt, 1 bag | 110 | 7 | 10 |
| **Jolly Time:** | | | |
| **Blast O Butter,** 1 cup | 45 | 3 | 4 |
| **Light Butter,** 1 cup | 25 | 1 | 4 |
| **Xtra Butter:** 1 cup | 40 | 2.5 | 4 |
| 4 cups | 160 | 10 | 16 |
| **Newman's Own:** | | | |
| **Butter Flavor,** Microwave: | | | |
| Regular, 3½ cups | 130 | 5 | 18 |
| Light, 3½ cups | 120 | 4 | 19 |
| **Butter Boom,** 3½ cups | 130 | 5 | 18 |
| **Orville Redenbacher's:** | | | |
| **Family Favorites:** | | | |
| Butter: 4 cups | 170 | 12 | 17 |
| Light, 5½ cups | 120 | 5 | 19 |
| Movie Theater Butter, 4 cups | 160 | 9 | 19 |
| Ultimate Butter, 5 cups | 170 | 12 | 16 |
| **Natural,** Lime & Salt, 5 cups | 220 | 15 | 21 |
| **Sweet & Savory,** | | | |
| Cheddar Cheese, 4½ cups | 180 | 14 | 16 |
| **Pop Secret:** *Per Cup* | | | |
| 94% Fat-Free, Butter | 20 | 0 | 3 |
| Double Butter | 40 | 2.5 | 3 |

## Bagged Popcorn | C | F | Cb |

*Average All Brands (Ready-to-Eat)*

| | C | F | Cb |
|---|---|---|---|
| **Regular/Plain:** ½ oz package | 80 | 5 | 8 |
| 1 oz package | 160 | 10 | 16 |
| 4 oz package | 640 | 40 | 64 |
| 2 oz Box (store/airport) | 320 | 16 | 32 |
| 3 oz Bag (9" high x 5" wide) | 480 | 24 | 48 |
| **Caramel Popcorn,** | | | |
| with nuts, 1 cup, 1.5 oz | 230 | 12 | 39 |

## Bagged Popcorn ~ Brands

| | C | F | Cb |
|---|---|---|---|
| **Boston's,** Lite, 3½ cups, 1 oz | 130 | 4.5 | 20 |
| **Cracker Jack:** Original, 1 cup, 2 oz | 240 | 4 | 46 |
| Chocolate & Caramel, 1 cup, 2 oz | 220 | 1 | 50 |
| **Crunch 'N Munch:** | | | |
| **Buttery Toffee:** ⅔ cup, 1 oz | 150 | 6 | 22 |
| 1 cup, 1.6 oz | 220 | 9 | 32 |
| **Caramel:** ⅔ cup, 1 oz | 160 | 8 | 20 |
| 1 cup, 1.6 oz | 230 | 12 | 29 |
| 12 oz box | 1745 | 87 | 218 |
| **Fiddle Faddle:** | | | |
| Average all varieties: 1 oz | 120 | 2 | 24 |
| 1 cup, 2 oz | 240 | 4 | 48 |
| 6 oz box | 720 | 12 | 144 |
| **Popcorn Indiana:** | | | |
| **Kettlecorn,** | | | |
| Original, 2 cups, 1 oz | 130 | 5 | 21 |
| **Popcorn:** | | | |
| Aged White Cheddar, 2.5 cups, 1 oz | 150 | 9 | 14 |
| Chicago Style, | | | |
| Caramel & Cheese, 1 cup, 1 oz | 140 | 6 | 20 |
| Movie Theater, 2 cups, 1 oz | 160 | 12 | 13 |
| Seasalt, 3.5 cups, 1 oz | 130 | 6 | 17 |
| **Poppycock:** | | | |
| Original/Pecan Delight, av: | | | |
| ½ cup, 1 oz | 155 | 8 | 20 |
| 1 cup, 2 oz | 310 | 16 | 40 |
| Cashew Lovers, ½ cup, 1 oz | 150 | 6 | 20 |
| Chocolate Lovers, ½ cup, 1.2 oz | 160 | 7 | 22 |

## Movie Theater Popcorn

| | C | F | Cb |
|---|---|---|---|
| **Small,** (7 cups): Plain | 385 | 21 | 44 |
| with Butter (3 pumps, 0.8 oz) | 570 | 42 | 44 |
| **Medium,** (15 cups): Plain | 825 | 45 | 94 |
| with Butter (4 pumps, 1 oz) | 1075 | 73 | 94 |
| **Large,** (20 cups): Plain | 1100 | 60 | 124 |
| with Butter (6 pumps, 1.5 oz) | 1485 | 102 | 124 |
| **Butter:** 1 Pump, 0.3 oz | 65 | 7 | 0 |
| 4 Pumps (2 Tbsp), 1 oz | 250 | 28 | 0 |

## Corn & Tortilla Chips    C  F  Cb

### Average All Brands
**Corn Chips:**

| | C | F | Cb |
|---|---|---|---|
| Average all types: 1 oz | 150 | 8 | 18 |
| 8 oz bag | 1200 | 64 | 144 |
| *Fritos*, Original, 32 chips, 1 oz | 160 | 10 | 15 |
| **Tortilla Chips:** Average, 1 oz | 140 | 7 | 18 |
| (1 oz = approx. 12 chips or 13 strips) | | | |
| *Doritos:* Original, 1 oz | 140 | 7 | 18 |
| Nacho Chse/ Salsa Verde, av., 1 oz | 140 | 8 | 18 |
| *Popchips:* Chili Limon, 1 oz | 120 | 4 | 19 |
| Nacho Cheese, 1 oz | 130 | 5 | 18 |
| *Snyder's:* | | | |
| El Restaurante, all flavors, 1 oz | 150 | 8 | 17 |
| Yellow Corn/White, av., 1 oz | 135 | 5 | 21 |
| *Tostitos:* | | | |
| Average all flav., 1 oz | 145 | 7 | 19 |
| Baked! Scoops, 1 oz | 120 | 3 | 22 |
| *Utz:* Multigrain, 1 oz | 150 | 8 | 16 |
| Baked, 1 oz | 120 | 2 | 23 |
| Other flavors, 1 oz | 140 | 8 | 18 |

## Potato Chips/Crisps

### Average All Brands
**Regular:**

| | C | F | Cb |
|---|---|---|---|
| Plain or flavored, (4 chips) | 30 | 2 | 3 |
| 1 oz package (20 chips) | 150 | 10 | 15 |
| 4 oz quantity | 600 | 40 | 60 |
| 14 oz package | 2100 | 140 | 210 |

## Chips/Crisps ~ Brands

| | C | F | Cb |
|---|---|---|---|
| **Lay's** *(Fritolay):* | | | |
| Air Pops, av. all flavors, 1 oz | 125 | 4 | 21 |
| Regular; Wavy, av. all flavors, 1 oz | 160 | 10 | 15 |
| Kettle Cooked, 1 oz | 135 | 6 | 19 |
| **Pringles:** | | | |
| All Flavors, 1 oz | 150 | 9 | 15 |
| Large can, 6 oz | 900 | 54 | 90 |
| Reduced Fat, all flavors, 1 oz | 140 | 7 | 17 |
| Fat Free, all flavors, 15 crisps, 1 oz | 70 | 0 | 15 |
| Multi Grain, av. all flavors, 1 oz | 140 | 8 | 17 |
| Snack Stacks, all flav., 1 tub | 110 | 7 | 11 |
| Cheez Ummms, all flavors, 1 oz | 150 | 9 | 15 |
| **Ruffles:** Regular, av. all flavors, 1 oz | 160 | 11 | 15 |
| Baked!, average all flavors, 1 oz | 120 | 3.5 | 21 |
| **Simply7,** Hummus/Lentil Chips, | | | |
| average all flavors, 1 oz | 135 | 5 | 19 |
| **Sun Chips,** Original, 16 crisps, 1 oz | 140 | 6 | 18 |

## Pretzels    C  F  Cb

### Average All Brands
**Hard-Baked Pretzels:** *Each*

| | C | F | Cb |
|---|---|---|---|
| 1 oz quantity | 110 | 1 | 23 |
| Sticks, thin, 2¼" (9/oz) | 12 | 0 | 3 |
| Twists, thin, ¼" thick, (5/oz) | 25 | 0 | 5 |
| Dutch (2¾"x 2⅝"), 0.5 oz | 55 | 1 | 11 |
| *Snyders*, Sourdough, 0.8oz | 100 | 0 | 22 |
| **Soft Pretzel Twists,** average: *Each* | | | |
| Plain: Small, 2 oz | 210 | 2 | 43 |
| Medium, 4 oz | 390 | 3.5 | 80 |
| Large, 5 oz | 485 | 4.5 | 100 |
| Big Cheese, 1.8 oz | 130 | 3 | 22 |
| New York Street Vendors, 7 oz | 660 | 6 | 135 |
| *Trader Joe's*, Peanut Butter filled, 1 oz | 140 | 8 | 14 |
| *Snyder's:* Milk Chocolate Dips, 1 oz | 140 | 6 | 19 |
| White Creme Dips, 1 oz | 130 | 6 | 19 |

## Pretzels ~ Brands

| | C | F | Cb |
|---|---|---|---|
| **Flipz:** Milk Choc, 8 pieces, 1 oz | 130 | 5 | 20 |
| White Fudge, 7 pcs, 1 oz | 130 | 5 | 20 |
| **Rold Gold** *(Frito-Lay):* | | | |
| Braided Twists, | | | |
| Honey Wheat (8), 1 oz | 110 | 1 | 24 |
| Pretzel, Sourdough (1) | 90 | 1 | 19 |
| Pretzel Dippers, 1 pkg | 230 | 12 | 29 |
| Pretzel Thins, 1 oz | 120 | 2 | 23 |
| Rods/Tiny Twists, av., 1 oz | 110 | 1 | 23 |
| Sticks, 1 oz | 100 | 0 | 23 |
| **Snyder's of Hanover:** | | | |
| Gluten Free Pretzel Sticks (30) | 110 | 1.5 | 25 |
| Homestyle (4), 1 oz | 120 | 1 | 25 |
| Pieces, Bacon Cheddar , 1 oz | 140 | 7 | 17 |
| Rods (3), 1 oz | 120 | 1 | 24 |
| Sticks (28), 1 oz | 110 | 1 | 23 |
| Thins (11), 1 oz | 110 | 0 | 23 |
| **Special K:** | | | |
| **Cracker Chips,** av., all flavors, 1 oz | 120 | 4 | 22 |
| **Popcorn Chips,** av. all flavors, 1 oz | 120 | 2.5 | 23 |
| **SuperPretzel:** | | | |
| **Soft:** Original (1), 2.3 oz | 160 | 1 | 34 |
| Sweet Cinnamon (1), | | | |
| with topping, 2.5 oz | 200 | 2 | 42 |
| Bites (5), 1.9 oz | 140 | 0.5 | 32 |
| Softstix, av. all flavors, (2), 1.8 oz | 125 | 3 | 22 |
| **Utz:** Sourdough, Hard (1) | 90 | 0 | 18 |
| Cinnamon, 1 oz | 120 | 1.5 | 24 |

## Snacks | C | F | Cb

Note: Actual weight of packaged snacks is usually 5-10% more than label Net Wt. For accuracy, weigh snack and allow extra calories, fat and carbs for any extra weight.

| | C | F | Cb |
|---|---|---|---|
| **Apple Chips** (Seneca), av., 1 oz | 140 | 7 | 20 |
| **Bagel Crisps** (N.Y. Style), 6 crisps, 1 oz | 130 | 6 | 17 |
| **Baguette Chips** (Pillsbury), av., (21) | 130 | 5 | 20 |
| **Banana Chips** (T.Joe's), 13 chips, 1 oz | 160 | 11 | 13 |
| **Beef Jerky** (Jack Link's), av., 1 oz | 80 | 1 | 4 |
| **Beef Sticks** (Slim Jim), Orig., 2 oz | 150 | 3 | 10 |
| Jack Links, Original, 1.5 oz | 160 | 13 | 2 |
| **BodyKey** (Amway): | | | |
| Mixed Nuts & Pumpkin Seeds, 1 bag | 200 | 16 | 8 |
| Whole Grain Tortilla Chips, 1 bag | 210 | 11 | 24 |
| **Bugles,** Original; Nacho Cheese, 1 oz | 160 | 9 | 18 |
| **Cheese Balls** (Utz), 1 oz serving | 150 | 9 | 16 |
| **Cheese Nips,** 1.3 oz package | 170 | 7 | 22 |
| **Cheese Puffs,** average, 1 oz | 160 | 10 | 15 |
| **Cheese Twists,** 1 oz | 140 | 8 | 15 |
| **Cheerios,** Snack Mix, average, ⅔ cup, 1 oz | 120 | 3 | 21 |
| **Cheetos:** | | | |
| Crunchy: Av. all flavors, 1 oz | 155 | 11 | 13 |
| 4 oz package | 640 | 40 | 60 |
| Baked!; Fantastix, all varieties, av., 1 oz | 130 | 5 | 19 |
| Simply Puffs, White Cheddar, 1 oz | 150 | 9 | 16 |
| **Cheez-It Crackers** (Sunshine): | | | |
| Original, 1.3 oz package | 180 | 9 | 20 |
| Original Big (13), 1 oz | 150 | 8 | 17 |
| Colby, 0.8 oz pouch | 110 | 6 | 12 |
| Mozzarella (25), 1 oz | 150 | 7 | 19 |
| Reduced Fat: Original, 1 oz | 130 | 4.5 | 20 |
| White Cheddar, 1 oz | 130 | 4 | 22 |
| **Chester's:** Fries, Flamin' Hot, 1 pkg | 140 | 8 | 16 |
| Puffcorn, Cheese, 1 oz | 160 | 11 | 14 |
| **Chex Mix,** (General Mills), Traditional, 1 oz | 120 | 3.5 | 21 |
| **Chips Ahoy!,** Choc Chip Cookies: | | | |
| 1.4 oz Single Serve Pack | 190 | 9 | 27 |
| Minis: Go-Pak!, 1 package, 3.5 oz | 525 | 25 | 70 |
| Snak Sak, 1 package, 8 oz | 1050 | 49 | 147 |
| **Chicharrones** ~ See Pork Skins | | | |
| **Churros** (Rubio's), 9", 1.6 oz | 170 | 8 | 22 |
| **Combos,** Crackers, av. all flavors, ⅓ cup, 1 oz | 140 | 6 | 18 |
| **Cool Cuts,** Carrot & Ranch, 2.3 oz | 70 | 5 | 5 |
| **Corn Chips** ~ See Page 149 | | | |
| **Corn Nuts:** Av all flav., 1 oz | 130 | 4.5 | 20 |
| 1.7 oz bag | 210 | 8 | 34 |
| **Corn Puffs/Twists,** (32 approx), 1 oz | 160 | 11 | 15 |

## Snacks (Cont) | C | F | Cb

| | C | F | Cb |
|---|---|---|---|
| **Dunkin Stix** (Dolly Madison), (3) | 490 | 25 | 63 |
| **Edamame,** | | | |
| Seapointe, Dry Roasted, 1 oz | 130 | 4 | 10 |
| **Fritos:** Corn Chips, all varieties, av., 1 oz | 150 | 10 | 15 |
| Flavor Twists, Honey BBQ, 1 oz | 150 | 9 | 16 |
| **Fruit Snacks** ~ See Page 102 | | | |
| **Funyuns,** Onion Flavored, 1 oz | 140 | 7 | 18 |
| **Goldfish,** av. all flavors 1 oz | 140 | 5 | 20 |
| **Gold-n-Chees** (Lance): | | | |
| Snack Mix, 1 oz | 150 | 8 | 17 |
| Tube, 1 oz | 130 | 6 | 18 |
| **Gripz,** (Sunshine), Mighty Tiny, 0.9 oz | 120 | 6 | 15 |
| **Hot Peanuts** (Munchies), 1.7 oz | 310 | 25 | 10 |
| **Lance:** | | | |
| Cracker Creations, Granola, av. all ,(2) | 190 | 9 | 24 |
| Sandwich Crackers, av. all, 6 crackers | 200 | 9 | 25 |
| **Munchies** (Frito-Lay), Snack Mix, all flavors, 1 oz | 140 | 7 | 18 |
| **Munchos,** all flavors, 16 pieces, 1 oz | 160 | 10 | 16 |
| **Newtons:** | | | |
| Single Serve: 2 oz pkg | 200 | 4 | 40 |
| Fat-Free, 2 oz package | 200 | 0 | 46 |
| **Nutter Butter,** Sandwich Cookies: | | | |
| Singles, 1.9 oz pkg | 250 | 10 | 37 |
| Bites, Go-Pak, 3.5 oz | 490 | 21 | 74 |
| **Onion Rings** (T.G.I. Friday), 1 oz | 140 | 7 | 16 |
| **Oreo Cookies,** all Creme Fillings: | | | |
| Double Stuf (2), 1 oz | 140 | 7 | 21 |
| Mini Bite Size: 1.3 oz pkg | 170 | 7 | 25 |
| Go-Pak, 3.5 oz | 455 | 21 | 74 |
| **Oreo Cakesters,** soft, 2 oz | 250 | 12 | 36 |
| **Oriental Mix Rice Snacks,** 1 oz | 125 | 3.5 | 21 |
| **Peanut Butter Nuggets,** (10), 1 oz | 140 | 6 | 15 |
| **Pepitas,** dried or roasted, ¼ cup, 1 oz | 155 | 14 | 3 |
| **Pirate's Booty:** | | | |
| Aged White Cheddar, 4 oz bag | 520 | 20 | 76 |
| Fruity Booty, 4 oz bag | 520 | 20 | 68 |
| **Pita Chips,** (9), average, 1 oz | 130 | 4 | 18 |
| **Plaintain Chips,** Goya, 34 chips, 1 oz | 150 | 8 | 19 |
| **PopCorners,** Butter/Kettle, 1 oz | 125 | 3.5 | 20 |
| **Popcorn** ~ See Page 148 | | | |
| **Pork Cracklins,** 1 oz | 160 | 12 | 0 |
| **Pork Skins/Rinds:** 1 oz | 160 | 10 | 0 |
| Baken-ets, Traditional, 0.5 oz | 80 | 5 | 0 |
| Mission, Chiccarones, 4 oz package | 640 | 40 | 0 |
| **Potato Chips** ~ See Page 149 | | | |
| **Potato Skins** (TGI Friday), all flavors, 16 chips, 1 oz | 140 | 8 | 15 |
| **Puffed Wheat,** Sabritones, Chili & Lime, 1 oz | 150 | 10 | 13 |
| **Pretzels** ~ See Page 149 | | | |

## Snacks (Cont)

| | C | F | Cb |
|---|---|---|---|
| **Puffed Wheat,** | | | |
| Sabritones, Chili & Lime, 1 oz | 150 | 10 | 13 |
| **Pretzels ~** See Page 149 Rice Cakes: | | | |
| Lundberg, (1), average, 0.7 oz | 75 | 0.5 | 16 |
| Quaker: Plain, lightly salted, 0.3 oz | 35 | 0 | 7 |
| Chocolate (1), 0.5 oz | 60 | 1 | 12 |
| **Rice Chips:** | | | |
| Lundberg, average, 1 oz | 140 | 7 | 18 |
| Quaker, Popped White Cheddar & Herb, 16 chips, 1 oz | 130 | 5 | 19 |
| **Sandwich Crackers:** | | | |
| Austin, Cheese Crackers: | | | |
| with Cheddar, 1.4 oz | 190 | 10 | 23 |
| with Peanut Butter, 1.3 oz | 190 | 10 | 23 |
| PB & J Flavored, 1.4 oz | 190 | 8 | 26 |
| Lance: | | | |
| Nip Chee, 6 pieces | 190 | 9 | 24 |
| Toasty, 6 pieces | 180 | 8 | 21 |
| Toast Chee, 6 pieces | 210 | 10 | 25 |
| Ritz Bits: | | | |
| Cheese: 1.5 oz package | 220 | 12 | 25 |
| Go-Pak: 13 crackers, 1 oz | 150 | 8 | 16 |
| 3.5 oz Pak | 520 | 29 | 58 |
| P'nut Butter: 1.3 oz pkg | 170 | 10 | 20 |
| Big Bag, 3 oz | 450 | 25 | 50 |
| **Sesame Sticks,** | | | |
| SunRidge Farm, 1 oz | 170 | 12 | 14 |
| **Smart Puffs,** | | | |
| Pirates Booty, 1 oz | 140 | 7 | 16 |
| **Snack Mix,** | | | |
| Quaker, Baked Cheddar, 1 package | 230 | 8 | 34 |
| **Soy Crisps,** average, 1 oz | 120 | 3 | 17 |
| **Soy Nuts:** Dry Roasted, ¼ cup, 1 oz | 130 | 6 | 9 |
| Choc-coated, 1 oz | 140 | 7 | 13 |
| **Sun Chips,** | | | |
| Fritolay, average, 1 oz | 140 | 6 | 19 |
| **Takis:** Fajitas, 1 oz | 140 | 7 | 17 |
| 4 oz package | 560 | 28 | 68 |
| **Tings,** | | | |
| Robert's, 2 oz bag | 300 | 16 | 36 |
| **Toasted Chips** (Ritz), av. all, 1 oz | 130 | 5.5 | 20 |
| **Tortilla Chips/Tostitos ~** Page 149 | | | |
| **Trail Mix (Nuts/Seeds/Dried Fruit):** | | | |
| Regular, 3 Tbsp, 1 oz | 140 | 9 | 13 |
| Tropical, 3 Tbsp, 1 oz | 130 | 7 | 16 |
| **Turkey Jerky:** Teriyaki, 1 oz | 80 | 1 | 9 |
| Trader Joe's, Original, 1 oz | 60 | 0.5 | 6 |
| **Veggie Crisps,** | | | |
| Snyder's, 1 oz | 140 | 7 | 18 |
| **Wheat Thins** (Nabisco), av. all, 1 oz | 135 | 5 | 19 |
| **Yogurt Pretzels,** 1.5 oz | 190 | 8 | 28 |
| **Yogurt Raisins,** | | | |
| Sun-Maid, 1 oz | 120 | 4.5 | 20 |

## Fruit Snacks

| | C | F | Cb |
|---|---|---|---|
| **Betty Crocker:** Fruit Gushers, 0.9 oz | 90 | 1 | 20 |
| Fruit by the Foot, 1 roll, 0.8 oz | 80 | 1 | 17 |
| Fruit Roll Ups, 1 roll, 0.5 oz | 50 | 1 | 12 |
| Fruit Flavored Shapes, all varieties, 0.9 oz | 80 | 0 | 19 |
| **Sunkist:** Fruit Snacks, 1 pouch | 80 | 0 | 19 |
| Fruit Smoothie Blitz, 1.3 oz | 140 | 1 | 32 |
| **Fruit Snack Cups ~** See Page 102 | | | |

## Vending Machines

| | C | F | Cb |
|---|---|---|---|
| **Bugles,** Nacho Cheese, 1 oz | 160 | 9 | 18 |
| **Cheese Balls** (Utz), 1 oz | 150 | 9 | 16 |
| **Cheetos,** Crunchy, 1 oz | 150 | 10 | 13 |
| **Cheeze-It,** Snack Mix, 1.5 oz | 195 | 6.5 | 30 |
| **Chex Mix,** Cheddar, 1 oz | 120 | 3.5 | 22 |
| **Chester's,** Flamin' Hot Fries, 1 oz | 140 | 8 | 16 |
| **Choc Chip Cookies:** | | | |
| Chips Ahoy, 1.4 oz | 190 | 9 | 27 |
| Famous Amos, (4), 1 oz | 150 | 8 | 18 |
| Grandma's, (2), 2.5 oz | 340 | 28 | 55 |
| **Chocolate Bars:** | | | |
| Hershey's, Milk Choc.,1.6 oz | 210 | 13 | 26 |
| Kit Kat, 1.5 oz | 210 | 11 | 27 |
| Snickers, 1.9 oz bar | 250 | 12 | 33 |
| **Donut,** plain cake, 1.4 oz | 160 | 9 | 18 |
| **Doritos,** av. all flavors, 1 oz | 145 | 8 | 18 |
| **Fritos,** Corn Chips, Orig., 1.8 oz | 280 | 17 | 26 |
| **Fruit Pie,** | | | |
| Hostess, 4.5 oz | 480 | 20 | 68 |
| **Granola/Cereal Bars,** av., 1 oz | 140 | 3 | 26 |
| **M & M's:** | | | |
| Milk Chocolate, 1.7 oz | 240 | 10 | 34 |
| Peanuts, 1.8 oz | 250 | 13 | 30 |
| **Oreo Cookies,** 2 oz | 270 | 11 | 41 |
| **Peanut Butter Cups,** | | | |
| Reese's, 1.5 oz | 210 | 13 | 24 |
| **Popcorn,** plain, 1 oz | 160 | 10 | 16 |
| **Pop Chips,** 0.8 oz | 100 | 3 | 16 |
| **Pork Skins,** 1.5 oz | 240 | 15 | 0 |
| **Potato Chips:** 1 oz | 150 | 10 | 15 |
| Baked! (Ruffles), Orig.,1 oz | 160 | 10 | 15 |
| **Potato Skins** (TGI Friday's), all flavors, 1 oz | 140 | 8 | 15 |
| **Pretzels** (Snyder's), Old Time, 1 oz | 120 | 1 | 24 |
| **Raisins,** 0.5 oz package | 45 | 0 | 11 |
| **Rice Krispies Treat** | 90 | 2 | 17 |
| **Skittles,** 2 oz | 230 | 2.5 | 52 |
| **Starburst,** Fruit Chews, Orig., 1.4 oz | 160 | 3.5 | 33 |
| **Tortilla Chips,** 1 oz | 140 | 7 | 18 |

# S Soups

## Homemade & Restaurant

| Restaurant & Take-Out: | C | F | Cb |
|---|---|---|---|
| *Average All Preparations: Per 8 fl.oz* | | | |
| Bean Medley | 200 | 3 | 34 |
| Beef Consomme | 30 | 0 | 2 |
| Borscht, with Sour Cream | 130 | 8 | 14 |
| Bouillabaisse | 400 | 15 | 10 |
| Chicken & Corn | 290 | 14 | 20 |
| Chicken & Wild Rice | 80 | 4 | 9 |
| Chicken Consomme | 50 | 0 | 2 |
| Chicken Curry | 180 | 8 | 18 |
| Chicken Jambalaya | 160 | 7 | 8 |
| Chicken Noodle | 80 | 2 | 12 |
| With Chicken | 160 | 4 | 12 |
| Chicken Soup | 80 | 2 | 6 |
| Chili with Beans | 250 | 12 | 25 |
| Clam Chowder | 240 | 15 | 17 |
| Corn & Crab | 120 | 3 | 18 |
| Corn Chowder | 150 | 8 | 16 |
| Cream of Broccoli | 200 | 12 | 20 |
| Cream of Potato | 150 | 6.5 | 17 |
| Cream of Mushroom | 200 | 13 | 15 |
| Fish Chowder | 220 | 15 | 6 |
| French Onion | 420 | 15 | 25 |
| Gazpacho | 50 | 0 | 5 |
| Lentil Soup | 250 | 9 | 28 |
| Lobster Bisque | 320 | 15 | 10 |
| Matzo Ball, with 1 large ball | 180 | 7 | 24 |
| Minestrone | 125 | 2.5 | 20 |
| Mulligatawny | 300 | 15 | 8 |
| Pea & Ham | 240 | 10 | 25 |
| Potato & Bacon | 170 | 7 | 19 |
| Pumpkin, Creamy | 210 | 10 | 26 |
| Shark Fin Soup | 100 | 4 | 8 |
| Spicy Shrimp Soup, 1 bowl | 160 | 7 | 10 |
| Split Pea Soup | 180 | 2.5 | 30 |
| Vegetable (Fat Free) | 75 | 0 | 18 |
| Vegetable Beef | 80 | 2 | 16 |
| Vichyssoise | 200 | 9 | 15 |
| Watercress | 90 | 4 | 13 |

**Other Soups ~** *See International & Fast-Foods Sections (Arby's, Au Bon Pain, Boston Market, Dunkin' Donuts, Denny's, Schlotzsky's, Sizzler, Souplantation, Sweet Tomatoes, Zoup!)*
**Homemade Soups:** *Calculate calories, fat and carbohydrates from recipe ingredients.*

## Bouillon Cubes & Powders

| | C | F | Cb |
|---|---|---|---|
| **Bouillon Cubes:** *Average all types* | | | |
| Regular, 1 cube | 5 | 0 | 1 |
| Extra Large, 1 cube | 20 | 1 | 1 |
| **Powders**, average, 1 tsp | 10 | 0 | 1 |
| **Herb-Ox:** | | | |
| Instant Broth & Seasoning, | | | |
| Beef, 1 envelope, 0.14 oz | 5 | 0 | 1 |
| Chicken, 1 envelope, 0.14 oz | 5 | 0 | 1 |

## Soup ~ Brands

| | C | F | Cb |
|---|---|---|---|
| **Amy's:** | | | |
| **Heat & Serve (Organic):** *Per 1 Cup, Unless Indicated* | | | |
| Alphabet | 80 | 0 | 16 |
| Chunky Vegetable | 60 | 0 | 13 |
| Cream of M'shrm, ¾ cup | 150 | 9 | 13 |
| Curried Lentil | 230 | 8 | 30 |
| Fire Roasted Sthwestern Veggie | 140 | 3 | 21 |
| Lentil | 180 | 5 | 25 |
| Lentil Vegetable | 160 | 4 | 24 |
| Rustic Italian Vegetable | 140 | 6 | 18 |
| Split Pea | 100 | 0 | 19 |
| Thai Coconut | 140 | 10 | 9 |
| Tuscan Bean & Rice | 160 | 4.5 | 25 |
| **Andersen's:** *Per 1 Cup* | | | |
| Split Pea | 130 | 0 | 24 |
| Split Pea flavored with Bacon | 140 | 1 | 23 |
| **Bertoli:** *Per ½ Carton, 12 oz* | | | |
| **Meal Soups:** Chicken Minestrone | 370 | 18 | 32 |
| Roasted Chicken & Rotini Pasta | 290 | 12 | 28 |
| Ricotta & Lobster Ravioli, | | | |
| in Seafood Bisque | 380 | 16 | 41 |
| Tomato Florentine | | | |
| & Tortellini with Chicken | 410 | 19 | 36 |
| Tuscan-Style Beef & Vegetables | 360 | 20 | 26 |
| **Campbell's:** | | | |
| **Chunky:** *Per 8 fl.oz Cup* | | | |
| Baked Potato w/ Ched. & Bacon Bits | 190 | 9 | 23 |
| BBQ Seasoned Pork | 160 | 1 | 28 |
| Beef Burrito | 190 | 9 | 21 |
| Beer–n–Cheese, with Beef & Bacon | 190 | 9 | 21 |
| Chicken Corn Chowder | 190 | 10 | 20 |
| Classic Chicken Noodle | 110 | 3 | 14 |
| Healthy Request: | | | |
| Beef w/ Country Veggies | 110 | 1.5 | 17 |
| Chicken Corn Chowder | 140 | 3 | 22 |
| Chicken Noodle | 100 | 1 | 16 |
| New England Clam Chowder | 130 | 3 | 20 |
| Split Pea & Ham, Smoke Flavor | 160 | 2.5 | 22 |
| Mushroom Swiss Burger | 160 | 7 | 17 |
| Sausage & Pepper Rigatoni | 190 | 8 | 22 |

**Campbell's (Cont):**
**Chunky (Cont):**

| | C | F | Cb |
|---|---|---|---|
| Hearty: Beef Noodle | 120 | 2 | 17 |
| Italian Style Wedding, with M'balls & Spinach | 120 | 3 | 15 |
| Wicked Thai Style Chicken, with Rice & Vegetables | 160 | 6 | 21 |

**Condensed Soup:** *Per ½ Cup, 4 fl.oz*

| | C | F | Cb |
|---|---|---|---|
| Bean with Bacon | 160 | 3 | 26 |
| Beef with Veggies & Barley | 80 | 1 | 15 |
| Chicken Noodle | 60 | 2 | 8 |
| Cream of Broccoli | 90 | 5 | 9 |
| Cream of Celery/Mushroom | 100 | 7 | 9 |
| Cream of Potato | 90 | 2 | 16 |
| Homestyle Chicken Noodle | 70 | 2 | 10 |
| Old Fashioned Tomato Rice | 130 | 1.5 | 26 |
| Split Pea w/ Ham & Bacon | 180 | 2 | 29 |
| Tomato | 90 | 0 | 20 |

**Go Soups:** *Per 8 fl.oz Cup*

| | C | F | Cb |
|---|---|---|---|
| Chicken & Quinoa with Chilies | 150 | 2.5 | 20 |
| Coconut Curry w/ Chicken & Shitaki Mushrooms | 150 | 5 | 17 |
| Creamy Red Pepper with Smoked Gouda | 220 | 15 | 15 |
| Golden Lentil w/ Madras Curry | 140 | 6 | 18 |
| Moroccan Style Chicken & Chickpeas | 180 | 2.5 | 26 |
| Spicy Chorizo, Chkn & Black Beans | 230 | 8 | 29 |

**Gourmet Bisques:** *Per 8 fl.oz Cup*

| | C | F | Cb |
|---|---|---|---|
| Golden Butternut Squash | 110 | 2 | 21 |
| Sweet Potato Tomatillo | 160 | 8 | 19 |
| Thai Tomato Coconut | 170 | 5 | 27 |
| Tomato Rstd Garlic Bacon | 210 | 8 | 31 |

**Homestyle:** *Per 8 fl.oz Cup*

| | C | F | Cb |
|---|---|---|---|
| Butternut Squash Bisque | 110 | 3 | 19 |
| Chicken Noodle | 90 | 2.5 | 10 |
| Creamy Chicken & Herb Dumplings | 160 | 9 | 14 |
| Creamy Gouda Bisque with Chicken | 190 | 11 | 16 |
| Harvest Tomato with Basil | 110 | 1 | 23 |
| Italian-Style Wedding | 120 | 3.5 | 15 |
| Maryland-Style Crab Soup | 80 | 0.5 | 14 |
| Mexican-Style Chkn Tortilla | 130 | 2 | 20 |
| Minestrone | 100 | 1 | 18 |
| New England Clam Chwdr | 170 | 10 | 15 |
| Potato Broccoli Cheese | 170 | 10 | 16 |
| Southwest-Style White Chkn Chili | 130 | 2.5 | 20 |
| Zesty Tomato Bisque | 110 | 2 | 19 |
| **Light:** Chicken Noodle | 70 | 1 | 9 |
| New England Clam Chowder | 120 | 4 | 15 |
| Italian-Style Wedding | 80 | 1.5 | 11 |
| Southwestern-Style Vegetable | 50 | 0 | 10 |

**Campbell's (Cont):**
**Slow Kettle Style:** *Per 8 fl.oz*

| | C | F | Cb |
|---|---|---|---|
| Braised Beef Stew | 150 | 3 | 19 |
| Portobello Mushroom & Madeira Bisque | 240 | 18 | 16 |
| Southwest Style Chicken Chili with Black Beans | 190 | 2 | 28 |
| Tomato & Sweet Basil Bisque | 290 | 16 | 33 |
| Tuscan Style Chicken & White Bean | 140 | 2.5 | 17 |

**Health Valley Organics:**
**Creamed:** *Per 8 fl.oz Cup*

| | C | F | Cb |
|---|---|---|---|
| Cream of Chicken | 110 | 3 | 15 |
| Cream of Celery | 100 | 2 | 17 |
| Cream of Mushroom | 90 | 2 | 14 |

**Fat Free, 40% Less Sodium:** *Per 8 fl.oz Cup*

| | C | F | Cb |
|---|---|---|---|
| Black Bean Vegetable | 110 | 0 | 25 |
| Corn & Vegetable | 100 | 0 | 22 |
| Lentil & Carrot | 110 | 0 | 24 |
| Split Pea & Carrots | 120 | 0 | 26 |
| Tomato Vegetable | 70 | 0 | 17 |

**Healthy Choice:**
**Canned:** *Per Cup*

| | C | F | Cb |
|---|---|---|---|
| Bean & Ham, 8.8 oz | 180 | 2.5 | 28 |
| Chicken & Dumplings, 8.9 oz | 150 | 3 | 22 |
| Chicken Tortilla, 8.4 oz | 140 | 1.5 | 23 |
| Chicken with Rice, 8.4 oz | 110 | 2 | 17 |
| Country Vegetable, 8.7 oz | 100 | 0 | 19 |
| New England Clam Chowder | 110 | 1.5 | 20 |
| Split Pea & Ham, 8.4 oz | 160 | 2.5 | 27 |
| Tomato Basil, 8.8 oz | 100 | 0 | 22 |

**Microwaveable Bowls:** *Per Cup*

| | C | F | Cb |
|---|---|---|---|
| Beef Pot Roast, 8.6 oz | 110 | 1.5 | 17 |
| Chicken Tortilla, 8.6 oz | 140 | 1.5 | 23 |
| Chicken with Rice, 8.5 oz | 90 | 2 | 13 |
| Country Vegetable, 8.6 oz | 100 | 0 | 20 |
| Hearty Vegetable Barley, 8.8 oz | 140 | 1 | 30 |

**Imagine:**
**Broths, Organic:** *Per Cup*

| | C | F | Cb |
|---|---|---|---|
| Beef Flavor | 20 | 1 | 2 |
| Free Range Chicken | 20 | 0.5 | 2 |
| Vegetable | 20 | 0 | 4 |
| Vegetarian, No-Chicken | 15 | 0 | 2 |

**Chunky Style, Organic:** *Per Cup*

| | C | F | Cb |
|---|---|---|---|
| Chicken & Dumplings | 130 | 4.5 | 18 |
| Cream of Mushroom | 100 | 3.5 | 15 |
| Ital. Vegetables & Beans | 120 | 1.5 | 24 |

*Continued Nex Page...*

| Imagine (Cont): | C | F | Cb |
|---|---|---|---|
| **Creamy:** *Per 8 fl.oz Cup* | | | |
| Acorn Squash & Mango | 70 | 1 | 15 |
| Portobello Mushroom | 70 | 2.5 | 12 |
| Potato Leek | 80 | 2.5 | 13 |
| Sweet Pea | 80 | 1.5 | 14 |
| Tomato Basil | 110 | 2 | 21 |
| **Kettle Cuisine:** *Per 8 oz* | | | |
| Angus Steak Chili with Beans | 250 | 7 | 20 |
| Aztec Chili with Ancient Grains | 170 | 2 | 29 |
| Broccoli Cheddar | 320 | 24 | 15 |
| Caribbean Jerk Chicken | 220 | 5 | 31 |
| Carrot Ginger | 110 | 4 | 18 |
| Chicken Tortilla | 120 | 3 | 15 |
| Chipotle Sweet Potato | 140 | 7 | 20 |
| Cream of Crab | 290 | 22 | 15 |
| Lobster Bisque | 270 | 18 | 18 |
| Manhattan Clam Chowder | 120 | 3 | 16 |
| North Atlantic Haddock Chowder | 260 | 17 | 14 |
| **Knorr:** | | | |
| **Cubes:** *Per ½ Cube, 1 Cup, Prepared* | | | |
| Beef; Chicken, average | 15 | 1.5 | 1 |
| Vegetable | 20 | 1 | 1 |
| **Homestyle Stock:** *Per 1 Tsp* | | | |
| Beef | 10 | 1 | 0 |
| Chicken | 10 | 2 | 0 |
| **Lipton:** | | | |
| **Cup-a-Soup:** *Per Envelope* | | | |
| Chicken Noodle, Original | 50 | 1 | 8 |
| Cream of Chicken | 60 | 1.5 | 12 |
| **Recipe Secrets:** *Per 1 Tbsp Dry Mix* | | | |
| Onion | 20 | 0 | 4 |
| Onion Mushroom | 25 | 0 | 7 |
| Savory Herb with Garlic | 25 | 0 | 6 |
| **Manischewitz:** | | | |
| **Canned:** *Per 1 cup* | | | |
| Broth: Beef | 15 | 0.5 | 1 |
| Turkey | 20 | 1 | 1 |
| Vegetable | 5 | 0 | 1 |
| Chicken Consomme, Clear | 30 | 0 | 4 |
| Chicken Noodle | 180 | 2 | 20 |
| **Glass Jar:** *Per 1 Cup* | | | |
| Matzo Ball | 120 | 5 | 15 |
| Reduced Sodium | 130 | 6 | 16 |
| Matzo Ball in Broth | 180 | 8 | 23 |
| Reduced Sodium | 180 | 8 | 21 |
| **Maruchan:** | | | |
| **Instant Lunch,** | | | |
| average all flavors, 1 pkg | 290 | 12 | 38 |
| **Ramen,** all flavors, 1 pkg, 3 oz | 380 | 14 | 52 |

| Nissin: | C | F | Cb |
|---|---|---|---|
| **Souper Meal:** *Per ½ of 4.3 oz Ctn* | | | |
| Chicken Flavor, with Vege Medley | 280 | 13 | 37 |
| Picante Shrimp Flavor, Hot & Spicy | 290 | 13 | 37 |
| **Top Ramen,** all flavors, 3 oz pkg | 380 | 14 | 53 |
| **Pacific Foods:** | | | |
| **Condensed:** | | | |
| Cream of Chicken, ½ cup | 90 | 3.5 | 10 |
| Cream of Mushroom, ½ cup | 100 | 2.5 | 18 |
| **Hearty Organic:** *Per 1 Cup* | | | |
| Butternut Squash Bisque | 110 | 3.5 | 18 |
| Cashew Carrot Ginger Bisque | 130 | 5 | 20 |
| Spicy Black Bean & Kale | 120 | 0 | 24 |
| Split Pea & Uncured Ham | 160 | 2.5 | 26 |
| Vegetable Quinoa | 90 | 2 | 18 |
| **Progresso:** | | | |
| **Broths:** Beef, 1 cup | 20 | 0 | 3 |
| Chicken, 1 cup | 20 | 0 | 1 |
| **Heart Healthy:** *Per Cup* | | | |
| Creamy Tomato with Basil | 120 | 3 | 22 |
| Creole Style Chkn Gumbo | 110 | 2 | 18 |
| Homestyle Vegetable Beef | 120 | 2 | 19 |
| Savory Garden Vegetable | 90 | 0 | 21 |
| S'West Style Black Bean & Vegetable | 110 | 2 | 21 |
| **Rich & Hearty:** *Per 1 Cup* | | | |
| Chkn & Hm'style Noodles | 110 | 3 | 14 |
| Chicken Corn Chowder | 200 | 9 | 23 |
| New Engl. Clam Chowder | 180 | 8 | 22 |
| Savory Beef Barley Vegetables | 110 | 2 | 16 |
| **Traditional:** *Per ½ Can, 1 Cup* | | | |
| Chickarina with Meatballs | 130 | 5 | 14 |
| Chicken & Sausage Gumbo | 120 | 3.5 | 17 |
| Creamy Tomato w/ Bacon & Cheese | 150 | 5 | 21 |
| **Vegetable Classic:** *Per 1 Cup* | | | |
| French Onion | 50 | 1 | 9 |
| Garden Vegetable | 90 | 0 | 20 |
| Minestrone | 100 | 2 | 20 |
| Tomato Basil | 150 | 3 | 29 |
| **Light:** *Per 1 cup* | | | |
| Beef Pot Roast | 80 | 2 | 10 |
| Chicken Pot Pie Style | 100 | 3 | 16 |
| Creamy Potato w/ Bacon & Cheese | 100 | 3 | 18 |
| Italian Style Vegetable | 70 | 0 | 16 |

## Safeway (Vons):

| | C | F | Cb |
|---|---|---|---|
| **Signature Soups:** *Per Cup* | | | |
| Broccoli & Cheesy Cheddar | 250 | 18 | 12 |
| Chunky Chicken Noodle | 160 | 5 | 14 |
| Fiesta Chicken Tortilla | 110 | 2 | 15 |
| Italian-Style Wedding | 120 | 4 | 14 |
| Pacific Coast Clam Chowder | 320 | 20 | 27 |
| Tuscan Tomato & Basil Bisque | 290 | 22 | 20 |

## Swanson:

| | C | F | Cb |
|---|---|---|---|
| **Broth:** *Per 8 fl.oz Cup* | | | |
| Beef | 15 | 0 | 1 |
| Chicken | 10 | 0.5 | 1 |
| Organic Chicken | 15 | 0.5 | 1 |
| Vegetable | 15 | 0 | 3 |
| **Flavor Boost:** *Per Pouch* | | | |
| Beef | 10 | 0 | 2 |
| Chicken | 35 | 2 | 3 |
| Vegetable | 20 | 0 | 4 |

## Tabatchnick:
### Frozen:

| | C | F | Cb |
|---|---|---|---|
| **Dairy:** *Per 7.5 oz Pouch* | | | |
| Corn Chowder | 130 | 4.5 | 21 |
| Cream of Mushroom | 100 | 5 | 11 |
| **Gluten Free:** *Per 7.5 oz Pouch* | | | |
| Southwest Bean | 220 | 5 | 36 |
| Split Pea | 140 | 0 | 34 |
| Vegetarian Chili | 180 | 3.5 | 28 |
| **Low Sodium:** *Per 7 .5oz Pouch* | | | |
| Barley & Mushroom | 80 | 1 | 17 |
| Split Pea | 140 | 0 | 34 |
| Vegetable | 90 | 1.5 | 17 |
| **Meat:** *Per 7.5 oz Pouch* | | | |
| Frenchman's Onion | 60 | 1.5 | 11 |
| Wilderness Wild Rice | 90 | 0.5 | 19 |
| **Parve:** *Per 7.5 oz Pouch* | | | |
| Black Bean | 220 | 2.5 | 38 |
| Minestrone | 110 | 1.5 | 20 |
| **Shelf Stable:** *Per ⅔ Cup, 5.3 fl.oz* | | | |
| **Broth:** Classic Chicken | 5 | 0 | 0 |
| Other Chicken Flavors | 10 | 0 | 1 |
| Gourmet Beef | 5 | 0 | 0 |
| **Soup:** Creamy Tomato | 70 | 2 | 14 |
| Rstd Red Pepper & Tomato | 70 | 2.5 | 13 |

## Thai Kitchen:

| | C | F | Cb |
|---|---|---|---|
| **Rice Noodle Soup Bowls:** *Per Bowl* | | | |
| Hot & Sour | 250 | 4 | 51 |
| Lemongrass & Chili | 250 | 3.5 | 52 |
| Roasted Garlic | 250 | 3 | 52 |
| Spring Onion | 260 | 4.5 | 50 |
| Thai Ginger | 260 | 3 | 52 |

## Trader Joe's:

| | C | F | Cb |
|---|---|---|---|
| **28 fl.oz Cans:** *Per Cup* | | | |
| Chunky, Low Fat: | | | |
| Lentil with Vegetables | 140 | 3 | 21 |
| Minestrone | 110 | 2.5 | 19 |
| **14.5 oz Cans:** *Per 1 Cup* | | | |
| Organic: Black Bean | 140 | 1.5 | 26 |
| Lentil Vegetable | 160 | 4 | 24 |
| Split Pea | 100 | 0 | 19 |
| **10.75 oz Can,** | | | |
| Low Sodium, Minestrone | 200 | 4 | 37 |
| **15 oz Can,** | | | |
| Low Fat, Chicken Noodle, 1 cup | 90 | 1 | 14 |
| **32 fl. oz. Cartons:** *Per 1 Cup* | | | |
| Butternut Squash | 90 | 2 | 16 |
| Carrot & Ginger | 80 | 1 | 17 |
| Creamy Corn & Rstd Pepper | 110 | 2 | 23 |
| Latin Style Black Bean | 70 | 1 | 12 |
| Sweet Potato Bisque | 130 | 1 | 28 |
| Organic: Butternut Squash | 70 | 0 | 17 |
| Tomato & Rstd Red Pepper | 100 | 3.5 | 15 |
| Low Sodium, Creamy Tomato | 90 | 3.5 | 15 |
| **17.6 fl.oz Cartons:** *Per Cup* | | | |
| Beef, Barley with Veggies | 100 | 0.5 | 16 |
| Chicken Noodle with Veggies | 100 | 1 | 16 |

## Whole Foods: *Per Cup*
### 365 Organic:

| | C | F | Cb |
|---|---|---|---|
| Chicken Noodle | 100 | 1.5 | 12 |
| Lentil | 70 | 0 | 15 |
| Minestrone | 140 | 1.5 | 23 |
| Southwestern Black Bean | 120 | 1 | 23 |
| Tomato Basil | 90 | 2 | 16 |

## Wolfgang Puck: *Per Cup*
### Organic:

| | C | F | Cb |
|---|---|---|---|
| Butternut Squash | 140 | 11 | 10 |
| Chicken & Dumplings | 140 | 7 | 14 |
| Classic Minestrone | 120 | 2.5 | 20 |
| Corn Chowder | 210 | 13 | 20 |
| Free Range Chicken with Rice | 110 | 4 | 15 |
| New Engl. Clam Chowder | 150 | 7 | 18 |
| Signature Tortilla | 160 | 3.5 | 27 |
| Thick Hearty Lentil & Vegetable | 160 | 1 | 29 |
| Thick Hearty Garden Vegetable | 130 | 5 | 19 |
| Tomato with Basil | 150 | 6 | 21 |

## Soybean Products  **C** **F** **Cb**

**Cheeses (Soy)** ~ *See Page 78*

**Miso Soy Bean Paste:**

| | C | F | Cb |
|---|---|---|---|
| *Cold Mountain:* Light Yellow, 1 tsp | 10 | 0 | 1 |
| Mellow Red, 1 tsp | 15 | 0 | 3 |
| Red, 1 tsp | 10 | 0 | 1 |
| **Miso Soup (dry mix):** | | | |
| 1 Tbsp., dry mix | 35 | 1 | 5 |
| 1 cup, prepared | 35 | 1 | 5 |
| **Natto**, ½ cup, 3 oz | 160 | 7 | 14 |
| **Okara (Tofu fiber residue)**, ½ c., 2 oz | 47 | 1 | 8 |
| **Tempeh:** 1 piece, 3 oz | 180 | 8 | 12 |
| Fried, 3 oz | 250 | 14 | 14 |
| **Seitan** *(Westsoy)*, Strips, 3 oz | 120 | 2 | 4 |
| **Soybean Protein** *(TVP)*, 1 oz | 95 | 0 | 8 |
| **Soy Bean Paste**, 1 tsp | 10 | 0 | 2 |

**Soy Beans** ~ *See Page 160*

**Soy Drinks** ~ *See Page 49*

## Tofu ~ Brands

**Azumaya Tofu:**

| | C | F | Cb |
|---|---|---|---|
| Extra Firm; Firm, av., 3 oz | 70 | 4 | 2 |
| Soft (Silken), 3.2 oz | 45 | 2 | 1 |
| **House Foods:** *Per 3 oz* | | | |
| **Premium Tofu:** Extra Firm | 80 | 4.5 | 2 |
| Firm | 70 | 4 | 2 |
| Medium Firm | 60 | 3.5 | 2 |
| Soft (Silken) | 60 | 3 | 2 |
| **Organic Tofu:** Firm | 70 | 4 | 2 |
| Extra Firm | 70 | 3.5 | 2 |
| **Ethnic:** Tokusen Kinugoshi, Extra Soft | 80 | 4 | 3 |
| Sukui; Soon (Extra Soft) | 45 | 2 | 2 |
| Yaki Tofu (Broiled) | 90 | 5 | 2 |

**Mori-Nu Tofu:**

**Morinaga Silken:**

| | C | F | Cb |
|---|---|---|---|
| Soft, 3 oz, 1" slice | 45 | 2.5 | 2 |
| Firm, 3 oz, 1" slice | 50 | 2.5 | 2 |
| Extra Firm, 3 oz, 1" slice | 45 | 1.5 | 2 |
| Organic, Silken 3 oz, 1" slice | 50 | 2.5 | 2 |
| Lite, Firm, 3 oz, 1" slice | 30 | 1 | 2 |
| **Nasoya:** Extra Firm, 3 oz | 80 | 4 | 3 |
| Firm, 3 oz | 70 | 3.5 | 2 |
| Silken, 3.2 oz | 45 | 2 | 1 |
| Soft, 2.8 oz | 60 | 3 | 1 |
| **Tofuplus:** | | | |
| Extra Firm, 3 oz | 80 | 4 | 2 |
| Firm, 3 oz | 70 | 3 | 2 |
| Sprouted, Super Firm, 3 oz | 100 | 5 | 3 |

## Supplements  **C** **F** **Cb**

| | C | F | Cb |
|---|---|---|---|
| **Aloe Vera Juice**, undiluted, 2 fl.oz | 5 | 0 | 1 |
| **Brewer's Yeast:** Tablets, 2 tabs | 4 | 0 | 0.5 |
| Flakes, 1 heaping Tbsp, 0.3 oz | 30 | 0.5 | 4 |
| Powder, 1 heaping Tbsp, 0.5 oz | 50 | 0.5 | 6 |
| **Calcium Chews**: *CVS*, 1 chew | 20 | 0 | 3 |
| *Trader Joe's*, Chocolate,1 chew | 20 | 1 | 3 |
| **Cod Liver Oil**, 1 Tbsp | 125 | 13 | 0 |
| *Fiber Choice*, 2 tabs | 15 | 0 | 4 |
| **Fiber**, | | | |
| *Fibersure*, 1 heaping tsp | 25 | 0 | 6 |
| **Fish Oil Capsules**, (1), av. | 10 | 1 | 0 |
| **Flax Oil:** | | | |
| Capsules (2) | 10 | 1 | 0 |
| *Barlean's*, softgels (3) | 110 | 11 | 0 |
| **Garlic Tablets/Capsules**, each | 3 | 0 | 1 |
| **Glowelle:** | | | |
| Beauty Drink, 8 fl.oz | 100 | 0 | 24 |
| Powder Stick (1) | 50 | 0 | 12 |
| **Lecithin Granules**, 1 Tbsp | 55 | 4 | 0.5 |
| *Metamucil*, Powder: | | | |
| Orange (Smooth Texture), | | | |
| 1 rounded Tbsp | 45 | 0 | 12 |
| Sugar-Free, 1 rounded tsp | 20 | 0 | 5 |
| Pink Lemonade, Sugar-Free, | | | |
| 1 rounded tsp | 20 | 0 | 5 |
| **Capsules:** Heart & Digestive (6) | 10 | 0 | 3 |
| Strong Bones (5) | 10 | 0 | 3 |
| **Meta**, Fiber Wafers (2) | 100 | 4.5 | 16 |
| **Protein**, Powders, av., 1 oz | 100 | 0.5 | 0 |
| **Seaweed:** Dried, 1 oz | 85 | 0.5 | 22 |
| Soaked, drained, 1 oz | 15 | 0.5 | 3 |
| **Spirulina**, 1 tablet | 2 | 0 | 0.5 |
| **Vitamins/Minerals:** Tabs/Caps (1) | 2 | 0 | 0 |
| Vitamin E Capsules, each | 5 | 0.5 | 0 |
| **Viactiv Chews**, Choc. (1) | 20 | 0.5 | 4 |

## Cough & Pharmaceutical

| | C | F | Cb |
|---|---|---|---|
| **Antacids:** Av., 1 tablet | 4 | 0 | 1 |
| Liquid, 1 Tbsp | 6 | 0 | 1 |
| **Antacid Sodium Counts** ~ *See Page 280* | | | |
| **Cough/Cold Syrups:** | | | |
| Regular: With sugar, 1 Tbsp | 35 | 0 | 9 |
| With alcohol, 1 Tbsp | 46 | 0 | 9 |
| *Diabetic Tussin*, Sugar Free, 1 T. | 0 | 0 | 0 |
| **Cough Drops/Lozenges** ~ *See Page 75* | | | |
| *Sudafed*, Syrup 1 tsp | 14 | 0 | 3 |
| *Tylenol*, Liquid: Child, 1 tsp | 17 | 0 | 4 |
| Extra Strength, 1 tsp | 11 | 0 | 3 |

## Sugar

**C  F  Cb**

**White Sugar, granulated:**

| | C | F | Cb |
|---|---|---|---|
| 1 level teaspoon, 4g | 15 | 0 | 4 |
| 1 heaping teaspoon, 6g | 25 | 0 | 6 |
| 1 Tablespoon, 12g | 50 | 0 | 12 |
| 1 ounce, 1 oz | 110 | 0 | 28 |
| 1 cup, 7 oz | 775 | 0 | 200 |
| 1 lb (16 oz) | 1760 | 0 | 454 |
| Single Portion Packages: | | | |
| 1 stick | 15 | 0 | 4 |
| 1 packet | 15 | 0 | 4 |
| 1 cube | 10 | 0 | 2.5 |
| **Brown Sugar:** 1 Tbsp | 50 | 0 | 13 |
| 1 ounce, 1 oz | 110 | 0 | 28 |
| 1 cup, not packed, 5 oz | 550 | 0 | 140 |
| 1 cup, packed, 7.8 oz | 835 | 0 | 216 |
| **Powdered Sugar:** | | | |
| Sifted, 1 cup, 3.5 oz | 390 | 0 | 100 |
| Unsifted, 1 cup, 4¼ oz | 470 | 0 | 120 |
| **Coconut Palm Sugar,** 1 tsp, 4g | 15 | 0 | 4 |
| **Dextrose,** 1 tsp | 12 | 0 | 3 |
| **Fructose,** powder, 1 tsp | 12 | 0 | 3 |
| **Glucose Powder,** 1 oz | 110 | 0 | 27 |
| **Glucose Tablets,** (1) | 20 | 0 | 5 |
| **Palm Sugar,** 3 Tbsp | 45 | 0 | 11 |
| **Piloncillo,** (Brown Sugar), 3oz | 325 | 0 | 81 |
| **Turbinado Sugar,** 2 Tbsp, 1 oz | 110 | 0 | 27 |

## Sugar Substitutes

| | C | F | Cb |
|---|---|---|---|
| **Agave,** 1 Tbsp, 0.7 oz | 60 | 0 | 16 |
| **DiabetiSweet,** 1 teaspoon | 9 | 0 | 4.5 |
| *Note: Carb figure includes 4.5 g sugar alcohol* | | | |
| **Domino,** Light, ½ tsp | 5 | 0 | 2 |
| **Equal:** Tablet (2) | 0 | 0 | 0 |
| Granular, 1 tsp | 0 | 0 | 0 |
| Packet (1) | 0 | 0 | 0 |
| **Next,** 1 packet | 0 | 0 | 0 |
| **Nectresse,** 1 packet | 0 | 0 | 0 |
| **NutraSweet,** 1 tsp | 0 | 0 | 0 |
| **Splenda,** Granulated No Calorie Sweetener: | | | |
| 1 tsp | 0 | 0 | 0 |
| 1 cup | 95 | 0 | 24 |
| Packets, all flavors | 0 | 0 | 0 |
| Sugar Blend, Orig/Brown, ½ cup | 385 | 0 | 96 |
| **Stevia,** single serving | 0 | 0 | 0 |
| **Sugar Twin,** 1 packet | 0 | 0 | 0 |
| **Sweet 'N Low,** 1 packet | 0 | 0 | 0 |
| **Truvia,** 1 packet | 0 | 0 | 0 |
| **Walgreens,** Wal-Sweet, 1 packet | 0 | 0 | 0 |
| **Whey Low,** 1 tsp | 4 | 0 | 1 |

## Syrups, Molasses, Agave

**Syrups· Plain:** *Average All Brands (Corn/Rice/Maple/Pancake/Sundae/Waffle) Includes Aunt Jemima, Cary's, Karo, Hershey's, Hungry Jack, IHOP, Log Cabin, Mrs Butterworth's*

**Regular/Dark/Light Color:**

| | C | F | Cb |
|---|---|---|---|
| 1 Tbsp, 0.5 fl.oz | 55 | 0 | 14 |
| ¼ cup (4 Tbsp) | 220 | 0 | 55 |
| Single Portion, 1.5 oz pkg | 170 | 0 | 42 |
| **Lite,** 1Tbsp, 1 oz | 25 | 0 | 6 |
| **Sugar-Free:** 2 Tbsp, 1 oz | 18 | 0 | 5 |
| *Maple Grove,* Cozy Cottage, 2 Tbsp | 10 | 0 | 3 |
| *IHOP,* 4 Tbsp, 2 oz | 20 | 0 | 7 |
| **Fruit Syrups,** (IHOP), ¼ cup, 2 oz | 200 | 0 | 52 |
| **Honey Cream Syrup,** ¼ cup, 2 oz | 220 | 0 | 55 |
| **Molasses:** Dark/Light: 1 T, 0.7 oz | 60 | 0 | 15 |
| 1 cup, 12 oz | 975 | 0.5 | 252 |
| **Blackstrap,** 1 Tbsp, 0.8 oz | 47 | 0 | 13 |
| **Agave Nectar,** av. all flavors, | | | |
| 1 Tablespoon, 0.8 oz | 60 | 0 | 15 |

## Flavored Syrups/Ice Cream Toppings

**Hershey's:** *Per 2 Tbsp*

| | C | F | Cb |
|---|---|---|---|
| Average all flavors | 105 | 0 | 26 |
| Lite | 45 | 0 | 12 |
| **Smuckers:** *Per 2 Tbsp* | | | |
| **Magic Shell,** average all flavors | 220 | 17 | 16 |
| **Spoonables:** Reg., average all flavors | 115 | 1 | 28 |
| Sugar Free: Caramel; Chocolate | 90 | 0 | 24 |
| Strawberry | 25 | 0 | 9 |
| *Note: Carb figures include 9g-17g sugar alcohol* | | | |
| **Sundae Syrups:** Regular, av. all flavors | 105 | 0 | 25 |
| Sugar Free, average all flavors | 90 | 0 | 24 |
| *Note: Carb figures includes 15g sugar alcohol* | | | |

## Honey, Jam, Preserves

### Average all Brands

**Honey:** 1 tsp, 0.3 oz

| | C | F | Cb |
|---|---|---|---|
| **Honey:** 1 tsp, 0.3 oz | 20 | 0 | 5.5 |
| 1 Tbsp, 0.8 oz | 65 | 0 | 17 |
| 1 ounce, 1 oz | 85 | 0 | 23 |
| 1 cup, 12 oz | 1030 | 0 | 269 |
| Single Portion, 0.5 oz package | 45 | 0 | 11 |
| **Jams/Jellies/Marmalade/Preserves:** | | | |
| Regular: 1 tsp, 0.3 oz | 20 | 0 | 5 |
| 1 Tbsp, 0.8 oz | 55 | 0 | 14 |
| 1 ounce, 1 oz | 80 | 0 | 20 |
| Single Portion, 0.5 oz pkg | 40 | 0 | 11 |
| **Apple/Fruit Butters,** 1 T., 0.6 oz | 20 | 0 | 6 |
| **Fruit Spreads:** Regular, 1 tsp | 15 | 0 | 4 |
| Low Sugar, 1 tsp | 8 | 0 | 2 |
| **Jelly:** Regular, average, 1 tsp | 18 | 0 | 4.5 |
| Imitation, Low Calorie, 1 tsp | 4 | 0 | 1 |

# V — Vegetables & Legumes ~ Fresh

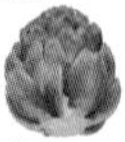

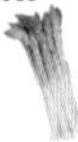

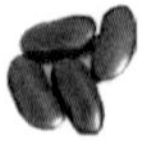

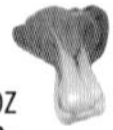

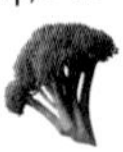

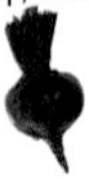

| Vegetables | C | F | Cb |
|---|---|---|---|
| **Alfalfa Sprouts**, ½ cup, 0.5 oz | 5 | 0 | 0.5 |
| **Artichokes**, Globe/French: | | | |
| 1 medium, 4.5 oz | 60 | 0 | 13 |
| 1 large, 5.7 oz | 75 | 0 | 17 |
| **Artichoke Heart**, plain, 2 pieces | 15 | 0 | 3 |
| **Asparagus**, raw/frozen: | | | |
| Cuts & Tips, ½ cup, 4.3 oz | 20 | 0 | 3 |
| Spears, 3 medium | 10 | 0 | 2 |
| **Bamboo Shoots**, cooked, ½ cup, 2 oz | 7 | 0 | 1 |
| **Beans**, Green/Snap/String: | | | |
| 10 beans (4" long), 2 oz | 20 | 0 | 4 |
| Pieces, ½ cup, 3 oz | 30 | 0 | 7 |
| Dried Beans (Kidney, Brown, Lima, Navy, Pinto, White): | | | |
| Raw: 2 Tbsp, 1 oz | 95 | 0.5 | 18 |
| 1 cup, 7 oz | 665 | 3 | 126 |
| Cooked: 1 cup | 35 | 0 | 7 |
| ½ cup, 3 oz | 105 | 0 | 21 |
| **Bean Sprouts**, average, ½ cup, 2 oz | 15 | 0 | 3.5 |
| **Beets (Beetroot):** | | | |
| Raw, 1 beet (2" diam.), 4 oz | 35 | 0 | 8 |
| Cooked, 1 cup, slices, 3 oz | 35 | 0 | 8 |
| **Canned ~** See Page 161 | | | |
| **Beet Greens**, cooked, ½ cup, 2.5 oz | 20 | 0 | 4 |
| **Bell Pepper ~** See Peppers | | | |
| **Bitter Melon/Gourd**, 1 cup, 1.5 oz | 15 | 0 | 1.5 |
| **Blackeye Peas**, cooked, ½ cup, 3 oz | 100 | 0.5 | 18 |
| **Bok Choy (Chinese Chard)**, | | | |
| cooked, 3 oz | 10 | 0 | 1.5 |
| **Breadfruit**, ¼ small fruit, 3 oz | 100 | 0 | 26 |
| **Broadbeans (Fava Beans):** | | | |
| Green, raw, (in pod): 4 pods | | | |
| (3.5 oz with shells, 1.2 oz beans) | 30 | 0 | 6 |
| 1 cup beans, without shell, 4.5 oz | 110 | 1 | 22 |
| Mature Seeds: Raw, 1 cup, 5.3 oz | 510 | 2.5 | 87 |
| Cooked, ½ cup, 3 oz | 95 | 0 | 17 |
| **Broccoflower**, ⅕ head, 3.5 oz | 35 | 0 | 7 |
| **Broccoli:** Raw, chopped,1 cup, 3 oz | 30 | 0 | 6 |
| 3 Florets, 2.5 oz | 25 | 0 | 5 |
| 1 Spear (5" long), 1.oz | 10 | 0 | 2 |
| 1 Whole: Medium, 14 oz | 135 | 1.5 | 26 |
| Large, 21 oz | 205 | 2 | 40 |
| 1 Head (no stalk), 11 oz | 105 | 1 | 21 |
| 1 Stalk, small (5" long), 5.3 oz | 50 | 0.5 | 10 |
| **Brocco Sprouts**, ½ cup, 1 oz | 15 | 0 | 2 |
| **Brussels Sprouts:** Cooked, ½ cup, 2.8 oz | 30 | 0.5 | 6 |
| 2 Sprouts, 1.5 oz | 15 | 0 | 3 |
| **Butterbeans**, cooked, ½ cup, 3 oz | 90 | 0 | 16 |
| **Cabbage**, average other flavors: | | | |
| Raw: 1 leaf, large, 2 oz | 5 | 0 | 2 |
| Shredded, 1 cup, 2.5 oz | 15 | 0 | 4 |
| ½ large head (7" diam), 22 oz | 150 | 1 | 35 |
| Cooked, shredded, ½ cup, 2.5 oz | 15 | 0.5 | 3.5 |

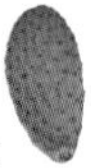

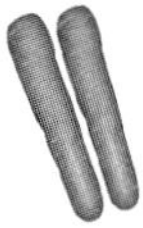

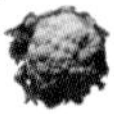

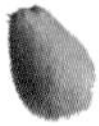

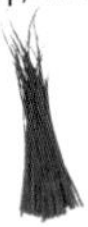

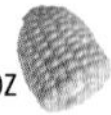

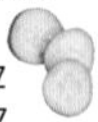

| Vegetables (Cont) | C | F | Cb |
|---|---|---|---|
| **Cactus Leaf (Nopales):** | | | |
| 1 leaf, 4.5 oz | 20 | 0 | 4 |
| 1 cup (slices), 3 oz | 15 | 0 | 3 |
| **Carrots**, regular thick variety: | | | |
| 1 small, 4 oz | 45 | 0 | 11 |
| 1 medium, 6 oz | 70 | 0 | 16 |
| 1 large, 8 oz | 95 | 0 | 22 |
| Chopped, 1 cup, 4.5 oz | 50 | 0 | 12 |
| Grated, 1 cup, 4 oz | 45 | 0 | 11 |
| Slices, 1 cup, 4.5 oz | 50 | 0 | 12 |
| Sticks (4"), 4-5, 1.5 oz | 20 | 0 | 4 |
| Long thin variety, 1 medium, 2.2 oz | 25 | 0 | 6 |
| Baby: Snack size, 3 medium, 1 oz | 10 | 0 | 2.5 |
| Snack Pack, 3 oz | 30 | 0 | 7 |
| **Cassava**, raw, 1 cup, 2.5 oz | 330 | 0.5 | 78 |
| **Cauliflower**, raw: Pieces, 1 cup, 3.5 oz | 25 | 0 | 5 |
| ½ medium head, 10 oz | 70 | 0 | 15 |
| Cooked, 3 florets, 2 oz | 10 | 0 | 2 |
| **Celeriac**, ½ cup, raw, 2.8 oz | 35 | 0 | 7 |
| **Celery:** 1 large stalk, 11", 2.2 oz | 10 | 0 | 2 |
| 4 Strips, thin sticks, 0.5 oz | 5 | 0 | 1 |
| Chopped, 1 cup, 3.5 oz | 15 | 0 | 3 |
| **Chard (Swiss)**, ½ cup, cooked, 3 oz | 20 | 0 | 3.5 |
| **Chayote Squash:** 1 medium, 7 oz | 40 | 0 | 9 |
| Pieces, 1 cup, 4.5 oz | 25 | 0 | 6 |
| **Chickpeas**, (Garbanzo Beans): | | | |
| Dry, 1 cup, 7 oz | 730 | 12 | 121 |
| Cooked, 1 cup, 5.8 oz | 270 | 4 | 45 |
| **Chicory Greens**, 1 cup, 1 oz | 7 | 0 | 1.5 |
| **Chili Peppers ~** See Peppers | | | |
| **Chinese Long Bean**, slices, 1 cup, 3.2 oz | 45 | 0 | 8 |
| **Chives**, chopped, 1 Tbsp | 1 | 0 | 0 |
| **Choy Sum**, 3 oz | 15 | 0 | 3 |
| **Cilantro**, (Coriander), 1 cup | 5 | 0 | 0.5 |
| **Collards**, cooked, ½ cup, 3 oz | 25 | 0 | 5 |
| **Corn**, Yellow/White: | | | |
| Raw: Kernels, ½ cup, 3 oz | 80 | 0.5 | 19 |
| Ear (5"x 1¾"), 5.5 oz | 155 | 1 | 37 |
| Cooked: Kernels, ½ cup, 3 oz | 77 | 0.5 | 18 |
| Cob, small, 2.3 oz | 60 | 0.5 | 14 |
| Ear, large, 5.5 oz | 120 | 1 | 28 |
| **Courgette ~** See Zucchini | | | |
| **Cowpeas ~** See Blackeye Peas | | | |
| **Cress**, garden, raw, 1 cup, 1.8 oz | 15 | 0 | 3 |
| **Cucumber**, average other flavors: | | | |
| Slices, ½ cup, 2 oz | 10 | 0 | 2 |
| Green, 1 medium (9"), 11 oz | 45 | 0 | 11 |
| Persian, 1 medium (8"), 6 oz | 25 | 0 | 5 |
| **Daikon Radish**, ½ cup, slices, 2 oz | 9 | 0 | 2 |
| **Dandelion Greens**, raw, ½ cup, 1 oz | 10 | 0 | 2.5 |
| **Edamame**, (Immature green soybeans): | | | |
| Shelled, ½ cup, 2.6 oz | 110 | 5 | 8 |
| With shells, 10 pods, 1.3 oz | 30 | 1 | 3 |

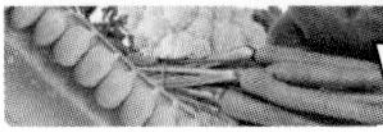

## Vegetables (Cont)

| | C | F | Cb |
|---|---|---|---|
| **Eggplant**, raw: 4 oz | 30 | 0 | 7 |
| ½ cup, 1" pieces, 1.5 oz | 10 | 0 | 2 |
| 1 slice, fried, 1 oz | 75 | 4 | 10 |
| **Endive**, Belgian/French: Raw, | | | |
| 1 medium head (6"), 2.5 oz | 12 | 0 | 3 |
| **Fennel**, 1 cup, sliced, 3 oz | 25 | 0 | 7 |
| **Gai Choy Cabbage**, cooked, 1 cup, 6 oz | 20 | 0 | 3 |
| **Gai Lan**, (Chinese Kale), cooked, 1 cup | 35 | 0.5 | 7 |
| **Garbanzo Beans** ~ See Chick Peas | | | |
| **Garlic**, 1 clove | 4 | 0 | 1 |
| **Ginger**: ¼ cup slices, 1 oz | 20 | 0 | 5 |
| Crystallized (sugared), 7 pieces, 1.5 oz | 130 | 0 | 35 |
| **Horseradish**, raw, 1 pod, 0.5 oz | 5 | 0 | 1 |
| **Jerusalem Artichoke**, raw, ½ cup | 55 | 0 | 13 |
| **Jicama**, raw, sliced, ½ cup, 2.3 oz | 25 | 0 | 6 |
| **Kale**, 1 cup, chopped, 2.5 oz | 35 | 0.5 | 7 |
| **Kohlrabi**, cooked, ½ cup, 1.8 oz | 17 | 0 | 5 |
| **Leek**, cooked, 1 whole, 4.5 oz | 40 | 0 | 9 |
| **Lentils**, green/brown: Dry, 1 oz | 100 | 0.5 | 17 |
| 1 cup, 6.8 oz | 675 | 3 | 115 |
| Cooked, ½ cup, 3.5 oz | 115 | 0.5 | 20 |
| **Lettuce:** 1 cup, chopped/shredded, 2 oz | 7 | 0 | 1 |
| Butterhead, 2 leaves, 0.5 oz | 2 | 0 | 0.5 |
| Cos/Romaine, shredded, 1 cup | 10 | 0 | 2 |
| Iceberg: 1 outer leaf, 0.5 oz | 2 | 0 | 0.5 |
| 1 medium head, 16 oz | 75 | 1 | 16 |
| **Lima Beans**, baby, cooked, ½ cup, 3 oz | 105 | 0 | 20 |
| **Lotus Root**, cooked, 10 slices, 3 oz | 60 | 0 | 14 |
| **Mung Bean Sprouts**, ½ cup, 2 oz | 15 | 0 | 3 |
| **Mushrooms**, average all varieties: | | | |
| Raw, diced/sliced, 1 cup, 3 oz | 20 | 0 | 3 |
| Pieces, 1 cup, 1.3 oz | 8 | 0 | 1 |
| Fried/Sauteed, 6 oz | 220 | 16 | 10 |
| Grilled, pieces, ½ cup, 2.5 oz | 20 | 0.5 | 4 |
| Shitake, dried, 1 oz package | 90 | 0 | 22 |
| **Mustard Greens**, raw, ½ cup, 1 oz | 7 | 0 | 2 |
| **Okra:** Raw, 8 pods, 4 oz | 30 | 0 | 7 |
| Cooked, ½ cup, 2.8 oz | 20 | 0 | 4 |
| **Onions:** Raw, 1 small, 2.5 oz | 30 | 0 | 7 |
| 1 medium, 4 oz | 50 | 0 | 11 |
| 1 large, 5.5 oz | 65 | 0 | 15 |
| 1 jumbo, 16 oz | 190 | 0.5 | 46 |
| Chopped: ½ cup, 3 oz | 35 | 0 | 8 |
| 1 Tbsp, 0.4 oz | 5 | 0 | 1 |
| Slices: 1 cup, 4 oz | 50 | 0 | 12 |
| 1 medium slice (⅛"), 0.5 oz | 5 | 0 | 1 |
| 1 large slice (¼"), 1.3 oz | 15 | 0 | 4 |
| Flakes, dried ⁄4 cup, 0.5 oz | 50 | 0 | 12 |
| Rings, breaded & fried, 2 rings | 80 | 5 | 9 |
| Scallions, ½ cup, 2 oz | 15 | 0 | 3 |
| Spring, chopped, ½ cup, 2 oz | 15 | 0 | 3 |

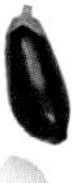

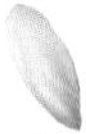

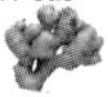

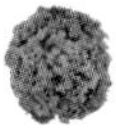

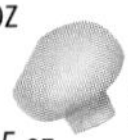

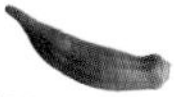

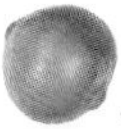

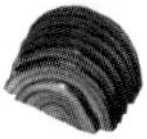

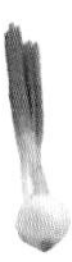

## Vegetables (Cont)

| | C | F | Cb |
|---|---|---|---|
| **Parsley**, chopped, ½ cup, 1 oz | 10 | 0 | 2 |
| **Parsnip:** 1 medium, 4 oz | 85 | 0 | 20 |
| Cooked, slices, ½ cup, 2.8 oz | 55 | 0 | 13 |
| **Peas:** Green, raw, ¼ cup, 1.5 oz | 30 | 0 | 5 |
| With pods, 0.5 lb | 70 | 0 | 13 |
| Snow Peas, 10 pods, 1.2 oz | 15 | 0 | 3 |
| Split: Dry, hulled, 1 oz | 100 | 0.5 | 17 |
| Cooked, 1 cup, 7 oz | 230 | 1 | 42 |
| **Peppers:** | | | |
| Sweet, 1 medium, 4.2 oz | 30 | 0 | 7 |
| Bell: 1 medium, 4.2 oz | 30 | 0 | 7 |
| raw, chopped, ½ cup, 2.5 oz | 20 | 0 | 5 |
| 2 rings (5" diam. x ¼" thick) | 3 | 0 | 1 |
| Chili: Green/Red, 1.5 oz | 20 | 0 | 5 |
| Habanero, 1 only, 0.3 oz | 10 | 0 | 2 |
| **Pigeon Peas**, cooked, ½ cup, 3 oz | 95 | 1 | 17 |
| **Pimientos**, 3 medium, 3.5 oz | 25 | 0 | 5 |
| **Poi**, ½ cup, 4.2 oz | 135 | 0 | 33 |
| **Potatoes:** | | | |
| Raw (with skin): | | | |
| 1 baby, 2 oz | 45 | 0 | 10 |
| 1 small, 6 oz | 135 | 0 | 30 |
| 1 medium, 8 oz | 180 | 0 | 40 |
| 1 large, 12 oz | 270 | 0 | 60 |
| 1 extra large, 16 oz | 360 | 0 | 80 |
| Baked, (no added fat), large, 10 oz (raw wt): | | | |
| Plain: With skin, 7 oz (cooked wt) | 185 | 0 | 42 |
| W/o skin, 5.5 oz (cooked wt) | 145 | 0 | 34 |
| With Skin/Toppings: | | | |
| With 2 tsp fat | 270 | 8 | 58 |
| With Grated Cheese, 1 oz | 370 | 9 | 58 |
| With Plain Yogurt, 2 Tbsp | 260 | 1 | 60 |
| With Sour Crm & Chives, 2 Tbsp | 320 | 6 | 60 |
| Mashed: | | | |
| With milk plus fat, ½ cup, 4 oz | 120 | 4.5 | 18 |
| KFC Style without gravy, 4 oz | 90 | 3 | 15 |
| Loaded (fat/cream/cheese/bacon): | | | |
| Side serving, 6 oz | 180 | 9 | 22 |
| Large serving, 12 oz | 360 | 18 | 44 |
| Potato Skins, baked w/ cheese topping, | | | |
| ½ whole, 4 oz | 240 | 13 | 22 |
| French Fries: Small serving, 2.6 oz | 250 | 13 | 30 |
| Medium serving, 4 oz | 380 | 20 | 47 |
| Frozen, uncooked, 18 fries, 4 oz | 165 | 5.5 | 28 |
| Oven-heated, 18 fries, 4 oz | 165 | 5.5 | 28 |
| Take-Out, 1 cup, 5 oz | 440 | 25 | 60 |
| Au Gratin, ½ cup, 4.3 oz | 160 | 9 | 14 |
| Pancakes, 2 small, 2 oz | 120 | 6.5 | 12 |
| Puffs, fried, 4 puffs, 1 oz | 55 | 2.5 | 8 |
| Scalloped, 8.5 oz | 220 | 9 | 26 |

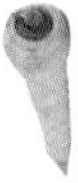

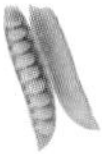

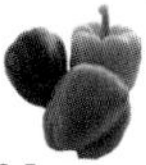

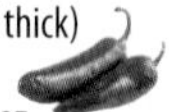

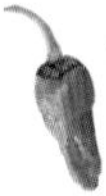

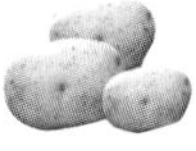

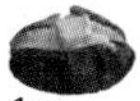

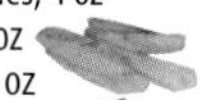

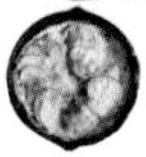

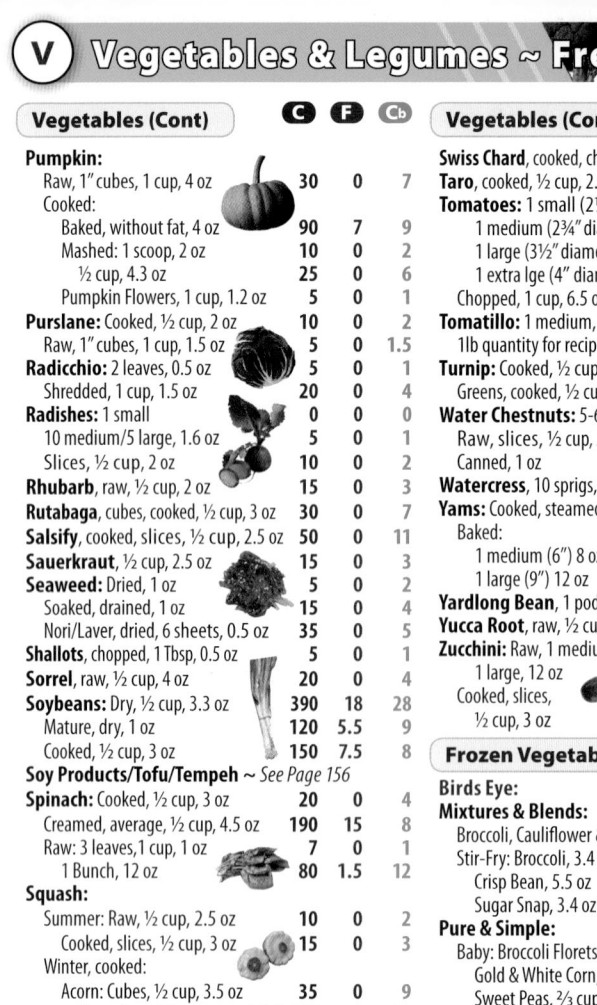

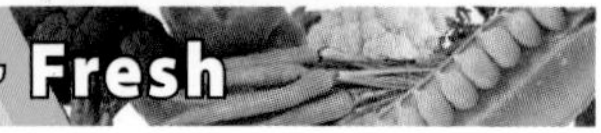

## Vegetables (Cont) — C F Cb

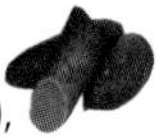

| | C | F | Cb |
|---|---|---|---|
| **Pumpkin:** | | | |
| Raw, 1" cubes, 1 cup, 4 oz | 30 | 0 | 7 |
| Cooked: | | | |
| Baked, without fat, 4 oz | 90 | 7 | 9 |
| Mashed: 1 scoop, 2 oz | 10 | 0 | 2 |
| ½ cup, 4.3 oz | 25 | 0 | 6 |
| Pumpkin Flowers, 1 cup, 1.2 oz | 5 | 0 | 1 |
| **Purslane:** Cooked, ½ cup, 2 oz | 10 | 0 | 2 |
| Raw, 1" cubes, 1 cup, 1.5 oz | 5 | 0 | 1.5 |
| **Radicchio:** 2 leaves, 0.5 oz | 5 | 0 | 1 |
| Shredded, 1 cup, 1.5 oz | 20 | 0 | 4 |
| **Radishes:** 1 small | 0 | 0 | 0 |
| 10 medium/5 large, 1.6 oz | 5 | 0 | 1 |
| Slices, ½ cup, 2 oz | 10 | 0 | 2 |
| **Rhubarb,** raw, ½ cup, 2 oz | 15 | 0 | 3 |
| **Rutabaga,** cubes, cooked, ½ cup, 3 oz | 30 | 0 | 7 |
| **Salsify,** cooked, slices, ½ cup, 2.5 oz | 50 | 0 | 11 |
| **Sauerkraut,** ½ cup, 2.5 oz | 15 | 0 | 3 |
| **Seaweed:** Dried, 1 oz | 5 | 0 | 2 |
| Soaked, drained, 1 oz | 15 | 0 | 4 |
| Nori/Laver, dried, 6 sheets, 0.5 oz | 35 | 0 | 5 |
| **Shallots,** chopped, 1 Tbsp, 0.5 oz | 5 | 0 | 1 |
| **Sorrel,** raw, ½ cup, 4 oz | 20 | 0 | 4 |
| **Soybeans:** Dry, ½ cup, 3.3 oz | 390 | 18 | 28 |
| Mature, dry, 1 oz | 120 | 5.5 | 9 |
| Cooked, ½ cup, 3 oz | 150 | 7.5 | 8 |
| **Soy Products/Tofu/Tempeh ~** *See Page 156* | | | |
| **Spinach:** Cooked, ½ cup, 3 oz | 20 | 0 | 4 |
| Creamed, average, ½ cup, 4.5 oz | 190 | 15 | 8 |
| Raw: 3 leaves, 1 cup, 1 oz | 7 | 0 | 1 |
| 1 Bunch, 12 oz | 80 | 1.5 | 12 |
| **Squash:** | | | |
| Summer: Raw, ½ cup, 2.5 oz | 10 | 0 | 2 |
| Cooked, slices, ½ cup, 3 oz | 15 | 0 | 3 |
| Winter, cooked: | | | |
| Acorn: Cubes, ½ cup, 3.5 oz | 35 | 0 | 9 |
| ½ medium (10 oz raw weight) | 115 | 0 | 30 |
| Butternut: Cubes, ½ cup, 3.5 oz | 40 | 0 | 10 |
| ¼ medium (9 oz raw weight) | 115 | 0 | 30 |
| Spaghetti, ½ cup, 1.8 oz | 15 | 0 | 3 |
| **Succotash,** cooked, ½ cup, 3.3 oz | 110 | 1 | 23 |
| **Sweetcorn ~** *See Corn* | | | |
| **Sweet Potatoes:** | | | |
| Cooked with skin (w/o fat), | | | |
| 1 medium, 4 oz | 105 | 0 | 24 |
| Without skin, mashed, ½ cup, 5.5 oz | 125 | 0 | 29 |
| Fries (Alexia, Julienne syle), | | | |
| approximately 12 pieces, 3 oz | 140 | 5 | 24 |

## Vegetables (Cont) — C F Cb

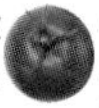

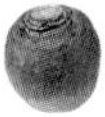

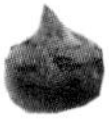

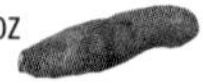

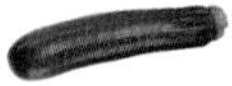

| | C | F | Cb |
|---|---|---|---|
| **Swiss Chard,** cooked, chopped, 1 c., 6 oz | 35 | 0 | 7 |
| **Taro,** cooked, ½ cup, 2.3 oz | 95 | 0 | 23 |
| **Tomatoes:** 1 small (2¼" diam.), 3 oz | 15 | 0 | 3 |
| 1 medium (2¾" diameter), 5 oz | 25 | 0 | 5 |
| 1 large (3½" diameter), 8 oz | 40 | 0.5 | 9 |
| 1 extra lge (4" diam.), 12 oz | 60 | 0.5 | 14 |
| Chopped, 1 cup, 6.5 oz | 35 | 0.5 | 7 |
| **Tomatillo:** 1 medium, 1.2 oz | 10 | 0 | 2 |
| 1lb quantity for recipe | 135 | 4.5 | 27 |
| **Turnip:** Cooked, ½ cup, 2.8 oz | 15 | 0 | 4 |
| Greens, cooked, ½ cup, 2.5 oz | 15 | 0 | 3 |
| **Water Chestnuts:** 5-6 nuts, 1 oz | 56 | 0.5 | 13 |
| Raw, slices, ½ cup, 2.3 oz | 60 | 0 | 15 |
| Canned, 1 oz | 15 | 0 | 3 |
| **Watercress,** 10 sprigs, 1 oz | 3 | 0 | 0.5 |
| **Yams:** Cooked, steamed, ½ cup, 2.5 oz | 80 | 0 | 19 |
| Baked: | | | |
| 1 medium (6") 8 oz | 265 | 0.5 | 63 |
| 1 large (9") 12 oz | 400 | 0.5 | 94 |
| **Yardlong Bean,** 1 pod, 0.5 oz | 5 | 0 | 1 |
| **Yucca Root,** raw, ½ cup, 3.5 oz | 165 | 0 | 39 |
| **Zucchini:** Raw, 1 medium, 7 oz | 30 | 0.5 | 7 |
| 1 large, 12 oz | 60 | 1 | 12 |
| Cooked, slices, | | | |
| ½ cup, 3 oz | 15 | 0 | 4 |

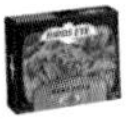

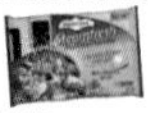

## Frozen Vegetables

| | C | F | Cb |
|---|---|---|---|
| **Birds Eye:** | | | |
| **Mixtures & Blends:** | | | |
| Broccoli, Cauliflower & Carrots, 3 oz | 35 | 0 | 5.5 |
| Stir-Fry: Broccoli, 3.4 oz | 35 | 0 | 6 |
| Crisp Bean, 5.5 oz | 60 | 0 | 11 |
| Sugar Snap, 3.4 oz | 40 | 0 | 7.5 |
| **Pure & Simple:** | | | |
| Baby: Broccoli Florets, 1 cup, 3 oz | 35 | 0.5 | 5 |
| Gold & White Corn, ⅔ cup, 3.2 oz | 105 | 1 | 22 |
| Sweet Peas, ⅔ cup, 3 oz | 80 | 0 | 14 |
| **Recipe Ready:** | | | |
| Chopped Green Peppers & Onions, 2.8 oz | 25 | 0 | 5 |
| Southwest Blend, 3.3 oz | 80 | 0.5 | 15 |
| **Sauced & Seasoned:** *Per 1 Cup* | | | |
| Green Beans & Spaetzle, | | | |
| in Bavarian Sauce | 95 | 4.5 | 10 |
| Pasta & Veggies in Creamy Cheese Sauce | 125 | 3 | 20 |
| **Steamfresh:** | | | |
| Pure & Simple Blends: | | | |
| Baby Broccoli Blend, 1 cup | 65 | 1.5 | 8 |
| Baby Potato Blend, ¾ cup | 50 | 0 | 10 |
| Brocc. & Cauliflower, 1 cup, 3.4 oz | 30 | 0.5 | 4.5 |

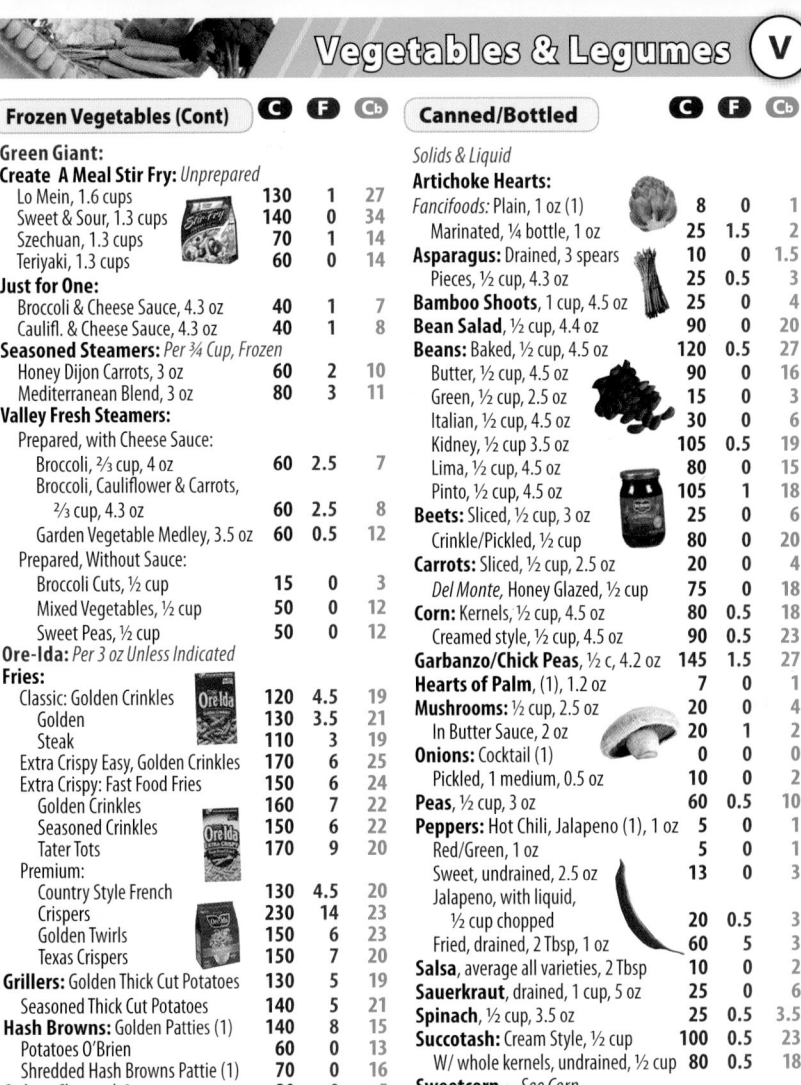

### Frozen Vegetables (Cont) — C F Cb

**Green Giant:**

**Create A Meal Stir Fry:** *Unprepared*

| | C | F | Cb |
|---|---|---|---|
| Lo Mein, 1.6 cups | 130 | 1 | 27 |
| Sweet & Sour, 1.3 cups | 140 | 0 | 34 |
| Szechuan, 1.3 cups | 70 | 1 | 14 |
| Teriyaki, 1.3 cups | 60 | 0 | 14 |

**Just for One:**

| | | | |
|---|---|---|---|
| Broccoli & Cheese Sauce, 4.3 oz | 40 | 1 | 7 |
| Caulifl. & Cheese Sauce, 4.3 oz | 40 | 1 | 8 |

**Seasoned Steamers:** *Per ¾ Cup, Frozen*

| | | | |
|---|---|---|---|
| Honey Dijon Carrots, 3 oz | 60 | 2 | 10 |
| Mediterranean Blend, 3 oz | 80 | 3 | 11 |

**Valley Fresh Steamers:**

Prepared, with Cheese Sauce:

| | | | |
|---|---|---|---|
| Broccoli, ⅔ cup, 4 oz | 60 | 2.5 | 7 |
| Broccoli, Cauliflower & Carrots, ⅔ cup, 4.3 oz | 60 | 2.5 | 8 |
| Garden Vegetable Medley, 3.5 oz | 60 | 0.5 | 12 |

Prepared, Without Sauce:

| | | | |
|---|---|---|---|
| Broccoli Cuts, ½ cup | 15 | 0 | 3 |
| Mixed Vegetables, ½ cup | 50 | 0 | 12 |
| Sweet Peas, ½ cup | 50 | 0 | 12 |

**Ore-Ida:** *Per 3 oz Unless Indicated*

**Fries:**

| | | | |
|---|---|---|---|
| Classic: Golden Crinkles | 120 | 4.5 | 19 |
| Golden | 130 | 3.5 | 21 |
| Steak | 110 | 3 | 19 |
| Extra Crispy Easy, Golden Crinkles | 170 | 6 | 25 |
| Extra Crispy: Fast Food Fries | 150 | 6 | 24 |
| Golden Crinkles | 160 | 7 | 22 |
| Seasoned Crinkles | 150 | 6 | 22 |
| Tater Tots | 170 | 9 | 20 |
| Premium: | | | |
| Country Style French | 130 | 4.5 | 20 |
| Crispers | 230 | 14 | 23 |
| Golden Twirls | 150 | 6 | 23 |
| Texas Crispers | 150 | 7 | 20 |

| | | | |
|---|---|---|---|
| **Grillers:** Golden Thick Cut Potatoes | 130 | 5 | 19 |
| Seasoned Thick Cut Potatoes | 140 | 5 | 21 |
| **Hash Browns:** Golden Patties (1) | 140 | 8 | 15 |
| Potatoes O'Brien | 60 | 0 | 13 |
| Shredded Hash Browns Pattie (1) | 70 | 0 | 16 |
| **Onion:** Chopped, 3 oz | 20 | 0 | 5 |
| Gourmet Rings, 2.7 oz | 185 | 9 | 24 |
| Onion Ringers, 3 oz | 180 | 10 | 21 |

**Simply:** Cracked Pepper & Sea Salt,

| | | | |
|---|---|---|---|
| Country Style French Fries | 130 | 4.5 | 22 |
| Homestyle Wedges, all varieties | 120 | 3.5 | 20 |
| **Steam n' Mash**, Cut Russet, 3.5 oz | 70 | 0 | 16 |
| **Tater Tots:** Regular | 160 | 8 | 20 |
| Crispy Crowns | 170 | 10 | 19 |

### Canned/Bottled — C F Cb

*Solids & Liquid*

**Artichoke Hearts:**

*Fancifoods:* Plain, 1 oz (1) | 8 | 0 | 1

| | C | F | Cb |
|---|---|---|---|
| Marinated, ¼ bottle, 1 oz | 25 | 1.5 | 1 |
| **Asparagus:** Drained, 3 spears | 10 | 0 | 1.5 |
| Pieces, ½ cup, 4.3 oz | 25 | 0.5 | 3 |
| **Bamboo Shoots**, 1 cup, 4.5 oz | 25 | 0 | 4 |
| **Bean Salad**, ½ cup, 4.4 oz | 90 | 0 | 20 |
| **Beans:** Baked, ½ cup, 4.5 oz | 120 | 0.5 | 27 |
| Butter, ½ cup, 4.5 oz | 90 | 0 | 16 |
| Green, ½ cup, 2.5 oz | 15 | 0 | 3 |
| Italian, ½ cup, 4.5 oz | 30 | 0 | 6 |
| Kidney, ½ cup 3.5 oz | 105 | 0.5 | 19 |
| Lima, ½ cup, 4.5 oz | 80 | 0 | 15 |
| Pinto, ½ cup, 4.5 oz | 105 | 1 | 18 |
| **Beets:** Sliced, ½ cup, 3 oz | 25 | 0 | 6 |
| Crinkle/Pickled, ½ cup | 80 | 0 | 20 |
| **Carrots:** Sliced, ½ cup, 2.5 oz | 20 | 0 | 4 |
| *Del Monte*, Honey Glazed, ½ cup | 75 | 0 | 18 |
| **Corn:** Kernels, ½ cup, 4.5 oz | 80 | 0.5 | 18 |
| Creamed style, ½ cup, 4.5 oz | 90 | 0.5 | 23 |
| **Garbanzo/Chick Peas**, ½ c, 4.2 oz | 145 | 1.5 | 27 |
| **Hearts of Palm**, (1), 1.2 oz | 7 | 0 | 1 |
| **Mushrooms:** ½ cup, 2.5 oz | 20 | 0 | 4 |
| In Butter Sauce, 2 oz | 20 | 1 | 2 |
| **Onions:** Cocktail (1) | 0 | 0 | 0 |
| Pickled, 1 medium, 0.5 oz | 10 | 0 | 2 |
| **Peas**, ½ cup, 3 oz | 60 | 0.5 | 10 |
| **Peppers:** Hot Chili, Jalapeno (1), 1 oz | 5 | 0 | 1 |
| Red/Green, 1 oz | 5 | 0 | 1 |
| Sweet, undrained, 2.5 oz | 13 | 0 | 3 |
| Jalapeno, with liquid, ½ cup chopped | 20 | 0.5 | 3 |
| Fried, drained, 2 Tbsp, 1 oz | 60 | 5 | 3 |
| **Salsa**, average all varieties, 2 Tbsp | 10 | 0 | 2 |
| **Sauerkraut**, drained, 1 cup, 5 oz | 25 | 0 | 6 |
| **Spinach**, ½ cup, 3.5 oz | 25 | 0.5 | 3.5 |
| **Succotash:** Cream Style, ½ cup | 100 | 0.5 | 23 |
| W/ whole kernels, undrained, ½ cup | 80 | 0.5 | 18 |
| **Sweetcorn ~** *See Corn* | | | |
| **Sweet Potato**, ½ cup, 3.5 oz | 90 | 0 | 24 |
| **Tomatoes**, Sundried: Nat., 5-6 pieces | 20 | 0 | 5 |
| In Oil, drained, 6 pieces, 0.5 oz | 40 | 2.5 | 4 |
| **Tomato Products ~** *See Page 144* | | | |
| **Vegetables**, mixed, ½ cup, 4 oz | 45 | 0 | 8 |
| **Yams:** In Light Syrup, ½ cup, 4 oz | 105 | 0 | 25 |
| Candied, ½ cup, 5 oz | 170 | 0 | 46 |
| **Zucchini**, in Tomato Sauce, ½ cup, 4 oz | 30 | 0 | 8 |

## Quick Guide

**C**  **F**  **Cb**

**Yogurt:** *Average All Brands: Per 8 oz Container*

| | C | F | Cb |
|---|---|---|---|
| **Plain Yogurt:** Whole | 140 | 8 | 10 |
| Low-Fat | 145 | 3.5 | 16 |
| Fat-Free | 125 | 0.5 | 17 |
| **Fruit Flavored:** Whole | 225 | 8 | 32 |
| Low-Fat | 230 | 3 | 43 |
| Fat-Free, regular | 215 | 0.5 | 43 |
| Fat-Free, no sugar added | 80 | 0 | 15 |
| **Yogurt Parfait/Deli Cups:** | | | |
| **With Fruit Pieces:** (⅔ Yogurt + ⅓ Fruit) | | | |
| Small, 8 oz cup | 140 | 3 | 20 |
| Large, 12 oz cup | 210 | 4.5 | 30 |
| **With Fruit + Granola:** | | | |
| Small, 8 oz cup (+ 0.75 oz Granola) | 235 | 7 | 30 |
| Large, 12 oz cup (+ 1.3 oz Granola) | 400 | 13 | 58 |

## Yogurt ~ Brands

| | C | F | Cb |
|---|---|---|---|
| **Activia:** *Per 4 oz Container Unless Indicated* | | | |
| Fiber with Fruit, average | 110 | 2 | 20 |
| Light flavors, fat free, all flav. | 60 | 0 | 10 |
| Greek: Av. all flavors, 5.3 oz | 130 | 0 | 20 |
| Light, Fruit/Vanilla, av., 5.3 oz | 80 | 0 | 8 |
| **Almond Dream** *(Non Dairy): Per 6 oz Container* | | | |
| **Low-Fat:** Plain | 150 | 3 | 30 |
| Mixed Berry; Strawberry; Vanilla | 160 | 3 | 33 |
| **Alpina:** | | | |
| **Greek**, Non-Fat, av., 5.3 oz | 125 | 0 | 19 |
| **Artisan Granolas**, av., 6 oz | 200 | 4 | 29 |
| **All-Stars:** | | | |
| Cookies & Cream, 4 oz | 120 | 2 | 21 |
| Choc. Mini Gems, 4 oz | 120 | 3 | 21 |
| Dunkers, 4 oz | 130 | 3 | 20 |
| **Cafe Selections**, av. 5.3oz | 120 | 0 | 18 |
| **Amande:** | | | |
| **Almond Milk Yogurt:** Plain, 8 oz | 170 | 9 | 19 |
| Fruit Flavors, 6 oz | 150 | 6 | 23 |
| Vanilla, 8 oz | 220 | 8 | 26 |
| **Axelrod:** | | | |
| **Plain**, (32 oz Ctn): Regular, 8 oz | 160 | 8 | 15 |
| Low Fat, Plain, 8 oz | 140 | 2.5 | 18 |
| Nonfat, Plain, 8 oz | 140 | 0 | 21 |
| **6 oz Containers:** | | | |
| Low Fat, Fruit flavors, average | 180 | 1.5 | 36 |
| NonFat, Fruit flavors, average | 90 | 0 | 17 |
| **Brown Cow:** *Per 6 oz Container* | | | |
| **Cream Top Fruit On Bottom:** | | | |
| Apricot Mango | 170 | 6 | 23 |
| Cherry-Vanilla; Strawb. | 180 | 6 | 28 |
| Chocolate | 190 | 6 | 28 |
| **Cream Top Smooth & Creamy:** | | | |
| Plain | 130 | 7 | 9 |
| Average other flavors | 165 | 7 | 20 |
| **Greek:** Fruit On Bottom, av. | 125 | 0 | 19 |
| Smooth & Creamy, Plain, nonfat | 125 | 0 | 19 |

| | C | F | Cb |
|---|---|---|---|
| **Cabot:** *Per 8 oz Serving* | | | |
| **Greek Style**, 32 oz Containers: Plain | 310 | 22 | 12 |
| Lowfat (2%): Plain | 180 | 5 | 12 |
| Strawberry; Vanilla Bean | 240 | 4 | 34 |
| **Chobani Greek Yogurt:** *Per 5.3 oz Containers* | | | |
| **Ancient Grains**, average | 170 | 2 | 27 |
| **Blended:** Coconut | 150 | 4.5 | 16 |
| Coffee | 160 | 2.5 | 23 |
| Fruit Flavors, average | 145 | 3 | 17 |
| **Plain:** Whole Milk | 130 | 6 | 7 |
| Non Fat | 90 | 0 | 7 |
| **Flip:** Almond Coco Loco | 240 | 10 | 26 |
| Coffee Break; PB Dream, av. | 200 | 6 | 26 |
| **Fruit On The Bottom:** | | | |
| 2% Fat, Fruit Flavors, av. | 140 | 3 | 18 |
| Fat Free, Fruit Flavors, av. | 125 | 0 | 20 |
| **Indulgent:** Cherry & Dark Choc, 3.5 oz | 120 | 5 | 13 |
| Other Flavors, av., 3.5 oz | 140 | 6 | 14 |
| **Kids:** 3.5 oz pouch | 100 | 2 | 12 |
| 2 oz Tube, all flavors | 50 | 1 | 7 |
| **Oats**, av. all flavors, 5.3 oz | 170 | 2 | 27 |
| **Simply 100:** Fruit flav., av., | 100 | 0 | 15 |
| Crunch, average | 100 | 1.5 | 15 |
| **Coconut Dream** *(Non Dairy): Per 6 oz Container* | | | |
| **Regular:** Plain | 120 | 4 | 24 |
| **Low-Fat:** Blueb.; Raspb. | 130 | 3 | 28 |
| Strawberry; Vanilla, av. | 130 | 3 | 28 |
| **Dannon:** | | | |
| **Activia** ~ *See Activia* | | | |
| **All Natural:** Plain, reg., 8 oz | 150 | 8 | 11 |
| Lowfat, 6 oz | 100 | 2.5 | 12 |
| Nonfat, 6 oz | 80 | 0 | 12 |
| **Classic**, Coffee; Van., av., 6 oz | 155 | 2.5 | 26 |
| **Danimals:** Nonfat, Strawberry, 4 oz | 80 | 0 | 16 |
| Greek, all flavors, 4 oz | 110 | 1.5 | 15 |
| Squeezables, all flavors, 1 Pouch, 4 oz | 100 | 1.5 | 18 |
| **Fruit On The Bottom**, | | | |
| av. all flavors, 6 oz | 150 | 1.5 | 29 |
| **Light & Fit:** | | | |
| 50-Calorie Packs, av. all flavors, 4 oz | 50 | 0 | 9 |
| Regular: 6 oz Cup, average all flavors | 80 | 0 | 14 |
| Quarts Cont., av. all flavors, 8 oz | 105 | 0 | 19 |
| Greek, all flavors, 5.3 oz cup | 80 | 0 | 9 |
| Carb & Sugar Control, 4- Pack, 4 0z | 45 | 1.5 | 3 |
| **Fage:** | | | |
| **Crossovers:** | | | |
| Coconut w/ Dark Choc, 5.3 oz | 220 | 7 | 26 |
| Maple Syrup w/ Granola, 5.3 oz | 190 | 5 | 21 |
| **Fruyo Greek:** Reg., av. all flav., 6 oz | 195 | 7 | 20 |
| Fat free, av. all flavors, 6 oz | 140 | 0 | 21 |
| **Total Classic:** Plain, Single Serve, 7 oz | 190 | 10 | 8 |
| Split Cup, Fruit Flavors, 5.3 oz | 170 | 6 | 17 |

## Yogurt Brands (Cont)

| | C | F | Cb |
|---|---|---|---|
| **Fage (Cont):** | | | |
| **Total 2%:** Plain, Single Serve, 7 oz | 150 | 4 | 8 |
| Split Cup, Fruit Flavors, 5.3 oz | 140 | 2.5 | 17 |
| **Total 0%:** Plain, 6 oz | 100 | 0 | 7 |
| Split Cup, Fruit Flavors, 5.3 oz | 120 | 0 | 17 |
| **Great Value** (Walmart): | | | |
| **Original**, average: 6 oz ctn | 150 | 1.5 | 29 |
| 32 oz ctn, 8 oz | 200 | 2 | 38 |
| **Plain**, 0% fat, 32 oz ct, 8 oz | 120 | 0 | 18 |
| **Light/Nonfat**, av. all flav., 6 oz ctn | 80 | 0 | 15 |
| **Greek:** Blueberry, fat free, 5.3 oz ctn | 140 | 0 | 21 |
| Plain, Nonfat, 32oz ctn, 8 oz | 120 | 0 | 9 |
| Blends, Toasted Coconut Vanilla, 6 oz | 160 | 4.5 | 20 |
| **Horizon Organic:** Per 8 oz Cup | | | |
| **Cream On Top:** | | | |
| Whole Milk: Plain | 170 | 8 | 16 |
| Vanilla | 230 | 6 | 33 |
| **Fat-Free:** Plain | 110 | 0 | 17 |
| Vanilla | 190 | 0 | 35 |
| **Tuberz**, all flavors, 1 tube | 60 | 0.5 | 11 |
| **Kemps:** | | | |
| **Greek Style:** | | | |
| Fat Free: Vanilla, 5.3 oz | 140 | 0 | 22 |
| Average Fruit Flavors, 5.3 oz | 130 | 0 | 18 |
| Snack Mousse, all flavors, 4.8 oz | 190 | 2.5 | 31 |
| **Light**, 80 Calories, av. all flav., 6 oz | 80 | 0 | 16 |
| **La Yogurt:** Per 6 oz Container | | | |
| **Low Fat:** Original, av. | 155 | 1.5 | 29 |
| Rich & Creamy, av. | 180 | 1.5 | 35 |
| **Sabor Latino**, Low Fat, av. | 185 | 1.5 | 37 |
| **LALA:** | | | |
| **32 oz Tubs**, Plain, 8 oz | 130 | 2.5 | 17 |
| **Single Serve:** | | | |
| Fruit Flavors, av., 6 oz | 150 | 1.5 | 30 |
| Pina Colada, 6 oz | 160 | 2 | 30 |
| **Lucerne:** Per 6 oz Container | | | |
| **Low-Fat**, av. all flavors | 170 | 2 | 32 |
| **Fat-Free:** Plain | 80 | 0 | 13 |
| Light Fat-Free, fruit, 6 oz | 90 | 0 | 18 |
| **Mountain High:** Per 8 oz | | | |
| **32 oz Containers:** | | | |
| Original Style: Plain | 170 | 6 | 19 |
| Vanilla | 200 | 6 | 28 |
| Lowfat: Plain | 140 | 2.5 | 18 |
| Honey; Vanilla | 185 | 2.5 | 30 |
| Fat-Free: Plain | 120 | 0 | 18 |
| Vanilla | 160 | 0 | 30 |
| **Nancy's:** | | | |
| **Natural:** Per 8 oz Container | | | |
| Whole Milk: Honey Yogurt, Plain | 180 | 8 | 17 |
| With Fruit on Top, av. | 235 | 5 | 40 |
| Lowfat: Lemon; Van., av. | 145 | 3 | 16 |
| Average other flavors | 175 | 2.5 | 28 |

## Nancy's (Cont):

| | C | F | Cb |
|---|---|---|---|
| **Organic:** Per 8 oz Unless Indicated | | | |
| Whole Milk, Plain | 175 | 8 | 15 |
| Low Fat, Plain | 140 | 3 | 16 |
| Nonfat: Fruit-On-Top | 150 | 0 | 28 |
| Maple; Vanilla, 6 oz | 120 | 0 | 21 |
| **Oikos** (Dannon): Per 5.3 oz Container | | | |
| **Chocolate On Top:** Raspberry Truffle | 150 | 4 | 18 |
| Choc. Covered Strawberry | 210 | 4.5 | 32 |
| **Traditional**, Fruit flavors | 160 | 4.5 | 19 |
| **Triple Zero**, all flavors | 120 | 0 | 15 |
| **Non-Fat Yogurt:** Plain, 5.3 oz | 80 | 0 | 14 |
| Fruit On Bottom, av., 5.3 oz | 130 | 0 | 21 |
| **O Organics**, Blended Low-Fat, av. 8 oz | 160 | 2.5 | 26 |
| **Publix:** Fat Free, Light, av., 6 oz | 110 | 0 | 18 |
| Premium Greek, av., 5.3 oz | 130 | 0 | 18 |
| **Schnucks,** Light/Nonfat, av., 6 oz | 110 | 0 | 20 |
| **Siggi's:** 0%: Plain, 5.3 oz | 80 | 0 | 5 |
| Fruit Flavors, av., 5.3 oz | 110 | 0 | 12 |
| Vanilla, 5.3 oz | 100 | 0 | 11 |
| **2%:** Coconut, 5.3 oz | 190 | 8 | 17 |
| Fruit Flavors, av., 5.3 oz | 140 | 2.5 | 15 |
| **4%:** Plain, 4.4 oz | 140 | 2.5 | 15 |
| Mixed Berries; Lemon Zest, 4.4 oz | 120 | 5 | 9 |
| **Silk** (Dairy Free): Plain, 8 oz cup | 140 | 5 | 13 |
| Vanilla, 8 oz cup | 190 | 4 | 30 |
| Fruit flavors, 5.3 oz cup | 140 | 3.5 | 21 |
| **So Delicious:** | | | |
| **Cultured Almond Milk:** | | | |
| Chocolate, 6 oz | 150 | 6 | 24 |
| Vanilla, 6 oz | 120 | 5 | 18 |
| **Cultured Coconut Milk:** | | | |
| Plain, unsweetened, 4 oz | 50 | 4 | 6 |
| Blueberry, 4 oz | 140 | 6 | 24 |
| Greek: Plain, 5.3 oz | 130 | 5 | 22 |
| Vanilla, 6 oz | 140 | 4.5 | 27 |
| **Stonyfield Organic:** | | | |
| **Chocolate Underground**, 6 oz | 170 | 0 | 36 |
| **Fruit On Bottom**, av., 6 oz | 115 | 0 | 22 |
| **Greek:** Plain, 5.3 oz | 80 | 0 | 6 |
| Chocolate, 5.3 oz | 140 | 0 | 23 |
| Fruit Flavors, av., 5.3 oz | 120 | 0 | 19 |
| **Smooth & Creamy (32 oz Ctn):** | | | |
| Fat Free: Plain, 8 oz | 100 | 0 | 16 |
| French Vanilla, 8 oz | 170 | 0 | 33 |
| Low Fat: Plain, 8 oz | 120 | 2 | 15 |
| French Vanilla, 8 oz | 170 | 2 | 29 |
| **Stop & Shop:** | | | |
| **Greek:** Non-Fat Fruit flav., av., 5.3 oz | 130 | 0 | 20 |
| Vanilla, 8 oz | 160 | 0 | 21 |

## Yogurt Brands (Cont) — C F Cb

**Trader Joes:**

| | C | F | Cb |
|---|---|---|---|
| **Organic:** Banana; Vanilla, 4 oz | 100 | 3 | 15 |
| Cream Top, Whole Milk, Plain, 8 oz | 160 | 9 | 9 |
| Low Fat, Fruit Flavors, 6 oz cup | 145 | 2.5 | 25 |
| Nonfat: Plain + Vit D, 8 oz | 100 | 0 | 16 |
| Strawberry + Vit D, 4 oz | 90 | 0 | 17 |
| Vanilla, 5.3 oz cup | 120 | 0 | 16 |
| **Fruits & Cream**, average, 4 oz cup | 140 | 6 | 20 |
| **Low Fat**, Fruit Flavors, 8 oz | 220 | 3 | 40 |
| **European:** Lowfat, Choc./Mocha, 5.3 oz | 135 | 3 | 21 |
| Smth & Crmy: Whole Milk, Plain, 8 oz | 170 | 7 | 14 |
| Nonfat, Plain, 8 oz | 120 | 0 | 17 |
| **French Village:** Cream Line, Plain, 8 oz | 180 | 10 | 13 |
| Nonfat: Apricot Mango/Strawb., 6 oz | 130 | 0 | 25 |
| 32 oz Ctn, Plain, 8 oz | 120 | 0 | 17 |
| Vanilla, 6 oz cup | 130 | 0 | 26 |
| **Greek:** 2% Low Fat, Plain, 8 oz | 170 | 4.5 | 10 |
| Whole Milk: Plain, 8 oz | 280 | 22 | 12 |
| Apricot Mango; Honey, av., 8 oz | 300 | 18 | 27 |
| Strawberry Vanilla, 8 oz | 320 | 18 | 32 |
| 0% Non Fat: Plain, 8 oz | 120 | 0 | 7 |
| Fruit Flavors; Honey, 5.3 oz cup | 120 | 0 | 17 |
| Vanilla Bean, 5.3 oz cup | 130 | 0 | 20 |
| **Goats Milk**, Plain ¾ cup, 6 oz | 100 | 4.5 | 7 |
| **Voskos:** Original, Plain, 8 oz | 280 | 20 | 15 |
| **Fruit On Bottom, Nonfat:** 6 oz cup | 140 | 0 | 19 |
| 5.3 oz cup, average | 115 | 0 | 17 |
| **Greek:** 16 oz Ctn, Orig. Honey, 8 oz | 290 | 14 | 32 |
| Fat Free Honey , 5.3 oz cup | 120 | 0 | 17 |
| **Wallaby Organic, Blended,** | | | |
| Low-Fat, Fruit Flavors, average, 6 oz | 140 | 2.5 | 24 |
| **Wegmans:** Per 6 oz Container | | | |
| **Blended Lowfat**, Fruit Flavors | 170 | 1.5 | 33 |
| **Fruit On The Bottom, Lowfat:** | | | |
| Strawberry | 180 | 2 | 35 |
| Average other Fruit Flavors | 165 | 2 | 31 |
| **Greek**, Non-Fat: Plain | 90 | 0 | 8 |
| Fruit flavors, average | 140 | 0 | 20 |
| Vanilla Flavored | 120 | 0 | 15 |
| **Whole Foods (365):** | | | |
| **32 oz Ctn, Plain:** Whole Milk, 8oz | 160 | 9 | 13 |
| Low-Fat, 8 oz | 120 | 2 | 15 |
| Fat-Free, 8 oz | 120 | 0 | 17 |
| **6 oz Ctn:** Blueberry Lemon | 160 | 1.5 | 31 |
| Peach Melba | 140 | 1 | 27 |
| **Greek**, 0% Nonfat, Plain,  6 oz | | | |
| **Whole Soy:** Plain, 6 oz | 150 | 4.5 | 19 |
| Av. other flavors, 6 oz | 170 | 3.5 | 33 |
| **YoCrunch:** With Toppings | | | |
| **M&M's:** Strawb./Vanilla , av., 6 oz ctn | 190 | 4 | 33 |
| Banana/Strawb./Vanilla, av., 4 oz | 140 | 3 | 24 |
| Vanilla/Peanut/Butter, av., 4 oz ctn | 180 | 6 | 25 |
| **Snickers**, Vanilla, w/ pieces, 6 oz ctn | 180 | 4 | 31 |

## Yogurt Brands (Cont) — C F Cb

**Yoplait:**

| | C | F | Cb |
|---|---|---|---|
| **Original**, 25% less sugar | 150 | 2 | 25 |
| **Light:** Fruit flavors, 6 oz | 90 | 0 | 16 |
| Thick & Creamy, 6 oz | 100 | 0 | 21 |
| **Lactose Free**, all flavors, 6 oz | 170 | 1.5 | 33 |
| **GoGurt:** All flavors, | | | |
| 2.3 oz tube | 60 | 0.5 | 12 |
| **Greek:** Per 5.3 oz Carton | | | |
| 100 Calories, all flavors | 100 | 0 | 18 |
| 2% Fat, all flavors | 150 | 3 | 20 |
| **Plenti:** Fruit flavors, 5.5 oz | 140 | 1.5 | 21 |
| Oatmeal: Fruit flavors,  5.5 oz | 180 | 2 | 29 |
| Vanilla; Maple Brn Sugar, 5.5 oz | 170 | 2 | 28 |
| **Thick & Creamy**, av., 6 oz | 180 | 2.5 | 31 |
| **Trix**, all flavors, av., 4 oz cup | 100 | 0.5 | 20 |
| **Whips!:** Choc. flav., 4 oz | 160 | 4 | 25 |
| Fruit flavors, 4 oz cup | 140 | 2.5 | 25 |
| Greek 100, all flav., 4 oz | 100 | 0 | 15 |
| **Yoplait Kids:** All flavors, 3 oz cup | 70 | 1 | 12 |
| 4 oz Cups, all flavors | 100 | 0.5 | 20 |

## Yogurt Drinks & Probiotics

**Dannon:**

| | C | F | Cb |
|---|---|---|---|
| **Activia**, av. all flavors, 7 fl oz | 165 | 3 | 27 |
| **DanActive**, fruit flavors, 3.1 fl.oz | 70 | 1 | 14 |
| **Danimals Smoothies:** | | | |
| Av. all flavors, 3.1 fl.oz | 60 | 0 | 10 |
| Max, all flavors, 7 fl.oz | 120 | 1.5 | 23 |
| **Dan-o-nino**, all flav., 3.1 fl.oz | 70 | 0.5 | 15 |
| **Light & Fit**, Protein Shake, 10 fl.oz | 140 | 0 | 23 |
| **Glen Oaks,** av. all flavors, 8 fl.oz | 150 | 3 | 28 |
| **Kemps,** Smoothie To Go, | | | |
| average all flavors, 4 fl.oz | 105 | 1 | 18 |
| **LaLa:** | | | |
| **Lalacult**, 5-pack, 1 bottle | 35 | 0 | 9 |
| **Proactive:** Prune, 6.3 oz bottle | 180 | 3 | 36 |
| Average other flavors, 6.3 oz bottle | 155 | 3.5 | 30 |
| **Yogurt Smoothies**, fruit flav., 7 fl.oz | 175 | 4.5 | 29 |
| **Lifeway Kefir:** | | | |
| **Original**, 8 fl.oz | 150 | 8 | 12 |
| **Lowfat:** Plain, 8 fl.oz | 110 | 2 | 12 |
| Chocolate Truffle, 8 fl.oz | 160 | 2 | 25 |
| Other flavors, 8 fl.oz | 140 | 2 | 20 |
| **Stonyfield Organic:** | | | |
| **Smoothies**, av. all flav., 10 oz | 230 | 3 | 40 |
| **Yobaby**, av. all flavors, 6 oz | 185 | 7 | 24 |
| **Yakult:** Reg., 2.7 oz bottle | 50 | 0 | 12 |
| Light, 2.7 fl.oz | 30 | 0 | 6 |
| **Yoplait,** Yogurt & Juice, av., 8 fl.oz | 115 | 0 | 21 |

## Cafeteria-Style Foods — C F Cb

*Average All Preparations:*

| | C | F | Cb |
|---|---|---|---|
| **Beef Stroganoff**, 5 oz | 195 | 13 | 7 |
| **Beef Stroganoff**, with 4 oz noodles | 350 | 14 | 36 |
| **Chicken Lasagna**, 1 piece | 300 | 11 | 32 |
| **Chicken Chop Suey**, with 4 oz rice | 245 | 4 | 37 |
| **Deep Dish Burrito**, 7 oz | 265 | 13 | 20 |
| **Ground Beef Casserole**, 2 scps, 6 oz | 245 | 13 | 17 |
| **Italian Meat Sce**, for Spaghetti, 5 oz | 150 | 9 | 9 |
| with 5 oz Spaghetti | 350 | 10 | 49 |
| **Lasagna**, 1 piece | 275 | 11 | 25 |
| **Meatloaf**, 3 oz | 205 | 13 | 4 |
| **Ranch Beans**, 2 scoops, 6 oz | 350 | 11 | 45 |
| **Red Beans & Rice**, 7 oz | 280 | 9 | 37 |
| **Scalloped Potato/Ham**, 2 scoops, 6 oz | 160 | 6 | 20 |
| **Stuffed Shells in Sauce**, (1) | 105 | 3 | 17 |
| **Swedish Meatballs**, (3) | 205 | 12 | 9 |
| **Sweet & Sour Pork/Rice**, 9 oz | 240 | 3 | 40 |
| **Swiss Steak**, w/ Mushroom Gravy, 6 oz | 280 | 11 | 4 |
| **Tator Tot Casserole**, 2 scoops, 6 oz | 260 | 15 | 20 |
| **Tenderloin Tips/Mshrm Gravy:** 5 oz | 210 | 13 | 3 |
| With 5 oz noodles | 395 | 15 | 38 |
| **Tuna Noodle Casserole**, 2 scoops, 6 oz | 180 | 6 | 17 |
| **Turkey Tetrazzini**, 2 scoops, 6 oz | 195 | 7 | 17 |
| **Vegetable Lasagna**, 1 piece | 250 | 13 | 21 |

### Croissants

| | C | F | Cb |
|---|---|---|---|
| **Unfilled,** medium 1.5 oz | 180 | 10 | 21 |
| **Filled:** With Ham (2 oz), garnish | 280 | 14 | 24 |
| With Ham (2 oz), Cheese (2 oz) | 470 | 30 | 20 |
| With Chick (2 oz) Cheese (2 oz) | 470 | 30 | 20 |
| With Turkey/Ham/Cheese (2 oz ea.) | 580 | 36 | 20 |
| *Au Bon Pain:* Ham & Cheese | 390 | 21 | 35 |
| Spinach & Cheese | 290 | 17 | 28 |
| **7-Eleven** ~ *See Page 236* | | | |

### Bagels

| | C | F | Cb |
|---|---|---|---|
| **Plain:** Large, 4 oz (without filling) | 320 | 2 | 65 |
| With 2 oz Cream Cheese | 500 | 27 | 54 |
| With 2 oz Lox (Smoked Salmon) | 400 | 4 | 65 |
| **Also see Bagels Section** ~ *Page 54* | | | |
| **Fast-Foods Restaurants** ~ *Page 175* | | | |
| **Au Bon Pain** ~ *Page 179* | | | |
| **Bruegger's** ~ *Page 185* | | | |
| **Einstein Bros Bagels** ~ *Page 199* | | | |

## Sandwiches — C F Cb

*No Spreads Unless Indicated:*
*Includes 2 Slices Bread ~ 3 oz*

| | C | F | Cb |
|---|---|---|---|
| **BLT**, (5 strips Bacon, 2 Tbsp Mayo) | 600 | 40 | 46 |
| **Breaded Chicken & Garnish** | 540 | 28 | 46 |
| **Chicken Salad**, with Mayo., 5 oz | 580 | 30 | 49 |
| **Chopped Liver, Egg Mayonnaise** | 630 | 25 | 44 |
| **Corned Beef with Mustard**, 5 oz | 560 | 28 | 44 |
| **Egg Salad**, with Mayonnaise | 570 | 29 | 49 |
| **Egg Salad Club**, with Bacon & Mayo, | 780 | 53 | 49 |
| **Grilled Cheese**, (3 oz) | 540 | 30 | 44 |
| **Ham**, (4 oz), Cheese (4 oz), & Mayo. | 910 | 56 | 44 |
| **Lobster Salad**, (4 oz), w/ Mayo. | 530 | 25 | 45 |
| **Overstuffed Tuna Salad**, (7 oz) | 870 | 39 | 75 |
| **Philly Cheese Steak Sandwich** | 550 | 23 | 42 |
| **Reuben**, (6 oz Beef/Pastrami, 2 oz Cheese, 2 Tbsp Dressing) | 920 | 60 | 28 |
| **Roast Beef**, (4 oz), with Mustard | 460 | 12 | 45 |
| **Roast Pork**, (4 oz), with Apple Sauce | 500 | 16 | 55 |
| **Shrimp Salad Club**, w/ Bacon & Mayo | 800 | 57 | 48 |
| **Sloppy Joe with Sauce**, (7 oz) | 600 | 30 | 45 |
| **Steak Sandwich**, (5 oz cooked) | 680 | 32 | 41 |
| **Triple Cheese Melt**, (4 oz) | 720 | 45 | 46 |
| **Tuna Salad**, (5 oz), with Mayonnaise | 610 | 30 | 49 |
| **Turkey Breast**, (5 oz), w/ Mayo. | 460 | 18 | 44 |
| **Turkey Breast**, (5 oz,) with Mustard | 360 | 7 | 44 |
| **Turkey Club**, with Bacon & Mayo. | 830 | 38 | 31 |
| **Vegetarian**, with Avocado & Cheese | 820 | 49 | 72 |
| **7-Eleven** ~ *Page 236* | | | |
| **Schlotzsky's** ~ *Page 237* | | | |
| **Subway** ~ *Page 245* | | | |

### Wraps & Roll-Ups

*Average All Types*
**Meat/Chicken/Fish/Veggie:**

| | C | F | Cb |
|---|---|---|---|
| Small, approximately 9 oz | 500 | 25 | 48 |
| Regular, approximately 15 oz | 830 | 40 | 80 |
| Large, approximately 22 oz | 1400 | 70 | 134 |
| **Fast-Foods Restaurants** ~ *Page 175* | | | |
| **Au Bon Pain** ~ *Page 179* | | | |
| **Sonic Drive-In** ~ *Page 241* | | | |
| **Subway** ~ *Page 245* | | | |
| **WAWA** ~ *Page 254* | | | |

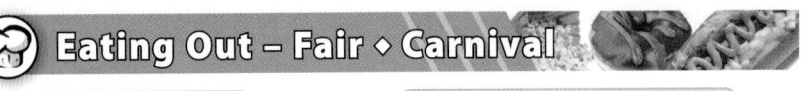

## Fair & Carnival Foods   **C**  **L**  **Cp**

| | C | L | Cp |
|---|---|---|---|
| **Barbeque Chicken/Meats:** | | | |
| **Chicken,** ½ chicken, 15 oz | 740 | 24 | 34 |
| **Grilled Chicken Pita,** with dressing | 680 | 19 | 82 |
| **Teriyaki Chicken,** on stick, w/ dress. | 250 | 6 | 4 |
| **Pork Ribs,** 18 oz | 1360 | 68 | 21 |
| **Turkey Leg:** Regular, 19 oz | 1135 | 54 | 0 |
| Caveman (2lb Turkey Leg, with 1lb Bacon) | 2360 | 177 | 3 |
| **Bacon:** Fried, on-a-stick, with syrup | 230 | 16 | 5 |
| Choc-covered Bacon, 4.5 oz dish | 640 | 43 | 30 |
| **Beef Stew over Rice,** 2 cups | 440 | 14 | 61 |
| **Butter Balls,** deep fried, 4 Balls | 460 | 38 | 24 |
| **Cheese Curds,** Breaded & fried, *Culver's,* 6.7 oz | 670 | 38 | 54 |
| **Corn Dogs:** Regular, 4 oz | 250 | 14 | 23 |
| Jumbo, 6 oz | 375 | 21 | 36 |
| Pretzel-Wrapped Dog | 300 | 16 | 30 |
| Papa Pup, on-a-stick | 400 | 24 | 32 |
| Pronto Pup, on-a-stick | 170 | 9 | 16 |
| **Corn On The Cob,** 8″ (1), 16 oz | 200 | 1 | 42 |
| **Finger Foods:** | | | |
| **Artichoke,** fried, 9 pieces | 250 | 14 | 24 |
| **Chicken Nuggets,** (6) | 340 | 17 | 26 |
| **Chicken Strips,** (4), 4.5 oz | 445 | 21 | 33 |
| **Onion Rings,** 3 rings | 310 | 13 | 40 |
| **Onion Flower** | 1320 | 72 | 140 |
| **Shrimp,** Fried, 10-12 pieces, 5 oz | 555 | 30 | 36 |
| **Spam,** deep-fried in batter, 2 pieces | 330 | 24 | 18 |
| **Gator:** | | | |
| **Big Gator,** Nuggets/Hushpuppies | 550 | 31 | 54 |
| **Stick Gator,** 1 sausage | 250 | 20 | 4 |
| **Greek:** | | | |
| **Baklava,** 2″ square | 245 | 13 | 32 |
| **Falafel,** 11.6 oz | 660 | 27 | 85 |
| **Greek Salad,** 14 oz | 520 | 48 | 17 |
| **Gyro,** 7.5″, 12 oz | 680 | 40 | 55 |
| **Spanakopita,** 8 oz | 200 | 7.5 | 23 |
| **Hamburgers:** | | | |
| **⅓ Pound Burger,** 7.5 oz | 670 | 41 | 26 |
| **Cheeseburger,** 6 oz | 550 | 36 | 25 |
| **Hot Dogs:** *With Bun* | | | |
| **Regular:** No extras | 215 | 14 | 28 |
| With Chili, 6 oz | 450 | 32 | 32 |
| With Chili & Cheese, 7.3 oz | 500 | 36 | 31 |
| **⅓ Pound Hot Dog** | 550 | 41 | 31 |
| **Foot Long Hot Dog** | 470 | 26 | 41 |
| **Jumbo,** Bratwurst/Kielbasa, average | 800 | 60 | 28 |

## Fair & Carnival Foods (Cont)

| | C | F | Cb |
|---|---|---|---|
| **Mexican:** | | | |
| **Burrito,** with Bean/Beef, 17 oz | 1100 | 41 | 104 |
| **Carne Asada,** 14.5 oz | 820 | 44 | 58 |
| **Cheese Quesadilla,** 1.8 oz | 480 | 27 | 40 |
| **Chicken Taco,** 3.3 oz | 210 | 12 | 16 |
| **Fish Taco,** 5 oz | 270 | 13 | 31 |
| **Jalapeno Pepper,** choc-covered (3) | 270 | 15 | 31 |
| **Nachos with Cheese,** 9″ plate | 860 | 59 | 70 |
| **Tamale,** 3.5 oz | 180 | 8 | 21 |
| **Taquito,** 5 oz | 370 | 17 | 43 |
| **Pizza:** | | | |
| **Pizza Bread,** Pepperoni, ½ loaf, 12 oz | 1115 | 32 | 151 |
| **Pizza on-a-stick,** 1 piece | 535 | 28 | 55 |
| **Personal Pizza:** *Per 7″* | | | |
| Cheese | 670 | 24 | 80 |
| Pepperoni | 795 | 35 | 80 |
| Ham & Pineapple | 800 | 31 | 87 |
| **Potatoes & Fries:** | | | |
| **Australian Battered Potatoes** | 1290 | 66 | 155 |
| **Baked Potato,** 14 oz | 435 | 0.5 | 100 |
| **Fries:** French, 7 oz | 560 | 24 | 79 |
| Cheese Fries, 10 oz | 645 | 38 | 62 |
| Chili Fries, 10 oz | 700 | 36 | 83 |
| Curly Fries, 7 oz | 620 | 30 | 78 |
| Jamaican Jerk Fries, 7 oz | 640 | 34 | 77 |
| **Sweet Potato,** baked, 14 oz | 405 | 0.5 | 97 |
| **Tornado,** on-a-stick | 210 | 15 | 18 |
| **Salads/Sides:** | | | |
| **Chili,** 1 cup | 280 | 11 | 24 |
| **Cole Slaw,** 5 oz | 350 | 21 | 37 |
| **Pickle,** whole (6″) | 30 | 0 | 8 |
| **Potato Salad,** 5 oz | 290 | 15 | 35 |
| **Sandwiches:** *7½″ Roll* | | | |
| **Ham,** 11 oz | 645 | 39 | 47 |
| **Hot Pastrami,** 9 oz | 760 | 17 | 62 |
| **Roast Beef,** 11 oz | 620 | 36 | 46 |
| **Philadelphia Cheese Steak,** 13 oz | 680 | 36 | 49 |
| **Turkey,** 11 oz | 665 | 24 | 65 |
| **Drinks:** | | | |
| **Icee,** 16 fl.oz | 235 | 0 | 59 |
| **Shakes,** average, 16 fl.oz | 690 | 33 | 85 |
| **Slushies:** Horchata, 16 fl.oz | 280 | 8 | 50 |
| Lemonade, 18 fl.oz | 210 | 0 | 52 |
| Orange Julius, 20 fl.oz | 490 | 10 | 96 |
| Strawberry Julius, 20 fl.oz | 430 | 0 | 98 |
| **Soft Frozen Lemonade,** 12 fl.oz | 300 | 0 | 78 |
| **Smoothies,** Berry Flavors, 16 fl.oz | 350 | 1 | 80 |

## Fair & Carnival Foods (Cont)

| | C | F | Cb |
|---|---|---|---|
| **Cakes, Pastries:** | | | |
| **Funnel Cake,** Plain (1) | 760 | 44 | 80 |
| **Toppings:** | | | |
| Apple Cinnamon, 2 oz | 85 | 3 | 16 |
| Cinnamon & Sugar, 2 tsp | 40 | 0 | 10 |
| Strawberry & Cream, 2 oz | 70 | 0 | 16 |
| **Cheesecake on-a-stick,** 6 oz | 655 | 47 | 56 |
| **Churro,** (1), 9", 1.6 oz | 170 | 8 | 22 |
| **Cream Puff,** 4.3 oz | 500 | 43 | 22 |
| **Fried Twinkie,** (1) | 420 | 34 | 45 |
| **Puff-on-a-Stick,** (4), 8.6 oz | 995 | 86 | 44 |
| **Strawberry Crepe,** 4.3 oz | 280 | 14 | 36 |
| **Twinkie Dog,** (Sundae) | 500 | 14 | 89 |
| **Candied Apple,** 7 oz | 330 | 0 | 80 |
| **Cookies:** | | | |
| **Sweet Martha,** (1), 0.8 oz | 90 | 4 | 14 |
| **Deep Fried: Oreos,** tray (5) | 890 | 48 | 108 |
| Cookie Dough on stick, 3 pieces | 670 | 32 | 89 |
| **Cotton Candy:** | | | |
| Small, 1 oz | 110 | 0 | 27 |
| Large, 2.3 oz | 250 | 0 | 62 |
| Family Size, 5.5 oz | 610 | 0 | 151 |
| **Dirt Dessert,** 1 cup, 9.3 oz | 405 | 12 | 69 |
| **Donuts,** Jumbo Twist, (1), 7.5 oz | 905 | 49 | 109 |
| **Fried Dough/FryBread:** | | | |
| **Plain:** 7", 3.7 oz | 390 | 19 | 47 |
| 9", 4¾ oz | 510 | 25 | 61 |
| **Toppings:** Cinnamon Sugar, 2 tsp | 40 | 0 | 10 |
| Butterscotch; Caramel, 2 Tbsp | 115 | 0 | 29 |
| Hot Fudge, average, 2 Tbsp | 110 | 4 | 22 |
| Cheese Powder, 2 tsp | 70 | 3 | 2 |
| Honey, 1 Tbsp, 0.8 oz | 65 | 0 | 17 |
| **Fudge,** 1.5 oz | 200 | 11 | 25 |
| **Ice Cream & Frozen Treats:** | | | |
| **Deep-fried Klondike Bar,** w/ syrup | 430 | 16 | 18 |
| **Dippin' Dots Ice Cream,** 6 oz cup | 380 | 20 | 46 |
| **Frozen Banana,** choc. coated, 5 oz | 240 | 4 | 53 |
| **Frozen Yogurt,** in sugar cone, 14 oz | 475 | 2 | 94 |
| **Ice Cream:** Small, sugar cone, 10 oz | 775 | 42 | 83 |
| Large, sugar cone, 14 oz | 935 | 54 | 96 |
| **Sherbet,** 8 oz | 270 | 4 | 59 |
| **Snow Cone,** with 3 oz syrup | 270 | 0 | 68 |
| **Strawberry,** Choc. Dipped, 1 piece | 125 | 7 | 15 |
| **Popcorn:** | | | |
| **Plain:** Small, 3 oz | 450 | 24 | 48 |
| Large, 6 oz | 900 | 48 | 96 |
| **Kettle Corn:** Small, 5 oz | 600 | 15 | 110 |
| Large, 10 oz | 1200 | 30 | 220 |
| **Pretzels,** Soft, 4.5 oz | 340 | 2 | 70 |
| **S'more,** on stick | 275 | 16 | 27 |

## Stadium Foods

| | C | F | Cb |
|---|---|---|---|
| **Burgers:** | | | |
| **Bacon Burger,** 8.3 oz | 470 | 25 | 34 |
| **Cheeseburger,** 8.3 oz | 450 | 23 | 33 |
| **Hamburger,** 7.8 oz | 400 | 19 | 33 |
| **French Fries,** 6.4 oz | 470 | 34 | 39 |
| **Fruit Cup,** 6 oz | 80 | 0 | 20 |
| **Hot Dogs:** | | | |
| **Chili Dog,** 7.7 oz | 520 | 29 | 45 |
| **Hot Dog,** 6.4 oz | 465 | 21 | 50 |
| **Jumbo Dog,** 6 oz | 440 | 25 | 38 |
| **Kraut Dog with Sauerkraut,** 7.8 oz | 490 | 27 | 41 |
| **Individual Pan Pizza (6"):** *Per Pizza* | | | |
| **BBQ Chicken** | 630 | 24 | 71 |
| **Cheese** | 630 | 27 | 71 |
| **Pepperoni** | 660 | 30 | 70 |
| **Nachos,** 40 chips, with 4 oz cheese | 1100 | 59 | 132 |
| **Sandwiches:** | | | |
| **Chicken:** With Bacon, 8.3 oz | 530 | 31 | 41 |
| With Cheese, 8.3 oz | 510 | 29 | 40 |
| Without Cheese, 7.7 oz | 460 | 25 | 40 |
| **Polish Sausage Sandwich,** 7 oz | 565 | 33 | 46 |
| **Snacks:** | | | |
| **Brownie,** 2.5" x 4.5" | 360 | 18 | 44 |
| **Cheese Sauce,** 1.3 oz | 100 | 8 | 4 |
| ***Cheetos***, 2.8 oz package | 440 | 28 | 42 |
| **Chocolate Chip Cookie,** 2.3 oz | 280 | 12 | 40 |
| **Churro,** (1), 10", 2 oz | 210 | 10 | 26 |
| ***Doritos***, Nacho, 2.8 oz package | 390 | 20 | 48 |
| **King Size Candy:** | | | |
| *Butterfinger*, 3.8 oz | 480 | 18 | 75 |
| *Nestle Crunch*, 2.8 oz | 390 | 21 | 85 |
| ***Lay's***, Chips, 2.8 oz package | 440 | 28 | 42 |
| **Peanuts,** in shell, 8 oz | 930 | 80 | 24 |
| **Popcorn:** Small (9 cup size) | 575 | 35 | 56 |
| Large (15 cup size) | 950 | 58 | 93 |
| **Pretzel,** Soft, Reg., 5.5 oz | 490 | 3.5 | 101 |
| **Red Vines,** 5 oz box | 500 | 0 | 117 |
| **Snow Cone:** With 3 oz syrup | 270 | 0 | 68 |
| With 6 oz syrup | 540 | 0 | 136 |
| **Beverages:** | | | |
| **Orange Juice,** 12 fl.oz | 180 | 0 | 2 |
| **Beer:** | | | |
| *Heineken*, 16 fl.oz | 200 | 0 | 16 |
| *Miller*: Draft, 16 fl.oz | 195 | 0 | 17 |
| Lite, 16 fl.oz | 125 | 16 | 4 |
| *Jack Daniels*, Punch, 12 fl.oz | 235 | 0 | 34 |
| **Wine,** White, 9 fl.oz | 190 | 0 | 6 |
| **Soda,** (with ½ ice), average: | | | |
| 20 fl.oz | 160 | 0 | 40 |
| 32 fl.oz | 260 | 0 | 65 |
| ***Starbuck's,*** Coffee, Frappuccino, 9.5 fl.oz | 200 | 3 | 37 |

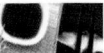

## Asian & Chinese Dishes | C | F | Cb

**Appetizers:**

| | C | F | Cb |
|---|---|---|---|
| **Crab Cake,** 2.3 oz | 125 | 10 | 1 |
| **Dumplings:** *Per Dumpling* | | | |
| Pork: Steamed | 80 | 4.5 | 5 |
| Fried | 90 | 6 | 5 |
| Vegetable, steamed | 35 | 1 | 5 |
| **Egg Rolls,** Mini, 3 rolls | 100 | 3 | 11 |
| **Spring Roll:** | | | |
| Small, 1.5 oz | 85 | 4 | 9 |
| Medium, 3 oz | 170 | 8 | 17 |
| Large, 5 oz | 290 | 15 | 29 |
| **Wonton,** 1 only | 75 | 4 | 5 |
| **Soup:** Egg Flower, bowl 12 oz | 90 | 2 | 16 |
| Hot & Sour Soup, bowl 12 oz | 110 | 3.5 | 14 |
| **Rice:** Plain, 1 cup, 6.5 oz | 320 | 2 | 66 |
| 2 Cups, 13 oz | 640 | 4 | 132 |
| Fried: 1 cup, 5 oz | 365 | 11 | 55 |
| Large dish, 16 oz | 950 | 28 | 67 |
| **Noodles,** Chinese Egg, cooked, 1 cup | 200 | 4 | 37 |
| **Entrees & Mains:** *Per Serving* | | | |
| **Almond Chicken,** 6 oz | 270 | 10 | 21 |
| **BBQ Pork,** 5.5oz | 440 | 23 | 15 |
| **Beef in Black Bean Sauce,** 8.5 oz | 390 | 17 | 17 |
| **Broccoli Beef,** 6 oz | 370 | 21 | 13 |
| **Chicken & Broccoli,** 5.5 oz | 160 | 8 | 10 |
| **Chicken Skewers,** 3 oz | 210 | 9 | 18 |
| **Chop Suey:** | | | |
| Chicken, 5 oz | 140 | 9 | 2 |
| Pork, 5 oz | 170 | 12 | 3 |
| **Chow Mein,** Beef/Chicken, 8 oz | 390 | 12 | 59 |
| **Crab Puff/Rangoon,** 1 dumpling | 190 | 11 | 13 |
| **Crispy Fried Chicken,** 8 oz | 485 | 33 | 12 |
| **Egg Drop Soup:** With Noodles, 1 cup | 110 | 3 | 16 |
| Without Noodles, 1 cup | 60 | 3 | 4 |
| **Egg Foo Yung with Sauce,** 1 cup | 270 | 15 | 16 |
| **Kung Pao Chicken,** 5.5 oz | 240 | 15 | 12 |
| **Lemon Chicken,** 5 oz | 525 | 21 | 57 |
| **Lo Mein,** stir-fried, 8 oz | 705 | 42 | 49 |
| **Omelet,** Chicken/Shrimp, 16 oz | 990 | 82 | 10 |
| **Orange Chicken,** 5.5 oz | 500 | 27 | 42 |
| **Steamed Whole Fish,** | | | |
| ½ Sockeye Salmon | 646 | 36 | 23 |
| **Sweet & Sour:** | | | |
| Fish, 20 oz | 1160 | 58 | 106 |
| Pork, 5.5 oz | 400 | 23 | 35 |
| **Vegetable Combo,** with oil, 6 oz | 367 | 5 | 66 |
| **Vegetables,** Steamed, without oil, 6 oz | 135 | 1 | 29 |
| **Sauces:** Mandarin Sauce 1.5 oz | 70 | 0 | 17 |
| Potsticker Sauce, 1.5 oz | 35 | 0 | 8 |
| **Bubble Tea,** average, 12 fl oz | 280 | 0.5 | 68 |
| **Fortune Cookie,** each | 32 | 0.5 | 7 |

## Cajun & Creole | C | F | Cb

| | C | F | Cb |
|---|---|---|---|
| **Alligator,** cooked, 4 oz | 160 | 2 | 0 |
| **Baked Herb Chicken,** 1 serving | 850 | 53 | 2 |
| **Bouillabaisse** | 400 | 15 | 10 |
| **Cajun Fried Turkey,** 1 serving | 630 | 25 | 0 |
| **Cocktail Sauce,** 2 Tbsp | 30 | 0 | 6 |
| **Couche-Couche,** ½ cup | 80 | 0 | 17 |
| **Crawfish Bisque,** 1 serving | 500 | 10 | 10 |
| **Crawfish,** cooked, 2 oz | 45 | 0.5 | 0 |
| **Creole Jambalaya,** | | | |
| 1 serving | 550 | 30 | 15 |
| **Frog Legs,** steamed (2) | 45 | 0 | 0 |
| **Guinea Fowl,** flesh, 4 oz, cooked | 160 | 4 | 0 |
| **Hogshead Cheese,** ¼ cup | 80 | 5.5 | 0 |
| **Jambalaya,** Shrimp & Crabmeat | 520 | 14 | 12 |
| **Red Beans & Rice,** 1 serving | 400 | 17 | 52 |
| **Roasted Quail,** with Bacon, on Toast | 550 | 25 | 15 |
| **Remoulade Sauce,** 2 Tbsp, 1 oz | 110 | 11 | 2 |
| **Shrimp Creole,** 1 serving | 450 | 20 | 10 |
| **Stuffed Smothered Steak,** | | | |
| with 1 cup Rice | 890 | 50 | 50 |
| **Turtle,** cooked, 3 oz | 120 | 3 | 0 |

## Canadian

| | C | F | Cb |
|---|---|---|---|
| **Bagels,** Montreal-Style: | | | |
| Plain, 100g/3.5 oz | 300 | 2 | 60 |
| Poppyseed, 100g/3.5 oz | 310 | 4 | 58 |
| Sesame, 100g/3.5 oz | 320 | 6 | 56 |
| **Bannock:** Plain 33g/1.2 oz | 120 | 3 | 20 |
| With currants/raisins, 85g/3 oz | 215 | 9 | 32 |
| **Meals:** | | | |
| **Baked Beans in Maple Syrup,** | | | |
| 1 cup, 250g/8.8 oz | 320 | 1 | 62 |
| **Donnairs** (*Pizza Delight*): | | | |
| Famous, regular, 250g/8.8 oz | 510 | 21 | 60 |
| Super, regular, 310g/11 oz | 685 | 34 | 62 |
| **Poutine:** | | | |
| *A&W,* 330g/12 oz | 610 | 33 | 58 |
| *Boston Pizza,* regular, 400g/14 oz | 610 | 30 | 67 |
| *Burger King,* Classic, 330g/11.6 oz | 680 | 36 | 72 |
| *Harvey's,* 240g/8.5 oz | 730 | 41 | 63 |
| *McDonald's,* 1 serving | 510 | 29 | 44 |
| *Swiss Chalet,* | | | |
| Chalet -Style, 340g/12 oz | 150 | 12 | 195 |
| **Shish Taouk:** | | | |
| Chicken: 1 skewer, 200g/7 oz | 270 | 25 | 9 |
| Wrap, 455g/16 oz | 1150 | 12 | 195 |
| **Tassot:** | | | |
| Beef, 283g/10 oz | 430 | 28 | 12 |
| Goat, 100g/3.5 oz | 360 | 36 | 9 |
| **Toutiere,** 170g/6oz | 600 | 42 | 35 |

## Canadian (Cont)

| | C | F | Cb |
|---|---|---|---|
| **Pastries:** | | | |
| **Beaver Tails:** | | | |
| Cheese & Garlic, 80g/2.8 oz | 390 | 30 | 28 |
| Cinnamon & Sugar, 80g/2.8 oz | 315 | 13 | 30 |
| **Butter Tart**, mini, 1 tart | 120 | 3 | 16 |
| **May West,** | | | |
| Original, 54g/1.9 oz | 240 | 11 | 34 |
| **Nanaimo Bar**, 56g/2 oz | 270 | 16 | 30 |
| **Snacks:** Maple Syrup Taffy, 40g/1.4 oz | 130 | 0 | 33 |
| Potato Chips: Dill Pickle Flav., 40g | 160 | 10 | 15 |
| Ketchup Flavor, 50g/1.8 oz | 260 | 16 | 26 |

## French Foods

| | C | F | Cb |
|---|---|---|---|
| **Blanquette d'Agneau,** (Lamb Stew) | 800 | 30 | 17 |
| **Brioche,** 1 cake | 280 | 14 | 34 |
| **Bouillabaisse** | 400 | 15 | 10 |
| **Coq au Vin,** leg/thigh | 700 | 28 | 31 |
| **Coquilles St. Jacques** | 320 | 13 | 36 |
| **Crème Brulée,** 1 serving | 460 | 40 | 21 |
| **Baguette,** 3 slices, 2.2 oz | 150 | 1 | 35 |
| **Creme Caramel,** (Caramel Custard) | 260 | 10 | 38 |
| **Crepe Suzette,** 1x6" crepe with sauce | 220 | 10 | 13 |
| **Duck a l'Orange,** ¼ duck, 22 oz | 970 | 44 | 19 |
| **Escargot,** (Snails), in garlic butter (6) | 200 | 10 | 4 |
| **Frog Legs,** fried, 4 medium pairs | 400 | 20 | 10 |
| **Lamb Noisettes,** fried, 2 chops | 500 | 40 | 1 |
| **Potage Creme Crecy,** (Carrot Soup) | 360 | 18 | 14 |
| **Salade Nicoise,** (Tuna/Olives/Vegs) | 450 | 13 | 14 |
| **Veal Cordon Bleu,** (Veal/Ham) | 650 | 25 | 18 |
| **Vichyssoise,** (Potato /Leek Soup), 1 c. | 200 | 9 | 15 |
| **Baguette & French Stick ~** Page 54 | | | |

## German

| | C | F | Cb |
|---|---|---|---|
| **Beef:** Goulash with Veggies | 520 | 20 | 46 |
| Weiner Schnitzel, 1 medium | 750 | 35 | 38 |
| **Chicken:** Fried, Viennese-style | 530 | 20 | 28 |
| Livers with Apple/Onion, 6 oz | 460 | 28 | 10 |
| **Herring,** pickled: Rollmops, 4 oz | 260 | 16 | 3 |
| With Sour Cream, 4 oz | 310 | 20 | 3 |
| **Pork,** Sauerbraten (Pot Roast) | 650 | 35 | 15 |
| **Sausage:** Bratwurst, grilled, 6 oz | 450 | 37 | 2 |
| Hot Sausage Curry | 300 | 7 | 6 |
| **Cakes:** | | | |
| **Black Forest,** 1 slice | 380 | 16 | 30 |
| **Bavarian Bread Dumpling,** 3 small | 330 | 10 | 28 |
| **Kugelhupf Cake,** 1 large slice, 4 oz | 400 | 23 | 40 |
| **Torte:** Linzer (Almond/Raspb. Jam) | 430 | 18 | 58 |
| Sacher (Chocolate/Apricot Jam) | 260 | 12 | 23 |

## Greek

| | C | F | Cb |
|---|---|---|---|
| **Baklava Pastry:** Small | 240 | 13 | 32 |
| Large, 3.8 oz | 400 | 21 | 45 |
| **Calamari,** deep fried, 1 cup | 300 | 13 | 17 |
| **Chicken Kebob Plate** | 345 | 13 | 8 |
| **Dolmades,** 2 rolls, 6 oz | 200 | 5 | 13 |
| **Galactobureko,** 1 only | | | |
| (Filo, Custard, Pastry in Syrup) | 360 | 15 | 48 |
| **Greek Chicken Salad** | 400 | 18 | 9 |
| **Gyros:** 6" Pita, 8 oz | 475 | 32 | 35 |
| 7½" Pita, 12 oz | 680 | 40 | 55 |
| **Hummus & Pita,** 4 oz | 260 | 12 | 30 |
| **Kataifi,** (Filo, Nut, Pastry in Syrup) | 350 | 11 | 56 |
| **Moussaka:** Small serving, 8 oz | 350 | 22 | 22 |
| Large serving, 16 oz | 700 | 44 | 44 |
| **Soup,** Avgolemono (Egg & Lemon | | | |
| with Chicken & Rice), 1 cup | 85 | 6 | 5 |
| **Souvlaki,** (Lamb), each, 2 oz | 120 | 6 | 1 |
| **Stuffed Tomatoes,** (2) | 250 | 12 | 17 |
| **Taramosalata,** 1 T., 0.5 oz | 40 | 3 | 2 |
| **Tyropita,** (Filo/Egg/Cheese Pastry) | 350 | 26 | 31 |

## Hawaiian

| | C | F | Cb |
|---|---|---|---|
| **Ahi Tuna,** grilled w/o fat, 6 oz fillet | 220 | 2 | 0 |
| **Chicken Long Rice,** 1 cup, 7 oz | 240 | 14 | 12 |
| **Gyoza,** 1 only | 55 | 2 | 6 |
| **Haupia,** (Coconut Pudd.), 1 pce, (4"x 2½") | 120 | 6 | 17 |
| **Hawaiian Sweet Bread,** ½" slice, 2 oz | 180 | 4.5 | 29 |
| **Kalua:** Chicken, 4 oz | 280 | 16 | 0 |
| Pork, 4 oz | 350 | 24 | 0 |
| **Kim Chee,** (pickled cabbage), ½ cup, 4 oz | 20 | 0 | 5 |
| **Kulolo,** (Taro Pudding), 1 slice | 125 | 5 | 19 |
| **Lau Lau:** | | | |
| Chicken (1), 7 oz | 280 | 21 | 3 |
| Pork (1), 7 oz | 320 | 26 | 5 |
| **Loco Moco,** (rice/burger/egg/gravy) | 650 | 27 | 63 |
| **Lomi Salmon,** ¼ cup, 4 oz | 20 | 1 | 2 |
| **Malasadas,** (Donut), 2 oz | 240 | 13 | 26 |
| **Manapua,** (Char Siu Pork Bun), 2.3 oz | 180 | 8 | 25 |
| **Poi ,**(mashed cooked taro), 1 cup, 8.5 oz | 270 | 0.5 | 65 |
| **Poke,** average all types, 3 oz | 90 | 1 | 0 |
| **Portuguese Sausage,** 2 oz | 180 | 15 | 2 |
| **Potato Salad,** ½ cup, 5 oz | 170 | 10 | 17 |
| **Shave Ice,** (Matsumoto), all flavors: | | | |
| With Ice Cream, 1 large | 300 | 4 | 64 |
| With Beans, 1 large | 290 | 0 | 72 |
| **Spam Musubi:** | | | |
| With Regular Spam | 265 | 11 | 34 |
| (4 oz rice+1.3 oz Spam/7-Eleven Hawaii) | | | |
| Homemade, w/ Lite Spam (50% less fat) | 220 | 5 | 34 |
| **Taro Pancake Mix,** ⅓ cup (makes 2) | 140 | 2 | 26 |

## Hawaiian (Cont)   **C  F  Cb**

**Plate Lunches:**

| | C | F | Cb |
|---|---|---|---|
| **Chicken Katsu**, (9 oz:) With Rice | 1110 | 48 | 108 |
| + Macaroni Salad, ¾ cup | 1360 | 68 | 123 |
| or Tossed Salad + 2Tbsp Fr. Dress. | 1240 | 61 | 111 |
| **Hamburger**, (5 oz): With Rice | 710 | 24 | 81 |
| Gravy + Macaroni Salad | 1135 | 49 | 112 |
| **Mahi Mahi**, (7 oz): With Rice | 650 | 12 | 90 |
| + Macaroni Salad + Tartar Sce | 1150 | 58 | 109 |
| or Macaroni Salad, w/o Tartar ce | 935 | 34 | 108 |
| or Tossed Salad + 3 Tbsp Fr. Dress. | 815 | 27 | 96 |
| or Tossed Salad, without dressing | 670 | 12 | 93 |
| **Teri Beef, (5 oz):** With 2 scoops Rice | 790 | 23 | 94 |
| + Macaroni Salad, ¾ cup | 1095 | 47 | 113 |
| or Tossed Salad, without dressing | 800 | 23 | 95 |

## Indian & Pakistani

*Per Serving, Meat dishes allow 4 oz meat/serving*

| | C | F | Cb |
|---|---|---|---|
| **Aloo Samosa**, each | 155 | 12 | 12 |
| **Alu Gosht Kari**, (Meat/Potato Curry) | 600 | 40 | 23 |
| **Chicken Korma** | 500 | 35 | 6 |
| **Chicken Pilaf** | 700 | 53 | 50 |
| **Chicken Tikka** | 260 | 16 | 2 |
| **Chicken Vindaloo** | 400 | 20 | 8 |
| **Chapati/Roti**, 7" diameter, 1 piece | 60 | 0.5 | 11 |
| **Dahl**, (Lentil Puree): | | | |
| 1 cup, without oil | 230 | 1 | 37 |
| 1 Tbsp Tadka (oil topping) | 120 | 13 | 0 |
| **Dhakla**, (Lentil Dish), 1" square, 1 oz | 105 | 5 | 13 |
| **Dhansak**, ½ cup | 105 | 3.5 | 11 |
| **Gosht Kari** | 460 | 25 | 17 |
| **Lamb Pilaf** | 520 | 35 | 40 |
| **Lassi**, (Sweet or Mango), 1 cup, 8 oz | 160 | 4 | 24 |
| **Masala Gosht**, (Beef/Tomato/Gravy) | 400 | 25 | 18 |
| **Mulligatawney Soup** | 300 | 15 | 8 |
| **Murgh Tikka**, 1 cup | 300 | 4 | 7 |
| **Naan Flatbread**, 2 oz | 160 | 3.5 | 29 |
| **Pappadum**, 1 large/2 small | 50 | 3 | 5 |
| **Pesrattu**, (Lentil Crepe), 9", 2.6 oz | 130 | 5 | 15 |
| **Pork Vindaloo Curry**, without Rice | 620 | 47 | 3 |
| **Rajmah**, 1 cup | 225 | 5 | 35 |
| **Rogan Josh**, | | | |
| without Rice/Potatoes | 500 | 30 | 3 |
| **Shahi Korma**, (Braised Lamb) | 430 | 28 | 3 |
| **Tandoori Chicken:** | | | |
| Breast | 260 | 13 | 5 |
| Leg/Thigh portion | 300 | 17 | 6 |

## Italian Dishes   **C  F  Cb**

**Entrees:**

| | C | F | Cb |
|---|---|---|---|
| **Baked Ziti:** Small | 370 | 27 | 32 |
| Regular | 575 | 42 | 49 |
| **Breadstick**, 2 oz piece | 120 | 2.5 | 25 |
| **Broccoli Fettucine Alfredo**, regular | 815 | 23 | 125 |
| **Bruschetta**, 2 slices | 380 | 17 | 53 |
| **Calzones**, av. all varieties | 840 | 34 | 101 |
| **Cannelloni**, 1 tube, 6 oz | 280 | 15 | 18 |
| **Cheese Breadstick**, 2.4 oz piece | 180 | 8 | 20 |
| **Cheese Ravioli**, with sauce | 495 | 17 | 65 |
| **Chicken Alfredo** | 775 | 29 | 82 |
| **Chicken Parmigiana**, 11 oz | 520 | 22 | 16 |
| **Chicken Scallopine**, dinner | 1110 | 71 | 68 |
| **Eggplant Parmigiana** | 900 | 39 | 78 |
| **Fettucine Alfredo:** Lunch, 9 oz | 885 | 65 | 63 |
| Dinner, 15 oz | 1475 | 108 | 104 |
| **Linquine & Seafood**, dinner | 1130 | 71 | 79 |
| **Manicotti Formaggio** | 800 | 38 | 57 |
| **Meat Lasagne:** | | | |
| Small, 10 oz | 440 | 23 | 39 |
| Large, 16 oz | 700 | 36 | 60 |
| **Meat Ravioli** | 725 | 22 | 102 |
| **Minestrone Soup**, 1 bowl | 110 | 2 | 18 |
| **Penne Rustica:** Lunch | 1300 | 71 | 76 |
| Dinner | 1540 | 80 | 101 |
| **Ravioli**, over-stuffed, average | 990 | 67 | 57 |
| **Panini Sandwich:** | | | |
| Chicken, 16 oz | 900 | 38 | 81 |
| Meats, average, 18 oz | 940 | 39 | 81 |
| Vegetarian, 15 oz | 750 | 31 | 83 |
| **Pizza, Ready-To-Eat** ~ *See Page 135* | | | |
| **Spaghetti & Meatballs:** | | | |
| With Tomato Sauce: Kids | 500 | 20 | 58 |
| Medium/Lunch | 1080 | 63 | 89 |
| Large/Dinner | 1430 | 81 | 119 |
| With Meat Sauce: Kids | 550 | 25 | 56 |
| Medium/Lunch | 1300 | 79 | 84 |
| Large/Dinner | 1700 | 103 | 110 |
| **Veal Marsala**, dinner | 1320 | 66 | 132 |
| **Veal Parmigiana**, dinner | 1270 | 65 | 116 |
| **Vegetable Primavera** | 610 | 8 | 116 |
| **Salad,** | | | |
| **Caprese** , 11 oz | 445 | 34 | 10 |
| **Desserts:** | | | |
| **Gelato:** Vanilla (Milk Base), ½ cup | 200 | 15 | 18 |
| Choc. Hazelnut (Milk), ½ cup | 370 | 29 | 26 |
| Water Base, ½ cup | 100 | 0 | 25 |
| **Lemon Ice,** | 180 | 0 | 45 |
| **Tiramisu**, 1 piece, 5 oz | 400 | 29 | 30 |
| **Further listings** ~ *See Fast-Foods Section* | | | |

### Japanese

**C  F  Cb**

**Sashimi:** (Sliced Raw Seafood/Beef)

| | C | F | Cb |
|---|---|---|---|
| Ika (Squid), 4 oz | 105 | 2 | 0 |
| Hamachi (Yellowtail), 4 oz | 165 | 6 | 0 |
| Maguro (Yellowfin Tuna), 4 oz | 120 | 1 | 0 |
| Niku (Beef), 5 oz | 200 | 10 | 0 |
| Saba (Mackerel), 4 oz | 160 | 7 | 0 |
| Suzuki (Sea Bass), 4 oz | 110 | 0.5 | 0 |
| Tako (Octopus), 4 oz | 95 | 1 | 0 |
| **Sushi Rice:** Cooked, 1 Tbsp | 25 | 0 | 5 |
| 1 cup, 5.3 oz | 380 | 3 | 82 |

**Sushi (Maki) Rolls:** *Per Piece*
Average all types (California Rolls; Cream Cheese with Crab; Eel; Salmon; Shrimp; Tuna; Yellowtail; Vegetable)

| | C | F | Cb |
|---|---|---|---|
| Small (1.2" diam. x 1.2" high), 0.8 oz | 25 | 0.5 | 3.5 |
| Medium (1¾" diam. x 1¾" high), 1.6 oz | 50 | 1 | 7 |
| Large (2¼" diam. x ⅞" high), 2 oz | 60 | 1.5 | 9 |

**Sushi Packs:** *Per Pack*

| | C | F | Cb |
|---|---|---|---|
| Average all types: 6 large pieces | 370 | 5 | 55 |
| 9 medium pieces | 360 | 6 | 60 |
| 12 small pieces | 265 | 3 | 45 |
| Futomaki (thick roll), 6 pieces | 380 | 5 | 72 |
| Hand Roll (Cone), 4 oz | 120 | 2 | 18 |
| Inari (rice filled soybean pocket), 4 pces | 420 | 9 | 73 |

**Sushi-Nigiri,** (fish on rice),

| | C | F | Cb |
|---|---|---|---|
| average all varieties, 1 piece | 70 | 0.5 | 12 |
| **Sushi Plate,** Assorted: 6 pieces | 420 | 3 | 36 |
| Combination (Sushi & Sushi Rolls) 2 Sushi + 6 small & 3 medium rolls | 400 | 7 | 72 |
| **Dipping Sauces:** Average, 2 Tbsp | 30 | 0 | 7 |
| Ginger Vinegar Dressing, 2 Tbsp | 20 | 0 | 5 |

**Edamame:** (young green soybeans):

| | C | F | Cb |
|---|---|---|---|
| Boiled beans (no pods), 4 oz | 160 | 7 | 12 |
| Steamed (in pods), 4 oz | 60 | 3 | 5 |
| **Katsu-don,** Pork with Rice | 1100 | 39 | 141 |
| **Miso Soup,** with Tofu pieces, 1 cup | 85 | 3 | 11 |
| **Sake Wine,** (16% alcohol), 3 fl.oz | 115 | 0 | 7 |
| **Seaweed Salad,** 1.5 oz | 20 | 2 | 0 |
| **Sukiyaki,** (Beef/Tofu/Veggies), 8 oz | 400 | 24 | 32 |

**Tempura:**

| | C | F | Cb |
|---|---|---|---|
| 3 large shrimp & veggies | 320 | 18 | 25 |
| 1 shrimp only | 60 | 4 | 3 |

**Teppan Yaki,** (Steak, Seafood & Veggies),

| | C | F | Cb |
|---|---|---|---|
| 10 oz serving | 470 | 30 | 15 |
| **Teriyaki:** Beef, 4 oz | 350 | 25 | 4 |
| Chicken, 4 oz | 260 | 9 | 7 |
| Salmon, medium, 6 oz | 270 | 8 | 3 |
| **Yakatori,** 1 skewer, 2.5 oz | 140 | 5 | 1 |

### Kosher/Deli Foods

**C  F  Cb**

| | C | F | Cb |
|---|---|---|---|
| **Bagel/Bialy,** 1 small, 2 oz | 160 | 2 | 32 |
| **Beiglach,** (Cheese Knish) | 350 | 17 | 35 |
| **Blintzes:** Average, 1 only | 120 | 1 | 25 |
| With Sour Cream & Preserves | 370 | 10 | 30 |
| **Borscht,** (Without Sour Cream): 1 cup | 85 | 3 | 14 |
| Diet/Reduced Calorie, 1 cup | 30 | 1 | 7 |
| **Cabbage Roll,** (meat/rice), 5 oz | 170 | 6 | 21 |
| **Chicken Broth:** 1 cup | 80 | 8 | 0 |
| With vegetables | 100 | 8 | 5 |
| With noodles | 150 | 9 | 16 |
| Lowfat, plain, 1 cup | 25 | 1 | 0 |
| **Cholent,** 1 medium serving, 1 cup | 350 | 16 | 48 |
| **Chopped Liver:** 1 serving, 3 oz | 110 | 6 | 5 |
| With Egg Salad, ¼ cup | 100 | 7 | 3 |
| **Farfel,** dry, ½ cup | 90 | 0.5 | 21 |

**Gefilte Fish Balls:**

| | C | F | Cb |
|---|---|---|---|
| Regular, 2 oz | 55 | 2 | 4 |
| With Jelled Broth | 80 | 2 | 5 |
| Cocktail size, 1 oz | 30 | 1 | 2 |
| Sweet: Medium, 2 oz | 65 | 2 | 4 |
| With Jelled Broth | 95 | 2 | 5 |
| **Hallah,** (Yeast Bread), 1 slice, 1 oz | 85 | 2 | 14 |
| **Herring:** Smoked, 2 oz | 120 | 8 | 0 |
| In Sour Cream, 2 oz | 150 | 10 | 0 |
| **Kasha,** cooked, ½ cup | 100 | 0.5 | 20 |
| **Kipfel,** (Vanilla/Almond Cookie), 1 pce | 60 | 2 | 7 |
| **Knaidlach** ~ *See Matzo Balls* | | | |
| **Knish:** Kasha/Potato, 1 only | 130 | 4 | 22 |
| Cheese, 1 only | 350 | 17 | 35 |
| **Kreplach,** beef, 1 piece | 40 | 1 | 6 |
| **Kugel,** potato/noodle, 1 serving | 300 | 20 | 25 |
| **Latkes,** (Potato Pancake): 2 oz | 200 | 11 | 22 |
| 3 Latkes w/ Sour Cran Apple Sauce | 750 | 25 | 95 |
| **Lochshen:** Plain, 1 cup | 130 | 2 | 26 |
| Pudding, 1 cup | 380 | 13 | 48 |
| **Lox,** (Smoked Salmon), 2 oz | 65 | 2 | 0 |
| **Mandelbrot,** (Almond Bread), 1 slice, ¼" thick | 45 | 2 | 5 |
| **Matzo,** 1 oz/board | 110 | 0.5 | 21 |
| **Matzo Balls:** 2 small, or 1 large, 2" | 90 | 3 | 12 |
| Extra large ball, 3" | 180 | 6 | 24 |

**Matzo Ball Soup:**

| | C | F | Cb |
|---|---|---|---|
| Cup w/ 2 small or 1 large ball | 150 | 5 | 27 |
| Bowl w/ Chkn & Noodles | 325 | 13 | 34 |
| *Jerry's Deli,* large bowl | 560 | 17 | 56 |
| **NY Cheesecake,** 4 oz | 350 | 24 | 26 |
| **Pierogi,** potato/cheese, 1 piece | 90 | 4 | 11 |
| **Reuben S'wich,** w/ ½ lb Corned Beef | 920 | 60 | 28 |
| **Schmaltz,** (Rend'd Chicken Fat), 1 T. | 90 | 10 | 0 |

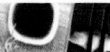

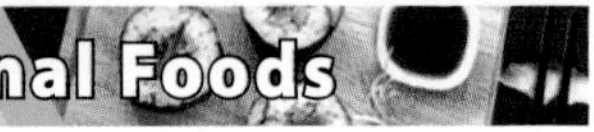

## Korean Food

| | C | F | Cb |
|---|---|---|---|
| **Bibimbab**, (Veg. & Beef on Rice), 1 cup | 565 | 15 | 89 |
| **Bulgogi**, (Barbeque Beef), 3.5 oz | 325 | 12 | 15 |
| **Galbi (Short Ribs)**, 16 oz | 975 | 61 | 16 |
| **Gujeolpan**, (Pancake with Meat & Vegetables), 1 cup with 1 pancake | 340 | 11 | 39 |
| **Japchae**, (Noodle w/ Veggies & Meat), 1¼ cups | 365 | 19 | 34 |
| **Sides:** | | | |
| **Kimchee**, (Cabbage Relish), ½ cup | 30 | 0 | 6 |
| **Namool**, (Assorted Vegetables), 1 cup | 125 | 6.5 | 9 |
| **Soups:** *Per Serving* | | | |
| **Muguk**, (Radish & Chive Soup), 6 oz | 105 | 7 | 6 |
| **Samgyetang**, (Ginseng Chkn Soup): | | | |
| Without Chicken Skin, 1 cup | 520 | 11 | 60 |
| With Chicken Skin, 1 cup | 725 | 35 | 60 |
| **Yuk Gae Jang**, (Spicy Beef Soup), 1¼ cups | 180 | 13 | 5 |

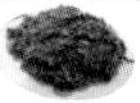

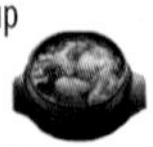

## Lebanese/Middle East

| | C | F | Cb |
|---|---|---|---|
| **Baba Ghannouj**, 2 Tbsp, 1 oz | 70 | 6 | 2 |
| **Baklava**, (Pastry, Nuts, Syrup), 1 pastry, 1¾ oz | 245 | 18 | 18 |
| **Cabbage Rolls**, (Cabb. Leaf, Meat, Rice), 1 roll, 3 oz | 100 | 3 | 12 |
| **Cous Cous**, (Semolina, Milk, Fruit, Nuts), 1 cup | 400 | 21 | 43 |
| **Falafel**, (Chick Pea Fritter), Fried, 1 medium, 1 oz | 60 | 4 | 4 |
| **Hummus**, ¼ cup, 2.2 oz | 105 | 3 | 5 |
| **Fried Kibbi**, (Wheat, Meat Pinenuts), 1 piece, 3 oz | 180 | 8 | 15 |
| **Kafta**, (Ground Lamb, Ssge on Skewer), 1 skewer, 1.5 oz oz | 85 | 5 | 2 |
| **Kibbeh Naye**, (raw Lamb, Bulgur & Spice) 1 cup, 9 oz | 450 | 18 | 28 |
| **Lebanese Omelet**, 1 serving, 4 oz (Egg, Spinach, Pinenuts, Onion) | 200 | 12 | 13 |
| **Pilaf**, (Rice, Onion, Raisins, Apr., Spice) 1 cup | 400 | 11 | 60 |
| **Shawourma**, (Spit-Roast Beef), 4 oz serving | 280 | 15 | 2 |
| **Shish Kabob**, 1 stick, 2.5 oz | 130 | 7 | 2 |
| **Spinach Pie**, 1 piece, 3.5 oz | 290 | 21 | 20 |
| **Sweet Almond Sanbusak**, (Pastry, Almonds, Spices), 1 piece | 200 | 15 | 11 |
| **Tabouli**, 1 serving, 4 oz | 125 | 7 | 13 |
| **Tahini Sauce**, average, 1 Tbsp | 90 | 8 | 2 |

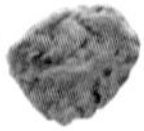

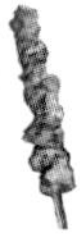

## Mexican

| | C | F | Cb |
|---|---|---|---|
| **Burritos** *(Taco Bell):* Bean | 370 | 10 | 56 |
| Supreme Beef | 420 | 16 | 53 |
| **Chili**, plain, ¼ cup | 90 | 6 | 8 |
| **Chili con Carne:** With Beans, 1 cup | 310 | 17 | 15 |
| Without Beans, 1 cup | 370 | 28 | 10 |
| **Chimichangas**, Beef, 5 oz | 400 | 19 | 43 |
| **Chorizo Sausage**, 2 oz | 265 | 23 | 0 |
| **Churro**, (1), 1.5 oz | 150 | 8 | 18 |
| **Corn Chips**, ½ cup, 1 oz | 160 | 10 | 17 |
| **Enchilada**, average | 330 | 10 | 49 |
| **Fajitas**, Chicken | 200 | 7 | 20 |
| **Guacamole**, average, 2 Tbsp, 1 oz | 45 | 4 | 2 |
| **Horchata:** *(Don Jose),* 1 cup, 8 fl.oz | 140 | 4 | 25 |
| *Cacique,* 1 pint bottle, 16 fl.oz | 320 | 7 | 62 |
| **Margarita**, with 1.5 oz Tequila | 160 | 0 | 6 |
| **Masa**, (Pre-mixed for Tamales), 1 oz | 80 | 5 | 9 |
| **Menudo:** | | | |
| With Hominy, 1 cup | 240 | 9 | 19 |
| Without Hominy, 1 cup | 170 | 9 | 2 |
| **Nachos:** With cheese, peppers, 1 portion, 6-8 nachos, 7 oz | 600 | 33 | 60 |
| With cheese, beans, beef, peppers, 1 portion, 6-8 nachos, 9 oz | 570 | 31 | 56 |
| *Del Taco:* Regular, 4 oz | 300 | 19 | 30 |
| Macho Nachos, 17 oz | 1000 | 56 | 94 |
| *Taco Bell,* BellGrande®, 10.8 oz | 780 | 40 | 84 |
| **Nopal Cactus Salad**, 1 cup | 130 | 9 | 11 |
| **Papas Fritas**, (1), 6 oz | 325 | 18 | 40 |
| **Piloncillo**, (Brown Sugar): | | | |
| 1 Tbsp, 0.5 oz | 50 | 0 | 13 |
| Cone, small, 3", 3 oz | 325 | 0 | 81 |
| **Quesadilla**, Cheese | 490 | 28 | 39 |
| **Queso Fresco**, ¼ cup | 80 | 4.5 | 8 |
| **Refried Beans**, ¾ cup, 6 oz | 160 | 3 | 26 |
| **Rice Pudding**, (Arroz Con Leche), 4 oz | 140 | 3 | 24 |
| **Soup**, Black Bean, 1 bowl | 200 | 3 | 34 |
| **Tacos** *(Taco Bell):* | | | |
| Crunchy: Regular | 170 | 10 | 12 |
| Supreme | 200 | 12 | 15 |
| Soft: Crispy Potato | 270 | 13 | 31 |
| Grilled Steak | 250 | 14 | 19 |
| Taco Salad with Salsa | 840 | 52 | 85 |
| **Taco Sauce**, average, ¼ cup | 15 | 0 | 3 |
| **Taco Shell**, regular | 50 | 2 | 8 |
| **Tamales**, Beef/Chicken, av. 4.5 oz | 250 | 11 | 27 |
| **Taquitos**, Beef & Cheese, 4.5 oz | 330 | 15 | 36 |
| **Tostada** (*Taco Bell*) | 250 | 10 | 29 |
| **Tortilla**, Corn, 6" diameter | 70 | 1 | 14 |
| **Tortilla Chips**, 1 oz | 150 | 8 | 18 |
| **Soup**, Black Bean, 1 bowl | 200 | 3 | 34 |

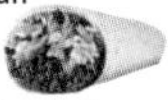

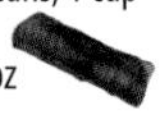

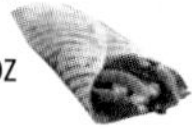

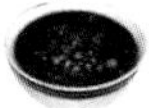

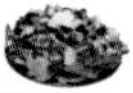

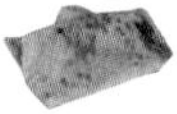

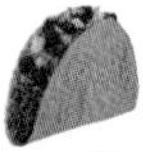

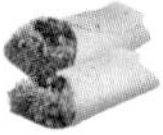

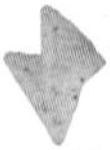

*Extra Food Listings ~ See Fast Food Section*
*(Examples: Del Taco, Taco Bell, Taco Cabana, Taco Time)*

## Mexican (Cont)

**C** **F** **Cb**

**Breads:**

| | C | F | Cb |
|---|---|---|---|
| **Bolillos**, 1 roll, 3.5 oz | 240 | 4 | 42 |
| **Mexican Cornbread**, 4" square | 210 | 11 | 19 |
| **Pan de Leche**, 1 roll, 1.3 oz | 110 | 2.5 | 20 |
| **Telera**, 2 oz | 150 | 1.5 | 19 |

**Cakes, Cookies, Pastries Pan Dulce:**

| | C | F | Cb |
|---|---|---|---|
| **Banderilla**, 1 piece | 140 | 10 | 8 |
| **Bigotes**, 7" | 570 | 22 | 44 |
| **Capirotada**, (Bread Pudding), 10 oz | 810 | 38 | 107 |
| **Cinnamon Cookies**, 2 | 125 | 8 | 13 |
| **Concha**, av. all varieties: | | | |
| Small (3" diameter), 2.5 oz | 250 | 8 | 38 |
| Medium (4" diameter), 3.5 oz | 350 | 11 | 53 |
| Large (5" diameter), 5.5 oz | 550 | 18 | 84 |
| **Cream Puff**, with Custard, 4.3 oz | 255 | 14 | 25 |
| **Cuernos**, (Horns), 3 oz | 340 | 17 | 41 |
| **Donut**, large, 4", 3.5 oz | 440 | 21 | 58 |
| **Elotes**, 3.5 oz | 450 | 24 | 51 |
| **Empanadas**, average all varieties: | | | |
| Medium, 3 oz | 300 | 14 | 42 |
| Large, 4 oz | 400 | 19 | 56 |
| **Fiesta Cookie**, (1), 2.3 oz | 280 | 8 | 47 |
| **Galletas Mixtas:** | | | |
| Small, 1 oz | 100 | 2.5 | 16 |
| Medium, 2 oz | 200 | 5 | 32 |
| Large, 3 oz | 300 | 7.5 | 48 |
| **Guayaba**, 3.3 oz | 360 | 14 | 53 |
| **Jelly Roll**, (1), 3.3 oz | 240 | 4 | 46 |
| **Mantecadites**, 4.5 oz | 670 | 42 | 64 |
| **Mini Cupcake**, (1),1.8 oz | 180 | 8 | 25 |
| **Muffins/Nino Enbuelto**, large, 6 oz | 465 | 11 | 48 |
| **Nuez**, 3.3 oz | 380 | 17 | 52 |
| **Ojo de Buey**, 4 oz | 360 | 15 | 55 |
| **Orejas**, 1 medium, 3 oz | 310 | 15 | 38 |
| **Pan Dulce**, 1 bun | 330 | 10 | 45 |
| **Panquecitos**, 2.5 oz | 260 | 11 | 36 |
| **Piedras**, 4 oz | 470 | 15 | 76 |
| **Polvorones:** Small, 1.5 oz | 180 | 9 | 24 |
| 1 large, 3 oz | 370 | 18 | 48 |
| **Pound Cakes**, mini, 3.5 oz | 380 | 16 | 52 |
| **Puerquitos**, 3.5 oz | 350 | 12 | 55 |
| **Rebanadas**, 3.5 oz | 390 | 18 | 51 |
| **Roles De Canela**, (Cinn. Roll), 4.5 oz | 490 | 15 | 81 |
| **Roscas**, 1 piece, 2.8 oz | 360 | 18 | 44 |
| **Semitas** (Bimbo), 1 piece, 2.2 oz | 210 | 6 | 33 |
| **Sopapillas**, (flaky pastry puffs): 1 piece | 100 | 7 | 10 |
| With Honey & Cream | 200 | 14 | 18 |
| **Strawberry Crema Roll**, 2.5 oz slice | 240 | 5 | 45 |

**Extra Food Listings** ~ *See CalorieKing.com*

## Polish

**C** **F** **Cb**

| | C | F | Cb |
|---|---|---|---|
| **Cabbage Rolls**, w/ Sour Cream, 2 small | 220 | 10 | 30 |
| **Chicken Casserole**, w/ Mshrms, 1 cup | 520 | 27 | 5 |
| **Kielbasa**, (Sausages, Onions, fried), 2 large | 350 | 28 | 2 |
| **Meatballs**, in sour cream, 3 x 1½" balls | 300 | 16 | 11 |
| **Pierogi**, Fruit/Vegetables, 3" ball | 80 | 2 | 15 |
| **Pork Goulash**, (Pork/Vegetable Stew) | 550 | 21 | 38 |
| **Pot Roast**, with Vegetables | 630 | 21 | 28 |

## Soul Foods

| | C | F | Cb |
|---|---|---|---|
| **Breakfast Sausage**, fried, 2 patties | 250 | 17 | 0 |
| **Brunswick Stew**, 1 cup, 8.5 oz | 320 | 14 | 19 |
| **Cornbread**, homemade, 3 oz | 200 | 7.5 | 28 |
| **Fatback**, 0.5 oz | 110 | 11 | 0 |
| **Ham Hock**, pickled, 3 oz | 200 | 12 | 0 |
| **Hog Maw**, 1 oz | 70 | 4.5 | 0 |
| **Hominy**, cooked, ¾ cup | 110 | 0.5 | 25 |
| **Hush Puppies**, 5 pieces | 260 | 12 | 35 |
| **Kale**, cooked, ½ cup | 20 | 0.5 | 4 |
| **Opossum**, roasted, without bone, 3 oz | 190 | 9 | 0 |
| **Oxtail**, cooked, without bone, 2 oz | 85 | 4.5 | 0 |
| **Pig's Ear**, ¼ ear | 50 | 3 | 0 |
| **Pig's Foot**, ½ foot | 70 | 4.5 | 0 |
| **Pig's Tail**, ⅓ tail | 115 | 10 | 0 |
| **Poke Salad**, cooked, ½ cup | 16 | 0.5 | 3 |
| **Pork Brains**, braised, 3 oz | 115 | 8 | 0 |
| **Pork Chitterlings**, simmered, 3 oz | 260 | 25 | 0 |
| **Pork Cracklings**, 0.5 oz | 80 | 6 | 0 |
| **Pork Neck Bones**, cooked, no bone, 2 oz | 100 | 4.5 | 0 |
| **Pork Skin**, 1 cup | 70 | 4.5 | 0 |
| **Pork Tongue**, ⅓ tongue | 75 | 5.5 | 0 |
| **Sousemeat**, 1 oz | 60 | 4.5 | 0 |
| **Succotash**, ½ cup | 80 | 1 | 17 |
| **Sweet Potato Pie**, ⅛ of 9" pie | 250 | 12 | 34 |
| **Tripe**, 2 oz | 55 | 2 | 0 |
| **Vienna Sausage:** | | | |
| 2 small, 1 oz | 90 | 8 | 1 |
| 1 small, 0.5 oz | 45 | 4 | 0.5 |

OLD McDONALDS FARM
128 FOR PEOPLE WHO WANT BETTER

Brooklyn

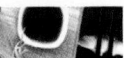

## Spanish

|  | C | F | Cb |
|---|---|---|---|
| **Arroz Abanda**, (Fish with Rice) | 340 | 8 | 31 |
| **Arroz Con Pollo**, (Rice/Chkn Salad) | 500 | 23 | 50 |
| **Clams Marinara**, 8 clams | 330 | 16 | 22 |
| **Cochifrito**, (Lamb with Lemon/Garlic) | 650 | 25 | 5 |
| **Cochinillo Asado**, (Rst Suckling Pig), 2 slices | 300 | 15 | 3 |
| **Cocido Madrileno**, (Madrid-Style Boiled Dinner) | 450 | 27 | 18 |
| **Flan de Leche**, (Caramel Custard) | 325 | 9 | 52 |
| **Fritadera de Ternera**, (Sauteed Veal) | 450 | 27 | 2 |
| **Gazpacho**, 1 bowl | 60 | 0 | 15 |
| **Mole Poblano**, ½ cup | 205 | 14 | 16 |
| **Paella a la Valenciana**, (Chicken & Shellfish Rice) | 900 | 42 | 70 |
| **Pollo a la Espanola**, (Chicken) | 475 | 30 | 4 |
| **Ternera al Jerez**, (Veal with Sherry) | 660 | 29 | 6 |
| **Zarzuela**, (Fish & Shellfish Medley) | 530 | 27 | 40 |

## Thai Foods

|  | C | F | Cb |
|---|---|---|---|
| **Appetizers:** Satay Pork, 1 oz | 100 | 4 | 2 |
| Spring Roll, 1.3 oz | 110 | 6 | 13 |
| **Soups,** Tom Yam (Hot & Sour): | | | |
| Spicy Shrimp/Seafood: | | | |
| 1 cup | 100 | 4 | 6 |
| 1 bowl | 160 | 7 | 10 |
| Vegetarian, 1 cup | 50 | 0 | 11 |
| **Curries:** Chicken with Ginger, 1 cup | 390 | 34 | 4 |
| Thick Red Curry with Beef, 1 cup | 600 | 50 | 7 |
| Thai Chicken Curry, 1 cup | 340 | 23 | 4 |
| Massaman Curry, 1 cup | 680 | 57 | 8 |
| Green Curry with Pork, 1 cup | 480 | 44 | 5 |
| **Pad Thai,** large serving, 18 oz | 990 | 38 | 125 |
| **Fish:** Steamed with Spicy Thai Sce | 450 | 8 | 46 |
| Crispy Fried, 5 oz | 290 | 15 | 9 |
| **Spicy Chicken,** stir-fry | 450 | 22 | 14 |
| **Spicy Garlic Tofu,** stir-fry | 340 | 18 | 18 |
| **Sticky Thai Rice:** Plain 1 cup, 6 oz | 170 | 0.5 | 36 |
| With Coconut & Sesame Seeds, 1 cup | 880 | 28 | 120 |
| **Stir-fried Rice Noodles,** 1 cup 5.5 oz | 270 | 9 | 40 |
| **Stir-fried Vegetables,** 1 cup | 100 | 3 | 18 |
| **Salads:** Green Papaya Salad | 160 | 0 | 40 |
| Spicy Prawn, 9 shrimp | 170 | 3 | 15 |
| Thai Beef Salad, 1 serving | 260 | 9 | 15 |
| Thai Chicken, 1 serving | 330 | 9 | 17 |
| Thai Noodle, 1 serving | 410 | 13 | 45 |
| **Satay Chicken & Peanut Sauce,** 1 satay stick | 390 | 24 | 20 |
| **Sauce,** Peanut Satay, ½ cup, 4 oz | 160 | 10 | 13 |

## Vietnamese

|  | C | F | Cb |
|---|---|---|---|
| **Banh Cuon**, (Steam Rice w/ Pork), 1 roll | 105 | 7 | 8 |
| **Bo Nuong**, (Beef Satay), 2 sticks | 265 | 9 | 4 |
| **Bo Xao Dau Phong**, (Ginger Beef with Onion, Fish Sce) | 750 | 30 | 10 |
| **Ca Chien Gung**, (Whole Snapper/Ginger) | 600 | 16 | 6 |
| **Canh Chay**, (Vegetable/Tofu Soup) | 80 | 3 | 13 |
| **Cari Chicken**, 1 cup | 475 | 29 | 16 |
| **Cari Chicken**, with Rice Noodle, 1 cup curry & 1 cup noodles | 660 | 29 | 60 |
| **Cari Chicken**, with Steamed Rice, 1 cup curry & 1 cup rice | 650 | 29 | 55 |
| **Cuu Xao Lan**, (Curried Lamb and Veggies in Coconut) | 900 | 40 | 80 |
| **Ga Chien**, (Crisp Chick + Plum Sauce) | 900 | 40 | 105 |
| **Ga Nuong**, (Chicken Satay + Sauce) | 240 | 10 | 4 |
| **Ga Xao Rau**, (Marinated Chicken Braised with Vegetables) | 800 | 26 | 100 |
| **Gio Lua**, (Lean Pork Pie), ⅙ of pie | 245 | 12 | 0 |
| **Goi Cuon**, (Cold Spring Rolls), 1 roll | 60 | 1 | 7 |
| **Rau Cai Xao Chay**, (Stir Fried Veggies) | 400 | 15 | 65 |
| **Thit Bo Vien**, (Beef Balls), 6 balls | 225 | 14 | 2 |
| **Thit Heo Goi Baup Cai**, (Spicy Cabb. Rolls with Pork), 1 roll | 200 | 7 | 11 |
| **Soup:** Per Bowl, ½ Cup | | | |
| Bun Bo Hue, (Hot & Spicy Soup): | | | |
| Without Pork Feet | 340 | 9 | 35 |
| With Pork Feet | 830 | 45 | 35 |
| Chicken & Rice Noodle Soup | 400 | 3 | 55 |
| Pho Bo, (Beef Noodle Soup) | 410 | 7 | 59 |
| Pho Ga, (Chicken Noodle Soup) | 460 | 6 | 58 |
| Pho Tai, (Rare Beef & Noodle Soup) | 440 | 7 | 73 |
| **Salad:** Goi Du Du, (Green Papaya), ½ cup | 155 | 3 | 29 |
| **Sauce,** Nuoc Cham (Hot Sauce) | 5 | 0 | 1 |

## Gourmet & Miscellaneous

|  | C | F | Cb |
|---|---|---|---|
| **Ants Eggs/Larvae,** 1 Tbsp | 20 | 0 | 0 |
| **Ants,** chocolate coated, 3 Tbsp | 140 | 7 | 2 |
| **Bee Maggots,** canned, 3 Tbsp | 65 | 2 | 0 |
| **Caviar,** black/red, 1 Tbsp | 40 | 3 | 0 |
| **Caterpillars,** canned, 2 oz | 60 | 2 | 0 |
| **Frog Legs,** fried, 1 pair (large) | 125 | 7 | 0 |
| **Haggis,** boiled, 4 oz | 350 | 24 | 22 |
| **Locusts,** roasted, 1 oz | 35 | 1 | 0 |
| **Silkworms,** raw, 1 oz | 60 | 2 | 0 |
| **Snails in garlic butter,** 6 large | 200 | 10 | 4 |
| **Snake,** roasted, 4 oz | 160 | 6 | 0 |

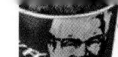

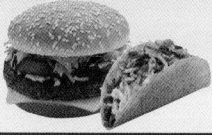

# Fast - Foods & *Restaurants*

©2017 Allan Borushek

*Nutritional data is based on U.S. outlets*

*For More Restaurants &*
*Full Nutritional Data*
*~ See CalorieKing.com*

## A&W® (Aug '16)

| | C | F | Cb |
|---|---|---|---|
| **Burgers:** | | | |
| Hamburger | 340 | 16 | 39 |
| Cheeseburger | 400 | 21 | 39 |
| Double Cheeseburger | 455 | 26 | 40 |
| Original: Bacon Cheeseburger | 440 | 25 | 41 |
| Bacon Double Cheeseburger | 645 | 41 | 42 |
| Papa Burger | 550 | 33 | 43 |
| **Sandwiches:** | | | |
| Crispy Chicken | 440 | 18 | 51 |
| Grilled Chicken | 400 | 15 | 40 |
| **Chicken Tenders,** breaded, 3 pcs | 260 | 9 | 5 |
| **Corn Dog Nuggets:** Kid's 5 pieces | 180 | 8 | 20 |
| 10 pieces | 350 | 17 | 40 |
| **Hot Dogs:** Plain | 310 | 19 | 23 |
| Coney Chili Dog | 340 | 20 | 26 |
| Coney Cheese Dog | 380 | 23 | 28 |
| **Fries/Sides:** | | | |
| **Cheese Curds,** 5 oz | 570 | 40 | 27 |
| **Chili Cheese Fries,** 7 oz | 410 | 17 | 52 |
| **French Fries:** | | | |
| Small/Kids, 2.5 oz | 200 | 8 | 29 |
| Regular, 4 oz | 310 | 13 | 45 |
| Large, 5.5 oz | 430 | 17 | 61 |
| **Onion Rings,** 7-9 rings | 350 | 16 | 45 |
| **Sauces:** Per 1.25 oz | | | |
| BBQ | 90 | 0 | 22 |
| Honey Mustard | 140 | 11 | 10 |
| Papas, Regular/Spicy | 170 | 15 | 8 |
| Spicy Ketchup | 60 | 0 | 15 |
| **A & W Root Beer:** Kids, 12 fl.oz | 150 | 0 | 43 |
| Small, 16 fl.oz | 220 | 0 | 58 |
| Regular, 20 fl.oz | 270 | 0 | 72 |
| Large, 32 fl.oz | 440 | 0 | 116 |
| **Famous Floats:** | | | |
| **A&W Root Beer Float:** | | | |
| 16 oz Cup | 330 | 5 | 70 |
| 20 oz Cup | 350 | 6 | 77 |
| 32 oz Cup | 640 | 10 | 136 |
| **Diet Root Beer,** 16 oz | 170 | 5 | 30 |
| **Orange Float,** 16 oz | 320 | 5 | 74 |
| **Freeze:** | | | |
| **A&W Root Beer:** 16 oz | 370 | 8 | 68 |
| 32 oz | 820 | 18 | 150 |
| **Diet Root Beer,** 16 oz | 270 | 8 | 39 |
| **Orange,** 16 oz | 420 | 8 | 82 |
| **Polar Swirls:** Oreo/M&M's, av. 12 oz | 700 | 25 | 107 |
| Reese's, 12 oz | 740 | 31 | 97 |
| **Shakes:** Strawberry, 16 oz | 670 | 29 | 90 |
| Chocolate/Vanilla, av. 16 oz | 710 | 30 | 100 |
| 20 oz Cup | 890 | 38 | 123 |
| **Soft Serve:** Includes Cone | | | |
| Small, 4 oz | 200 | 5 | 32 |
| Large, 5.5 oz | 260 | 7 | 41 |
| **Sundaes:** Choc./Strawberry, av. | 310 | 8 | 50 |
| Caramel/Hot Fudge, av. | 350 | 10 | 56 |

## Applebees® (Aug '16)

| | C | F | Cb |
|---|---|---|---|
| **Appetizers:** As Served | | | |
| Boneless Wings, w/out Dressing | 680 | 35 | 52 |
| **Dressings:** Bleu Cheese | 240 | 25 | 1 |
| Ranch | 200 | 21 | 2 |
| **Sauce:** Honey BBQ | 230 | 0 | 55 |
| Sweet Asian Chili | 250 | 2 | 56 |
| Brew Pub Pretzels & Beer Cheese Dip | 1050 | 44 | 130 |
| Chicken Quesadillas | 980 | 58 | 61 |
| Chips & Salsa | 500 | 22 | 69 |
| Mozzarella Sticks | 920 | 51 | 79 |
| Salsa Verde Beef Nachos | 1800 | 122 | 109 |
| Spinach & Artichoke Dip | 960 | 58 | 91 |
| Sriracha Shrimp | 680 | 44 | 55 |
| Steak Quesadilla | 1000 | 61 | 61 |
| Sweet Potato Fries & Dip | 1070 | 63 | 118 |
| **Burgers:** Without Sides | | | |
| Classic Burger: No cheese or bacon | 780 | 50 | 44 |
| + American or Swiss, average | 155 | 12 | 1 |
| + Cheddar; Monterey Jack, av. | 85 | 8 | 0 |
| + Bacon | 100 | 8 | 1 |
| Quesadilla Burger | 1410 | 106 | 47 |
| The All Day Brunch | 1190 | 81 | 61 |
| The American Standard | 1030 | 71 | 48 |
| The Blazin' Texan | 1060 | 66 | 61 |
| Triple Bacon | 1190 | 84 | 47 |
| **Chicken:** Includes Standard Sides | | | |
| Bourbon Street Chkn & Shrimp | 640 | 31 | 40 |
| Chicken Tenders, Basket | 1160 | 66 | 102 |
| Crispy Brewhouse Chicken | 1090 | 63 | 82 |
| Fiesta Lime Chicken | 1140 | 62 | 91 |
| **Handhelds:** Without Sides | | | |
| Battered Fish Sandwich | 770 | 51 | 56 |
| Brew Pub Philly | 1130 | 69 | 73 |
| Chicken Fajita Rollup | 1100 | 63 | 66 |
| Clubhouse Grille | 1120 | 63 | 87 |
| **Lighter Fare:** Includes Standard Sides | | | |
| Cedar Grilled Lemon Chicken | 570 | 25 | 47 |
| Grilled Onion Sirloin with Stout Gravy | 550 | 24 | 44 |
| Hot Shot Whisky Chicken | 640 | 30 | 42 |
| Shrimp Wonton Stir Fry | 590 | 12 | 95 |
| Thai Shrimp Salad | 380 | 19 | 32 |
| **Pasta:** As Served | | | |
| 4-Cheese Mac & Cheese, w/ Honey Pepper Chicken Tenders | 1580 | 78 | 154 |
| Three- Cheese Chicken Cavatappi | 1170 | 72 | 82 |
| **Seafood:** As Served | | | |
| Blackened Tilapia | 510 | 26 | 41 |
| Double Crunch Shrimp | 1240 | 59 | 146 |
| Hand-Battered Fish & Chips | 1530 | 102 | 108 |
| New England Fish & Chips | 2010 | 138 | 138 |

Updated Nutrition Data ~ www.CalorieKing.com
Persons with Diabetes ~ See Disclaimer (Page 22)

## Applebees® cont... (Aug '16)

*Wood-Fired Grill:* Without Sides

| | C | F | Cb |
|---|---|---|---|
| Butcher's Reserve 12 Top Sirloin | 380 | 11 | 1 |
| Cedar Grilled Salmon | 340 | 22 | 2 |

**Chef's Selection:**

| | C | F | Cb |
|---|---|---|---|
| Cedar Salmon w/ Maple Mustrd | 540 | 32 | 28 |
| Shrimp 'N Parmesan Sirloin, 8 oz | 580 | 37 | 6 |
| Smokin' double Steak & Egg | 470 | 21 | 15 |

Double Glazed Baby Back Ribs:

| | C | F | Cb |
|---|---|---|---|
| Full Rack, without Sauce | 850 | 57 | 21 |
| Half Rack, without Sauce | 430 | 28 | 10 |
| Sauce: Honey BBQ, Full Rack | 150 | 0 | 37 |
| Half Rack | 80 | 0 | 18 |
| Smokey Chipotle, Full Rack | 170 | 1.5 | 38 |
| Half Rack | 60 | 1.5 | 12 |
| Grilled Chicken Breast | 190 | 3 | 1 |
| Hand-Cut Bone-In Pork Chop | 370 | 18 | 3 |
| Top Sirloin: 6 oz | 230 | 9 | 2 |
| 8 oz | 280 | 10 | 2 |

*Salads:* Regular, with Dressing

| | C | F | Cb |
|---|---|---|---|
| Fiesta Chicken, Chopped | 860 | 42 | 84 |
| Grilled Chicken Caesar | 790 | 56 | 26 |
| Oriental Grilled Chicken | 1280 | 84 | 84 |
| Pecan Crusted Chicken | 1340 | 80 | 115 |

*Sides:* As Served

| | C | F | Cb |
|---|---|---|---|
| 4-Cheese Mac & Cheese | 510 | 28 | 41 |
| Baked Potato | 390 | 24 | 41 |
| BBQ Spiced Fries | 440 | 20 | 60 |
| Classic Fries | 440 | 20 | 59 |
| Crunchy Onion Rings | 530 | 29 | 60 |
| Garlic Mashed Potatoes | 270 | 14 | 30 |
| Garlic Mashed Potatoes, loaded | 490 | 33 | 34 |
| Garlicky Green Beans | 180 | 15 | 11 |
| Hearty Grains & Rice | 250 | 2 | 53 |
| House Salad, w/out Dressing | 190 | 12 | 11 |
| Sweet Potato Fries | 340 | 12 | 57 |
| Wood-Fired Grilled Veggies | 160 | 13 | 11 |

*Soup:*

| | C | F | Cb |
|---|---|---|---|
| Chicken Tortilla Soup | 200 | 9 | 22 |
| Chili | 320 | 18 | 14 |
| French Onion Soup | 330 | 20 | 20 |
| Tomato Basil Soup | 190 | 12 | 16 |

*Desserts:* As Served

| | C | F | Cb |
|---|---|---|---|
| Apple Chimi Cheesecake | 930 | 36 | 138 |
| Butter Pecan Blondie | 1180 | 62 | 139 |
| Churro S'mores | 580 | 10 | 120 |
| Triple Choc. Meltdown | 980 | 52 | 125 |

## Arby's® (Aug '16)

*Sandwiches:*

| | C | F | Cb |
|---|---|---|---|
| **Beef 'n Cheddar:** Classic | 450 | 20 | 45 |
| Mid | 560 | 27 | 45 |
| Reuben | 680 | 31 | 62 |
| **Roast Beef:** Classic | 360 | 14 | 37 |
| Mid | 460 | 20 | 37 |
| Max | 560 | 27 | 38 |

**Chicken:**

| | C | F | Cb |
|---|---|---|---|
| Chicken Bacon Swiss, Crispy | 610 | 30 | 52 |
| Chicken Cordon Bleu , Crispy | 650 | 34 | 49 |
| Crispy Chicken | 500 | 25 | 49 |

**Turkey:**

| | C | F | Cb |
|---|---|---|---|
| Roast Turkey & Swiss | 710 | 28 | 79 |
| Roast Turkey, Ranch & Bacon | 800 | 34 | 79 |

**Wraps:**

| | C | F | Cb |
|---|---|---|---|
| Roast Turkey & Swiss | 520 | 27 | 39 |
| Roast Turkey, Ranch & Bacon | 620 | 34 | 39 |

*Sliders:*

| | C | F | Cb |
|---|---|---|---|
| Chicken Tender 'N Cheese | 290 | 12 | 30 |
| Corned Beef 'N Cheese | 220 | 9 | 21 |
| Ham & Cheddar | 230 | 9 | 22 |
| Jalapeno/Roast Beef 'N Cheese | 240 | 11 | 21 |

*Chicken:*

| | C | F | Cb |
|---|---|---|---|
| **Chicken Tenders,** 3 tenders | 360 | 17 | 28 |
| **Chicken Tenders,** 5 tenders | 600 | 28 | 47 |

*Optional/Regional Menu:*

| | C | F | Cb |
|---|---|---|---|
| **Homestyle Fries:** Kids | 240 | 11 | 33 |
| Small | 350 | 16 | 49 |
| Medium | 480 | 21 | 67 |
| Large | 600 | 26 | 84 |
| **Melts:** Arby's | 330 | 12 | 39 |
| Ham & Swiss | 300 | 8 | 37 |

*Kids Meals:*

| | C | F | Cb |
|---|---|---|---|
| Curly Fries, 2.75 oz | 250 | 13 | 29 |
| Prime Cut Chkn Tenders, (2), 3 oz | 240 | 11 | 19 |
| Roast Beef 'n Cheese Slider | 240 | 11 | 21 |

*Fries:*

| | C | F | Cb |
|---|---|---|---|
| **Curly Fries:** Small, 4.5 oz | 410 | 22 | 49 |
| Medium, 6 oz | 550 | 29 | 65 |
| Large, 7 oz | 650 | 35 | 77 |

*Snack 'N Save:*

| | C | F | Cb |
|---|---|---|---|
| **Jalapeno Bites:** | | | |
| 5 bites | 290 | 17 | 31 |
| 8 bites | 470 | 27 | 50 |
| **Mozzarella Sticks:** 4 sticks | 440 | 23 | 37 |
| 6 sticks | 650 | 35 | 56 |
| **Potato Cakes:** 3 cakes | 370 | 21 | 35 |
| 4 cakes | 490 | 28 | 46 |
| **Steakhouse Onion Rings,** 5 rings | 420 | 21 | 52 |

*Continued Next Page...*

## Arby's® cont... (June '16)

*Salads: Without Dressing*

| | C | F | Cb |
|---|---|---|---|
| **Chopped Farmhouse:** | | | |
| Crispy Chicken | 430 | 24 | 26 |
| Roast Turkey | 230 | 13 | 8 |
| **Dressings:** *Per 1.5 oz packet* | | | |
| Balsamic Vinaigrette | 130 | 12 | 4 |
| Buttermilk Ranch | 210 | 22 | 2 |
| Dijon Honey Mustard | 180 | 16 | 8 |
| Light Italian | 20 | 1 | 2 |
| **Breakfast:** *Per Serving* | | | |
| **Biscuits:** Bacon, Egg & Cheese | 490 | 29 | 38 |
| Ham, Egg & Cheese | 470 | 25 | 39 |
| Sausage, Egg & Cheese | 620 | 43 | 36 |
| **Croissants:** Bacon, Egg & Cheese | 440 | 27 | 29 |
| Ham, Egg & Cheese | 420 | 23 | 30 |
| Sausage, Egg & Cheese | 590 | 44 | 30 |
| **Sourdoughs:** | | | |
| Bacon, Egg & Cheese | 490 | 23 | 46 |
| Ham, Egg & Cheese | 470 | 19 | 47 |
| Sausage, Egg & Cheese | 640 | 39 | 47 |
| **Wraps:** Bacon, Egg & Cheese | 500 | 27 | 41 |
| Ham, Egg & Cheese | 440 | 22 | 42 |
| Sausage, Egg & Cheese | 630 | 41 | 42 |
| **Sauces:** Arby's, 0.5 oz | 15 | 0 | 3 |
| Bronco Berry, 1 oz | 60 | 0 | 15 |
| Cheddar Cheese, 1.5 oz | 50 | 3.5 | 4 |
| Horsey, 0.5 oz | 60 | 5 | 3 |
| Marinara, 1 oz | 20 | 0 | 4 |
| Spicy Three Pepper, 0.5 oz | 25 | 1 | 3 |
| Tangy BBQ, 1 oz | 40 | 0 | 9 |
| **Dipping Sauces:** Buffalo, 1 oz | 10 | 1 | 2 |
| Honey Mustard, 1 oz | 140 | 13 | 5 |
| Ranch, 1 oz | 100 | 11 | 2 |
| **Dessert:** | | | |
| **Turnovers:** Apple with Icing | 430 | 18 | 65 |
| Cherry Turnover with Icing | 390 | 13 | 65 |
| **Shakes:** *Per Regular 22 oz* | | | |
| Chocolate; Jamocha | 570 | 15 | 99 |
| Vanilla | 470 | 15 | 75 |
| **Sodas:** *Without Ice* | | | |
| **Mountain Dew:** | | | |
| Small, 16 oz | 200 | 0 | 54 |
| Medium, 22 oz | 280 | 0 | 75 |
| Large, 29 oz | 360 | 0 | 96 |
| **Dr Pepper/Pepsi, average:** | | | |
| Small, 16 fl.oz | 180 | 0 | 48 |
| Medium, 22 oz | 250 | 0 | 68 |
| Large, 28 oz | 325 | 0 | 88 |

## Atlanta Bread Co® (Aug '16)

| | C | F | Cb |
|---|---|---|---|
| **Breakfast Sandwiches:** | | | |
| Egg & Cheese | 410 | 13 | 55 |
| Egg, Cheese & Ham | 460 | 15 | 56 |
| Egg, Cheese & Turkey Sausage | 520 | 20 | 56 |
| *Side,* Breakfast Potatoes | 170 | 9 | 20 |
| **Sandwiches:** Chicken Salad | 630 | 27 | 59 |
| Honey Maple Ham | 420 | 7 | 66 |
| Roast Beef | 400 | 6 | 57 |
| Roasted Turkey | 380 | 3 | 58 |
| Veggie | 460 | 17 | 59 |
| **Half Sandwich/Panini & Half Salad Options:** | | | |
| *Without Salad Dressing or Sandwich Condiments* | | | |
| Hummus & Edamame S'wch & Greek Salad | 370 | 24 | 24 |
| Italian Veggie Panini w/ Caesar Salad | 330 | 22 | 23 |
| Roast Beef S'wich w/ MontAmore Salad | 300 | 10 | 34 |
| Tuna Salad S'wch w/ Bals Blue Salad | 520 | 25 | 56 |
| Veggie Sandwich with Greek Salad | 360 | 17 | 38 |
| **Salads:** *Without Dressing or Bread* | | | |
| Buffalo Chicken Salad | 280 | 12 | 14 |
| Chardonnay Brie Salad | 260 | 16 | 18 |
| Salsa Fresca Salmon Salad | 280 | 11 | 23 |
| **Sides:** Edamame | 150 | 4.5 | 14 |
| Black Beans & Corn | 190 | 9 | 24 |

## Au Bon Pain® (Aug '16)

| | C | F | Cb |
|---|---|---|---|
| **Bagels:** *Per Bagel* | | | |
| Asiago Cheese, 3.9 oz | 330 | 7 | 50 |
| Cinnamon Crisp, 3.9 oz | 370 | 6 | 71 |
| Everything, 3.3 oz | 260 | 2 | 52 |
| Honey 9 Grain, 3.6 oz | 280 | 2.5 | 56 |
| Onion Dill, 3.6 oz | 260 | 1 | 53 |
| Plain Bagel, 3.2 oz | 250 | 1 | 51 |
| Whole Wheat Skinny , 1.6 oz | 90 | 1 | 21 |
| **Breakfast Sandwiches:** | | | |
| 2 Eggs on a Bagel | 390 | 11 | 51 |
| with Bacon | 470 | 17 | 51 |
| with Cheese | 450 | 16 | 51 |
| Egg Whites, Cheddar w/ Skinny Bagel | 210 | 7 | 22 |
| Smoked Salmon & Wasabi on Bagel | 380 | 9 | 58 |
| **Fruit Cup,** Large, 12 oz | 140 | 0 | 36 |
| **Yogurt/Parfait:** Blueberry | 380 | 8 | 71 |
| Greek Vanilla/Blueberry | 340 | 6 | 51 |
| **Oatmeal:** Classic, Medium, 12 oz | 260 | 5 | 47 |
| Blueberry Chia, Medium, 12 oz | 270 | 9 | 39 |
| **Sandwiches:** *Whole* | | | |
| **Cafe:** BLT | 500 | 23 | 52 |
| Black Angus Rst Beef & Cheddar | 560 | 20 | 62 |
| Classic Chicken Salad | 440 | 12 | 59 |
| Tuna Salad | 450 | 9 | 60 |
| Turkey & Swiss | 660 | 28 | 66 |
| **Signature:** Caprese, with Chicken | 670 | 30 | 54 |
| Chipotle Turkey & Avocado | 670 | 30 | 61 |
| Turkey Club | 610 | 24 | 53 |

## Au Bon Pain® cont... (Aug '16)

*Harvest Hot Bowls:*

| | C | F | Cb |
|---|---|---|---|
| Mayan Chicken | 600 | 16 | 81 |
| Roasted Vetetarian | 790 | 41 | 85 |
| Teriyaki Steak | 550 | 12 | 78 |
| *Macaroni & Cheese,* medium, 12 oz | 880 | 43 | 92 |
| *Meat Lasagna,* 11 oz | 470 | 24 | 41 |
| *Soups:* Chicken Gumbo, 12 oz | 200 | 9 | 23 |
| French Onion, 12 oz | 110 | 5 | 15 |
| Harvest Pumpkin, 12 oz | 230 | 13 | 24 |
| Lobster & Corn Bisque, 12 oz | 280 | 16 | 25 |
| Minestrone, 12 oz | 180 | 6 | 24 |
| *Vegetarian Chili,* 12 oz | 260 | 2 | 46 |
| *Salads: Without Dressing* | | | |
| Chicken Caesar Asiago | 270 | 10 | 20 |
| Chicken Cobb, w/ Avocado | 440 | 26 | 15 |
| Harvest Turkey | 390 | 15 | 35 |
| Vegetarian Deluxe | 270 | 13 | 29 |
| *Dressings:* Bleu Cheese, 2 oz | 310 | 33 | 2 |
| Caesar, 2 oz | 250 | 25 | 3 |
| Lite Buttermilk Ranch, 2 oz | 120 | 2 | 5 |
| *Cakes, Cookies, Croissants : Per Item* | | | |
| **Brownie Bites,** 5 oz | 600 | 25 | 82 |
| **Cakes:** Red Velvet Cupcake, 3 oz | 400 | 22 | 46 |
| Pound Cakes: Iced Lemon, 4.5 oz | 470 | 21 | 66 |
| Marble, 4 oz | 450 | 24 | 54 |
| **Cookies:** Chocolate Chip | 370 | 18 | 54 |
| Oatmeal Raisin | 290 | 11 | 46 |
| **Croissants:** Almond, 4 oz | 500 | 31 | 48 |
| Apple & Cinn., 3.4 oz | 240 | 8 | 38 |
| Chocolate, 4 oz | 480 | 25 | 57 |
| Ham & Cheese Croissant | 410 | 22 | 35 |
| **Danish,** Blueb./Cherry, av. 3.7 oz | 380 | 15 | 53 |
| **Muffins:** Blueberry, 4.7 oz | 490 | 19 | 73 |
| Berry, Low-Fat, 4.5 oz | 290 | 3 | 61 |
| Carrot Walnut, 5 oz | 540 | 25 | 73 |
| Raisin Bran, 5.5oz | 420 | 11 | 78 |
| **Palmier,** 2.6 oz | 380 | 20 | 46 |
| **Pecan Roll,** 6 oz | 740 | 43 | 85 |
| **Scone,** Blueberry, 3.7 oz | 410 | 21 | 50 |
| **Beverages:** Caffe Latte, 16 fl.oz | 140 | 7 | 12 |
| Caramel Macchiato, 16 fl.oz | 270 | 7 | 43 |
| Hot Chocolate, 16 fl.oz | 360 | 8 | 50 |
| Raspberry Iced Tea, 24 fl.oz | 180 | 0 | 50 |
| Strawberry Smoothie, 16 fl.oz | 290 | 0 | 68 |

*Extra Menu Items ~ See CalorieKing.com*

## Auntie Anne's® (Aug '16)

*Pretzels:* With Butter

| | C | F | Cb |
|---|---|---|---|
| Cinnamon Sugar | 470 | 12 | 84 |
| Jalapeno | 330 | 5 | 63 |
| Original | 340 | 5 | 65 |
| Original Stix, 6 sticks | 340 | 5 | 65 |
| Pepperoni | 480 | 16 | 65 |
| Sour Cream & Onion | 360 | 5 | 68 |
| Sweet Almond | 390 | 6 | 74 |
| *Dipping Sauces:* | | | |
| Caramel Dip, 1.5 oz | 130 | 3 | 23 |
| Cheese Dip; Hot Salsa Cheese, av., 1 oz | 95 | 8 | 3 |
| Light Cream Cheese, 1.3 oz | 80 | 6 | 1 |
| Marinara, 2 oz | 45 | 1 | 7 |
| Sweet Glaze, 1.4 oz | 130 | 0 | 32 |
| Sweet Mustard, 1.3 oz | 60 | 2 | 10 |
| *Pretzel Dogs:* Original | 360 | 20 | 33 |
| Cheese | 370 | 20 | 33 |
| Jalapeno & Cheese | 370 | 20 | 34 |
| Jumbo | 610 | 29 | 67 |
| *Beverages:* Per 16 fl.oz | | | |
| **Frozen Lemonade Mixer,** | | | |
| Blue Raspberry; Strawberry, av. | 235 | 0 | 60 |

## Back Yard Burgers® (Aug '16)

*Black Angus Burgers:*

| | C | F | Cb |
|---|---|---|---|
| ⅓ lb Bacon Cheddar Burger | 840 | 57 | 37 |
| Back Yard: Classic Burger | 650 | 40 | 36 |
| Double Classic | 1040 | 70 | 36 |
| Black Jack Burger | 860 | 64 | 34 |
| Black & Bleu Burger | 880 | 63 | 36 |
| Chipotle Burger | 910 | 60 | 34 |
| Junior Back Yard Burger | 440 | 22 | 34 |
| Mushroom Swiss Burger | 760 | 50 | 35 |
| *Chicken Sandwiches:* | | | |
| Blackened Chicken | 500 | 25 | 41 |
| Black Jack Chicken Club | 670 | 43 | 38 |
| Grilled Chicken | 370 | 12 | 36 |
| Hawaiian Chicken | 420 | 12 | 48 |
| *Chicken Tenders:* Basket | 465 | 25 | 33 |
| Crispy Tenders, Kids | 310 | 17 | 22 |
| *Turkey Burgers:* Classic | 565 | 38 | 36 |
| Wild Turkey Burger | 675 | 50 | 35 |
| *Veggie Burger,* Regular | 410 | 15 | 57 |
| *Specialties:* | | | |
| Back Yard Dog | 320 | 18 | 29 |
| Chili Cheese Dog | 640 | 145 | 32 |
| Loaded Smoked Sausage | 580 | 39 | 30 |
| Original Smoked Sausage | 450 | 28 | 32 |

*Continued Next Page ...*

## Back Yard Burgers® cont... (Aug '16)

*Fries:*

| | C | F | Cb |
|---|---|---|---|
| **Chili Cheese Fries,** regular | 660 | 48 | 48 |
| **Seasoned Fries:** Kid's, 3.5 oz | 350 | 25 | 32 |
| Regular, 6.5 oz | 510 | 36 | 46 |
| Large, 8 oz | 650 | 47 | 56 |
| **Sweet Potato Fries,** regular, 5 oz | 560 | 43 | 43 |
| **Waffle Fries:** Kid's, 3.5 oz | 380 | 25 | 35 |
| Regular, 4.5 oz | 570 | 37 | 52 |
| *Sides:* Coleslaw | 40 | 2 | 5 |
| **Fried Pickles,** 4 oz | 260 | 19 | 30 |
| **Back Yard Chili** | 375 | 23 | 22 |
| **Loaded Baked Potato** | 540 | 21 | 70 |
| **Panko Onion Rings,** regular, 4 oz | 300 | 14 | 37 |
| *Salads:* Side Salad | 190 | 11 | 30 |
| **Back Yard Salad:** w. Grilled Chkn | 490 | 26 | 22 |
| with Blackened Chicken | 590 | 38 | 22 |
| **Cranberry Pecan Chicken** | 760 | 42 | 55 |
| *Dressings:* Bleu Cheese | 220 | 24 | 1 |
| Gorgonzola Vinaigrette | 170 | 15 | 6 |
| Honey Mustard | 240 | 23 | 7 |
| Ranch, Homestyle | 150 | 15 | 2 |
| *Dessert/Cobblers:* Apple/Cherry, av. | 350 | 13 | 59 |
| Apple/Cherry A La Mode | 510 | 20 | 78 |
| *Ice Cream:* A La Carte | 150 | 8 | 20 |
| *Milk Shakes:* Choc./Strawb./Van., av. | 630 | 29 | 83 |
| Chocolate Oreo | 780 | 36 | 104 |

## Baja Fresh® (Aug '16)

| | C | F | Cb |
|---|---|---|---|
| *Baja Bowls:* Chicken | 640 | 7 | 97 |
| Shrimp | 630 | 7 | 100 |
| Steak/Carnitas, av. | 700 | 15 | 99 |
| Veggie & Cheese | 580 | 10 | 101 |
| *Burritos: With Standard Menu Board Components* | | | |
| **Baja:** with Carnitas | 830 | 45 | 67 |
| with Chicken | 790 | 38 | 65 |
| with Steak | 850 | 46 | 67 |
| **Bean & Cheese:** | | | |
| with Carnitas | 1010 | 42 | 98 |
| with Chicken | 970 | 35 | 96 |
| with Steak | 1030 | 43 | 97 |
| Vegetarian, without Meat | 840 | 33 | 96 |
| **Mexicano:** with Carnitas | 830 | 20 | 119 |
| with Chicken | 790 | 13 | 117 |
| with Steak | 860 | 21 | 118 |
| **Ultimo:** with Chicken | 880 | 38 | 84 |
| with Steak | 950 | 44 | 85 |
| **Vegetarian,** Grilled Veggie | 800 | 33 | 94 |
| *Fajitas: As Served, without Tortilla Chips* | | | |
| Chicken, with Corn Tortillas | 860 | 24 | 105 |
| Chicken, with Flour Tortillas | 1140 | 33 | 147 |

## Baja Fresh® cont... (Aug '16)

*Nachos: As Served*

| | C | F | Cb |
|---|---|---|---|
| **Regular:** with Cheese | 945 | 54 | 82 |
| with Chicken | 1010 | 55 | 82 |
| with Steak | 1060 | 59 | 82 |
| *Quesadillas:* | | | |
| with Cheese | 1200 | 78 | 84 |
| with Chicken | 1330 | 80 | 84 |
| with Steak | 1430 | 87 | 84 |
| Vegetarian | 1260 | 78 | 96 |
| *Tacos: With Standard Components, Without Dressing* | | | |
| **Americano, Soft Taco:** Carnitas | 250 | 12 | 21 |
| Chicken | 230 | 10 | 20 |
| **Crispy Wahoo** | 250 | 13 | 27 |
| **Grilled Wahoo,** with black beans | 180 | 1 | 30 |
| **Original Baja,** average all varieties | 215 | 6.5 | 28 |
| *Salads: With Standard Components, Without Dressing* | | | |
| **Baja Ensalada:** with Carnitas | 370 | 18 | 20 |
| with Chicken | 310 | 7 | 18 |
| with Shrimp | 230 | 6 | 18 |
| with Steak | 450 | 18 | 18 |
| **Tostada:** with Carnitas | 1180 | 62 | 100 |
| with Chicken | 1140 | 55 | 98 |
| with Shrimp | 1120 | 55 | 99 |
| with Steak | 1230 | 63 | 98 |
| *Sides:* Tortilla Chips, 1.5 oz | 210 | 9 | 29 |
| Tortilla Chips & Guacamole | 1340 | 83 | 141 |

*For Complete Nutritional Data ~ see CalorieKing.com*

## Baskin Robbins® (Aug '16)

*Cones:*

| | C | F | Cb |
|---|---|---|---|
| Cake | 25 | 0 | 5 |
| Fresh-Baked Waffle | 160 | 3.5 | 29 |
| Sugar | 45 | 0.5 | 9 |
| *Ice Creams: Per 4 oz Scoop* | | | |
| **Classic Flavors:** Cherries Jubilee | 220 | 11 | 26 |
| Chocolate Chip | 250 | 16 | 23 |
| Chocolate | 240 | 14 | 26 |
| Jamoca Almond Fudge | 260 | 15 | 28 |
| Mint Chocolate Chip | 250 | 16 | 23 |
| Old Fashioned Butter Pecan | 260 | 18 | 20 |
| Oreo Cookies 'n Cream | 260 | 15 | 28 |
| Peanut Butter 'n Chocolate | 300 | 20 | 25 |
| Pistachio Almond | 270 | 19 | 21 |
| Pralines 'n Cream | 270 | 14 | 32 |
| Rainbow Sherbet | 130 | 2 | 27 |
| Reese's P'nut Butter Cup | 300 | 17 | 32 |
| Vanilla | 240 | 16 | 21 |
| Very Berry Strawberry | 200 | 11 | 23 |
| World Class Chocolate | 260 | 16 | 25 |

**Updated Nutrition Data ~ www.CalorieKing.com**
Persons with Diabetes ~ See Disclaimer (Page 22)

## Baskin Robbins® cont... (Aug '16)

| Ice Creams (Cont): Per 4 oz Scoop | C | F | Cb |
|---|---|---|---|
| **Seasonal Flavors:** Bananas Foster | 250 | 13 | 31 |
| Black Walnut | 260 | 18 | 20 |
| Chocolate Fudge | 250 | 15 | 27 |
| Creole Cream Cheese | 230 | 13 | 24 |
| Strawberry Cheesecake | 250 | 13 | 29 |
| *Grab-N-Go:* | | | |
| Brownie a la Mode, 3 oz slice | 280 | 14 | 39 |
| Chocolate Ice Cream, ½ cup 2.6 oz | 170 | 9 | 21 |
| Choc. Chip Ice Cream, ½ cup, 2.6 oz | 170 | 10 | 18 |
| **Ice Cream Quarts:** Chocolate, ½ cup | 170 | 9 | 21 |
| Rainbow Sherbert, ½ cup, 3 oz | 100 | 2 | 22 |
| Vanilla, ½ cup, 2.6 oz | 170 | 10 | 17 |
| *Soft Serve:* | | | |
| **Cups:** Vanilla: Kid's, 3 oz | 110 | 4.5 | 14 |
| Regular, 6 oz | 230 | 9 | 29 |
| Large, 9 oz | 340 | 14 | 43 |
| **Parfaits:** M&M's, Mini | 400 | 15 | 56 |
| M&M's, Regular | 820 | 32 | 119 |
| Oreo, Regular | 920 | 60 | 75 |
| Reese's, Regular | 920 | 60 | 75 |
| *31 Below' Mix-In: Per 16 oz Medium Cup* | | | |
| Butterfinger | 850 | 34 | 120 |
| Choc. Chip Cookie Dough | 870 | 32 | 129 |
| Heath | 910 | 46 | 111 |
| M&M's | 1000 | 40 | 139 |
| Oreo | 720 | 29 | 99 |
| Reese's PB Cup | 910 | 45 | 109 |
| *Sundaes:* | | | |
| Banana Royale | 680 | 33 | 90 |
| Brownie | 800 | 43 | 95 |
| Chocolate Chip Cookie Dough | 1100 | 47 | 160 |
| Classic Banana | 970 | 39 | 146 |
| Made with Snickers | 1060 | 43 | 155 |
| Two Scoop | 570 | 33 | 63 |
| Warm Brownie | 800 | 43 | 95 |
| *Beverages:* | | | |
| **Fruit Blast:** | | | |
| Mango, 24 fl.oz | 500 | 1.5 | 123 |
| Strawb. Citrus, 24 fl.oz | 350 | 0 | 87 |
| Tropical, 24 fl.oz | 370 | 0.5 | 93 |
| **Milk Shakes:** *Per Medium, 24 fl.oz* | | | |
| Choc. with Choc. Ice Cream | 920 | 40 | 125 |
| Chocolate Chip | 880 | 43 | 106 |
| Mint Chocolate Chip | 880 | 44 | 106 |
| **Smoothie:** *Per Medium, 24 fl.oz* | | | |
| Mango Banana | 620 | 2 | 149 |
| Strawberry Banana | 520 | 1 | 124 |
| Tropical Banana | 540 | 1.5 | 130 |

## Big Apple Bagels® (Aug '16)

| Bagels: | C | F | Cb |
|---|---|---|---|
| **Regular,** average all flavors, 5 oz | 340 | 2 | 70 |
| **Bab's Choice Bagels,** av., 5 oz | 380 | 8 | 65 |
| *Cream Cheese: Per 2 Tbsp, 1 oz* | | | |
| Plain/Cheddar/Veg./Onion, av. | 90 | 9 | 2 |
| Plain, Lite | 60 | 4.5 | 3 |
| Strawberry | 90 | 7 | 5 |
| *Muffins:* | | | |
| **Regular:** Blueberry (2), 2 oz | 170 | 8 | 22 |
| Cinnamon Swirl Cheesecake (2) | 215 | 11 | 28 |
| Lemon Poppyseed (2), 2 oz | 200 | 10 | 25 |
| **Jumbo:** Blueberry, 6 oz | 510 | 24 | 66 |
| Chocolate Cheesecake, 6 oz | 600 | 36 | 66 |
| *Sandwiches:* | | | |
| **Breakfast:** BLT | 700 | 31 | 83 |
| Morning Classic | 490 | 11 | 73 |
| Lox & Cream Cheese | 600 | 21 | 78 |
| **Gourmet:** Classic Turkey | 550 | 14 | 74 |
| Kick-N Roast Beef | 580 | 15 | 79 |
| **Specialty:** Big Apple Club | 800 | 37 | 75 |
| Chicken Caesar | 610 | 19 | 78 |
| **Overstuffed:** Classic Reuben | 960 | 43 | 57 |
| Corned Beef/Pastrami | 660 | 19 | 77 |
| Manhattan Club | 1120 | 40 | 120 |
| **Toasted:** Chicken Melt | 815 | 32 | 80 |
| Spicy Italian Sub | 770 | 34 | 77 |
| Tuna Melt | 640 | 23 | 75 |

## Biggby Coffee® (Aug '16)

| Hot Drinks: Per Tall. 16 fl.oz, Without Whipped Cream & Sugar | C | F | Cb |
|---|---|---|---|
| **Caffe au Lait:** with 2% Milk | 100 | 4 | 9 |
| with Non-Fat Milk | 65 | 0 | 9 |
| with Soy | 90 | 3 | 11 |
| **Caffe Latte:** with 2% Milk | 175 | 7.5 | 16 |
| with Non-Fat Milk | 115 | 0 | 16 |
| with Soy | 160 | 5 | 19 |
| **Cappuccino:** with 2% Milk | 105 | 4.5 | 10 |
| with Non-Fat Milk | 70 | 0 | 10 |
| with Soy | 95 | 3 | 11 |
| **Chai Latte:** with 2% Milk | 315 | 7.5 | 51 |
| with Non-Fat Milk | 255 | 0 | 51 |
| **Dark Hot Chocolate:** with 2% Milk | 275 | 7 | 39 |
| with Non-Fat Milk | 215 | 0 | 39 |
| *Creme Freeze: Per Tall, With Whipped Cream* | | | |
| **Banana Berry,** 16 fl.oz | 535 | 15 | 95 |
| **Mango,** 16 fl.oz | 670 | 15 | 125 |
| **Pomaberry,** 16 fl.oz | 540 | 15 | 94 |
| **Red Bull,** 16 fl.oz | 480 | 15 | 83 |
| *Food:* Cinnamon Roll | 660 | 38 | 74 |
| Bragel, Ham & Cheese | 430 | 13 | 58 |
| Donut Holes, 1 donut | 80 | 3.5 | 10 |
| Muffin, Blueberry | 450 | 17 | 65 |
| Yogurt Parfait | 370 | 13 | 57 |

## BJ's Restaurant® (Sept '16)

| Shareable Appetizers: Full Order | C | F | Cb |
|---|---|---|---|
| Ahi Poke | 310 | 10 | 23 |
| Boneless Wings, Hot Spicy | 900 | 41 | 62 |
| Mozzarella Sticks | 810 | 39 | 76 |
| Root Beer Glazed Ribs | 490 | 21 | 61 |
| Sliders | 880 | 32 | 97 |

| Handcrafted Burgers: Includes Thin Fries | | | |
|---|---|---|---|
| All-Portobello Vegetarian-Style | 1120 | 59 | 108 |
| Bacon Cheeseburger | 1420 | 85 | 99 |
| BJ's Brewhouse Burger | 1040 | 52 | 95 |
| Black & Bleu-House Burger | 1200 | 65 | 97 |
| Classic Burger | 1250 | 71 | 98 |
| Portobello Swiss Burger | 1460 | 82 | 10 |

| Brunch: Baked Italian Omelette | 1170 | 63 | 93 |
|---|---|---|---|
| BJ's Buttermilk Pancakes, short stack | 910 | 32 | 136 |
| EnLIGHTened Veggie Omelette | 270 | 9 | 24 |
| Ham & 2 Eggs, with Toast | 710 | 25 | 85 |

| Entrees: Includes Menu Set Sides | | | |
|---|---|---|---|
| BJ's Brewhouse Blonde Fish 'n' Chips | 1150 | 40 | 148 |
| Cherry Chipotle Glazed Salmon | 590 | 26 | 40 |
| Mediterranean Chicken Pita Tacos | 670 | 20 | 79 |
| North Beach Mahi-Mahi & Shrimp | 560 | 18 | 42 |
| Parmesan Crusted Chicken | 1140 | 63 | 62 |
| Quinoa Bowls: Roasted Salmon | 1040 | 56 | 77 |
| Seared Ahi Salad | 580 | 31 | 43 |

| Pasta: Includes Garlic Knot | | | |
|---|---|---|---|
| Deep Dish Ravioli | 950 | 48 | 89 |
| Grilled Chkn Alfredo | 1380 | 69 | 129 |
| Italiano Veggie Penne | 740 | 31 | 93 |
| Jumbo Spaghetti & Meatballs | 1450 | 66 | 162 |
| Sriracha Chkn Bacon Mac 'n' Cheese | 1040 | 46 | 86 |

| Pizza, Deep Dish: Medium, Per Slice (⅛ Pizza) | | | |
|---|---|---|---|
| BBQ/Buffalo Chicken, av. | 310 | 10 | 35 |
| BJ's Classic/5-Meat/Pepperoni, av. | 340 | 17 | 32 |
| BJ's Favorite | 310 | 15 | 33 |
| Spicy Hawaiian Chkn | 330 | 13 | 35 |
| Sweet Pig; Vegetarian, av. | 270 | 9 | 35 |

| Pizza, Tavern-Cut: Per Slice (½ Pizza) | | | |
|---|---|---|---|
| Brewhouse/Chicken/Italian Mkt, av. | 110 | 6 | 9 |
| Spicy Pig/Old Country Tom.,av. | 80 | 3 | 9 |

| Sandwiches: Includes Crispy Thin Fries | | | |
|---|---|---|---|
| Barbeque Pulled Pork | 1460 | 54 | 174 |
| California Chicken Club/Rst Beef, av. | 1320 | 68 | 96 |
| Triple Decker Sandwich | 1310 | 67 | 99 |

| Ribs & Steaks: Without Sides | | | |
|---|---|---|---|
| Baby Back Pork Ribs: Half Rack | 710 | 34 | 75 |
| BJ's Classic Rib-eye | 1080 | 67 | 5 |
| House Top Sirloin | 500 | 32 | 2 |
| Fries: Crispy-Thin Fries | 390 | 23 | 42 |
| Wedge-Cut Seasoned Fries | 390 | 21 | 48 |

## BJ's Restaurant® Cont (Sept '16)

| Salads: Includes Dressings/Toppings | C | F | Cb |
|---|---|---|---|
| Caesar Salad | 810 | 64 | 44 |
| Derby-Style Chkn Cobb | 1000 | 70 | 17 |
| Honey-Crisp Chicken | 1370 | 103 | 77 |
| Kale & Roasted Brussels Sprouts | 440 | 20 | 54 |

| Soups: Chicken Tortilla, Bowl | 280 | 12 | 30 |
|---|---|---|---|
| Clam Chowder: Bowl | 430 | 26 | 33 |
| Sourdough Loaf | 1470 | 42 | 219 |

| Desserts: Baked Beignet | 630 | 25 | 91 |
|---|---|---|---|
| Pizookies w. Ice Cream, av. all flav. | 1200 | 60 | 160 |
| Soda Floats, average all flav. | 510 | 19 | 82 |

| Drinks: Cream Sodas, average | 165 | 0 | 41 |
|---|---|---|---|
| Lemonade | 210 | 0 | 53 |
| Root Beer Float | 200 | 0 | 51 |

*Extra Menu Items ~ See Calorieking.com*

## Blimpie® (Aug '16)

| Cold Deli Subs: | C | F | Cb |
|---|---|---|---|
| Per Regular, 6" White Sub, with Standard Menu Board Toppings | | | |
| Blimpie Best | 450 | 18 | 47 |
| BLT/Club | 410 | 13 | 49 |
| Ham & Swiss | 410 | 14 | 47 |
| Roast Beef & Provolone | 430 | 15 | 44 |
| Tuna without Cheese | 460 | 21 | 41 |
| Turkey & Provolone | 410 | 14 | 47 |

| Wraps: Chicken Caesar | 590 | 26 | 56 |
|---|---|---|---|
| Southwestern | 490 | 18 | 57 |

| Hot Deli Subs: Per 6" White Sub with Standard Menu Board Toppings | | | |
|---|---|---|---|
| Meatball Parmigiana | 560 | 29 | 47 |
| Pastrami | 430 | 16 | 42 |
| VegiMax | 520 | 21 | 55 |

| Salads: Regular, without Dressing | | | |
|---|---|---|---|
| Buffalo Chicken | 200 | 8 | 11 |
| Garden | 30 | 0 | 6 |
| Tuna | 270 | 19 | 6 |
| Ultimate Club | 270 | 14 | 11 |

| Dressings: Creamy Caesar, 1.5 oz | 210 | 21 | 2 |
|---|---|---|---|
| Creamy Italian, 1.5 oz | 180 | 18 | 4 |

| Soups: Per Cup | | | |
|---|---|---|---|
| Chicken Noodle | 130 | 4 | 18 |
| Cream of Broccoli. w.Cheese | 250 | 19 | 13 |
| Harvest Vegetable | 100 | 1 | 19 |
| New England Clam Chowder | 170 | 3 | 28 |
| Vegetable Beef | 80 | 2 | 13 |

| Breakfast: Cinnamon Roll | 450 | 20 | 60 |
|---|---|---|---|
| Biscuits: Bacon, Egg & Cheese | 440 | 25 | 37 |
| Sausage, Egg & Cheese | 520 | 33 | 37 |
| Bluffin, Egg & Cheese | 240 | 10 | 27 |
| Burritos: Ham, Egg & Cheese | 580 | 25 | 57 |
| Sausage, Egg & Cheese | 800 | 52 | 54 |
| Sandwich, Grilled Bacon | 480 | 23 | 44 |

## Bob Evans® (Sept '16)

| | **C** | **F** | **Cb** |
|---|---|---|---|
| *Starters:* | | | |
| Loaded Potato Wedges | 810 | 51 | 52 |
| Onion Petals | 1010 | 56 | 115 |
| Potato Chip Nachos | 480 | 30 | 46 |
| Twisted Cheese Sticks | 820 | 58 | 53 |
| *Burgers: Without Fries or Coleslaw* | | | |
| **Big Farm Burgers:** | | | |
| Hamburger | 910 | 61 | 48 |
| Bacon Cheeseburger | 1090 | 76 | 50 |
| Three Cheese Burger | 1090 | 76 | 50 |
| **Big Farm Sandwiches:** *Without Fries/Coleslaw* | | | |
| **Chicken Salad** Sandwich | 510 | 23 | 59 |
| **Farmhouse Chicken Club:** | | | |
| w/Crispy Chicken | 610 | 25 | 58 |
| w/Grilled Chicken | 520 | 19 | 47 |
| **Five Cheese Griddled** Sandwich | 950 | 57 | 73 |
| **Slow Roasted:** Ham & Cheese | 910 | 41 | 77 |
| Pot Roast Platter | 650 | 36 | 48 |
| Turkey Bacon Melt | 560 | 26 | 48 |
| Turkey Knife & Fork | 850 | 37 | 101 |
| *Sandwich Sides:* | | | |
| French Fries + Coleslaw | 450 | 23 | 55 |
| *Dinners: Without Sides or Bread* | | | |
| Beef, USDA Choice Sirloin, Blkn'd, 6 oz | 350 | 5 | 4 |
| Black Angus Chop'd Steak w/Mushr. | 810 | 72 | 5 |
| **Chicken:** Broasted, 1 breast | 315 | 9 | 5 |
| Grilled, 1 breast | 150 | 4 | 0 |
| **Chicken Pot Pie** | 880 | 57 | 64 |
| **Chicken Tenders:** *Without Sides* | | | |
| Broasted, 4 pcs | 540 | 28 | 30 |
| Grilled, 4 tenders | 140 | 3 | 0 |
| **Country Fried Steak Dinner** w/Gvy | 830 | 50 | 72 |
| **Seafood:** Salmon, grilled w/Veg. | 410 | 24 | 19 |
| Blk'd White Fish w/Tartare Sce | 460 | 36 | 11 |
| Potato Crusted Flounder w/Veg. | 360 | 17 | 30 |
| **Slow Roasted:** Pot Roast, entree | 590 | 39 | 43 |
| Turkey & Dressing, entree | 900 | 41 | 92 |
| *Farmhouse Sides:* | | | |
| **Baked Russet Potato** | 220 | 0 | 49 |
| **Bread & Celery Dressing,** 6 oz | 280 | 15 | 29 |
| **Broccoli,** steamed | 25 | 0 | 5 |
| **Coleslaw,** 3.5 oz | 210 | 14 | 19 |
| **French Fries** | 240 | 9 | 36 |
| **Hash Browns** | 400 | 26 | 28 |
| **Home Fries** | 390 | 23 | 33 |
| **Loaded Baked Potato** | 420 | 16 | 52 |
| **Macaroni & Cheese** | 280 | 15 | 24 |
| **Mashed Potatoes,** Plain | 190 | 9 | 24 |
| *Gravy:* Beef/Chicken, av. 2 oz | 20 | 2 | 3 |
| Country, 3 oz | 50 | 2 | 8 |

## Bob Evans® cont... (Sept '16)

| | **C** | **F** | **Cb** |
|---|---|---|---|
| *Sauces:* | | | |
| Bob Evans Wildfire, 1 ramekin | 60 | 0 | 15 |
| Garlic Herb Butter, 1 ramekin | 10 | 1 | 1 |
| Honey Mustard, 1 pkt | 140 | 13 | 6 |
| Old Route 35, 2 Tbsp | 140 | 14 | 3 |
| Spicy Chipotle, 2 Tbsp | 180 | 19 | 1 |
| *Soups: Per Bowl, with 2 Saltine Crackers* | | | |
| Cheddar Baked Potato | 380 | 20 | 34 |
| Chicken N Noodles, w/o Saltines | 230 | 5 | 31 |
| Farm Festival Bean | 220 | 4.5 | 33 |
| Hearty Beef Vegetable | 220 | 4.5 | 34 |
| Tomato Basil | 390 | 17 | 48 |
| *Cup + 1 Cracker: Halve Bowl Figures* | | | |
| *Salads: Without Dressing or Sides* | | | |
| Chicken Salad Plate | 700 | 35 | 84 |
| Cobb Salad | 300 | 17 | 6 |
| Cranb. Pecan Chicken | 370 | 23 | 21 |
| Wildfire Fried Chicken | 630 | 30 | 57 |
| *Dressings: Per Ramekin* | | | |
| Blue Cheese | 180 | 16 | 8 |
| Buttermilk Ranch | 130 | 13 | 1 |
| Sweet Italian | 160 | 15 | 7 |
| *Breakfast:* | | | |
| **Farm-Fresh Egg Combinations:** *Includes 2 Fried Eggs, 3 Sausage Links, Grits & 2 Slices Specialty Bread* | | | |
| BE Fit Breakfast, w/o Syrup | 450 | 9 | 74 |
| Big Breakfast | 1000 | 50 | 108 |
| Country Fried Steak & Eggs | 2260 | 115 | 268 |
| Homestead | 1430 | 93 | 104 |
| Rise & Shine | 1290 | 78 | 107 |
| Steak & Eggs | 1940 | 90 | 228 |
| Sunrise | 920 | 45 | 107 |
| **Omelets:** *Eggs, w/ Hash Browns & Bread* | | | |
| Border Scramble | 1440 | 82 | 123 |
| Western | 1250 | 69 | 111 |
| **Hotcakes:** *With Margarine & Syrup* | | | |
| Cinnamon (4) | 1010 | 30 | 175 |
| Chocolate Chip (4) | 1030 | 32 | 158 |
| Multigrain (4) | 1030 | 18 | 203 |
| **Sweet & Stacked Hotcakes:** | | | |
| Cinnamon Supreme, w/ Bacon | 1170 | 42 | 178 |
| Dble Blueb. w/ sausage links | 1440 | 65 | 187 |
| *Breakfast Sides:* | | | |
| Fresh Fruit Dish | 45 | 0 | 12 |
| Home Fries | 190 | 6 | 31 |
| Shredded Hash Browns | 200 | 10 | 26 |
| *Dessert:* Coconut Cream Pie, 1 slice | 590 | 36 | 63 |
| French Silk Pie, 1 slice | 650 | 43 | 59 |
| Peanut Butter Brownie Bites (8) | 880 | 40 | 120 |

## Bojangles® (Aug '16)

### Biscuit:

| | C | F | Cb |
|---|---|---|---|
| Plain | 320 | 17 | 37 |
| Bacon, Egg & Cheese | 460 | 28 | 38 |
| Cajun Filet | 570 | 30 | 54 |
| Country Ham | 430 | 24 | 37 |
| Egg & Cheese | 410 | 24 | 38 |
| Gravy Biscuits | 440 | 23 | 48 |
| Sausage | 520 | 35 | 37 |
| Steak | 590 | 38 | 47 |

### Chicken: *Per Piece Unless Indicated*

| | C | F | Cb |
|---|---|---|---|
| Breast | 290 | 12 | 10 |
| Leg | 130 | 7 | 5 |
| Thigh | 255 | 17 | 10 |
| Wing | 140 | 9 | 7 |
| Homestyle Tenders, 4 pieces | 495 | 24 | 38 |
| Supremes, 4 pieces | 455 | 20 | 39 |

### Sandwiches:

| | C | F | Cb |
|---|---|---|---|
| Cajun Filet: Regular | 600 | 32 | 56 |
| Club | 690 | 40 | 57 |
| Grilled Chicken: Regular | 470 | 22 | 41 |
| Club | 570 | 30 | 42 |

### Fixins': *Per Individual Serve*

| | C | F | Cb |
|---|---|---|---|
| Bo-Tato Rounds | 220 | 12 | 27 |
| Coleslaw | 170 | 11 | 20 |
| Green Beans | 40 | 0 | 8 |
| Macaroni & Cheese | 260 | 13 | 29 |
| Mashed Potatoes 'N Gravy | 120 | 4 | 17 |
| **Seasoned Fries:** Individual | 300 | 15 | 38 |
| Medium size | 410 | 21 | 51 |
| Picnic size | 740 | 37 | 92 |
| **Salads:** Chicken Supreme | 490 | 25 | 37 |
| Garden | 160 | 10 | 10 |
| Grilled Chicken | 290 | 14 | 11 |

### Sweets:

| | C | F | Cb |
|---|---|---|---|
| Bo-Berry Biscuit (1) | 350 | 16 | 48 |
| Cinnamon Twist (1) | 350 | 17 | 45 |
| Sweet Potato Pie | 370 | 21 | 40 |

*For Complete Nutritional Data ~ see CalorieKing.com*

## Boston Market® (Aug '16)

### Sandwiches:
*Per Whole with Set Menu Board Toppings*

| | C | F | Cb |
|---|---|---|---|
| All-White Chicken Salad | 910 | 53 | 72 |
| Meatloaf Carver | 910 | 35 | 98 |
| Roasted Turkey Carver | 870 | 44 | 71 |
| Rotisserie Chicken Carver | 790 | 34 | 72 |

### Individual Meals: *Without Sides Or Bread*

| | C | F | Cb |
|---|---|---|---|
| Meatloaf, regular | 450 | 26 | 23 |
| Rotisserie Chicken, half | 500 | 24 | 1 |
| St Louis Style BBQ Ribs, ½ rack | 990 | 75 | 22 |

## Boston Market® cont... (Aug '16)

### Salads: *Per Whole, with Dressing*

| | C | F | Cb |
|---|---|---|---|
| Chicken Caesar, 10.8 oz | 480 | 29 | 17 |
| Mediterranean, 13.4 | 510 | 34 | 17 |
| Southwest Santa Fe, 13.7 oz | 530 | 29 | 28 |

### Sides:

| | C | F | Cb |
|---|---|---|---|
| Creamed Spinach, 6.3 oz | 250 | 20 | 11 |
| Fresh Steamed Vegetables, 4.8 oz | 60 | 3.5 | 6 |
| Fresh Vegetable Stuffing, 5.5 oz | 220 | 10 | 28 |
| Garlic Dill New Potatoes, 4.5 oz | 130 | 2.5 | 24 |
| Green Beans, 4.3 oz | 80 | 4 | 7 |
| Macaroni & Chse, 7.4 oz | 270 | 9 | 36 |
| Mashed Potatoes, 7.oz | 240 | 10 | 32 |
| Southwest Rice | 250 | 9 | 38 |
| Sweet Corn | 130 | 5 | 19 |
| Sweet Potato Casserole, 7.4 oz | 440 | 12 | 80 |

### Soups:

| | C | F | Cb |
|---|---|---|---|
| Chicken Noodle | 220 | 8 | 21 |
| Chicken Tortilla | 320 | 18 | 19 |

### Desserts:

| | C | F | Cb |
|---|---|---|---|
| Apple Pie, 1 slice | 440 | 21 | 58 |
| Chocolate Brownie (1) | 490 | 20 | 77 |
| Chocolate Cake, 1 slice | 560 | 32 | 65 |
| Pecan Pie, 1 slice | 640 | 35 | 75 |

*For Complete Nutritional Data ~ see CalorieKing.com*

## Boston Pizza® Canada (Aug '16)

### Starters:

| | C | F | Cb |
|---|---|---|---|
| Oven Roasted Wings, 8.4 oz | 580 | 37 | 7 |
| Poutine, 14 oz | 610 | 30 | 67 |
| Spinach & Artichoke Dip, 13.7 oz | 660 | 35 | 65 |
| **Burgers:** Prime Rib with Bacon | 880 | 76 | 58 |
| Pepperoni & Bacon Pizzaburger | 1040 | 88 | 51 |
| Spicy Perogy Burger | 1200 | 107 | 64 |

### Gourmet Pastas: *Full Order, without Garlic Toast*

| | C | F | Cb |
|---|---|---|---|
| Boston's Lasagna | 790 | 23 | 107 |
| Montréal Smoked Meat Pasta | 890 | 16 | 142 |
| Spicy Sausage Arrabiata Penne | 1230 | 54 | 142 |

### Gourmet Pizza: *Per Individual Pizza*

**Classic Crust:**

| | C | F | Cb |
|---|---|---|---|
| Boston Royal | 710 | 30 | 69 |
| Deluxe | 730 | 33 | 65 |
| Hawaiian | 660 | 24 | 72 |
| Pepperoni | 630 | 30 | 60 |

**Thin Crust:**

| | C | F | Cb |
|---|---|---|---|
| Bacon Double Cheeseburger | 430 | 22 | 36 |
| The Meateor | 450 | 23 | 34 |

*Continued Next Page...*

## Boston Pizza® Canada cont... (Aug '16)

*Sandwiches: Without Sides*

| | C | F | Cb |
|---|---|---|---|
| BBQ Pulled Pork | 1070 | 57 | 92 |
| Boston Brute | 800 | 24 | 108 |
| Buffalo Chicken | 920 | 35 | 119 |
| Chipotle Chicken Club | 710 | 35 | 57 |
| NY Striploin Steak Sandwich | 1060 | 51 | 95 |
| Smoked Meat | 910 | 59 | 40 |

*Salads: Full Order with Dressing*

| | C | F | Cb |
|---|---|---|---|
| Crispy Chicken Pecan | 1170 | 88 | 46 |
| Santa Fe | 710 | 51 | 64 |

*Desssert:*

| | C | F | Cb |
|---|---|---|---|
| NY Cheesecake | 600 | 32 | 76 |
| The Panookie, with ice cream | 880 | 38 | 133 |

*For Complete Nutritional Data ~ see CalorieKing.com*

## Braum's® ~ see CalorieKing.com

## Bruegger's® (Aug '16)

*Bagels:*

| | C | F | Cb |
|---|---|---|---|
| Chocolate Chip, 4 oz | 330 | 3.5 | 65 |
| Jalapeno Cheddar, 5.5 oz | 440 | 9 | 75 |
| Plain, 4.1 oz | 300 | 2 | 60 |
| Sesame; Whole Wheat, av., 4 oz | 310 | 3.5 | 61 |

*Cream Cheese: Per 1.5 oz*

| | C | F | Cb |
|---|---|---|---|
| Bacon Scallion, Jalapeno, av. | 140 | 12 | 5 |
| Honey Walnut | 150 | 12 | 8 |
| Plain | 130 | 11 | 6 |
| Smoked Salmon | 150 | 13 | 3 |

*Breakfast Bagel S'wiches: With Standard Toppings*

| | C | F | Cb |
|---|---|---|---|
| Egg & Cheese | 430 | 18 | 63 |
| Egg White, Cheese & Bacon | 460 | 12 | 64 |
| Smoked Salmon | 460 | 10 | 66 |
| Spinach & Cheddar Omelet | 490 | 16 | 63 |
| Sriracha, Egg & Sausage | 680 | 33 | 72 |
| Western | 670 | 34 | 67 |

*Deli Sandwiches: With Standard Toppings*

| | C | F | Cb |
|---|---|---|---|
| BLT on Hearty White Bread | 720 | 42 | 62 |
| Chicken Breast on Plain Bagel | 550 | 6 | 81 |
| Garden Veggie on Plain Bagel | 360 | 2 | 72 |
| Ham On Honey Wheat Bread | 500 | 13 | 62 |

*Hot Paninis: On Ciabatta with Standard Toppings*

| | C | F | Cb |
|---|---|---|---|
| Four Cheese & Tomato | 570 | 26 | 59 |
| Harvest Turkey | 690 | 24 | 84 |
| Primo Pesto Chicken | 560 | 19 | 58 |
| Roast Beef Cheddar Melt | 630 | 26 | 72 |
| Turkey, Artichoke, Mozzarella | 520 | 14 | 61 |

*Signature & Classic Sandwiches: With Standard Toppings*

| | C | F | Cb |
|---|---|---|---|
| Herby Turkey on Sesame Bagel | 570 | 15 | 75 |
| Leon. da Veggie on Asiago Parm. Bagel | 490 | 14 | 70 |
| Thai Peanut Chicken on Plain Bagel | 580 | 11 | 91 |
| Turkey Chipotle Club on Wheat Bread | 400 | 17 | 36 |

## Bruegger's® cont... (Aug '16)

*Café Salads: wWthout Dressing*

| | C | F | Cb |
|---|---|---|---|
| Blue Apple, 7 oz | 300 | 14 | 20 |
| Chicken Almond, 11 oz | 260 | 14 | 8 |
| Chicken Caesar, 6 oz | 190 | 7 | 11 |

*Dressings: Balsamic Vinaig., 1 oz*

| | C | F | Cb |
|---|---|---|---|
| Balsamic Vinaig., 1 oz | 60 | 6 | 3 |
| Caesar, 1 oz | 80 | 7 | 2 |
| Ranch | 90 | 10 | 1 |

*Dessert Bars:*

| | C | F | Cb |
|---|---|---|---|
| Chocolate Chunk Brownie, 2.7 oz | 340 | 17 | 42 |
| Marshmallow Chew, 2.7 oz | 290 | 7 | 54 |
| Toffee Almond, 2.7 oz | 350 | 17 | 44 |

*For Complete Menu & Data ~ see CalorieKing.com*

## Burgerville® (Aug '16)

*Burgers: With Standard Ingredients*

| | C | F | Cb |
|---|---|---|---|
| Original: Hamburger | 330 | 17 | 30 |
| Cheeseburger | 380 | 21 | 30 |
| Colossal Cheseburger | 540 | 29 | 41 |
| Double Colossal Cheeseburger | 800 | 47 | 41 |
| Pepper Bacon Cheeseburger | 670 | 40 | 37 |
| Tillamook Cheeseburger | 600 | 34 | 39 |

*Fish & Chips: With Lemon & Tartar Sce*

| | C | F | Cb |
|---|---|---|---|
| Hallibut, 3 pieces | 1040 | 71 | 73 |
| Hallibut, 4 pieces | 1130 | 75 | 80 |

*Sandwiches: With Spread*

| | C | F | Cb |
|---|---|---|---|
| Crispy Chicken | 630 | 31 | 66 |
| Deluxe Crispy Chkn | 780 | 43 | 67 |
| Halibut Fish w/out fries | 450 | 27 | 38 |
| Turkey Club, all components | 630 | 40 | 36 |

*French Fries: Small, 2.8 oz*

| | C | F | Cb |
|---|---|---|---|
| Small, 2.8 oz | 220 | 11 | 28 |
| Regular, 5 oz | 400 | 19 | 50 |
| Large, 6.5 oz | 510 | 25 | 65 |

*Salads: Full Size, Without Dressing*

| | C | F | Cb |
|---|---|---|---|
| Blue Cheese & Apple | 250 | 8 | 36 |
| Grilled Chicken Club | 340 | 18 | 8 |
| Wild Smoked Salmon & Hazelnuts | 460 | 32 | 13 |

*Breakfast:*

| | C | F | Cb |
|---|---|---|---|
| Breakfast Platter, Bacon, Engl Mffn | 860 | 55 | 69 |
| Burger, with Bacon | 460 | 27 | 25 |
| Burrito | 680 | 45 | 41 |

*Ice Cream Sundaes: With Whipped Cream*

| | C | F | Cb |
|---|---|---|---|
| Caramel | 390 | 19 | 50 |
| Hot Fudge | 390 | 19 | 51 |
| Triple Berry | 340 | 18 | 39 |

**185**

## Burger King® (Aug '16)

### Whopper Sandwich:

| | C | F | Cb |
|---|---|---|---|
| Orginal | 630 | 38 | 49 |
| Original, w/out Mayo | 470 | 20 | 49 |
| Original, with Cheese | 710 | 45 | 50 |
| Bacon & Cheese Whopper | 750 | 49 | 46 |
| Double Whopper Sandwich | 850 | 54 | 49 |
| With Cheese | 930 | 61 | 50 |
| Whopper Jr | 310 | 18 | 27 |

### Flame Broiled Burgers:

| | C | F | Cb |
|---|---|---|---|
| A.1. Ultimate Bacon Chseburger | 750 | 45 | 40 |
| Bacon Cheeseburger | 280 | 13 | 27 |
| Cheeseburger | 270 | 12 | 27 |
| Double Cheeseburger | 350 | 18 | 27 |
| Extra Long BBQ Cheeseburger | 590 | 34 | 45 |
| Hamburger | 220 | 8 | 26 |
| Rodeo Burger | 310 | 12 | 38 |

### Grilled Dogs: Classic Dog

| | C | F | Cb |
|---|---|---|---|
| Grilled Dogs: Classic Dog | 310 | 16 | 32 |
| Chili Cheese Dog | 330 | 19 | 28 |

### Chicken:

| | C | F | Cb |
|---|---|---|---|
| A.1. Smoky Bacon TenderCrisp S'wich | 600 | 27 | 57 |
| Original Chicken S'wich | 660 | 40 | 48 |
| TenderGrill Chicken Sandwich | 420 | 18 | 35 |
| TenderCrisp Chicken Sandwich | 660 | 40 | 50 |
| Chicken Fries, 9 pcs, 3.6 oz | 280 | 17 | 20 |
| Chicken Nuggets: 4 pieces | 170 | 11 | 11 |
| 6 pieces | 260 | 16 | 16 |
| 10 pieces | 430 | 27 | 27 |

### Big Fish S'wich

| | C | F | Cb |
|---|---|---|---|
| Big Fish S'wich | 510 | 28 | 51 |

### Veggie Burger: M'Star

| | C | F | Cb |
|---|---|---|---|
| Veggie Burger: M'Star | 390 | 15 | 42 |
| Without Mayo | 310 | 7 | 42 |

### Dipping Sauces: BBQ

| | C | F | Cb |
|---|---|---|---|
| Dipping Sauces: BBQ | 40 | 0 | 11 |
| Buffalo | 80 | 8 | 2 |
| Chicken Fry | 140 | 13 | 6 |
| Ranch; Zesty Onion Ring, av. | 145 | 15 | 2 |

### French Fries: Small, 4.3 oz

| | C | F | Cb |
|---|---|---|---|
| French Fries: Small, 4.3 oz | 320 | 14 | 44 |
| Medium, 5.8 oz | 380 | 17 | 53 |
| Large, 7 oz | 430 | 19 | 60 |

### Mac N' Cheetos

| | C | F | Cb |
|---|---|---|---|
| Mac N' Cheetos | 310 | 13 | 37 |

### Onion Rings: Small

| | C | F | Cb |
|---|---|---|---|
| Onion Rings: Small | 320 | 16 | 41 |
| Medium | 410 | 21 | 53 |
| Large | 500 | 25 | 64 |

### Garden Fresh Salads:

**Bacon Cheddar Ranch Chicken:**

| | C | F | Cb |
|---|---|---|---|
| Tendercrisp, w/ Dressing | 720 | 50 | 32 |
| Tendergrill, w/ Dressing | 590 | 40 | 18 |

**Garden Grilled Chicken:**

| | C | F | Cb |
|---|---|---|---|
| Tendercrisp, w/out Dressing | 450 | 24 | 30 |
| Tendergrill, w/out Dressing | 320 | 14 | 16 |
| Garden Side Salad, w/out Dressing | 60 | 4 | 3 |
| Dressing, Ken's Ranch, 1.5 oz pkt | 260 | 28 | 2 |

## Burger King® cont... (Aug '16)

### Breakfast:

| | C | F | Cb |
|---|---|---|---|
| Biscuits: Bacon, Egg & Cheese | 380 | 23 | 29 |
| Ham, Egg & Cheese | 370 | 21 | 30 |
| Sausage | 390 | 25 | 28 |
| Saus., Egg & Cheese | 510 | 35 | 29 |
| Burrito: Egg-Normous Burrito | 930 | 57 | 67 |
| Hash Brown Burrito | 370 | 23 | 27 |

### Croissan'wich:

| | C | F | Cb |
|---|---|---|---|
| Bacon, Egg & Cheese | 340 | 18 | 30 |
| Egg & Cheese | 300 | 15 | 30 |
| Fully Loaded | 570 | 37 | 32 |
| Ham, Egg & Cheese | 340 | 16 | 31 |

### King Croissan'wich:

| | C | F | Cb |
|---|---|---|---|
| with Double Sausage | 700 | 51 | 31 |
| with Ham & Sausage | 530 | 34 | 31 |
| with Sausage & Bacon | 580 | 39 | 31 |
| French Toast Sticks: 5 pieces | 380 | 18 | 49 |
| with 1 oz Breakfast Syrup | 500 | 18 | 79 |
| Hash Browns: Small, 3 oz | 250 | 16 | 24 |
| Medium, 6 oz | 500 | 33 | 48 |
| Large, 8 oz | 670 | 44 | 65 |
| Oatmeal, Orig. Maple Flavored | 170 | 3 | 32 |
| Platters: Pancakes & Sausage | 610 | 31 | 72 |
| Ultimate Breakfast | 1190 | 66 | 123 |

### Sweets: Cinnamon Roll

| | C | F | Cb |
|---|---|---|---|
| Sweets: Cinnamon Roll | 280 | 11 | 41 |
| Cookie, Chocolate Chip (1) | 160 | 8 | 24 |
| Pies: Dutch Apple | 340 | 14 | 51 |
| Hershey's Sundae | 310 | 19 | 32 |
| Reese's P'nut Butter | 310 | 19 | 31 |
| Snickers | 300 | 16 | 36 |
| Sundaes: Caramel | 290 | 6 | 53 |
| Chocolate Fudge | 270 | 7 | 47 |
| Vanilla Soft Serve, in cone | 140 | 4 | 24 |

### Shakes: Dr Pepper

| | C | F | Cb |
|---|---|---|---|
| Shakes: Dr Pepper | 450 | 13 | 73 |
| Oreo | 730 | 21 | 121 |
| Oreo Chocolate | 610 | 19 | 99 |
| Hand Spun: Choc. | 760 | 21 | 131 |
| Strawberry | 640 | 15 | 113 |
| Vanilla | 580 | 15 | 98 |

### Smoothies: Strawb. Banana,16 fl.oz

| | C | F | Cb |
|---|---|---|---|
| Smoothies: Strawb. Banana,16 fl.oz | 280 | 1 | 65 |
| Tropical Mango, 16 fl.oz | 320 | 0 | 76 |
| Beverages: BK Frappe, av. | 410 | 16 | 62 |

### Coca Cola/Sprite: With 50% Ice

| | C | F | Cb |
|---|---|---|---|
| Value, 15 fl.oz | 140 | 0 | 39 |
| Small, 20 fl.oz | 190 | 0 | 51 |
| Medium, 30 fl.oz | 290 | 0 | 77 |
| Large, 40 fl.oz | 380 | 0 | 102 |
| Mellow Yellow, small, 20 fl.oz | 230 | 0 | 61 |
| Minute Maid Lemonade, medium | 280 | 0 | 77 |
| Icee, Coke/Fanta Cherry, 16 oz | 140 | 0 | 38 |
| Iced Coffee: Regular, 16 oz | 150 | 8 | 19 |
| Vanilla, 16 oz | 190 | 8 | 28 |
| Iced Tea, sweetened, 20 oz | 120 | 0 | 35 |

Updated Nutrition Data ~ www.CalorieKing.com
Persons with Diabetes ~ See Disclaimer (Page 22)

## Captain D's Seafood® (Aug '16)

| | C | F | Cb |
|---|---|---|---|
| **Fish:** *Without Sides* | | | |
| Battered Dipped Fish, 1 piece | 210 | 15 | 23 |
| Breaded Flounder, 1 piece | 230 | 15 | 30 |
| **From The Grill:** *Without Sides* | | | |
| Blackened Tilapia | 210 | 7 | 1 |
| Grilled Salmon | 220 | 10 | 1 |
| Grilled Steak Tips, 1 kabob | 110 | 4 | 2 |
| Grilled Whitefish Fillet | 180 | 8 | 2 |
| Shrimp Scampi, 1 serving | 980 | 67 | 70 |
| **Other Favorites:** | | | |
| Cheese Sticks, 1 order | 500 | 32 | 35 |
| Jalapeno Poppers, 1 order | 510 | 36 | 40 |
| **Seafood:** | | | |
| Butterfly Shrimp (6) | 360 | 24 | 24 |
| Popcon Shrimp | 490 | 27 | 48 |
| Stuffed Crab, 1 piece | 140 | 10 | 11 |
| **Side Dishes:** | | | |
| Baked Potato (1) | 210 | 0 | 48 |
| Cole Slaw, 1 order | 180 | 13 | 15 |
| French Fries, 1 serving | 330 | 22 | 28 |
| Hushpuppy (1) | 80 | 4 | 9 |
| **Dessert,** Chocolate Cake, 1 order | 300 | 11 | 49 |

## Caribou Coffee® (Aug '16)

*Without Whipped Cream Unless Indicated*

| | C | F | Cb |
|---|---|---|---|
| **Hot Coffees:** *Per Medium* | | | |
| **Classic:** Coffee Of The Day, 2% Milk | 90 | 3.5 | 9 |
| Espresso, 4 oz | 0 | 0 | 0 |
| Cappuccino, with 2% Milk | 110 | 4.5 | 10 |
| Latte, with 2% Milk | 180 | 7 | 17 |
| Macchiato, with 2% Milk | 20 | 1 | 1 |
| **Hot Chocolate:** *Per Medium, with Whipped Cream* | | | |
| Milk Chocolate, 2% Milk | 600 | 36 | 50 |
| **Specialty,** Mint Condition Mocha, | | | |
| Milk Choc., 2% Milk, medium | 630 | 27 | 48 |
| **Cold Beverages:** *Per Medium* | | | |
| **Blended:** *Without Whipped Cream* | | | |
| Fruit & Yogurt Smoothies: | | | |
| Mango Orange Key Lime | 450 | 0 | 113 |
| Strawberry Banana | 380 | 0 | 88 |
| White Peach Berry | 330 | 0 | 80 |
| Snowdrift, with Milk Chocolate: | | | |
| Cookies & Crm, with 2% Milk | 630 | 17 | 91 |
| Mint, with 2% Milk | 490 | 12 | 82 |
| **Classics:** Iced Americano | 5 | 0 | 0 |
| Iced Latte, with 2% Milk | 90 | 3.5 | 8 |
| Iced Mocha, Milk Choc., 2% Milk | 320 | 10 | 47 |
| **Specialty, Cooler:** *With Whipped Cream* | | | |
| Caramel High Rise | 690 | 26 | 108 |
| Mint Condition, Milk Chocolate | 780 | 26 | 123 |
| Turtle Mocha, Milk Chocolate | 890 | 32 | 137 |

## Carl's Jr.® (Aug '16)

*California menu only. Please check instore for further nutritional information.*

| | C | F | Cb |
|---|---|---|---|
| **Charbroiled Burgers:** | | | |
| Big Hamburger | 480 | 18 | 56 |
| Famous Star with Cheese | 670 | 37 | 57 |
| Kid's Hamburger | 270 | 10 | 33 |
| Super Star with Cheese | 930 | 56 | 59 |
| The Big Carl | 920 | 58 | 56 |
| Western Bacon Cheeseburger | 750 | 35 | 75 |
| **½ lb Thickburgers:** Original $6 | 1050 | 72 | 62 |
| Guacamole Bacon | 1230 | 90 | 58 |
| Low-Carb | 650 | 34 | 9 |
| Super Bacon | 1180 | 84 | 54 |
| **Chicken Sandwiches:** | | | |
| Bacon Swiss Crispy Chicken | 800 | 43 | 64 |
| Big Chicken Fillet | 680 | 35 | 62 |
| Charbroiled: BBQ Chicken | 390 | 7 | 50 |
| Chicken Club | 600 | 29 | 47 |
| Santa Fe Chicken | 560 | 27 | 46 |
| Spicy Chicken Sandwich | 490 | 29 | 43 |
| **Chicken Tenders,** hand breaded, | | | |
| 5 pieces, without Sauce | 440 | 21 | 21 |
| **Chicken Stars,** 6 pieces, w/o Sce | 260 | 16 | 18 |
| **Fish,** Beer Battered Cod Sandwich | 550 | 19 | 74 |
| **Breakfast:** | | | |
| Bacon & Egg Burrito | 590 | 35 | 39 |
| Breakfast Burger | 830 | 44 | 68 |
| Grilled Cheese & Sausage S'wich | 640 | 43 | 40 |
| Hash Brown Nuggets: Small, 3.8 oz | 350 | 23 | 32 |
| Medium, 4.2 oz | 390 | 26 | 36 |
| Large, 6 oz | 560 | 37 | 52 |
| Loaded Breakfast Burrito | 780 | 48 | 53 |
| Steak & Egg Burrito | 650 | 36 | 44 |
| **Fries:** CrissCut Fries, 5 oz | 450 | 29 | 42 |
| Natural Cut: Small, 3.5 oz | 300 | 15 | 39 |
| Medium, 6 oz | 430 | 21 | 55 |
| Large, 6.5oz | 460 | 22 | 59 |
| **Fried Zucchini,** 5 oz | 330 | 18 | 36 |
| **Onion Rings,** 4.5 oz | 530 | 28 | 61 |
| **Salads:** *Without Dressing* | | | |
| Charbroiled Chicken Salad | 320 | 11 | 27 |
| Garden, Side | 110 | 4.5 | 15 |
| **Dressings:** *Per 2 oz Package* | | | |
| Blue Cheese | 310 | 34 | 2 |
| House | 210 | 23 | 5 |
| Low-Fat Balsamic | 60 | 5 | 3 |
| **Malts,** with Ice Cream: | | | |
| Oreo Cookie | 780 | 40 | 94 |
| Other flavors, average | 770 | 36 | 99 |
| **Shakes,** with Ice Cream: | | | |
| Oreo Cookie | 710 | 39 | 79 |
| Vanilla; Chocolate; Strawberry, av. | 700 | 35 | 85 |

## Carvel® (Aug '16)

*Carvelanche:*

| | C | F | Cb |
|---|---|---|---|
| **Average all flavors:** Small, 12 oz | 600 | 30 | 70 |
| Regular, 16 oz | 870 | 46 | 100 |
| Large, 24 oz | 1300 | 70 | 150 |

*Classic Sundaes:* Per Small, 12 oz

| | | | |
|---|---|---|---|
| Caramel | 700 | 36 | 84 |
| Hot Fudge | 540 | 30 | 60 |
| Strawberry | 610 | 34 | 67 |

*Sundae Dashers:* Per Regular, 16 oz

| | | | |
|---|---|---|---|
| Banana's Foster | 1020 | 31 | 176 |
| Fudge Brownie | 1170 | 60 | 147 |
| Mint Chocolate Chip | 1230 | 64 | 157 |
| Peanut Butter Cup | 1850 | 105 | 163 |
| Strawberry Shortcake | 730 | 38 | 91 |

*Ice Cream:*

**Chocolate/Vanilla, average:**

| | | | |
|---|---|---|---|
| Junior Cup, 4.5 oz | 260 | 14 | 28 |
| with Carvelite | 180 | 4 | 30 |
| Small Cup, 7.5 oz | 430 | 24 | 47 |
| with Carvelite | 290 | 6 | 52 |
| Medium Cup, 9.5 oz | 550 | 30 | 60 |
| with Carvelite | 360 | 8 | 65 |

*Thick Shakes:* Per 16 oz

| | | | |
|---|---|---|---|
| Chocolate; Vanilla, av. | 650 | 27 | 93 |
| Strawberry | 600 | 31 | 70 |

## Checkers®

*Same Menu & Data as Rally's ~ See Page 231*

## Cheesecake Factory® (Apr '16)

*Cheesecake:* Per Slice

| | C | F | Cb |
|---|---|---|---|
| Original | 830 | n/a | 62 |
| Godiva Chocolate | 1280 | n/a | 96 |
| Reese's P.B. Chocolate Cake | 1510 | n/a | 153 |
| White Chocolate Raspb. Truffle | 1170 | n/a | 87 |

*Small Plates & Snacks:* Per Dish, As Served

| | | | |
|---|---|---|---|
| Crispy Crab Bites | 350 | n/a | 11 |
| Pretzel Crusted Chicken | 770 | n/a | 62 |
| Stuffed Mushrooms | 460 | n/a | 15 |

*Glamburgers & Sandwiches:* Without Sides

| | | | |
|---|---|---|---|
| Bacon Bacon Chseburger | 1590 | n/a | 74 |
| Factory Burger | 860 | n/a | 81 |
| Grilled Turkey Burger | 1160 | n/a | 72 |

*Specialties:* Per Dish, As Served

| | | | |
|---|---|---|---|
| Crispy Chicken Costoletta | 2590 | n/a | 103 |
| Famous Factory Meatloaf | 1630 | n/a | 117 |
| White Chicken Chili | 570 | n/a | 36 |

*Salads:* As Served, Includes Dressing

| | | | |
|---|---|---|---|
| Herb-Crusted Salmon | 760 | n/a | 22 |
| Santa Fe Salad | 1820 | n/a | 99 |
| Sheila's Chicken & Avocado | 1890 | n/a | 140 |

*n/a = not available*

*For Complete Menu & Data ~ see CalorieKing.com*

## Charley's Grilled Subs® (Aug '16)

*Subs:* Regular Size, Includes Standard Toppings, without Sauce or Dressings

| | C | F | Cb |
|---|---|---|---|
| Bacon 3 Cheese Steak | 720 | 31 | 56 |
| Chicken Buffalo | 610 | 18 | 60 |
| Chicken California | 690 | 28 | 52 |
| Chicken Teriyaki | 630 | 18 | 62 |
| Italian Deli Deluxe | 750 | 36 | 58 |
| Pepperoni Melt | 780 | 37 | 55 |
| Philly Cheesesteak | 640 | 24 | 58 |
| Philly Chicken | 590 | 17 | 58 |
| Turkey Cheddar Melt | 670 | 21 | 62 |
| Ultimate Club | 710 | 27 | 61 |

*Salads:* Cheese or Dressings not included

| | | | |
|---|---|---|---|
| Grilled Chicken; Grilled Steak, average | 130 | 3 | 8 |

*Fries:* Original

| | | | |
|---|---|---|---|
| Original | 400 | 22 | 46 |
| Cheese Gourmet | 550 | 31 | 62 |
| Ultimate Gourmet | 720 | 49 | 61 |

*Breakfast:*

**Hashbrowns** 460 | 29 | 45

*Omelet Platter:*

| | | | |
|---|---|---|---|
| Bacon, Egg & Cheese | 1010 | 63 | 74 |
| Sausage, Egg & Cheese | 1110 | 70 | 73 |
| Steak, Egg & Cheese | 1050 | 62 | 74 |

*Sandwiches:*

| | | | |
|---|---|---|---|
| Bacon, Egg & Cheese | 490 | 26 | 36 |
| Sausage, Egg & Cheese | 590 | 33 | 36 |
| Steak, Egg & Cheese | 520 | 25 | 36 |
| Toast, 2 slices | 130 | 2 | 24 |

*For Complete Menu & Data ~ see CalorieKing.com*

## Chevys Fresh Mex® (Apr '16)

*Burritos:* As Served

| | C | F | Cb |
|---|---|---|---|
| Fajita Carnitas | 1260 | 51 | 144 |
| Fajita Chicken | 1240 | 46 | 142 |
| Fajita Steak | 1300 | 54 | 142 |

*Fresh Mex Combos:* As Served

| | | | |
|---|---|---|---|
| Chevys Super Cinco | 1920 | 100 | 171 |
| Mar Y Tierra Combo | 1230 | 54 | 108 |
| Taste of Chevys | 1480 | 68 | 155 |

*Fresh Mex Innovations:* As Served

| | | | |
|---|---|---|---|
| Enchiladas: Chipotle Chicken | 1070 | 65 | 93 |
| Farmers' Market | 1130 | 72 | 101 |
| Shrimp & Crab | 1250 | 80 | 94 |

*Tacos:* As Served

| | | | |
|---|---|---|---|
| Mesquite Grilled: Chicken | 980 | 28 | 123 |
| Steak | 1050 | 38 | 123 |
| Fish | 920 | 27 | 123 |

*Grande Salads:* Without Dressing Unless Indicated

| | | | |
|---|---|---|---|
| Sizzling Fajita Chicken w/ dressing | 1220 | 90 | 51 |
| Santa Fe Chopped | 660 | 39 | 26 |
| Tostada Steak | 1560 | 100 | 91 |
| **Soup,** Tortilla, 1 bowl | 420 | 18 | 38 |
| **Tortilla,** El Machino, 6" | 140 | 4 | 22 |
| **Tortilla Chips** | 430 | 20 | 56 |

## Chick-fil-A® (Aug '16)

### Breakfast:

| | C | F | Cb |
|---|---|---|---|
| **Bagel,** Chicken, Egg & Cheese | 480 | 20 | 48 |
| **Biscuits:** Chicken | 440 | 20 | 48 |
| Bacon, Egg & Cheese | 460 | 23 | 44 |
| Sausage, Egg & Cheese | 670 | 44 | 44 |
| **Burritos:** Chicken | 460 | 20 | 43 |
| Sausage | 500 | 28 | 40 |
| **Chick-n-Minis,** 1 box, 3 pieces | 280 | 11 | 30 |
| **Cinnamon Cluster** | 430 | 17 | 63 |
| **Hash Browns,** 2.7 oz | 240 | 15 | 25 |
| **Oatmeal:** Multigrain w/ toppings | 290 | 10 | 50 |
| without toppings | 140 | 2.5 | 28 |

### Chick-fil-A Sandwiches: Without Sauce

| | C | F | Cb |
|---|---|---|---|
| Chicken | 440 | 18 | 41 |
| Chicken Salad | 500 | 20 | 53 |
| Grilled Chicken | 320 | 5 | 40 |
| Grilled Chicken Club | 440 | 14 | 41 |

### Cool Wrap, Grilled Chkn,

| | C | F | Cb |
|---|---|---|---|
| without dressing | 340 | 13 | 30 |

### Chicken:

| | C | F | Cb |
|---|---|---|---|
| **Chick-n-Strips,** breaded, 4 count | 470 | 24 | 21 |
| **Nuggets:** Breaded, 8 count | 270 | 13 | 10 |
| Grilled, 8 count | 140 | 3 | 4 |

### Salads: Without Dressing

| | C | F | Cb |
|---|---|---|---|
| Cobb | 500 | 27 | 27 |
| Grilled Market | 320 | 14 | 26 |
| Spicy Southwest | 420 | 19 | 32 |

### Dressings:

| | C | F | Cb |
|---|---|---|---|
| Avocado Lime Ranch | 310 | 32 | 3 |
| Creamy Salsa | 290 | 31 | 3 |
| Garlic & Herb Ranch | 280 | 29 | 2 |
| Light Italian | 25 | 2 | 3 |
| **Sauces:** BBQ | 45 | 0 | 10 |
| Buffalo, 0.8 oz | 10 | 0 | 1 |
| Buttermilk Ranch, 0.8 oz | 110 | 11 | 1 |
| Chick-fil-A, 1 oz | 140 | 13 | 6 |
| Honey Roasted BBQ, 0.5 oz | 60 | 5 | 3 |

### Sides:

| | C | F | Cb |
|---|---|---|---|
| Chicken Salad Cup, 6 oz | 360 | 24 | 7 |
| Fruit Cup, w/ Blueberries, medium | 50 | 0 | 13 |
| Hearty Brst of Chicken Soup, med. | 140 | 2.5 | 18 |
| Side Salad | 80 | 4.5 | 6 |
| Waffle Potato Fries: Small | 310 | 16 | 37 |
| Medium | 400 | 21 | 48 |
| Large | 520 | 27 | 63 |
| **Dessert,** Chocolate Chunk Cookie | 330 | 14 | 45 |
| **Milkshakes:** Chocolate, large | 710 | 26 | 108 |
| Vanilla, large | 620 | 25 | 86 |

## Chili's® (Aug '16)

### For The Table: As Served

| | C | F | Cb |
|---|---|---|---|
| Bottomless Tostada Chips w/ Salsa | 910 | 45 | 113 |
| **Classic Nachos:** Beef, lge | 1590 | 103 | 60 |
| Chicken, large | 1420 | 88 | 61 |
| Southwest Eggrolls | 800 | 41 | 82 |
| Texas Cheese Fries, full order | 1710 | 119 | 85 |

### Triple Dipper: Serving for One

| | C | F | Cb |
|---|---|---|---|
| Big Mouth Bites | 800 | 54 | 48 |
| Original Chicken Crispers | 570 | 37 | 31 |

### Burgers: As Served, without Fries

| | C | F | Cb |
|---|---|---|---|
| Classic Bacon | 930 | 60 | 48 |
| Oldtimer, with Cheddar Cheese | 760 | 45 | 47 |
| Southern Smokehouse Bacon | 1130 | 69 | 75 |

### Chicken: As Served, with Set Sides

| | C | F | Cb |
|---|---|---|---|
| Cajun Pasta with Grilled Chicken | 1270 | 60 | 111 |
| Crispy Crispers, without sauce | 1140 | 51 | 123 |

### Fresh Mex: As Served

| | C | F | Cb |
|---|---|---|---|
| **Bowls:** Chipotle | 880 | 39 | 79 |
| Margarita | 860 | 25 | 105 |
| Prime Rib | 860 | 40 | 86 |
| **Pairings:** Beef Enchilada | 300 | 17 | 22 |
| Beef Taco | 290 | 15 | 22 |
| Cheese Enchilada | 340 | 23 | 19 |
| Chicken Quesadilla | 690 | 48 | 34 |
| Rice & Black Beans | 240 | 2 | 47 |

### Lighter Choices: As Served

| | C | F | Cb |
|---|---|---|---|
| Ancho Salmon | 590 | 27 | 41 |
| Grilled Chicken Salad | 440 | 23 | 25 |
| Mango Chile Chicken/Tilapia, av. | 510 | 17 | 55 |
| Margarita Grilled Chicken | 580 | 14 | 64 |

### Top Shelf Tacos: Per Taco, without Sides

| | C | F | Cb |
|---|---|---|---|
| Grilled Fish | 270 | 16 | 20 |
| Por Carnitas | 330 | 19 | 17 |
| Prime Rib | 260 | 15 | 17 |
| Spicy Shrimp | 270 | 16 | 22 |

### Baby Back Ribs: Full Rack, without Sides

| | C | F | Cb |
|---|---|---|---|
| Original BBQ | 930 | 56 | 30 |
| Craft Beer BBQ | 480 | 28 | 16 |
| Dr Pepper | 930 | 56 | 34 |

### Steaks: Without Sides

| | C | F | Cb |
|---|---|---|---|
| Classic Sirloin, 6 oz | 260 | 13 | 1 |
| Classic Ribeye | 630 | 40 | 0 |
| Country-Fried Steak | 590 | 35 | 30 |

### Sides: Homestyle Fries

| | C | F | Cb |
|---|---|---|---|
| Sides: Homestyle Fries | 390 | 17 | 55 |
| Loaded Mashed Potatoes | 380 | 23 | 32 |
| Southwest Mac 'n' Cheese | 490 | 30 | 38 |
| Spiced Panko Onion Rings | 400 | 19 | 48 |

### Salads: Includes Dressing

| | C | F | Cb |
|---|---|---|---|
| Boneless Buffalo Chicken | 1040 | 72 | 50 |
| Caribbean with Seared Shrimp | 620 | 26 | 84 |
| Quesadilla Explosion | 1430 | 96 | 83 |

### Sweet Stuff: Per Slice

| | C | F | Cb |
|---|---|---|---|
| Cheesecake | 760 | 47 | 72 |
| Molten Chocolate Cake | 1180 | 62 | 150 |

*For Complete Menu & Data ~ see CalorieKing.com*

## Chipotle® (Aug '16)

| Tortillas: | C | F | Cb |
|---|---|---|---|
| Burrito Size Flour Tortillas (1) | 300 | 10 | 46 |
| Taco Size: Crispy Corn Tortilla (3) | 210 | 8 | 31 |
| Soft Corn Tortillas (Taco), (3) | 210 | 2 | 42 |
| Soft Flour Tortillas (Taco), (3) | 250 | 8 | 40 |
| **Meal Components:** | | | |
| Barbacoa, 4 oz | 165 | 7 | 2 |
| Black/Pinto Beans, average, 4 oz | 120 | 1 | 22 |
| Brown Rice, 4 oz | 210 | 5.5 | 36 |
| Carnitas, 4 oz | 210 | 12 | 0 |
| Cheese, 1 oz | 100 | 7.5 | 1 |
| Chicken, 4 oz | 180 | 7 | 0.5 |
| Fajita Vegetables, 2.5 oz | 20 | 0.5 | 4 |
| Guacamole, 3.5 oz | 230 | 22 | 8 |
| Lettuce, 1 oz | 5 | 0 | 0 |
| Sofritas, 4 oz | 145 | 10 | 9 |
| Steak, 4 oz | 190 | 6.5 | 2 |
| **Condiments:** | | | |
| Salsa: Chili Corn, 3.5 oz | 80 | 1.5 | 16 |
| Green Tomatillo, 2 oz | 15 | 0 | 4 |
| Red Tomatillo, 2 oz | 30 | 0 | 8 |
| Tomato, 3.5 oz | 20 | 0 | 4 |
| Sour Cream, 2 oz | 95 | 9 | 2 |
| **Extras,** Chips, serving, 4 oz | 570 | 27 | 73 |

## Chuck E. Cheese® (Aug '16)

| Appetizers: | C | F | Cb |
|---|---|---|---|
| Buffalo Wings, Traditional (1) | 125 | 9 | 1 |
| Boneless Wings, Plain (1) | 95 | 6 | 5 |
| **Oven Baked Sandwiches:** | | | |
| Ham & Cheese | 620 | 24 | 70 |
| Italian Sub | 910 | 53 | 75 |
| **Pizzas:** Per Medium Slice | | | |
| BBQ Chicken | 145 | 4 | 21 |
| Canadian Bacon & Pineapple | 160 | 4 | 22 |
| Cheese | 150 | 4 | 21 |
| Pepperoni | 180 | 7 | 21 |
| Super Combo | 180 | 7 | 22 |
| Veggie Combo | 160 | 5 | 22 |
| **Platters:** Sandwich, ½ Platter | 185 | 8 | 20 |
| Veggie, ⅛ Platter | 130 | 11 | 7 |
| **French Fries,** | | | |
| w/ Ketchup & Light Ranch, 8 oz | 655 | 38 | 75 |
| **Desserts:** Choc. Cake (8"), 1 slice | 290 | 13 | 41 |
| Van. Buttercream Cake, 1 slice | 310 | 14 | 41 |

## Church's Chicken® (Aug '16)

| Chicken: Per Serving | C | F | Cb |
|---|---|---|---|
| **Original:** Breast, 1 piece | 200 | 11 | 3 |
| Leg, 1 piece | 110 | 6 | 3 |
| Thigh, 1 piece | 330 | 23 | 8 |
| Wing, 1 piece | 300 | 18 | 7 |
| **Spicy:** Breast, 1 piece | 320 | 20 | 12 |
| Leg, 1 piece | 180 | 11 | 8 |
| Thigh, 1 piece | 480 | 35 | 20 |
| Wing, 1 piece | 430 | 27 | 17 |
| **Tender Strips,** average, 1 piece | 110 | 5 | 7 |
| **Sides:** Per Small Serving | | | |
| Baked Macaroni & Cheese, 4.7 oz | 210 | 12 | 19 |
| Cajun Rice, 4.8 oz | 230 | 14 | 21 |
| Cole Slaw, 4.2 oz | 170 | 11 | 16 |
| Dinner Roll (1), 1.7 oz | 60 | 1 | 11 |
| French Fries, 2.6 oz | 210 | 9 | 29 |
| Honey Butter Biscuits (1), 2.2 oz | 230 | 15 | 25 |
| Jalapeno Cheese Bombers (4) | 220 | 11 | 24 |
| Mashed Potatoes & Gravy, 4.5 oz | 110 | 1 | 24 |
| Okra, 3.4 oz | 260 | 15 | 30 |
| **Sauces:** Per Packet | | | |
| BBQ | 45 | 0 | 11 |
| Creamy Jalapeno | 120 | 13 | 2 |
| Honey Mustard/Ranch, av. | 140 | 15 | 2 |

## Cici's Pizza® (Aug '16)

| Large Pizzas: Per Slice | C | F | Cb |
|---|---|---|---|
| Alfredo | 150 | 5 | 22 |
| BBQ Pork; Buffalo Chicken, av. | 160 | 5 | 23 |
| Beef Topping | 190 | 7 | 24 |
| Cheese; Sausage, av. | 180 | 6 | 23 |
| Pepperoni & Jalapeno | 190 | 7 | 24 |
| Spin. Alfredo; Zesty Ham & Chedd. | 155 | 5.5 | 22 |
| **Extras:** Oven Roasted Wings (5) | 190 | 12 | 1 |
| Hot/Mild Sauce | 25 | 1 | 3 |

## Cinnabon® (Aug '16)

| | C | F | Cb |
|---|---|---|---|
| Cinnabon Classic Roll (1) | 880 | 37 | 127 |
| MiniBon Roll (1), 3.4 oz | 350 | 15 | 51 |
| Bites: Cinnabon Classic (4) | 430 | 16 | 63 |
| Caramel Pecan Bites (4) | 550 | 26 | 71 |
| Centre of The Roll Classic (1) | 750 | 34 | 105 |
| **Chillata:** Per 16 fl.oz | | | |
| Chocolate Mocha | 370 | 14 | 61 |
| Oreo | 810 | 38 | 109 |
| Strawberry/Strawb. Banana, av. | 520 | 11 | 105 |
| **MochaLatta Chill,** 16 oz | 360 | 15 | 52 |

**Updated Nutrition Data ~ www.CalorieKing.com**
**Persons with Diabetes ~ See Disclaimer (Page 22)**

## Claim Jumper® (Aug '16)

*Appetizers:* As Served

| | C | F | Cb |
|---|---|---|---|
| Southwest Eggrolls | 1190 | 53 | 114 |
| Three Cheese Potatocakes (3) | 1075 | 71 | 80 |

*Burgers & Sandwiches:* Without Sides

| | | | |
|---|---|---|---|
| Grilled Cobb Sandwich | 1210 | 78 | 78 |
| Widow Maker Burger | 1370 | 87 | 84 |
| *Calzones:* Specialty | 1430 | 80 | 137 |
| Traditional | 1350 | 66 | 140 |

*Meals:*

*Favorites:* With Menu Set Sides & Toppings

| | | | |
|---|---|---|---|
| Country Fried Steak | 2030 | 107 | 189 |
| Giant Stuffed Chicken Baker | 990 | 34 | 118 |
| Meatloaf & Mashed Potatoes | 1300 | 75 | 117 |
| *Pasta:* Black Tie Pasta | 1535 | 84 | 126 |
| Parmesan Crusted Chicken | 975 | 47 | 83 |
| *Pizza:* Calif. Works, Classic Crust | 1295 | 64 | 127 |
| Steakhouse, Flatbread | 820 | 47 | 65 |

*Specialties:*

| | | | |
|---|---|---|---|
| BBQ Baby Back Pork Ribs, Full Rack | 1745 | 111 | 111 |
| Roasted Tri-Tip with Demi Glaze | 800 | 47 | 19 |

*Seafood:* Atlantic Salmon,

| | | | |
|---|---|---|---|
| Blackened | 715 | 42 | 48 |
| Tilapia Bianca, with Shrimp, Artichoke Hearts & Sauce | 1165 | 80 | 56 |

*Entree Salads:* Without Dressing Or Bread

| | | | |
|---|---|---|---|
| Calif. Citrus Chkn, Charbroiled | 865 | 53 | 58 |
| Seared Ahi Spinach | 515 | 24 | 31 |

*Soups:* Per Bowl

| | | | |
|---|---|---|---|
| New England Clam Chowder | 525 | 45 | 23 |
| Potato Cheddar | 710 | 61 | 31 |
| *Sweets:* Choc. Motherlode Cake | 2770 | 144 | 340 |
| Italian Lemon Cake | 1240 | 62 | 158 |

## Coldstone Creamery® (Aug '16)

*Ice Creams:*

| | C | F | Cb |
|---|---|---|---|
| **Amaretto:** Like it | 330 | 20 | 33 |
| Love it | 530 | 31 | 53 |
| Gotta have it | 790 | 47 | 80 |
| **Chocolate:** Like it | 320 | 20 | 33 |
| Love it | 520 | 31 | 53 |
| Gotta have it | 780 | 48 | 79 |

*Hot Stone:*

| | | | |
|---|---|---|---|
| Brownie A La Cold Stone, 11 oz | 810 | 55 | 99 |
| Chocolate Lava Meltdown, 9 oz | 730 | 36 | 97 |
| Churro Caramel Crave, 8.6 oz | 700 | 33 | 98 |

*Sorbet:*

| | | | |
|---|---|---|---|
| **Strawberry Mango:** Like it | 220 | 0 | 55 |
| Love it | 350 | 0 | 87 |
| Gotta have it | 520 | 0.5 | 131 |

## Cosi® (Aug '16)

*Melts:* With Set Menu Components

| | C | F | Cb |
|---|---|---|---|
| Grilled Chicken TBM | 650 | 32 | 46 |
| Pesto Chicken | 580 | 17 | 49 |
| Steakhouse Gorgonzola | 780 | 44 | 65 |
| Tuna Melt | 790 | 42 | 54 |

*Bowls:* With Set Menu Components

| | | | |
|---|---|---|---|
| Adobo Chili Chicken | 555 | 21 | 67 |
| Brazilian Steak | 540 | 27 | 52 |
| Caribbean Chicken | 390 | 16 | 37 |
| Thai Curry Chicken | 540 | 17 | 65 |
| Thai Curry Tofu | 510 | 17 | 64 |

*Soup:* Per Regular

| | | | |
|---|---|---|---|
| Classic Clam Chowder | 315 | 20 | 25 |
| Tomato Basil | 400 | 31 | 20 |

*Salads:*

| | | | |
|---|---|---|---|
| Cobb, with Sherry Shallot Dressing | 740 | 56 | 20 |
| Greek, with Italian Vinaigrette | 535 | 47 | 20 |
| Signature, w/ Sherry Shallot Drsng | 620 | 45 | 40 |
| Steakhouse, with Blue Chse Drsng | 655 | 53 | 15 |

*Breakfast:*

| | | | |
|---|---|---|---|
| Ancient Grains Oatmeal, without toppings, large | 365 | 6 | 43 |
| Santa Fe Wrap, 8.8 oz | 470 | 29 | 30 |
| Squagel Sandwich Club Omelette on Plain Bagel, 7.1 oz | 600 | 15 | 73 |
| *Pastries:* Banana Nut Muffin | 500 | 31 | 47 |
| Chocolate Biscotti | 280 | 13 | 38 |

## Cousins Subs® (Aug '16)

*Subs:* Per 7.5", Standard Toppings

| | C | F | Cb |
|---|---|---|---|
| Chicken Bacon Cheddar, Mayo | 835 | 47 | 54 |
| Chicken Bacon Mshrm, Bistro Sce | 760 | 36 | 58 |
| Chicken Cheese Steak, Mayo | 870 | 51 | 52 |
| Club, with Mayo | 715 | 39 | 53 |
| Ham & Provolone, with Mayo | 680 | 38 | 51 |
| Italian Special, with Oil | 895 | 56 | 51 |
| Roast Beef & Cheddar, with Mayo | 730 | 37 | 52 |
| Tuna with Mayo | 890 | 63 | 50 |
| Turkey Breast w/ Mayo | 535 | 31 | 53 |

*Soup:* Per Regular

| | | | |
|---|---|---|---|
| Beef Steak with Noodle | 105 | 4 | 12 |
| Cheddar Cauliflower | 115 | 5 | 13 |
| Chicken Noodle | 115 | 3 | 16 |
| Cream of Broccoli | 165 | 10 | 13 |
| New England Clam Chowder | 150 | 3 | 25 |

*For Complete Nutritional Data ~ See CalorieKing.com*

*For Complete Nutritional Data ~ see CalorieKing.com*

## Culver's® (Aug '16)

| ButterBurgers: | C | F | Cb |
|---|---|---|---|
| **Original:** Single | 390 | 18 | 39 |
| Double | 560 | 32 | 39 |
| Triple | 730 | 44 | 39 |
| Cheddar with Bacon, Single | 510 | 28 | 39 |
| Cheese: Single | 460 | 24 | 40 |
| Double | 700 | 44 | 41 |
| Culver's Bacon Deluxe: Single | 610 | 38 | 42 |
| Double | 850 | 58 | 43 |
| Culver's Deluxe: Single | 570 | 36 | 42 |
| Double | 810 | 54 | 43 |
| Mushroom & Swiss, Single | 490 | 26 | 40 |
| Sourdough Melt, Single | 460 | 25 | 34 |
| Corn Dog, Kids | 230 | 14 | 17 |
| Chicken Tenders, Breaded, 2 pcs | 270 | 12 | 21 |
| **Sandwiches:** Beef Pot Roast | 410 | 14 | 41 |
| Crispy Chicken | 460 | 15 | 58 |
| Grilled Reuben Melt | 690 | 38 | 46 |
| North Atlantic Cod Filet | 600 | 32 | 49 |
| Pork Tenderloin | 630 | 26 | 73 |
| *Sides:* | | | |
| Chili Cheddar Fries | 670 | 32 | 78 |
| Crinkle Cut Fries, regular | 360 | 14 | 53 |
| Mashed Potatoes, w/ Gravy, reg. | 140 | 2 | 25 |
| Wisconsin Cheese Curds, 5.3 oz | 510 | 25 | 51 |
| ***Dinners:*** *With Fries, Cole Slaw & Bread Roll* | | | |
| Butterfly Jumbo Shrimp, 6 pieces | 1090 | 54 | 129 |
| Fried Chicken, 1 breast, 1 wing | 840 | 35 | 57 |
| North Atlantic Cod, Fried, 2 pieces | 1480 | 99 | 106 |
| *Soup:* | | | |
| Broccoli Cheese, 10.5 oz | 220 | 12 | 17 |
| Chicken Noodle, 10.5 oz | 110 | 2 | 14 |
| Potato with Bacon, 10.5 oz | 240 | 10 | 28 |
| ***Salads:*** *Without Dressing* | | | |
| Chicken Cashew w/ Gr. Chicken | 460 | 24 | 16 |
| Cranberry Bacon Bleu, with Grilled Chicken | 360 | 13 | 18 |
| Garden Fresco w/ Gr. Chicken | 360 | 14 | 16 |
| Side Salad | 60 | 2 | 6 |
| *Dressings:* | | | |
| Chunky Bleu Cheese, 1.8 oz | 310 | 33 | 2 |
| French Dressing, 1.8 oz | 190 | 13 | 19 |
| Ranch, 1.75 oz | 180 | 19 | 2 |
| Sesame Ginger, 2 oz | 70 | 0 | 16 |

## Culver's® cont... (Aug '16)

| Concrete Mixers: Per Regular | | | |
|---|---|---|---|
| Chocolate | 950 | 46 | 121 |
| Cookie Dough | 1010 | 56 | 113 |
| ***Sundaes:*** *Per 2 Scoops* | | | |
| Banana Split | 1060 | 60 | 122 |
| Caramel Cashew | 1000 | 51 | 121 |
| Fudge Pecan | 1040 | 64 | 107 |
| Turtle | 1040 | 62 | 112 |
| ***Beverages:*** Chocolate Malt, reg. | 880 | 39 | 120 |
| Chocolate Shake, regular | 820 | 38 | 108 |
| Strawberry Malt, regular | 770 | 38 | 96 |
| Strawberry Shake, regular | 730 | 38 | 86 |

## D'Angelo's® (Aug '16)

| | C | F | Cb |
|---|---|---|---|
| ***Toasted & Hot Sandwiches:*** *Per Medium Size, Menu Board Toppings Only, w/out Bread* | | | |
| Classic Veggie | 350 | 23 | 16 |
| Italian Toasted | 840 | 69 | 14 |
| Meatball & Cheese | 770 | 59 | 25 |
| **Add Sandwich Bread:** *Per Medium Size* | | | |
| Classic Italian Sub | 310 | 3.5 | 58 |
| Multigrain Sub | 310 | 3.5 | 60 |
| Pokket | 160 | 0 | 34 |
| ***Wraps:*** *Menu Board Toppings, without Wraps* | | | |
| Buffalo Chicken, Whole | 520 | 36 | 17 |
| Chicken Caesar, Whole | 620 | 42 | 25 |
| **Add Wraps:** Wheat, 4 oz | 310 | 8 | 55 |
| Tortilla Wrap, 4 oz | 310 | 9 | 49 |
| *Dressings:* Caesar, 1.5 oz | 200 | 21 | 3 |
| Greek, 1.5 oz | 210 | 24 | 1 |
| Ranch, 1.5 oz | 150 | 15 | 2 |
| ***Salads:*** *Entree Size, without Bread* | | | |
| Caesar, with Dressing | 630 | 53 | 28 |
| Chicken Caesar, with Dressing | 770 | 55 | 30 |
| Chicken Cobb, w/out Dressing | 310 | 17 | 11 |
| Greek, w/out Dressing | 240 | 13 | 17 |
| ***Soup:*** *Per Bowl* | | | |
| Extreme Broccoli & Cheddar | 370 | 28 | 18 |
| Hearty Beef Stew | 330 | 12 | 34 |
| Main Lobster Bisque | 540 | 43 | 24 |
| New England Clam Chowder | 480 | 27 | 46 |

*For Complete Menu & Data ~ see CalorieKing.com*

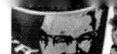 

## Dairy Queen® (Aug '16)

*Burgers & Sandwiches:*

|  | C | F | Cb |
|---|---|---|---|
| **Burgers:** | | | |
| Cheeseburger: Original | 400 | 18 | 34 |
| Double | 630 | 34 | 34 |
| **GrillBurgers:** | | | |
| ¼ lb Bacon Cheese | 630 | 37 | 44 |
| ½ lb Grillburger with Cheese | 800 | 51 | 44 |
| ½ lb Flame Thrower | 1000 | 74 | 40 |
| Mushroom Swiss | 570 | 35 | 39 |
| **Sandwiches:** Crispy Chicken | 600 | 30 | 59 |
| Grilled Chicken | 390 | 14 | 44 |
| **Baskets:** | | | |
| Chicken Strips: 4 pces w/ Ctry Gravy | 1030 | 53 | 105 |
| 6 piece, with Country Gravy | 1260 | 66 | 121 |
| **Hot Dogs:** Beef | 290 | 17 | 22 |
| Beef, Chili & Cheese | 380 | 24 | 23 |
| **Salads:** *Without Dressing* | | | |
| **Garden Green:** Crispy Chicken | 280 | 13 | 26 |
| Grilled Chicken | 150 | 2 | 10 |
| **Sides:** | | | |
| French Fries, regular, 4 oz | 310 | 13 | 43 |
| Onion Rings, 4 oz | 360 | 16 | 47 |
| **Desserts:** *Per Medium* | | | |
| **Blizzard Treats:** Banana Split | 570 | 17 | 93 |
| Butterfinger | 740 | 26 | 114 |
| Cookie Dough | 1020 | 40 | 148 |
| Heath | 920 | 41 | 126 |
| Oreo Cookies | 790 | 30 | 117 |
| Reese's Peanut Butter Cups | 740 | 31 | 101 |
| Salted Caramel Truffle | 1060 | 49 | 142 |
| Strawberry Cheesecake | 690 | 28 | 92 |
| **DQ Blizzard Cakes (10"):** | | | |
| Oreo, ⅒ cake | 760 | 33 | 104 |
| Reese's P'nut Butter Cup, ⅒ cake | 720 | 33 | 94 |
| **DQ Dipped Cone,** Chocolate, med. | 470 | 22 | 61 |
| **DQ Sundaes:** *Per Medium* | | | |
| Caramel | 430 | 11 | 74 |
| Hot Fudge | 440 | 15 | 67 |
| Strawberry | 350 | 10 | 56 |
| **Malts:** *Per Medium* | | | |
| Caramel | 830 | 25 | 134 |
| Chocolate | 790 | 23 | 130 |
| Strawberry | 700 | 22 | 107 |
| **Moo Latte:** *Per Medium, with Whipped Topping* | | | |
| Cappuccino | 570 | 19 | 90 |
| French Vanilla | 630 | 19 | 107 |
| Mocha | 660 | 25 | 102 |

*For Complete Nutritional Data ~ see CalorieKing.com*

## Daphne's Greek Cafe® (Aug '16)

*Starters:*

|  | C | F | Cb |
|---|---|---|---|
| Fire Feta & Warm Pita | 400 | 19 | 43 |
| Hummus & Warm Pita | 330 | 13 | 41 |
| **Pita Sandwiches:** *With Sides, without Tzatziki Sauce* | | | |
| with Chicken | 480 | 16 | 43 |
| with Crispy Shrimp | 450 | 19 | 51 |
| with Falafel | 560 | 25 | 72 |
| with Gyro | 730 | 47 | 52 |
| **Cali-Greek Bowls:** with Falafel | 840 | 33 | 115 |
| with Crispy Shrimp | 730 | 26 | 95 |
| with Falafel | 840 | 33 | 115 |
| with Grilled Chicken | 750 | 23 | 87 |
| with Grilled Shrimp | 710 | 26 | 86 |
| **Plate: Mediterranean Veggie,** | | | |
| with Rice & Greek Salad | 1050 | 60 | 110 |
| **Classic Greek Salads:** *With Dressing, w/o Pita & Sce* | | | |
| Crispy Shrimp | 440 | 31 | 25 |
| Falafel | 540 | 37 | 45 |
| Grilled Chicken | 460 | 28 | 18 |
| **Add:** Pita & Tzatziki | 150 | 4 | 21 |
| **Sides:** Cucumber-Tomato Salad | 120 | 11 | 5 |
| Fire Roasted Vegetables | 60 | 3 | 6 |
| French Fries | 320 | 16 | 40 |
| Greek Salad, small | 130 | 12 | 6 |
| Moroccan Carrot-Walnut Salad | 180 | 13 | 16 |
| Multigrain Pita Chips | 170 | 5 | 27 |
| Pita Bread | 240 | 5 | 39 |
| Seasoned Rice | 250 | 6 | 47 |
| Tabouli Salad | 220 | 15 | 20 |
| Tzatziki | 30 | 0 | 2 |

## Davanni's® (Aug '16)

*Half Hoagies: Inc. 6" White Bun & Standard Toppings*

|  | C | F | Cb |
|---|---|---|---|
| Assorted | 490 | 30 | 39 |
| Cheese | 500 | 31 | 39 |
| Chicken & Bacon w/ Honey Mstrd | 505 | 22 | 46 |
| Chicken Parmigiana | 445 | 16 | 40 |
| Club | 495 | 27 | 40 |
| Pastrami | 470 | 27 | 40 |
| Roast Beef | 470 | 25 | 39 |
| Southwestern Chicken | 535 | 26 | 43 |
| Tuna Melt | 645 | 44 | 42 |
| Turkey Bacon Chipotle | 565 | 33 | 39 |
| Veggie | 445 | 24 | 43 |
| **Pasta:** *As Served, with Garlic Toast* | | | |
| Chicken Florentine, half portion | 570 | 23 | 56 |
| Lasagna, half portion | 625 | 43 | 37 |

*continued next page...*

# Fast - Foods & Restaurants

## Davanni's® cont... (Aug '16)

| *Pizzas:* Per Slice | C | F | Cb |
|---|---|---|---|
| **Five Meat:** Thin Crust | 255 | 13 | 19 |
| Traditional Crust | 305 | 13 | 30 |
| Solo, Thin Crust | 655 | 36 | 44 |
| **Veggie:** Thin Crust | 220 | 10 | 19 |
| Traditional Crust | 275 | 10 | 30 |
| **Works:** Thin Crust | 265 | 14 | 19 |
| Traditional Crust | 315 | 15 | 30 |

## Del Taco® (Aug '16)

| *Breakfast:* | C | F | Cb |
|---|---|---|---|
| **Burritos:** Breakfast | 310 | 15 | 28 |
| Half Pounders: Bacon | 640 | 36 | 38 |
| ½ lb Chorizo/Steak, av. | 520 | 28 | 39 |
| **Hash Brown Sticks,** 5 pieces | 230 | 17 | 18 |
| **Quesadilla,** Bacon & Egg | 430 | 24 | 32 |
| **Tacos,** Egg & Cheese | 200 | 11 | 15 |
| **Burgers:** Cheeseburger | 430 | 22 | 40 |
| Double Del Cheeseburger | 720 | 48 | 40 |
| Bacon Double Cheeseburger | 770 | 52 | 40 |
| **Crinkle Cut Fries:** Kids, 3 oz | 160 | 10 | 17 |
| Regular, 4 oz | 210 | 13 | 22 |
| Medium, 6 oz | 320 | 19 | 34 |
| Macho, 8.8 oz | 470 | 28 | 49 |
| Chili Cheddar Fries, 10.5 oz | 570 | 34 | 41 |
| **Burritos:** ½ lb Bean & Cheese, av | 460 | 10 | 70 |
| Classic Grilled Chicken | 530 | 33 | 40 |
| Del Beef | 490 | 20 | 40 |
| Del Combo | 530 | 16 | 64 |
| Macho Combo | 940 | 34 | 100 |
| **Epic:** Bacon/Chicken/Avocado | 980 | 52 | 90 |
| Carne Asada | 750 | 24 | 90 |
| Gr/Chicken Avocado | 840 | 36 | 90 |
| **Macho Nachos:** | | | |
| Beef/Chicken/Steak, av | 950 | 8 | 98 |
| **Quesadillas:** Mini Bacon | 170 | 9 | 14 |
| Cheddar; Spicy Jack, average | 460 | 27 | 32 |
| Chicken Cheddar/Spicy Jack, av | 550 | 31 | 35 |
| **Tacos:** Beer Battered Fish | 230 | 12 | 26 |
| Del Taco: Crunchy | 310 | 20 | 14 |
| Soft | 300 | 16 | 17 |
| Grilled Chicken | 220 | 12 | 16 |
| Street Taco, Chicken/Steak, av. | 180 | 7 | 20 |
| **Salads:** Chicken, Bacon Avocado | 590 | 46 | 23 |
| Mexican Chopped Chicken | 510 | 23 | 39 |
| **Desserts:** Cinn. Churro (1) | 220 | 15 | 23 |
| Caramel Cheesecake Bites (2) | 460 | 28 | 43 |
| **Shakes:** Per 16 oz | | | |
| Chocolate | 560 | 11 | 105 |
| Strawberry; Vanilla, av. | 520 | 11 | 95 |

## Denny's® (Aug '16)

| *Breakfast:* | C | F | Cb |
|---|---|---|---|
| **Favorites:** *Without Side Choices* | | | |
| Banana Pecan Pancakes | 750 | 13 | 134 |
| Blueberry P'cakes w/ Scr. Eggs | 840 | 44 | 88 |
| Cinn. P'cakes, Hsh Brwns, Fr. Eggs | 990 | 48 | 117 |
| Moons Over My Hammy | 980 | 65 | 55 |
| Peanut Butter Cup Pancakes, | | | |
| Hash Browns & Fried Egg | 1510 | 90 | 147 |
| **Omelettes:** *With Hash Browns, without Bread* | | | |
| Loaded Veggie | 600 | 43 | 25 |
| Philly Cheesesteak | 1170 | 92 | 28 |
| Ultimate | 830 | 66 | 25 |
| **Skillets:** *As Served* | | | |
| Hearty Breakfast | 1090 | 85 | 40 |
| Loaded Bacon, Steak & Potato | 900 | 59 | 40 |
| Santa Fe | 720 | 53 | 31 |
| Ultimate | 720 | 54 | 33 |
| **Slams:** | | | |
| All American, w/ Hash Browns | 990 | 83 | 20 |
| French Toast | 810 | 48 | 66 |
| Honey Jalapeno Bacon Slam | 1060 | 65 | 84 |
| Lumberjack, w/out bread, 17oz | 1230 | 76 | 90 |
| Grand Slamwich & Hsh Brwns | 1390 | 96 | 82 |
| **Sides:** Buttermilk Biscuit (2) | 400 | 18 | 50 |
| English Muffin, w/out Margarine (1) | 140 | 1 | 29 |
| Hash Browns, 1 serve | 210 | 16 | 15 |
| **Pancakes:** | | | |
| Buttermilk, w/ Margarine, (2) | 370 | 8 | 68 |
| Hearty Wheat, 2 cakes | 310 | 2 | 64 |
| *Burgers & Sandwiches:* | | | |
| **Burgers:** *Without Sides, Unless Indicated* | | | |
| Bacon, Avocado Cheeseburger | 1030 | 75 | 50 |
| Bourbon Bacon Burger | 1060 | 65 | 77 |
| Chicken Bacon Classic | 920 | 56 | 48 |
| Double Cheeseburger | 1120 | 67 | 49 |
| Spicy Sriracha Burger | 860 | 54 | 51 |
| **Melts:** Chicken Philly | 800 | 49 | 56 |
| Pot Roast Melt | 710 | 44 | 59 |
| Prime Rib Philly | 970 | 57 | 60 |
| **Sandwiches:** *Without Sides* | | | |
| Cali Club | 1100 | 75 | 70 |
| Club | 810 | 39 | 75 |
| The Super Bird | 610 | 32 | 42 |
| **Lunch Sides:** Caesar Salad | 220 | 11 | 26 |
| French Fries | 510 | 28 | 59 |
| Garden Salad, without Dressing | 190 | 9 | 20 |
| Seasonal Fries | 630 | 47 | 48 |

## Denny's® cont... (Aug '16)

*Dinners: W/out Sides Unless Indicated* **C** **F** **Cb**

| | C | F | Cb |
|---|---|---|---|
| Bourbon Chicken Skillet | 840 | 26 | 78 |
| Brooklyn Spag. & M'balls & Bread | 1230 | 61 | 111 |
| Chicken Strips, with Bread | 780 | 40 | 64 |
| Fish & Chips | 1050 | 75 | 131 |
| Slow-Cooked Pot Rst | 1390 | 37 | 166 |
| T-Bone Steak: with Bread | 840 | 38 | 23 |
| with Shrimp & Bread | 1030 | 46 | 43 |

*Dinner Sides:*

| | | | |
|---|---|---|---|
| Broccoli, 3 oz | 25 | 0 | 4 |
| French Fries, salted, 6 oz | 510 | 28 | 59 |
| Golden-Fried Shrimp, 6 pieces | 190 | 8 | 20 |
| Hash Browns, 1 serving | 210 | 16 | 15 |
| Mashed Potatoes, 1 serving | 200 | 8 | 29 |
| Red-Skinned Potatoes, 4 oz | 200 | 9 | 27 |

*Soups: Per Bowl, without Bread*

| | | | |
|---|---|---|---|
| Broccoli & Cheddar | 370 | 16 | 48 |
| Chicken Noodle | 140 | 4 | 17 |
| Vegetable Beef | 170 | 4 | 23 |

*Salads: Without Bread*

| | | | |
|---|---|---|---|
| Avocado Chicken Caesar, | | | |
| with Caesar Drssng | 660 | 49 | 15 |
| Cranb. Apple Chicken | | | |
| with Balsamic Vinaigrette | 360 | 9 | 36 |
| Prime Rib Cobb, without Dressing | 630 | 46 | 18 |

*Dressings: Per 1.5oz*

| | | | |
|---|---|---|---|
| Bleu Cheese | 160 | 16 | 2 |
| Caesar | 210 | 23 | 0 |
| French | 110 | 7 | 12 |
| Honey Mustard | 165 | 14 | 11 |
| Ranch | 180 | 19 | 1 |

*Desserts: As Served*

| | | | |
|---|---|---|---|
| Banana Split | 810 | 31 | 125 |
| Caramel Apple Pie Crisp | 740 | 21 | 134 |
| Chocolate Lava Cake | 730 | 36 | 84 |
| NY Style Cheesecake, no topping | 500 | 34 | 43 |

*Beverages:*

| | | | |
|---|---|---|---|
| Hot Chocolate, 8 oz | 100 | 2 | 28 |
| Iced Cappuccino, 15 oz | 190 | 5 | 30 |
| Lemonade Iced Tea, 15 oz | 70 | 0 | 19 |
| Strawberry Lemonade, 15 oz | 200 | 0 | 50 |
| **Milk Shakes:** Chocolate, 16 oz | 860 | 44 | 104 |
| Vanilla, 16 oz | 870 | 44 | 107 |

*For Complete Nutritional Data ~ see CalorieKing.com*

## Dippin' Dots® (Aug '16)

*Flavored Ices: Per ½ Cup, 3 oz* **C** **F** **Cb**

| | C | F | Cb |
|---|---|---|---|
| Rockin' Cherry w/- Popping Candy | 130 | 0.5 | 30 |
| Sour Blue Razz | 100 | 0 | 26 |
| Other varieties | 100 | 0 | 26 |

*Frozen Yogurt: Per ½ Cup*

| | | | |
|---|---|---|---|
| Strawberry Cheesecake, ½ cup | 100 | 0 | 21 |
| YoDots: Cookies 'N Cream | 100 | 1.5 | 16 |
| Chocolate & Vanilla | 70 | 0 | 12 |
| Cookie Dough | 110 | 2 | 19 |

*Ice Cream: Per ½ Cup*

| | | | |
|---|---|---|---|
| Banana Split | 160 | 8 | 20 |
| Choc. Chip Cookie Dough | 230 | 11 | 32 |
| Mint Chocolate | 170 | 8 | 21 |
| Strawberry | 160 | 8 | 18 |

## Donatos Pizza® (Aug '16)

*Pizzas:* **C** **F** **Cb**

*Signature: Thin Crust, ¼ Large Pizza*

| | C | F | Cb |
|---|---|---|---|
| Classic Trio | 630 | 33 | 49 |
| Founder's Favorite | 670 | 34 | 50 |
| Hawaiian | 550 | 24 | 53 |

*Signatures: Thicker Crust, ¼ Large Pizza*

| | | | |
|---|---|---|---|
| Founder's Favorite | 720 | 34 | 66 |
| Mariachi Beef | 590 | 21 | 67 |
| Mariachi Chicken | 590 | 21 | 67 |
| Pepperoni | 660 | 31 | 64 |
| Serious Cheese | 640 | 28 | 64 |
| The Works | 700 | 33 | 69 |
| Vegy | 560 | 21 | 70 |

*Signature Subs: On White*

| | | | |
|---|---|---|---|
| Big Don: Italian | 660 | 33 | 60 |
| Marinara | 600 | 25 | 62 |
| Sausage Italian | 920 | 54 | 62 |
| Sausage Marinara | 870 | 46 | 65 |
| Buffalo Chicken | 650 | 27 | 64 |
| Chicken Bacon Cheddar | 770 | 38 | 61 |
| Meatball | 890 | 46 | 71 |

*Signature Subs: On Wheat*

| | | | |
|---|---|---|---|
| Buffalo Chicken | 620 | 27 | 60 |
| Steak Hoagie: Marinara Sauce | 610 | 27 | 58 |
| Mushroom Gravy | 610 | 27 | 58 |
| Turkey Club | 660 | 30 | 55 |
| **Stromboli:** Deluxe | 860 | 33 | 95 |
| Pepperoni | 980 | 45 | 94 |
| Three Meat | 970 | 42 | 94 |

*Desserts:*

| | | | |
|---|---|---|---|
| Apple Crisp Timpano, 1 slice | 390 | 7 | 72 |
| Cinnamon Crisp Timpano, 1 slice | 410 | 13 | 65 |
| Cinnamon Twists (2 sticks) | 210 | 2 | 42 |

*For Complete Nutritional Data ~ see CalorieKing.com*

## Domino's® (Aug '16)

**C  F  Cb**

### 12" Hand Tossed:
*Per Slice, ⅛ Pizza, Includes Base Sauce and Cheese*

| | C | F | Cb |
|---|---|---|---|
| Bacon, Beef & Sausage | 275 | 14 | 27 |
| Beef, Green Pepp., On. & Mshrm | 200 | 8 | 25 |
| Black Olives, Green Peppers, Onions, Mushrooms, Tomatoes | 190 | 7 | 25 |
| Ham & Pineapple | 200 | 6.5 | 26 |
| Pepperoni | 215 | 9 | 25 |
| Pepperoni & Sausage | 240 | 11 | 26 |
| Sausage | 230 | 10 | 26 |
| Sliced Ital. Saus., Beef & Pepperoni | 265 | 14 | 25 |

### 14" Thin Crust: *Per Slice, ⅛ Pizza, Includes Base Sauce and Cheese*

| | C | F | Cb |
|---|---|---|---|
| Bacon, Beef & Sausage | 325 | 19 | 21 |
| Beef, Green Pepp., On. & Mshrm | 220 | 12 | 19 |
| Black Olives, Green Peppers, Onions, Mushrooms & Tomatoes | 210 | 11 | 19 |
| Ham & Pineapple | 220 | 10 | 21 |
| Pepperoni | 240 | 13 | 19 |
| Pepperoni & Sausage | 275 | 16 | 20 |
| Sausage | 260 | 15 | 21 |

### 14" Brooklyn: *Per Slice, ⅙ Pizza, Includes Base Sauce and Cheese*

| | C | F | Cb |
|---|---|---|---|
| Beef, Green Pepp., On. & Mushroom | 270 | 13 | 26 |
| Black Olives, Green Peppers, Onions, Mushrooms, Tomatoes | 250 | 12 | 26 |
| Ham & Pineapple | 265 | 12 | 29 |
| Pepperoni | 290 | 15 | 26 |
| Pepperoni & Sausage | 340 | 19 | 27 |
| Sausage | 320 | 18 | 28 |

### 12" Feast Hand-Tossed: *Per Slice, ⅛ Pizza*

| | C | F | Cb |
|---|---|---|---|
| America's Favorite | 240 | 11 | 27 |
| Bacon Cheeseburger | 270 | 13 | 27 |
| Deluxe | 230 | 10 | 27 |
| ExtravaganZZa | 280 | 14 | 27 |
| MeatZZa | 270 | 13 | 27 |
| Ultimate Pepperoni | 260 | 14 | 26 |

### 14" Feast Hand Tossed: *Per Slice, ⅛ Pizza*

| | C | F | Cb |
|---|---|---|---|
| America's Favorite | 340 | 16 | 36 |
| Bacon Cheeseburger | 370 | 17 | 36 |
| Deluxe | 310 | 13 | 36 |
| ExtravaganZZa | 380 | 19 | 37 |
| MeatZZa Feast | 370 | 18 | 36 |
| Ultimate Pepperoni | 360 | 18 | 35 |

### 12" Legends Thin Crust: *Per ¼ Party Pizza*

| | C | F | Cb |
|---|---|---|---|
| Buffalo Chicken | 360 | 21 | 23 |
| Cali Chicken Bacon Ranch | 470 | 32 | 25 |
| Fiery Hawaiian | 370 | 21 | 29 |
| Memphis BBQ Chicken | 350 | 18 | 30 |
| Philly Cheese Steak | 340 | 20 | 23 |

## Domino's® cont... (Aug '16)

**C  F  Cb**

### Chicken Wings: *W/out Dipping Sauce*

| | C | F | Cb |
|---|---|---|---|
| Barbeque, 4 wings | 240 | 13 | 13 |
| Hot, 4 wings | 190 | 13 | 4 |

### Chicken Dipping Cups: *Per 1.5 oz Container*

| | C | F | Cb |
|---|---|---|---|
| Blue Cheese | 240 | 25 | 2 |
| Kicker Hot | 50 | 4.5 | 3 |
| Mango Habanero | 80 | 0 | 20 |
| Ranch | 200 | 21 | 2 |

### BreadBowl Pasta: *Per ½ Bowl*

| | C | F | Cb |
|---|---|---|---|
| Chicken Alfredo, 10.85 oz | 700 | 26 | 93 |
| Chicken Carbonara, 11.6 oz | 740 | 28 | 94 |
| Italian Sausage Marinara, 11.85 oz | 730 | 26 | 99 |
| Pasta Primavera, 11 oz | 670 | 24 | 94 |

### Oven Baked Sandwiches: *Per Sandwich*

| | C | F | Cb |
|---|---|---|---|
| Buffalo Chicken with Blue Cheese | 860 | 41 | 80 |
| Chicken Bacon Ranch | 880 | 44 | 77 |
| Chicken Parmesan | 780 | 31 | 79 |
| Italian | 860 | 42 | 77 |
| Italian Sausage & Peppers | 900 | 46 | 81 |
| Mediterranean Veggie | 720 | 30 | 70 |
| Philly Cheese Steak | 740 | 31 | 76 |
| Sweet & Spicy Chicken Habanero | 810 | 30 | 89 |

### Salads: *Per Serving without Dressing*

| | C | F | Cb |
|---|---|---|---|
| Chicken Apple Pecan | 190 | 6 | 20 |
| Classic Garden | 120 | 7 | 9 |
| Chicken Caesar | 190 | 7 | 15 |

### Salad Dressings: *Per 1.5 oz Package*

| | C | F | Cb |
|---|---|---|---|
| Balsamic Dressing | 120 | 12 | 4 |
| Caesar Dressing | 230 | 25 | 1 |
| Ranch Dressing | 220 | 24 | 2 |
| Raspberry Dressing, fat-free | 45 | 0 | 11 |

### Bread Side Items:

| | C | F | Cb |
|---|---|---|---|
| **Breadsticks:** 1 stick, without sauce | 110 | 6 | 11 |
| 8 sticks, without sauce | 880 | 48 | 88 |

### Stufed Cheesy Bread:

| | C | F | Cb |
|---|---|---|---|
| 1 stick, without sauce | 140 | 6 | 16 |
| 8 sticks, without sauce | 1120 | 48 | 128 |

### Bread Dipping Sauces: *Per Container*

| | C | F | Cb |
|---|---|---|---|
| Garlic, 1 oz | 250 | 28 | 0 |
| Marinara, 2 oz | 25 | 0 | 5 |

### Cinna Stix:

| | C | F | Cb |
|---|---|---|---|
| 1 stick, without icing | 120 | 6 | 14 |
| 8 sticks, without icing | 960 | 48 | 112 |

| | C | F | Cb |
|---|---|---|---|
| **Sweet Icing,** Dipping Cup | 250 | 2.5 | 57 |
| **Dessert,** Chocolate Lava Crunch Cake | 350 | 17 | 47 |

Updated Nutrition Data ~ www.CalorieKing.com
Persons with Diabetes ~ See Disclaimer (Page 22)

## Don Pablos® (Apr '16)

*Start The Fiesta: Per Entire Plate* **C** **F** **Cb**

| | C | F | Cb |
|---|---|---|---|
| **Don's Boneless Wings:** *Without Bleu Cheese Dressing* | | | |
| Buffalo | 750 | 48 | 49 |
| Chipotle Honey BBQ | 1010 | 59 | 94 |
| **Flautas,** without Guacamole | 505 | 29 | 40 |
| **Taquitos,** without Guacamole | 560 | 39 | 28 |
| **Optional Guacamole,** #30 scoop | 70 | 6 | 1 |
| **Nachos:** | | | |
| Cantina: with Chicken | 1060 | 46 | 108 |
| with Beef | 1185 | 55 | 109 |
| **Quesadillas:** *Without Guacamole* | | | |
| Cheese, small | 950 | 66 | 50 |
| Mesquite Grilled, Steak, small | 860 | 53 | 54 |
| **Dips:** *Without Chips or Tortillas* | | | |
| Bowls: Queso Blanco | 1080 | 88 | 14 |
| Prairie Fire Bean | 715 | 43 | 53 |
| **Entrees:** *Per Meal, without Sides* | | | |
| **Burritos:** Chicken | 1025 | 53 | 79 |
| Fajita Steak | 1025 | 50 | 79 |
| **Carnitas:** Pork | 815 | 31 | 88 |
| Cold Set, Side | 185 | 11 | 24 |
| **Chimichangas:** Chicken | 785 | 37 | 64 |
| Spicy Beef De Oro | 1360 | 79 | 89 |
| **Don's Combos:** *Without Sides* | | | |
| Cinco Combo | 1175 | 66 | 64 |
| El Matador | 960 | 54 | 59 |
| Mexicano | 715 | 43 | 31 |
| Numero uno Favorito | 870 | 45 | 65 |
| Presidente | 1010 | 54 | 70 |
| **Enchiladas:** Cadillac Chicken | 875 | 43 | 60 |
| Cadillac Steak | 1015 | 53 | 65 |
| **Sizzlin' Fajitas:** *With Proteins, Onions & Peppers* | | | |
| Combo - Steak & Chicken | 580 | 28 | 34 |
| Mesquite-Grilled: Chicken | 485 | 20 | 32 |
| Steak | 680 | 36 | 36 |
| **Fajita Fixin's:** 7" Flour Tortilla (3) | 375 | 11 | 60 |
| Corn Tortillas (4) | 60 | 1 | 12 |
| Guacamole, #30 scoop | 70 | 6 | 4 |
| Pico de Gallo, #30 scoop | 5 | 0 | 2 |
| Sour Cream, #30 scoop | 80 | 8 | 2 |
| **Fresh Salads:** *Without Dressing* | | | |
| **Caesar:** with Chicken | 815 | 27 | 96 |
| with Steak | 945 | 38 | 99 |
| **Southwest:** *Without Extra Dressing* | | | |
| with Buffalo Sauce | 950 | 57 | 73 |
| with Chipotle-Honey BBQ Sauce | 1215 | 67 | 118 |
| **Sides:** | | | |
| Mexican Rice, 3 oz | 120 | 2 | 23 |
| Refritos, 5 oz | 215 | 7 | 27 |
| Seasoned French Fries, 7 oz | 345 | 16 | 46 |
| Seasoned Vegetables, 6 oz | 110 | 5 | 16 |

## Dunkin' Donuts® (Aug '16)

*Bagels: Per Bagel* **C** **F** **Cb**

| | C | F | Cb |
|---|---|---|---|
| Plain; Onion, average | 310 | 1 | 64 |
| Cinnamon Raisin | 320 | 1 | 66 |
| Everything | 340 | 3 | 67 |
| Sesame Seed | 350 | 4.5 | 65 |
| Sour Cream & Onion | 330 | 1.5 | 66 |
| Whole Wheat | 320 | 2 | 61 |
| **Danish:** Apple Cheese | 400 | 19 | 53 |
| Cheese | 420 | 21 | 52 |
| Strawberry Cheese | 400 | 19 | 52 |
| **Donuts:** Apple 'n Spice | 260 | 14 | 29 |
| Bavarian Kreme | 270 | 15 | 31 |
| Boston Kreme | 300 | 16 | 37 |
| Bowtie Donut | 270 | 12 | 38 |
| Chocolate Frosted Cake | 350 | 19 | 40 |
| Double Chocolate | 350 | 20 | 39 |
| French Cruller | 260 | 18 | 21 |
| Jelly | 270 | 14 | 32 |
| Old Fashioned Cake | 320 | 22 | 33 |
| Powdered | 320 | 19 | 33 |
| Strawberry Frosted | 280 | 15 | 32 |
| Sugar Raised | 230 | 14 | 22 |
| Vanilla Creme | 330 | 20 | 35 |
| **Muffins:** | | | |
| Blueberry: Regular | 460 | 15 | 76 |
| Reduced Fat | 410 | 10 | 75 |
| Chocolate Chip | 550 | 21 | 83 |
| Coffee Cake | 590 | 24 | 87 |
| Corn; Honey Bran Raisin, av. | 450 | 15 | 73 |
| **Munchkins:** Cinnamon | 60 | 3.5 | 6 |
| Glazed | 70 | 4 | 7 |
| Jelly | 70 | 4 | 8 |
| Sugared Raised | 60 | 4 | 5 |
| Toasted Coconut | 90 | 5 | 10 |
| **Bakery Sandwiches:** | | | |
| Bacon Ancho Chicken | 640 | 25 | 70 |
| Chicken Salad Croissant | 580 | 39 | 42 |
| Deluxe Grilled Cheese with Bacon | 560 | 34 | 41 |
| Ham & Cheese Flatbread | 330 | 12 | 35 |
| Texas Toast Grilled Cheese | 500 | 29 | 41 |
| Tuna Salad on Plain Bagel | 580 | 25 | 68 |
| Turkey Cheddar Bacon Flatbread | 380 | 17 | 32 |

*Continued Next Page... ...*

## Dunkin' Donuts® cont... (Aug '16)

| Breakfast: | C | F | Cb |
|---|---|---|---|
| Hash Browns, 6 pieces | 140 | 8 | 17 |
| **Oatmeal:** | | | |
| Original, w/ Dried Fruit Topping | 270 | 4 | 54 |
| Brown Sugar Flavored Oatmeal, with Dried Fruit Topping | 300 | 4 | 61 |
| **Plain Bagels:** | | | |
| Bacon, Egg & Cheese | 470 | 12 | 67 |
| Egg & Cheese | 410 | 7 | 67 |
| Ham, Egg & Cheese | 440 | 8 | 67 |
| Sausage, Egg & Cheese | 620 | 26 | 67 |
| **Big N' Toasted** | 570 | 31 | 44 |
| **Biscuits:** Bacon, Egg & Cheese | 470 | 27 | 38 |
| Sausage, Egg & Cheese | 630 | 43 | 38 |
| **Croissants:** Bacon, Egg & Cheese | 490 | 29 | 40 |
| Egg & Cheese | 440 | 25 | 40 |
| Ham, Egg & Cheese | 470 | 26 | 40 |
| Sausage, Egg & Cheese | 650 | 44 | 41 |
| **English Muffins:** | | | |
| Bacon, Egg & Cheese | 300 | 12 | 32 |
| Ham, Egg & Cheese | 270 | 8 | 33 |
| Sausage, Egg & Cheese | 450 | 26 | 33 |
| **Multigrain Flatbreads:** | | | |
| Egg White | 320 | 13 | 33 |
| Turkey Sausage | 420 | 22 | 32 |
| **Wake-Up Wraps:** | | | |
| Bacon, Egg & Cheese | 180 | 9 | 14 |
| Egg & Cheese | 150 | 8 | 13 |
| Ham, Egg & Cheese | 170 | 8 | 14 |
| Turkey Sausage | 250 | 15 | 13 |
| *Hot Beverages: Per Medium Size* | | | |
| **Chocolate:** Original | 330 | 10 | 58 |
| Mint | 300 | 10 | 53 |
| **Dunkaccino** | 350 | 15 | 52 |
| *Cold Beverages: Per Medium Size* | | | |
| **Coolatta:** Orange, 24 fl.oz | 330 | 0 | 81 |
| Strawberry Fruit, 24 fl.oz | 370 | 0 | 88 |
| Vanilla Bean, 24 fl.oz | 630 | 9 | 138 |
| *Iced Coffee: Per Medium Size, without Cream* | | | |
| Regular, without sugar | 15 | 0 | 2 |
| Caramel Mocha | 180 | 0 | 41 |
| French Vanilla Swirl | 170 | 0 | 40 |
| *Iced Lattes: Per Medium, with Whole Milk* | | | |
| Caramel Mocha, 16 fl.oz | 330 | 9 | 52 |
| French Vanilla Swirl, 16 fl.oz | 340 | 9 | 53 |

## Eat 'N Park® (Aug '16)

| Breakfast: | C | F | Cb |
|---|---|---|---|
| Bananas Foster French Toast, 2 slices | 495 | 15 | 82 |
| **Omelettes:** Ham & Cheese | 535 | 35 | 5 |
| Meat Lover's | 725 | 55 | 3 |
| **Pancakes:** | | | |
| Buttermilk: Plain (1) | 75 | 1 | 15 |
| Blueberry (1) | 85 | 1 | 16 |
| **Scramblers:** | | | |
| All-American w/ sausage | 705 | 39 | 55 |
| Skinny | 355 | 14 | 32 |
| **Waffles:** Belgian (1) | 280 | 12 | 35 |
| Strawberry (1) | 375 | 17 | 48 |
| *Appetizers:* | | | |
| Fried Cheese Sticks | 535 | 36 | 26 |
| Fried Ravioli | 455 | 31 | 30 |
| Grilled Chicken Quesadilla | 905 | 56 | 52 |
| Onion Ring Basket | 365 | 24 | 34 |
| *Burgers:* | | | |
| **Black Angus:** | | | |
| American Grill | 615 | 37 | 30 |
| Mushroom & Onion | 575 | 31 | 31 |
| Superburger | 1085 | 73 | 28 |
| **Classic:** Black Angus | 455 | 22 | 28 |
| Black Angus Bacon Cheeseburger | 570 | 31 | 28 |
| Black Angus Cheeseburger | 505 | 26 | 28 |
| Garden Burger | 290 | 5 | 43 |
| **Original,** Superburger | 565 | 38 | 27 |
| *Sandwiches: With Menu Board Standard Add-Ins* | | | |
| BLT | 490 | 15 | 65 |
| Buffalo Chicken Wrap | 835 | 48 | 61 |
| Chargrilled Chicken | 345 | 7 | 31 |
| Gourmet Grilled Cheese | 795 | 58 | 27 |
| Hot Turkey | 500 | 8 | 71 |
| Santa Fe Turkey | 740 | 50 | 31 |
| Shredded Pot Roast | 530 | 31 | 28 |
| Turkey Club | 835 | 49 | 51 |
| Whale of a Cod Fish | 880 | 42 | 76 |
| *Dinners: Without Sides* | | | |
| **Baked Chicken Parmigiana:** | | | |
| with Marinara Sauce | 960 | 38 | 99 |
| with Meat Sauce | 985 | 41 | 95 |
| Baked Lemon Sole, 2 fillets | 390 | 19 | 11 |
| Chicken Fillets, 5 pieces | 530 | 26 | 28 |
| Cod Floridian, 2 fillets | 240 | 3 | 8 |
| Mile-High Meatloaf | 900 | 57 | 59 |
| Smothered Ground Sirloin Steak | 445 | 27 | 8 |
| Spaghetti Marinara | 695 | 8 | 129 |
| Spaghetti with Meat Sauce | 835 | 16 | 146 |
| Whitefish w/ Mac & Cheese 2 fillets | 750 | 34 | 58 |

*Continued Next Page....*

## Eat 'N Park® cont... (Aug '16)

**Salads:** *Without Dressing*

| | C | F | Cb |
|---|---|---|---|
| Buffalo Chicken | 610 | 33 | 42 |
| Garden | 95 | 3 | 16 |
| Grilled Chicken | 445 | 20 | 30 |
| Steak | 740 | 46 | 33 |

**Dressings:** *Per 2 oz*

| | | | |
|---|---|---|---|
| Bleu Cheese | 245 | 25 | 3 |
| Citrus Lime Vinaigrette | 70 | 6 | 13 |
| French, Fat Free | 75 | 0 | 18 |
| House Ranch | 215 | 21 | 4 |
| Poppy & Sesame Seed | 390 | 32 | 26 |

**Desserts:**

| | | | |
|---|---|---|---|
| Ice Cream, 2 scoops | 230 | 12 | 27 |

**Pies:** Apple Pie, 1 slice

| | | | |
|---|---|---|---|
| Apple Pie, 1 slice | 525 | 27 | 67 |
| Blackberry Pie, 1 slice | 565 | 28 | 75 |
| Coconut Cream Pie, 1 slice | 490 | 27 | 55 |
| Dutch Apple Pie, 1 slice | 375 | 14 | 61 |
| **Sundaes:** Caramel Fudge | 400 | 19 | 56 |
| Oreo | 505 | 21 | 74 |

## Edo Japan® (Aug '16)

**Bento Box:** *Without Teriyaki Sauce*

| | C | F | Cb |
|---|---|---|---|
| Beef Yakisoba, 20.3 oz | 840 | 29 | 102 |
| Chicken Yakisoba, 20.5 oz | 790 | 24 | 102 |
| Sizzling Shrimp, 22 oz | 790 | 15 | 122 |
| Sukiyaki Beef, 20.3 oz | 880 | 27 | 120 |

**Teriyaki Dishes:** *Without Teriyaki Sauce*

| | | | |
|---|---|---|---|
| Chicken, 15 oz | 570 | 11 | 80 |
| Chicken & Shrimp | 640 | 14 | 82 |
| Sukiyaki Beef, 14.8 oz | 580 | 15 | 80 |

**Soup:** *Per 33 oz Bowl*

| | | | |
|---|---|---|---|
| Beef Udon | 580 | 17 | 72 |
| Chicken Udon | 550 | 13 | 72 |

**Maki Sushi:** *Per 6 Pieces*

| | | | |
|---|---|---|---|
| California Roll, 7.6 oz | 430 | 17 | 61 |
| Spicy Tuna Roll, 6.5 oz | 300 | 2.5 | 54 |

**Nigiri Sushi:** *Per 1 Piece*

| | | | |
|---|---|---|---|
| Ebi (Steamed Prawn), 1.7 oz | 70 | 0.5 | 12 |
| Salmon Sashimi, 0.7 oz | 30 | 1.5 | 1 |

## Einstein Bros® (Aug '16)

**Bagels:**

| | C | F | Cb |
|---|---|---|---|
| **Bagels:** Asiago Cheese | 300 | 4 | 54 |
| Blueberry | 290 | 1 | 60 |
| Chocolate Chip | 290 | 3 | 58 |
| Cinnamon Sugar | 320 | 6 | 59 |
| Garlic | 270 | 2.5 | 56 |
| Honey Whole Wheat | 260 | 3 | 50 |
| Onion | 270 | 1 | 59 |
| Potato | 280 | 4 | 52 |
| Sesame | 290 | 3 | 54 |

**Gourmet Bagels:**

| | | | |
|---|---|---|---|
| Apple Cinnamon | 440 | 8 | 82 |
| Green Chile | 370 | 9 | 58 |
| Power Protein | 350 | 6 | 64 |
| Six-Cheese | 370 | 9 | 57 |
| Spinach Florentine | 380 | 11 | 58 |

**Bagel Dogs:**

| | | | |
|---|---|---|---|
| Original | 610 | 32 | 57 |
| Asiago | 620 | 33 | 58 |

**Egg Sandwiches:**

| | | | |
|---|---|---|---|
| Applewood Bacon & Spinach Panini | 790 | 49 | 60 |
| Cinnamon Toast | 270 | 30 | 73 |
| S'west Turkey Ssg | 400 | 13 | 45 |
| Spinach, M'shrm & Swiss, on Plain Bagel | 490 | 18 | 58 |
| **Flatbreads:** BBQ Chicken | 590 | 20 | 67 |
| Pepperoni | 590 | 31 | 51 |
| Roasted Veggie | 570 | 28 | 55 |

**Signature Sandwiches:**

| | | | |
|---|---|---|---|
| Albacore Tuna Salad | 570 | 24 | 62 |
| Harvest Chicken Salad | 570 | 21 | 69 |
| Honey Smoked Salmon | 560 | 16 | 65 |
| Hummus Veg Out | 440 | 12 | 72 |
| Tasty Turkey | 510 | 15 | 63 |

**Soup:**

| | | | |
|---|---|---|---|
| Broccoli Cheddar, 14 oz | 470 | 33 | 24 |
| Chicken Noodle, 14 oz | 170 | 5 | 22 |
| Turkey Chilli, 14 oz | 260 | 7 | 35 |
| **Tostinis:** BBQ Chicken | 560 | 13 | 74 |
| Buffalo Chicken & Bacon | 570 | 20 | 57 |
| Iltalian Chicken | 660 | 32 | 57 |
| Roasted Veggie | 560 | 24 | 63 |
| Turkey Club | 760 | 41 | 62 |
| **Wraps:** Buffalo Chicken | 600 | 28 | 60 |
| Santa Fe | 650 | 32 | 60 |

**Cream Cheese:** *Per 1.3 oz Schmear*

**Reduced Fat:**

| | | | |
|---|---|---|---|
| Garlic Herb/Garden Veggie | 130 | 10 | 6 |
| Honey Almond; Strawberry, av. | 150 | 10 | 13 |
| Plain | 150 | 14 | 2 |
| Onion and Chive | 140 | 12 | 5 |
| **Sweets:** Blueberry Muffin, 5.5 oz | 510 | 24 | 69 |
| Cinnamon Twist, 3.4 oz | 360 | 18 | 23 |
| Snickerdoodle Cookie, 2.9 oz | 350 | 14 | 31 |

# Fast - Foods & *Restaurants*

## El Pollo Loco® (Aug '16)

| | C | F | Cb |
|---|---|---|---|
| **Soup Starters:** *Per Small Serving* | | | |
| Chicken Tortilla w/ Tortilla Strips | 210 | 9 | 19 |
| without Tortilla Strips | 140 | 5 | 10 |
| **Bowl:** Original Pollo, 18.1 oz | 610 | 10 | 87 |
| Ultimate Double Chicken, 25.3 oz | 970 | 34 | 94 |
| **Burritos, Chicken/Shrimp:** | | | |
| Avocado, average | 950 | 53 | 74 |
| Poblano Avocado, average | 910 | 40 | 93 |
| Ranchero, average | 885 | 40 | 85 |
| Spicy Chipotle, average | 855 | 36 | 85 |
| **Flame-Grilled Chicken:** *Skin On* | | | |
| Breast; Thigh, av. | 220 | 12 | 0 |
| Leg; Wing, av. | 90 | 4.5 | 0 |
| **Quesadillas:** | | | |
| Avocado Chicken | 960 | 61 | 59 |
| Avocado Shrimp | 1020 | 63 | 67 |
| **Salads:** *Without Dressing* | | | |
| **Classic:** Chicken | 240 | 8 | 19 |
| Shrimp | 290 | 14 | 22 |
| **Mexican Cobb:** Chicken | 520 | 25 | 38 |
| Shrimp | 560 | 32 | 40 |
| **Tacos,** Avocado Chkn/Shrimp, av. | 315 | 18 | 20 |
| **Tostada:** *Without Dressing* | | | |
| Chicken | 860 | 42 | 77 |
| Shrimp | 910 | 49 | 80 |
| Ultimate Double: Chicken | 1030 | 50 | 82 |
| Shrimp | 1070 | 61 | 85 |
| **Under 500 Calories:** *Without Dressing* | | | |
| Chicken Avocado Tortilla Wrap | 480 | 20 | 46 |
| Chicken Enchiladas, 13.5 oz | 460 | 10 | 65 |
| Double Chicken Avocado Salad | 380 | 15 | 15 |
| **Dressings:** Creamy Cllantro: 3 oz | 440 | 46 | 3 |
| Light Creamy Cilantro, 1.5 oz | 70 | 5 | 5 |
| Ranch, 1.5 oz | 230 | 24 | 2 |
| **Sides:** Black Beans, 6 oz | 140 | 1 | 24 |
| Cole Slaw, 4 oz | 130 | 10 | 9 |
| Cut Corn with Red Peppers, 5 oz | 160 | 5 | 24 |
| Gravy, 1 oz | 10 | 0 | 2 |
| Macaroni & Cheese, 5.5 oz | 250 | 15 | 22 |
| Mashed Potatoes, 5 oz | 110 | 1.5 | 23 |
| Pinto Beans, 6 oz | 200 | 4 | 29 |
| **Condiments:** | | | |
| Pico de Gallo, 1.5 oz | 15 | 1 | 2 |
| **Salsa:** Avocado, 1.5 oz | 30 | 2.5 | 2 |
| House; Roja, av.,1.5 oz | 10 | 0 | 2 |
| Sour Cream, 1.3 oz | 80 | 7 | 1 |
| **Dessert,** Two Cinnamon Churros | 300 | 18 | 32 |

## Fatburger® (Aug '16)

| | C | F | Cb |
|---|---|---|---|
| **Burgers:** *Without Extras* | | | |
| Burgers: Small | 400 | 21 | 37 |
| Medium | 590 | 31 | 46 |
| Large | 850 | 41 | 69 |
| Turkeyburger | 480 | 21 | 50 |
| Veggieburger | 510 | 20 | 60 |
| **Hot Dogs:** *Without Extras* | | | |
| Chili Cheese | 480 | 27 | 35 |
| Regular Hot Dog | 320 | 15 | 32 |
| **Sandwiches:** *Without Extras* | | | |
| Chicken: Crispy | 560 | 27 | 53 |
| Grilled | 430 | 14 | 42 |
| Fish | 560 | 31 | 55 |
| **Fries:** Fat Fries | 380 | 18 | 47 |
| with Chili | 480 | 24 | 52 |
| with Chili & Cheese | 590 | 33 | 53 |
| Skinny Fries | 390 | 15 | 58 |
| with Chili Cheese | 600 | 30 | 64 |
| **Add-Ons:** American Cheese, 1 slice | 70 | 5 | 1 |
| Cheddar Cheese, 1 slice | 110 | 9 | 1 |
| Mayonnaise, 1 serving | 90 | 10 | 1 |
| Relish, 1 serving | 20 | 0 | 5 |
| **Sides:** Chili Cup | 200 | 11 | 10 |
| with Cheese & Onions | 320 | 20 | 12 |
| Onion Rings | 540 | 29 | 64 |
| **Shakes:** Chocolate | 910 | 45 | 115 |
| Cookies & Ice Cream | 1180 | 59 | 163 |
| Maui-Banana | 940 | 44 | 126 |
| Peanut Butter | 950 | 53 | 114 |
| Strawberry; Vanilla, average | 885 | 44 | 112 |

*For Complete Nutritional Data ~ see CalorieKing.com*

## Fazoli's® (Aug '16)

| | C | F | Cb |
|---|---|---|---|
| **Oven-Baked Pasta:** *Per Serving* | | | |
| Baked Ziti | 670 | 26 | 72 |
| Chicken Broccoli Penne | 830 | 37 | 75 |
| Chicken Parmigano | 870 | 35 | 91 |
| Penne Romano | 860 | 42 | 76 |
| Penne with Creamy Basil Chicken | 850 | 41 | 72 |
| Twice-Baked Lasagna | 710 | 31 | 72 |
| **Top It Options:** | | | |
| Bacon, 0.3 oz | 45 | 4 | 0 |
| Broccoli, 2.5 oz | 60 | 5 | 3 |
| Italian Meatballs, 3 oz | 250 | 18 | 6 |
| Italian Sausage, 2 oz | 200 | 16 | 3 |
| Roasted Chicken, 3 oz | 90 | 2.5 | 1 |

*Continued Next Page....*

## Fazoli's® cont... (Aug '16)

**Samplers:** *Per Serving*

| | C | F | Cb |
|---|---|---|---|
| Classic Sampler | 870 | 25 | 121 |
| Spicy Sampler | 1010 | 34 | 125 |
| Ultimate Sampler Platter | 1120 | 29 | 165 |

**Signature Pastas:**

| | C | F | Cb |
|---|---|---|---|
| Chicken Carbonara | 860 | 37 | 75 |
| Ultimate Fettuccine | 930 | 38 | 95 |
| Ultimate Spaghetti | 900 | 36 | 102 |

**Submarinos:**

| | C | F | Cb |
|---|---|---|---|
| Meatball da Vinci | 990 | 58 | 64 |
| Primo Italiano | 880 | 50 | 68 |
| Turkey Club Classico | 800 | 45 | 59 |

*For Complete Nutritional Data ~ see CalorieKing.com*

## Firehouse Subs® (Aug '16)

**Hot Subs:** *Per Medium White Sub, with Standard Toppings and Dressings*

| | C | F | Cb |
|---|---|---|---|
| Ham | 740 | 37 | 71 |
| Roast Beef | 710 | 36 | 54 |
| Turkey | 670 | 35 | 58 |
| Veggie | 720 | 45 | 60 |
| **Specialty:** Club on a Sub | 780 | 43 | 64 |
| Engineer | 685 | 35 | 61 |
| Hero | 770 | 37 | 64 |
| Hook & Ladder | 700 | 37 | 64 |
| Italian | 915 | 57 | 64 |
| Meatball | 815 | 50 | 60 |
| **Sides,** Chili, Bowl | 335 | 18 | 25 |

**Under 500 Calorie Salads:** *With Dressing*

| | C | F | Cb |
|---|---|---|---|
| **Chopped:** with Chicken Salad | 425 | 26 | 23 |
| with Grilled Chicken | 335 | 16 | 19 |
| with Honey Ham | 405 | 19 | 33 |
| with Turkey | 345 | 17 | 21 |
| Hook & Ladder | 375 | 18 | 27 |
| House, without meat | 240 | 16 | 17 |
| Italian, with Grilled Chicken | 485 | 32 | 18 |

## Five Guys® (Aug '16)

**Burgers:**

| | C | F | Cb |
|---|---|---|---|
| Bacon Burger | 780 | 50 | 39 |
| Bacon Cheeseburger | 920 | 62 | 40 |
| Cheeseburger | 840 | 55 | 40 |
| Hamburger | 700 | 43 | 39 |

**Little Burgers:**

| | C | F | Cb |
|---|---|---|---|
| **Little:** Bacon Burger | 560 | 33 | 39 |
| Bacon Cheeseburger | 630 | 39 | 40 |
| Cheeseburger | 550 | 32 | 40 |
| Hamburger | 480 | 26 | 39 |

## Five Guys® cont... (Aug '16)

**Dogs:**

| | C | F | Cb |
|---|---|---|---|
| Bacon Dog; Cheese Dog | 620 | 42 | 40 |
| Bacon Cheese Dog | 695 | 48 | 41 |
| Hot Dog | 545 | 35 | 40 |

**Fries:**

| | C | F | Cb |
|---|---|---|---|
| Cajun Style, 14.5 oz | 955 | 41 | 131 |
| Five Guys Style, 14.5 oz | 955 | 41 | 131 |

## Flame Broiler® (June '16)

**Bowls:** *With White Rice*

| | C | F | Cb |
|---|---|---|---|
| Beef | 620 | 11 | 74 |
| Chicken | 600 | 14 | 68 |
| Chicken & Veggie | 510 | 14 | 49 |
| Half & Half | 610 | 13 | 71 |
| The Works | 520 | 13 | 52 |

**Plates:** *With White Rice*

| | C | F | Cb |
|---|---|---|---|
| Beef | 840 | 18 | 94 |
| Rib | 1100 | 44 | 95 |
| The Works | 700 | 19 | 63 |

## Freshens® (Aug '16)

**Smoothies:** *100% Juice*

**Blended Fruit Classics:** *Per 20 fl.oz*

| | C | F | Cb |
|---|---|---|---|
| Bangin' Berry | 370 | 0 | 90 |
| Caribbean Craze; Maui Mango | 330 | 0 | 81 |
| Feelin' Peachy | 310 | 0 | 78 |
| Jmcn Jammer; Orge. Sunrise, av. | 320 | 2 | 70 |
| Peach On The Beach | 280 | 3 | 61 |
| Pom-Tastic; Purple Rein, av. | 320 | 0 | 80 |
| Tropical Therapy | 480 | 6 | 109 |
| Wild Strawberry | 340 | 0 | 87 |
| **Protein:** Peanut Butter | 500 | 12 | 76 |
| Power-Up | 560 | 14 | 73 |

**Crepes:**

| | C | F | Cb |
|---|---|---|---|
| Breakfast, Denver, with Bacon | 510 | 27 | 28 |

**Savory Golden Crepes:**

| | C | F | Cb |
|---|---|---|---|
| Chipotle Ranch Turkey | 430 | 24 | 27 |
| Pesto Chicken | 350 | 12 | 30 |

**Flatbreads:** BBQ Chicken, 10.4 oz

| | C | F | Cb |
|---|---|---|---|
| Flatbreads: BBQ Chicken, 10.4 oz | 550 | 13 | 75 |
| California Club, 11 oz | 600 | 35 | 32 |
| Roasted Vegie, 10 oz | 430 | 20 | 45 |

**Rice Bowls:** Buffalo Chicken

| | C | F | Cb |
|---|---|---|---|
| Rice Bowls: Buffalo Chicken | 510 | 14 | 71 |
| KC BBQ, 16.8 oz | 620 | 22 | 79 |
| Mediterranean, 16 oz | 650 | 37 | 71 |

**Dessert Crepes:**

| | C | F | Cb |
|---|---|---|---|
| Cheesecake Supreme | 450 | 23 | 51 |
| Nutella Supreme | 520 | 21 | 75 |

## Godfather's Pizza® (Aug '16)

*Golden Crust Pizza: Per Slice*

| | C | F | Cb |
|---|---|---|---|
| **Cheese:** Medium, ⅛ pizza | 220 | 8 | 25 |
| Large, ⅒ pizza | 250 | 9 | 28 |
| **Combo:** Medium, ⅛ | 290 | 13 | 27 |
| Large, ⅒ pizza | 330 | 15 | 30 |
| **Super Combo:** | | | |
| Medium, ⅛ pizza | 320 | 15 | 28 |
| Large, ⅒ pizza | 370 | 18 | 31 |

*Original Crust Pizza:*

| | C | F | Cb |
|---|---|---|---|
| **Cheese:** Mini, ¼ pizza | 150 | 4 | 20 |
| Medium, ⅛ pizza | 260 | 7 | 34 |
| Jumbo, 1/12 pizza | 350 | 10 | 44 |
| **Combo:** Mini, ¼ pizza | 200 | 8 | 21 |
| Medium, ⅛ pizza | 350 | 14 | 36 |
| Jumbo, 1/12 pizza | 480 | 20 | 47 |
| **Super Combo:** Mini, ¼ pizza | 220 | 9 | 22 |
| Medium, ⅛ pizza | 350 | 14 | 36 |
| Jumbo, 1/12 pizza | 520 | 23 | 48 |

*Thin Crust Pizza:*

| | C | F | Cb |
|---|---|---|---|
| **Cheese:** Medium, ⅛ pizza | 170 | 8 | 15 |
| Large, ⅒ pizza | 210 | 10 | 17 |
| **Combo:** Medium, ⅛ pizza | 240 | 13 | 17 |
| Large, ⅒ pizza | 280 | 16 | 20 |
| **Super Combo:** Medium, ⅛ pizza | 290 | 16 | 19 |
| Large, ⅒ pizza | 330 | 19 | 20 |

*Calzones: Per Medium Calzone*

| | C | F | Cb |
|---|---|---|---|
| Cheese | 1660 | 52 | 200 |
| Combo | 1450 | 40 | 200 |
| Pepperoni | 1410 | 39 | 195 |

*Sides:*

| | C | F | Cb |
|---|---|---|---|
| Breadstick (1) | 110 | 2 | 20 |
| Cheesestick, medium, ⅛ | 200 | 7 | 24 |
| **Garlic Toast:** 1 piece | 150 | 9 | 15 |
| with Cheese, 1 piece | 210 | 12 | 16 |
| Chicken Wings, Buffalo (4) | 180 | 13 | 6 |
| Potato Wedges, 4 oz | 175 | 8 | 24 |

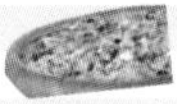

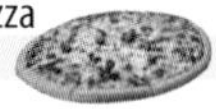

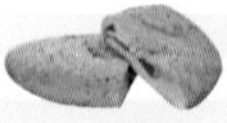

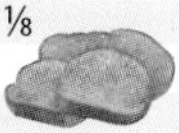

## Gold Star Chili® (Aug '16)

*Burritos & Burrito Bowls:*

| | C | F | Cb |
|---|---|---|---|
| Gold Star Chili Burrito | 970 | 33 | 126 |
| Grilled Chicken Bowl | 905 | 29 | 111 |

*Coneys:*

| | C | F | Cb |
|---|---|---|---|
| Cheese | 310 | 19 | 21 |
| Coney | 225 | 12 | 21 |
| Sriracha Coney | 315 | 19 | 22 |

*Ways,* Regular:

| | C | F | Cb |
|---|---|---|---|
| 2-Way | 395 | 10 | 54 |
| 3-Way | 680 | 34 | 55 |
| 4-Way, Bean | 825 | 34 | 81 |
| 5-Way | 840 | 33 | 87 |
| Super 5-Way | 1180 | 48 | 122 |

*Chili By The Bowl:*

| | C | F | Cb |
|---|---|---|---|
| Gold Star | 205 | 10 | 10 |
| Veggie | 200 | 3 | 34 |

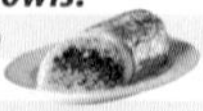

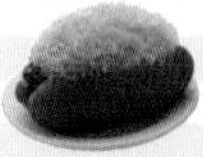

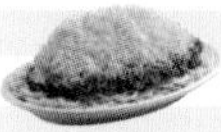

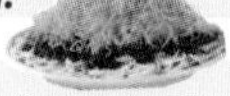

## Gold Star Chili® cont... (Aug '16)

*Double Deckers:*

| | C | F | Cb |
|---|---|---|---|
| Ham & Bacon | 515 | 29 | 40 |
| Ham & Turkey | 620 | 26 | 48 |
| Turkey & Bacon | 590 | 30 | 44 |
| **Sandwich,** Crispy Chicken | 355 | 20 | 24 |

*Salads: Without Dressing*

| | C | F | Cb |
|---|---|---|---|
| Cafe | 305 | 13 | 34 |
| Chili | 685 | 36 | 62 |
| Spring Harvest | 185 | 5 | 29 |
| **Fries:** French | 400 | 16 | 58 |
| Cheese | 575 | 30 | 59 |
| Chili Cheese | 680 | 36 | 63 |
| Sriracha | 425 | 16 | 64 |

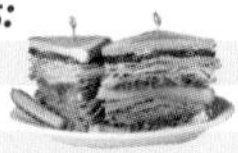

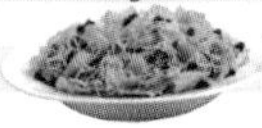

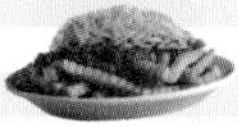

## Golden Corral® (Apr '16)

*Breakfast:*

| | C | F | Cb |
|---|---|---|---|
| Bacon & Cheese Quiche, 1 slice | 290 | 21 | 15 |
| Corned Beef Hash, Grilled, 1 cup | 440 | 28 | 26 |
| Creamed Chipped Beef, 1 cup | 320 | 18 | 20 |
| French Toast, Plain, 1 slice | 200 | 6 | 29 |
| Hash Brown Casserole, 1 cup | 260 | 10 | 28 |
| Sausage Links (1) | 120 | 11 | 1 |

*Meals: Without Sides*

**Hot Buffet:**

| | C | F | Cb |
|---|---|---|---|
| Awesome Pot Roast, 1 cup | 320 | 14 | 16 |
| Baked Fish w/ Shrimp & Sce, 3 oz | 160 | 10 | 2 |
| Baked Florentine Fish, 1 piece | 180 | 12 | 2 |
| BBQ: Chicken Leg Quarter, 1 pce | 490 | 22 | 21 |
| Pork, 3 oz | 170 | 8 | 5 |
| Bone-In Catfish, 3 oz | 210 | 14 | 7 |
| Bourbon Street Chicken, 3 oz | 170 | 9 | 4 |
| Lasagne, 1 piece | 430 | 26 | 21 |
| Pork Meatloaf, 1 sl. | 200 | 11 | 10 |
| Roast Beef, 3 oz | 110 | 3 | 0 |
| Salisbury Steak (1) | 130 | 4.5 | 9 |
| Sirloin Steak, 3 oz | 150 | 6 | 0 |

*Sides:* Baby Carrots; Baby Corn, av 45 | 1 | 8

| | C | F | Cb |
|---|---|---|---|
| Baby Carrots; Baby Corn, av | 45 | 1 | 8 |
| BBQ Baked Beans, ½ cup | 160 | 1 | 35 |
| Breaded Okra (10) | 110 | 7 | 10 |
| Creamed Corn, ½ cup | 110 | 0.5 | 25 |
| Flamed Broiled Mixed Veg., ½ cup | 15 | 0 | 3 |
| Fried Cubed Potatoes, ½ cup | 160 | 9 | 19 |

*Salad Buffet: Per ½ Cup Unless Indicated*

| | C | F | Cb |
|---|---|---|---|
| Caesar, without dressing, 1 cup | 110 | 8 | 8 |
| Cajun Potato | 230 | 17 | 15 |
| Chicken | 240 | 20 | 3 |
| Coleslaw | 110 | 9 | 6 |
| Seafood | 140 | 10 | 9 |
| Spinach Bacon, 1 cup | 120 | 9 | 4 |
| Tuna | 190 | 13 | 5 |

*Dressings:* Balsamic Vinaig., 2 T.

| | C | F | Cb |
|---|---|---|---|
| Balsamic Vinaig., 2 T. | 20 | 0 | 5 |
| Caesar, 2 Tbsp | 150 | 15 | 2 |
| Ranch, 2 Tbsp | 110 | 12 | 2 |

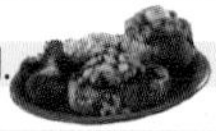

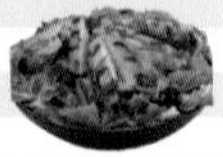

Updated Nutrition Data ~ www.CalorieKing.com
Persons with Diabetes ~ See Disclaimer (Page 22)

# (The) Great American Bagel Co® (Apr '16)

| | **C** | **F** | **Cb** |
|---|---|---|---|
| **Bagels:** | | | |
| Asiago Cheese | 520 | 16 | 72 |
| Cheddar Herb | 390 | 8 | 66 |
| Cinnamon Raisin | 380 | 3.5 | 76 |
| Jalapeno Cheddar | 370 | 7 | 63 |
| Plain | 360 | 4 | 71 |
| Spinach Tomazzo | 640 | 20 | 86 |
| Tomazzo | 520 | 13 | 77 |
| **Paninis:** *On Regular Baguette* | | | |
| Chicken Pesto | 770 | 35 | 70 |
| Ham & Swiss | 600 | 26 | 58 |
| Philly Beef | 920 | 40 | 92 |
| Turkey Club | 680 | 29 | 67 |
| **Sandwiches:** Asiago Omelet | 720 | 29 | 80 |
| BLT | 550 | 17 | 72 |
| Chicken Parmigiana | 740 | 22 | 81 |
| Ham | 460 | 9 | 71 |
| Roast Beef | 465 | 9 | 71 |
| Turkey | 435 | 5 | 72 |
| **Cream Cheese Filling:** *Per 1 oz* | | | |
| Plain | 100 | 10 | 1 |
| Strawberry; Vegetable, average | 90 | 8 | 4 |
| **Pastries:** | | | |
| **Cookies:** Chocolate Chunk, 4 oz | 110 | 3.5 | 19 |
| Oatmeal Raisin, 4 oz | 120 | 5 | 18 |
| **Muffins:** Blueberry, 4.25 oz | 430 | 16 | 64 |
| Banana Nut, 4.25 oz | 430 | 18 | 61 |

# Green Burrito® (Aug '16)

| | **C** | **F** | **Cb** |
|---|---|---|---|
| **Burritos:** | | | |
| Bean & Cheese | 440 | 15 | 56 |
| Beef, Bean & Cheese | 470 | 18 | 52 |
| **California:** Chicken | 470 | 21 | 45 |
| Steak | 480 | 21 | 44 |
| Chicken Especial | 550 | 22 | 59 |
| **Mexican:** Chicken | 520 | 20 | 57 |
| Steak | 540 | 19 | 56 |
| **Specialties:** | | | |
| **Super Nachos:** | | | |
| Chicken | 920 | 47 | 95 |
| Ground Beef | 970 | 51 | 95 |
| **Taco Salad:** Chicken | 800 | 43 | 70 |
| Ground Beef | 850 | 47 | 70 |
| Steak | 810 | 43 | 69 |
| **Tacos:** | | | |
| Ground Beef, hard taco | 210 | 12 | 16 |
| Southwest Chicken, soft taco | 310 | 21 | 19 |
| **Street Tacos:** Chicken | 150 | 7 | 15 |
| Steak | 160 | 7 | 14 |
| **Sides:** Beans, 6.25 oz | 250 | 6 | 35 |
| Chips, 2 oz | 300 | 17 | 35 |
| Guacamole, 1.4 oz | 60 | 5 | 3 |

# Great Steak® (Aug '16)

| | **C** | **F** | **Cb** |
|---|---|---|---|
| **Breakfast Sandwiches:** | | | |
| Bacon, Egg & Cheese | 600 | 36 | 39 |
| Sausage, Egg & Cheese | 700 | 47 | 39 |
| Steak, Egg & Chse | 590 | 31 | 41 |
| **Burgers:** | | | |
| Bacon Cheeseburger | 680 | 45 | 33 |
| BBQ Cheeseburger | 570 | 28 | 50 |
| Cheeseburger | 600 | 39 | 33 |
| Chili Burger | 550 | 27 | 47 |
| Hamburger | 550 | 34 | 32 |
| Philly Cheeseburger | 570 | 32 | 37 |
| **Sandwiches:** 7" | | | |
| Bacon Cheddar Cheesesteak | 620 | 23 | 60 |
| Buffalo Chicken Philly | 800 | 42 | 66 |
| Chicagoland Cheesesteak | 640 | 25 | 61 |
| Chicken Bacon Ranch | 700 | 45 | 36 |
| Great Steak Cheesesteak | 720 | 34 | 60 |
| Gyro | 600 | 32 | 53 |
| Orig. Philly Cheesesteak | 540 | 17 | 60 |
| Pastrami Philly | 830 | 46 | 62 |
| Reuben Philly | 770 | 39 | 61 |
| Super Steak Cheesesteak | 720 | 34 | 62 |
| Turkey Philly | 570 | 19 | 63 |
| Ultimate Chicken Philly | 620 | 23 | 65 |
| Veggie Delight | 530 | 21 | 67 |
| Wisconsin Inside-Out | 550 | 26 | 55 |
| **Baked Potatoes:** | | | |
| Bacon & Cheese | 430 | 23 | 29 |
| Broccoli & Cheese | 220 | 6 | 38 |
| **The Great Potato:** Chicken | 430 | 19 | 42 |
| Ham | 420 | 19 | 45 |
| Steak | 440 | 20 | 39 |
| Turkey | 390 | 16 | 41 |
| The King | 480 | 29 | 30 |
| **Fries:** | | | |
| **Great Fry:** Kids | 270 | 13 | 36 |
| Regular | 440 | 20 | 60 |
| Large | 540 | 25 | 72 |
| Coney Island Fry, Regular | 590 | 29 | 72 |
| King Fry, regular | 570 | 31 | 64 |
| Nacho Fry, regular | 490 | 23 | 64 |
| **Salads:** *Without Dressing* | | | |
| **Great Salad:** Chicken | 380 | 22 | 16 |
| Ham | 370 | 22 | 20 |
| Steak | 370 | 23 | 13 |
| Turkey | 340 | 19 | 15 |
| **Salad Dressings:** Ranch, 1 oz | 170 | 18 | 1 |
| Thousand Island, 1 oz | 130 | 12 | 4 |

## Haagen-Dazs® (Aug '16)

| *Classic Flavors:* Per ½ Cup | C | F | Cb |
|---|---|---|---|
| Butter Pecan | 300 | 22 | 20 |
| Caramel Cone | 320 | 20 | 30 |
| Chocolate Chocolate Chip | 300 | 19 | 26 |
| Chocolate Chip Cookie Dough | 300 | 18 | 30 |
| Chocolate Peanut Butter | 340 | 23 | 26 |
| Coffee; Green Tea | 250 | 17 | 20 |
| Dulce de Leche | 270 | 16 | 27 |
| Mint Chip | 250 | 16 | 23 |
| Pineapple Coconut | 210 | 12 | 23 |
| Rocky Road | 290 | 17 | 29 |
| Rum Raisin | 240 | 16 | 21 |
| Strawberry | 240 | 15 | 22 |
| Vanilla Swiss Almond | 290 | 19 | 24 |
| Vanilla Bean | 270 | 17 | 24 |
| White Chocolate Raspberry Truffle | 280 | 16 | 31 |
| *Frozen Yogurt:* Per ½ Cup | | | |
| Coffee | 180 | 2.5 | 31 |
| Vanilla | 170 | 2.5 | 29 |
| Vanilla Raspberry Swirl | 150 | 1 | 31 |
| *Gelato:* Per ½ Cup | | | |
| Black Cherry Amaretto | 240 | 9 | 35 |
| Dark Chocolae Chip | 270 | 12 | 36 |
| Sea Salt Caramel | 270 | 11 | 38 |
| Tiramisu | 260 | 11 | 35 |
| *Sorbet:* Per ½ Cup | | | |
| Mango | 150 | 0 | 38 |
| Orchard Peach | 130 | 0 | 33 |
| Raspberry; Zesty Lemon, av. | 115 | 0 | 29 |

*Ice Cream Bars/Cones ~ See Page 109*

## Hardee's® (Aug '16)

| *Burgers:* | C | F | Cb |
|---|---|---|---|
| Cheeseburgers: Small | 330 | 15 | 32 |
| Double, 7 oz | 420 | 22 | 33 |
| Hamburger, Small | 280 | 12 | 32 |
| **Thickburgers:** | | | |
| Original, ⅓ lb | 820 | 53 | 56 |
| Bacon Cheese: ⅓ lb | 900 | 59 | 54 |
| ½ lb | 1110 | 76 | 55 |
| ⅔ lb Double | 1140 | 79 | 58 |
| Frisco: ⅓ lb | 860 | 59 | 46 |
| ½ lb | 1060 | 75 | 47 |

## Hardee's® cont... (Aug '16)

| *Burgers (Cont):* | C | F | Cb |
|---|---|---|---|
| **Thickburgers (Cont):** | | | |
| Little Thick Cheeseburger, 6 oz | 450 | 25 | 33 |
| Little Thickburger, ¼ lb | 600 | 42 | 33 |
| Low-Carb, ⅓ lb | 440 | 35 | 9 |
| Mushroom 'N' Swiss: | | | |
| ⅓ lb | 690 | 40 | 52 |
| ½ lb | 890 | 56 | 53 |
| *Sandwiches:* | | | |
| Big Chicken Fillet | 750 | 42 | 63 |
| Big Hot Ham 'N' Cheese | 530 | 22 | 50 |
| Big Roast Beef | 500 | 23 | 48 |
| **Chicken:** Charbroiled BBQ Chicken | 340 | 4 | 42 |
| Charbroiled Chicken Club | 590 | 31 | 35 |
| Spicy Chicken | 450 | 24 | 44 |
| Regular Roast Beef | 300 | 14 | 28 |
| *Breaded Chicken Tenders:* Without Sauce | | | |
| 3 pieces, 4.5 oz | 260 | 13 | 13 |
| 5 pieces, 7.5 oz | 440 | 21 | 21 |
| *Fried Chicken Pieces:* | | | |
| Breast, 5.2 oz | 370 | 15 | 29 |
| Leg, 2.4 oz | 170 | 7 | 15 |
| Thigh, 4.3 oz | 330 | 15 | 30 |
| Wing, 2.3 oz | 200 | 8 | 23 |
| *Sides:* | | | |
| **Crispy Curls:** Small | 360 | 18 | 46 |
| Medium | 470 | 23 | 60 |
| Large | 570 | 28 | 72 |
| Side Salad, without Dressing | 120 | 7 | 7 |
| *Fries & Onion Rings:* | | | |
| Beer Battered Onion Rings, 4.5 oz | 410 | 24 | 45 |
| **Natural Cut Fries:** Small, 4 oz | 360 | 18 | 47 |
| Medium, 5.85 oz | 490 | 24 | 63 |
| Large, 6.8 oz | 530 | 26 | 69 |
| *Kids Meals:* Includes Kid's Fries | | | |
| Cheeseburger | 550 | 26 | 61 |
| Chicken Tenders | 400 | 19 | 37 |
| Hamburger | 500 | 22 | 61 |

*Continued Next Page...*

**Updated Nutrition Data ~ www.CalorieKing.com**
**Persons with Diabetes ~ See Disclaimer (Page 22)**

## Hardee's® cont... (Aug '16)

### Breakfast:

| | C | F | Cb |
|---|---|---|---|
| **Biscuits:** Bacon, Egg & Cheese | 480 | 27 | 39 |
| Bacon, Swiss with Egg | 740 | 45 | 50 |
| Biscuit 'N' Gravy | 460 | 26 | 49 |
| Chicken Fillet | 550 | 32 | 47 |
| Cinnamon 'N Raisin | 340 | 15 | 49 |
| Country Steak | 510 | 31 | 44 |
| Loaded Omelet | 490 | 28 | 40 |
| Made From Scratch | 300 | 15 | 36 |
| Monster | 750 | 50 | 40 |
| Sausage | 490 | 33 | 37 |
| Sausage and Egg | 560 | 37 | 39 |
| **Bowl,** Low Carb | 660 | 52 | 10 |
| **Burrito,** Loaded | 580 | 30 | 46 |
| **Frisco Sandwich** | 450 | 19 | 45 |
| **Platter,** with Bacon | 830 | 50 | 68 |
| **Sunrise Croissant,** with Ham | 400 | 23 | 29 |

### Breakfast Sides:

| | C | F | Cb |
|---|---|---|---|
| Grits | 100 | 3 | 16 |
| **Hash Rounds:** Small, 2.9 oz | 260 | 15 | 23 |
| Medium, 4.2 oz | 370 | 22 | 33 |
| Large, 5.8 oz | 510 | 30 | 45 |

### Desserts:

| | C | F | Cb |
|---|---|---|---|
| Apple Turnover w/o Cinn. Sugar | 270 | 13 | 35 |
| Chocolate Chip Cookie (2), 2 oz | 240 | 10 | 36 |
| Single Scoop Ice Cream: | | | |
| Vanilla: Bowl, 4 oz | 240 | 13 | 27 |
| Sugar Cone, 4.4 oz | 290 | 13 | 37 |

### Drinks:

| | C | F | Cb |
|---|---|---|---|
| **Hot Chocolate** | 150 | 3 | 18 |
| **Ice Cream Malts:** | | | |
| Chocolate, 14 oz | 780 | 35 | 99 |
| Strawberry, 14 oz | 770 | 35 | 97 |
| Vanilla, 14 oz | 780 | 35 | 98 |
| **Ice Cream Shakes:** | | | |
| Choc.; Strawb., av., 14 oz | 705 | 34 | 86 |
| Vanilla, 14 oz | 700 | 33 | 86 |

## Hissho Sushi® (Aug '16)

### Starters: With White Rice

| | C | F | Cb |
|---|---|---|---|
| Baby Octopus Salad, 4 oz | 170 | 3 | 20 |
| Chicken Gyoza, 4 oz | 180 | 6 | 20 |
| Pork Gyoza, 4 oz | 230 | 11 | 23 |
| Spring Rolls: Regular | 185 | 4 | 30 |
| Ocean | 180 | 2 | 29 |
| Squid Salad, 4 oz | 95 | 2 | 7 |

### Maki Sushi: With White Rice

| | C | F | Cb |
|---|---|---|---|
| **Rolls:** Blazing California, 7 oz | 405 | 12 | 65 |
| California, 7 oz | 295 | 3 | 59 |
| Dynamaite Roll, 7 oz | 470 | 13 | 66 |
| Eel, 7 oz | 375 | 1 | 69 |
| Hissho Healthy, 6 oz | 210 | 1 | 46 |
| Nippon Favorite, 6 oz | 300 | 4 | 45 |
| Philadelphia, 7 oz | 385 | 12 | 60 |
| Snow Crab, 7 oz | 280 | 3 | 56 |
| Spicy, 7 oz | 430 | 11 | 62 |
| Sushicado, 7 oz | 290 | 3 | 54 |
| Veggie Roll, 7 oz | 275 | 2 | 57 |

### Specialty Rolls: Per 7 oz Roll Unless Indicated

| | C | F | Cb |
|---|---|---|---|
| Caterpillar | 480 | 5 | 84 |
| Living Color | 370 | 5 | 51 |
| Mango Tango | 420 | 10 | 58 |
| Salmon Lover | 720 | 32 | 63 |
| Sriracha Party | 540 | 14 | 77 |
| Tempura Shrimp, 9 oz | 664 | 19 | 108 |
| TNT | 545 | 14 | 71 |
| Wasabi Crunch | 550 | 19 | 76 |

## Hot Dog on a Stick® (Aug '16)

### Menu Items:

| | C | F | Cb |
|---|---|---|---|
| American Cheese on a Stick | 260 | 16 | 21 |
| Beef Hot Dog on a Bun | 340 | 23 | 22 |
| Turkey Hot Dog on a Stick | 240 | 13 | 23 |
| Veggie Dog on a Stick | 220 | 8 | 24 |
| Pepperjack Cheese on a Stick | 240 | 14 | 19 |
| **Sides,** French Fries, 4.5 oz | 410 | 22 | 49 |
| **Dessert,** Funnel Cake Sticks, with Powdered Sugar, (10) | 210 | 8 | 31 |
| **Beverages:** Per Regular Size, 16 fl.oz | | | |
| Lemonade: Original | 150 | 0 | 38 |
| Cherry | 210 | 0 | 52 |
| Lime | 230 | 0 | 57 |

## Hungry Howie's Pizza® (Aug '16)

*Counts may vary in Florida.*

| | **C** | **F** | **Cb** |
|---|---|---|---|
| ***Specialty Pizza:** Per Slice* | | | |
| BBQ Chicken: Small, ⅙ pizza | 210 | 7 | 24 |
| Medium, ⅛ pizza | 240 | 8 | 30 |
| Large, ¹⁄₁₀ pizza | 260 | 9 | 31 |
| X-Large, ¹⁄₁₂ pizza | 300 | 10 | 37 |
| ***Calzones:** Per Regular 8" Calzone* | | | |
| Deluxe Italian | 660 | 23 | 81 |
| Ham & Cheese | 590 | 15 | 68 |
| Steak, Cheese & Mushroom | 610 | 18 | 81 |
| Turkey Club | 660 | 18 | 80 |
| Veggie | 610 | 19 | 83 |
| ***Wings:** Bone In, average, 5 pcs* | 440 | 29 | 10 |
| Boneless, Buffalo, 3 pieces | 280 | 11 | 21 |
| ***Salads:** Per Regular* | | | |
| Antipasto | 170 | 10 | 10 |
| Chef | 140 | 8 | 9 |
| Garden | 70 | 2 | 12 |
| Greek | 140 | 7 | 15 |
| ***Dressings:** Per 1 oz* | | | |
| Creamy Italian | 120 | 12 | 2 |
| Greek | 110 | 11 | 2 |
| Ranch | 140 | 14 | 1 |
| Thousand Island | 140 | 14 | 4 |

## In-N-Out Burger® (Aug '16)

| | **C** | **F** | **Cb** |
|---|---|---|---|
| ***Burgers:*** | | | |
| **Hamburger:** with Onion | 390 | 19 | 39 |
| with Mustard/Ketchup, w/o Spread | 310 | 10 | 41 |
| Protein Style w/ Lettuce Wrap, w/o Bun | 240 | 17 | 11 |
| **Cheeseburger:** with Onion | 480 | 27 | 39 |
| with Mustard/Ketchup, w/o Spread | 400 | 18 | 41 |
| Protein Style w/ Lettuce Wrap, w/o Bun | 330 | 25 | 11 |
| **Double Double:** with Onion | 670 | 41 | 39 |
| with Mustard/Ketchup, w/o Spread | 590 | 32 | 41 |
| Protein Style w/ Lettuce Wrap, w/o Bun | 520 | 39 | 11 |
| ***French Fries,** 4.5 oz* | 395 | 18 | 54 |
| ***Drinks:** Milk, 10 fl.oz* | 180 | 6 | 18 |
| Coca-Cola, 16 fl.oz | 195 | 0 | 54 |
| Dr Pepper; 7-Up, av., 16 fl.oz | 200 | 0 | 53 |
| Lemonade, 16 fl.oz | 180 | 0 | 40 |
| Root Beer, 16 fl.oz | 220 | 0 | 60 |
| ***Shakes:*** | | | |
| Chocolate, 15 fl.oz | 590 | 29 | 72 |
| Strawberry, 15 fl.oz | 590 | 27 | 81 |
| Vanilla, 15 fl.oz | 580 | 31 | 67 |

## IHOP® (Aug '16)

| | **C** | **F** | **Cb** |
|---|---|---|---|
| ***Pancakes:*** | | | |
| Chocolate Chocolate Chip: | | | |
| Buttermilk version (4) | 610 | 21 | 93 |
| Chocolate version (4) | 630 | 22 | 97 |
| Double Blueberry (4) | 600 | 15 | 101 |
| NY Cheesecake (4) | 940 | 35 | 135 |
| Orig. Buttermilk (3) | 430 | 17 | 57 |
| Strawberry Banana (4) | 670 | 15 | 121 |
| ***Condiments:*** | | | |
| Syrup: Blueb.; Butter Pecan,1 fl.oz | 110 | 0 | 27 |
| Boysenberry; Strawberry, 1 fl.oz | 100 | 0 | 26 |
| Sugar-Free Syrup, 1 fl.oz | 15 | 0 | 6 |
| ***French Toast & Waffles:** With Toppings* | | | |
| French Toast: Original | 730 | 29 | 94 |
| Bananas Foster Brioche | 940 | 41 | 123 |
| Cinnamon Swirl Brioche | 860 | 29 | 131 |
| Strawberry Banana | 860 | 24 | 140 |
| Waffle, Belgian | 520 | 27 | 60 |
| ***Crepes:*** | | | |
| Banana with Nutella | 960 | 44 | 121 |
| Chicken Florentine | 790 | 42 | 48 |
| German Crepes | 680 | 34 | 76 |
| Strawberries & Cream | 800 | 30 | 116 |
| Swedish | 660 | 30 | 81 |
| ***Made To Order Omelettes:** Without Pancakes or Sides* | | | |
| Big Steak | 1160 | 79 | 47 |
| Garden | 840 | 66 | 17 |
| Hearty Ham & Cheese | 940 | 68 | 17 |
| Spinach & Mushroom | 890 | 70 | 20 |
| ***Made to Build Combos:*** | | | |
| Biscuits & Gravy Combo, 2 Fried Eggs with Country Gravy | 1320 | 83 | 106 |
| Breakfast Sampler, w/out Eggs | 920 | 56 | 69 |
| Chicken Fried Chicken: | | | |
| 2 Fried Eggs, with Country Gravy | 1060 | 60 | 85 |
| 2 Fried Eggs, with Saus. Gravy | 1110 | 64 | 88 |
| T-Bone Steak & 3 Fried Eggs | 960 | 54 | 59 |
| ***Sandwiches:** Without Sides* | | | |
| Chicken Clubhouse Super Stacker | 1240 | 85 | 62 |
| Double BLT | 660 | 42 | 43 |
| Ham & Egg Melt | 1230 | 70 | 78 |
| Patty Melt | 1080 | 71 | 64 |
| Sandwich Sides: French Fries | 320 | 13 | 45 |
| Hash Browns | 280 | 18 | 28 |
| Onion Rings | 500 | 28 | 57 |
| ***Entrees:** With Menu Set Sides, without Garlic Bread, Soup or Salad* | | | |
| Chicken Fried Chicken, w/ Country Gravy | 620 | 29 | 68 |
| Pot Roast | 840 | 44 | 65 |
| T-Bone Steak, 12 oz | 880 | 54 | 41 |

*For Complete Menu & Data ~ see CalorieKing.com*

Updated Nutrition Data ~ www.CalorieKing.com
Persons with Diabetes ~ See Disclaimer (Page 22)

## Jack in the Box® (Aug '16)

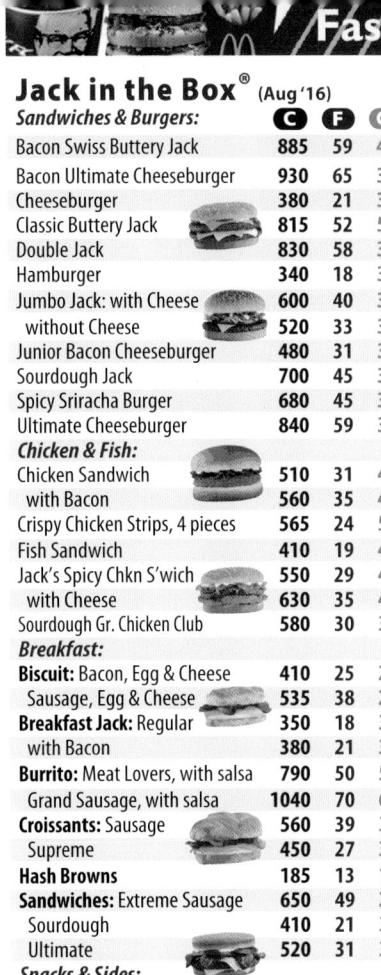

| Sandwiches & Burgers: | C | F | Cb |
|---|---|---|---|
| Bacon Swiss Buttery Jack | 885 | 59 | 48 |
| Bacon Ultimate Cheeseburger | 930 | 65 | 32 |
| Cheeseburger | 380 | 21 | 32 |
| Classic Buttery Jack | 815 | 52 | 50 |
| Double Jack | 830 | 58 | 34 |
| Hamburger | 340 | 18 | 32 |
| Jumbo Jack: with Cheese | 600 | 40 | 33 |
| without Cheese | 520 | 33 | 32 |
| Junior Bacon Cheeseburger | 480 | 31 | 32 |
| Sourdough Jack | 700 | 45 | 39 |
| Spicy Sriracha Burger | 680 | 45 | 38 |
| Ultimate Cheeseburger | 840 | 59 | 31 |
| **Chicken & Fish:** | | | |
| Chicken Sandwich | 510 | 31 | 42 |
| with Bacon | 560 | 35 | 42 |
| Crispy Chicken Strips, 4 pieces | 565 | 24 | 53 |
| Fish Sandwich | 410 | 19 | 45 |
| Jack's Spicy Chkn S'wich | 550 | 29 | 48 |
| with Cheese | 630 | 35 | 49 |
| Sourdough Gr. Chicken Club | 580 | 30 | 38 |
| **Breakfast:** | | | |
| Biscuit: Bacon, Egg & Cheese | 410 | 25 | 26 |
| Sausage, Egg & Cheese | 535 | 38 | 27 |
| Breakfast Jack: Regular | 350 | 18 | 30 |
| with Bacon | 380 | 21 | 30 |
| Burrito: Meat Lovers, with salsa | 790 | 50 | 50 |
| Grand Sausage, with salsa | 1040 | 70 | 68 |
| Croissants: Sausage | 560 | 39 | 32 |
| Supreme | 450 | 27 | 32 |
| Hash Browns | 185 | 13 | 17 |
| Sandwiches: Extreme Sausage | 650 | 49 | 29 |
| Sourdough | 410 | 21 | 35 |
| Ultimate | 520 | 31 | 30 |
| **Snacks & Sides:** | | | |
| Bacon Cheddar Potato Wedges | 680 | 41 | 58 |
| Chiquita Apple Bites, without dip | 30 | 0 | 8 |
| Egg Rolls (3), without sauce | 440 | 22 | 46 |
| French Fries: Small | 300 | 14 | 40 |
| Medium | 430 | 20 | 58 |
| Large | 550 | 25 | 75 |
| Onion Rings (8), 4.3 oz | 450 | 28 | 45 |
| Seasoned Curly Fries: Small | 280 | 16 | 30 |
| Medium | 430 | 25 | 46 |
| Large | 480 | 28 | 52 |
| Stuffed Jalapenos: 3 Pieces | 220 | 12 | 21 |
| 7 Pieces | 510 | 29 | 49 |

## Jack in the Box® cont... (Aug '16)

| Better For You: | C | F | Cb |
|---|---|---|---|
| Chicken Fajita Pita, without Salsa | 340 | 12 | 35 |
| Chicken Teriyaki Bowl | 690 | 6 | 134 |
| Grilled Chicken Salad, w/o drssng | 250 | 9 | 13 |
| **Salads:** *Without Dressing or Toppings* | | | |
| Chicken Club with Grilled Chicken | 370 | 20 | 11 |
| Side Salad | 20 | 0 | 4 |
| Southwest Chicken, with Grilled Chicken Strips | 350 | 15 | 27 |
| Croutons | 70 | 3 | 9 |
| Dressings: Creamy Southwest | 190 | 19 | 3 |
| Ranch | 250 | 25 | 5 |
| Low Fat Balsamic Vinaigrette | 25 | 1.5 | 3 |
| **Sauces:** | | | |
| Dipping Sauce: Barbecue, 1 oz | 40 | 0 | 10 |
| Buttermilk, 1 oz | 110 | 11 | 2 |
| Frank's Red Hot Buffalo, 1 oz | 10 | 0 | 1 |
| Sweet & Sour, 1 oz | 40 | 0 | 10 |
| Teriyaki | 50 | 1 | 11 |
| **Sandwich Sauce:** | | | |
| Creamy Bacon Mayo, 0.7 fl.oz | 120 | 13 | 1 |
| Mayo-Onion, 0.5 fl.oz | 90 | 10 | 0 |
| Peppercorn Mayo, 1.5 fl.oz | 280 | 31 | 1 |
| Tartar Sauce, 0.5 fl.oz | 50 | 4.5 | 2 |
| **Desserts:** | | | |
| Chocolate Overload Cake | 300 | 7 | 57 |
| Churros, Mini (5) | 345 | 18 | 42 |
| New York Style Cheesecake | 310 | 17 | 32 |
| **Shakes:** *16 fl.oz, with Whipped Topping* | | | |
| Chocolate | 780 | 38 | 103 |
| Oreo Cookie | 800 | 43 | 95 |
| Strawberry | 760 | 38 | 97 |
| Vanilla | 685 | 38 | 78 |

*For Complete Nutritional Data ~ see CalorieKing.com*

## Jack's® (Aug '16)

| Burgers & Sandwiches: | C | F | Cb |
|---|---|---|---|
| Big Bacon | 610 | 41 | 31 |
| Big Jack Burger | 530 | 33 | 35 |
| Cheeseburger | 380 | 21 | 31 |
| Chicken Fillet Sandwich | 490 | 24 | 40 |
| Double Big Jack Cheese Burger | 850 | 59 | 35 |
| Double Cheeseburger | 540 | 33 | 31 |
| Grilled Chicken Sandwich | 380 | 16 | 32 |
| Hamburger | 340 | 18 | 31 |
| **Chicken:** Breast | 480 | 29 | 20 |
| Fingers & Fries, 4 piece | 720 | 32 | 47 |
| **Fries,** regular | 310 | 13 | 42 |
| **Breakfast:** Egg & Cheese Biscuit | 360 | 21 | 31 |
| Sausage, Egg & Cheese Biscuit | 520 | 35 | 32 |
| Steak Biscuit | 480 | 28 | 43 |

*For Complete Menu & Data ~ see CalorieKing.com*

## Jamba Juice® (Aug '16)

*Freshly Squeezed Juice:* 16 fl.oz

| | C | F | Cb |
|---|---|---|---|
| Orange Berry Oxidant | 200 | 1 | 48 |
| Purely Carrot | 130 | 0.5 | 30 |
| Purely Orange | 220 | 1 | 52 |
| Tropical Kick-Start | 210 | 1 | 50 |

*Smoothies:* Per Small

| | | | |
|---|---|---|---|
| **Classic:** Banana Berry | 280 | 1 | 67 |
| Mango-A-Go-Go | 300 | 1.5 | 69 |
| Peach Pleasure | 280 | 1 | 65 |
| Razzamatazz | 290 | 1 | 67 |
| Strawberry Surf Rider | 320 | 1 | 78 |
| Strawberry Wild | 260 | 0 | 62 |
| **Make It Light:** | | | |
| Aloha Pineapple | 190 | 0 | 40 |
| Caribbean Passion | 150 | 0 | 34 |
| Razzmatazz | 180 | 0 | 41 |

*Tasty Bites:*

**Artisan Flat Bread:** *Per Flatbread*

| | | | |
|---|---|---|---|
| Four Cheese | 420 | 16 | 46 |
| Sweet 'n Spicy | 390 | 10 | 53 |
| **Baked Goods:** *Per Item* | | | |
| Apple Cinnamon Pretzel | 380 | 4 | 76 |
| Cheddar Tomato Twist | 240 | 4.5 | 41 |
| Sourdough Parmesan Pretzel | 410 | 10 | 67 |
| Sweet Belgian Waffle | 320 | 15 | 42 |
| **Breakfast Wraps:** | | | |
| Spinach 'n Cheese | 240 | 8 | 30 |
| Turkey Sausage 'n Cheese | 320 | 16 | 29 |

**Steel-Cut Oatmeal:** *With Soymilk*

| | | | |
|---|---|---|---|
| Plain | 180 | 2.5 | 35 |
| Add: Apple Cinnamon | 70 | 0 | 16 |
| Banana | 50 | 0 | 13 |
| Blueberries | 10 | 0 | 2 |
| Brown Sugar Crumble | 40 | 1 | 8 |
| Clover Honey | 30 | 0 | 9 |
| Strawberries | 5 | 0 | 1 |

**Toasted Bistro Sandwiches:**

| | | | |
|---|---|---|---|
| Ham, Jarlsberg & Dijon | 290 | 8 | 33 |
| Roast Chicken, Cheddar & Honey Dijon | 290 | 7 | 34 |
| Three Cheeses | 330 | 14 | 32 |

*Energy Bowls:* Per 16 fl.oz

| | | | |
|---|---|---|---|
| Acai Primo | 490 | 10 | 99 |
| Chunky Strawberry | 590 | 17 | 96 |
| Fruit & Greek Yogurt | 390 | 4 | 62 |

## Jersey Mike's Subs® (Aug '16)

*Cold Subs:* Per Regular, on White, without Vinegar, Oil or Mayo Unless Indicated

| | C | F | Cb |
|---|---|---|---|
| #1 BLT, with Mayo | 785 | 48 | 66 |
| #2 Jersey Shore Favorite | 550 | 15 | 69 |
| #3 American Classic | 495 | 13 | 67 |
| #5 Super Sub | 570 | 15 | 70 |
| #6 Roast Beef & Provolone | 710 | 24 | 66 |
| #7 Turkey Breast & Provolone | 530 | 12 | 66 |
| #8 Club Sub with Mayonnaise | 895 | 49 | 70 |
| #9 Club Supreme w/ Mayonnaise | 940 | 49 | 69 |
| #10 Albacore Tuna | 790 | 43 | 70 |
| #13 Original Italian | 680 | 24 | 72 |
| #14 Veggie | 705 | 27 | 70 |

*Hot Subs:* Per Regular on White Roll

| | | | |
|---|---|---|---|
| #15 Meatball & Cheese | 830 | 42 | 75 |
| #17: Chicken Philly | 720 | 23 | 71 |
| Steak Philly | 650 | 22 | 71 |
| #18 Grilled Chicken Parmesan | 680 | 22 | 75 |
| #19 BBQ Beef | 750 | 18 | 87 |
| #20 Reuben | 675 | 25 | 74 |
| #43: Chipotle Chicken, with Mayo | 1000 | 53 | 74 |
| Chipotle Steak, with Mayo | 930 | 52 | 74 |
| #56: Big Kahuna Steak | 710 | 26 | 73 |
| Big Kahuna Chicken | 770 | 27 | 72 |

*Signature Wraps:*

| | | | |
|---|---|---|---|
| Baja Chicken | 610 | 23 | 63 |
| Grilled Ham & Cheese | 740 | 41 | 63 |
| Grilled Veggie | 945 | 59 | 69 |
| Turkey with Honey Mustard Sauce | 540 | 20 | 63 |

*Salads:* Without Dressing

| | | | |
|---|---|---|---|
| Chef, 16 oz | 255 | 10 | 16 |
| Grilled Chicken Caesar, 12.5 oz | 510 | 35 | 11 |
| Tossed, 12 oz | 50 | 0.5 | 11 |
| Tuna, 18 oz | 690 | 60 | 15 |

*Dressings:* Per 2 Tbsp, 1 oz

| | | | |
|---|---|---|---|
| Caesar | 150 | 15 | 2 |
| Chipotle Mayo | 180 | 20 | 0 |
| Golden Italian | 110 | 11 | 3 |
| Ranch | 120 | 12 | 2 |
| Russian | 160 | 16 | 4 |
| **Desserts:** Cookie, Choc Chip, 1.5 oz | 190 | 9 | 26 |
| Chocolate Brownie, 4 oz | 470 | 21 | 79 |
| **Drinks:** Mountain Dew, 22 oz | 310 | 0 | 84 |
| Mug Root Beer, 22 oz | 290 | 0 | 79 |
| Tropicana Twister Orange, 22 oz | 360 | 0 | 96 |

Updated Nutrition Data ~ www.CalorieKing.com
Persons with Diabetes ~ See Disclaimer (Page 22)

## Jimmy John's® (Aug '16)

**Subs:** (8")
*Figures Based on French Bread w/ Standard Toppings & Mayo, Unless Indicated*

| | C | F | Cb |
|---|---|---|---|
| #1 Pepe | 630 | 31 | 58 |
| #2 Big John | 540 | 23 | 55 |
| #3 Totally Tuna, without mayo | 720 | 35 | 61 |
| #4 Turkey Tom | 510 | 21 | 56 |
| #5 Vito with Italian Vinaigrette | 645 | 32 | 60 |
| #6 Vegetarian | 690 | 39 | 60 |
| JJBLT | 600 | 32 | 55 |

**Giant Club Sandwiches:** *Figures Based on 8-Grain Bread w/ Standard Toppings & Mayo, Unless Indicated*

| | | | |
|---|---|---|---|
| #7 Gourmet Smoked Ham | 760 | 35 | 70 |
| #8 Billy Club | 790 | 37 | 68 |
| #9 Italian Night w/ Mayo & Vinaig. | 935 | 54 | 72 |
| #10 Hunter's Club | 800 | 38 | 66 |
| #11 Country Club | 750 | 34 | 69 |
| #12 Beach Club | 810 | 43 | 71 |
| #13 Gourmet Veggie Club | 970 | 60 | 72 |
| #14 Bootlegger | 660 | 27 | 66 |
| #15 Club Tuna w/o dressing | 1000 | 56 | 73 |
| #16 Club Lulu | 720 | 35 | 66 |
| #17 Ultimate Porker | 730 | 36 | 67 |

**Plain Slims:** *Figures Based on French Bread without Toppings, Dressing or Mayo*

| | | | |
|---|---|---|---|
| Slim 1 Ham & Cheese | 570 | 13 | 76 |
| Slim 2 Roast Beef | 480 | 5.5 | 73 |
| Slim 3 Tuna Salad | 815 | 36 | 78 |
| Slim 4 Turkey Breast | 450 | 3 | 74 |
| Slim 5 Salami Capicola & Cheese | 655 | 23 | 75 |
| Slim 6 Double Provolone | 610 | 21 | 75 |

**Sides:**

| | | | |
|---|---|---|---|
| **Jimmy Chips:** Average | 150 | 9 | 16 |
| Thinny, 1 oz | 130 | 5 | 19 |
| **Cookies:** Chocolate Chunk, 3 oz | 400 | 19 | 55 |
| Raisin Oatmeal, 3 oz | 365 | 13 | 57 |
| **Jumbo Kosher Dill Pickle,** 6.9 oz | 20 | 0 | 4 |

## Johnny Rockets® (June'16)

**Starters & Shareables:**

| | | | |
|---|---|---|---|
| Chili Bowl | 610 | 48 | 17 |
| **Fries:** American | 480 | 19 | 69 |
| Bacon Cheese | 830 | 44 | 82 |
| Cheese | 740 | 37 | 82 |
| Chili Cheese | 1000 | 56 | 93 |
| Sweet Potato | 590 | 31 | 75 |
| Onion Rings | 880 | 40 | 90 |
| Rocket Wings, traditional | 660 | 49 | 19 |

## Johnny Rockets® ...cont (Aug '16)

**Original Hamburgers:**

| | C | F | Cb |
|---|---|---|---|
| Hamburger #12 | 950 | 60 | 57 |
| Original Burger | 900 | 59 | 54 |
| **Rocket:** Single | 930 | 59 | 52 |
| Double | 1400 | 96 | 52 |
| Route 66 | 980 | 67 | 49 |
| **Smoke House:** Single | 1080 | 65 | 67 |
| Double | 1640 | 109 | 67 |
| Streamliner | 400 | 10 | 56 |
| **Chicken Tenders,** (6), w/o sauce | 880 | 56 | 42 |

**Chicken Philly Cheese Steak,**

| | | | |
|---|---|---|---|
| with American Cheese | 660 | 24 | 58 |
| **Hot Dogs:** Regular, w/out sauce | 410 | 22 | 34 |
| Chili Cheese Dog | 770 | 51 | 42 |

**Philly Cheese Steaks:**

| | | | |
|---|---|---|---|
| with Cheddar, 11.7 oz | 780 | 40 | 55 |
| with Swiss, 12 oz | 830 | 42 | 57 |

**Sandwiches:**

| | | | |
|---|---|---|---|
| BLT, on White Bread | 480 | 26 | 49 |
| Chicken Club, on White Bread | 920 | 36 | 77 |
| Grilled Chicken, on Hambger Bun | 590 | 26 | 52 |
| Tuna Salad, on White Bread | 750 | 48 | 47 |

**Salads:** *Without Dressing*

| | | | |
|---|---|---|---|
| Breaded Chicken Club | 660 | 45 | 23 |
| Egg Salad | 390 | 35 | 2 |
| Grilled Chkn Club | 510 | 28 | 12 |
| Garden Salad | 280 | 19 | 9 |
| Tuna Salad | 370 | 29 | 0 |

**Breakfast:** *With Menu Set Components*

| | | | |
|---|---|---|---|
| 2 French Toast with Bacon | 600 | 29 | 56 |
| 2 Pancakes with Bacon | 380 | 19 | 36 |
| Patty & 2 Eggs, Beef & Potatoes | 1150 | 86 | 46 |
| Sandwiches: Egg, Bacon, White | 810 | 60 | 46 |
| Egg, Bacon Rye | 850 | 61 | 50 |
| Egg, Ham, English Muffin | 820 | 54 | 55 |
| The Works | 1000 | 70 | 55 |

**Desserts:** Apple Pie | 620 | 34 | 74 |

| | | | |
|---|---|---|---|
| Super Sundae w/ Hot Fudge, Almonds & Wh. Cream, 11 oz | 660 | 41 | 65 |

**Beverages:**

| | | | |
|---|---|---|---|
| Coke, 20 oz | 240 | 0 | 67 |
| Fanta Orange, 20 oz | 270 | 0 | 74 |
| Minute Made Lemonade, 20 oz | 240 | 0 | 65 |

**Deluxe Shakes:**

| | | | |
|---|---|---|---|
| Black Forest, 18.5 oz | 910 | 50 | 103 |
| Butterfinger, 18.4 oz | 1030 | 61 | 110 |
| Chocolate Vanilla Twist, 18.3 oz | 910 | 50 | 102 |

*For Complete Menu & Data ~ see CalorieKing.com*

## KFC® (Aug '16)

| Chicken Pieces: Per Piece | C | F | Cb |
|---|---|---|---|
| **Original Recipe:** Breast, 5.3 oz | 320 | 16 | 9 |
| Drumstick, 2 oz | 160 | 10 | 5 |
| Thigh, 3.3 oz | 270 | 19 | 8 |
| Whole Wing, 1.4 oz | 120 | 7 | 4 |
| **Extra Crispy:** Breast, 5.6 oz | 390 | 23 | 10 |
| Drumstick, 1.9 oz | 130 | 7 | 4 |
| Tenders, 1 order | 140 | 7 | 8 |
| Thigh, 3.5 oz | 290 | 20 | 11 |
| Whole Wing, 1.7 oz | 170 | 11 | 6 |
| **Kentucky Grilled:** | | | |
| Breast, 4 oz | 180 | 6 | 0 |
| Drumstick, 1.3 oz | 60 | 3 | 0 |
| Thigh, 2 oz | 130 | 9 | 0 |
| Whole Wing, 1 oz | 60 | 3.5 | 0 |
| **Spicy Crispy:** | | | |
| Breast, 5.2 oz | 350 | 20 | 11 |
| Drumstick, 1.6 oz | 130 | 8 | 5 |
| Thigh, 2.8 oz | 270 | 20 | 10 |
| Whole Wing, 1.2 oz | 120 | 8 | 5 |
| **Go Cups:** Chicken Littles | 590 | 32 | 59 |
| Exta Crispy Tenders | 540 | 27 | 50 |
| Fiery Buff. Hot Wings | 480 | 25 | 49 |
| HBBQ Hot Wings | 540 | 25 | 61 |
| Hot Wings | 480 | 25 | 43 |
| Popcorn Nuggets | 570 | 32 | 53 |
| **Popcorn Nuggets:** Kids | 290 | 19 | 19 |
| Large | 620 | 39 | 39 |
| ***Wings:*** *Without Dipping Sauce* | | | |
| Fiery Buffalo, Hot | 70 | 4 | 5 |
| Honey BBQ, Hot | 90 | 4 | 9 |
| Hot | 70 | 4 | 3 |
| ***Dipping Sauces:*** *Per 0.9 oz Container* | | | |
| Buttermilk Ranch | 100 | 10 | 2 |
| Colonel's Buttery Spread | 30 | 3.5 | 0 |
| Creamy Buffalo | 70 | 7 | 2 |
| Honey Mustard | 120 | 10 | 6 |
| Summertime BBQ | 40 | 0 | 9 |
| Sweet & Tangy | 45 | 0 | 12 |

***Big Box Meals:*** *Includes Cole Slaw, Biscuit, Individual Mashed Potatoes & Gravy & Medium 16 oz Pepsi*

| | C | F | Cb |
|---|---|---|---|
| **Original Chicken:** 1 Breast, 1 Thigh | 1260 | 60 | 127 |
| 1 Breast, 1 Thigh, 1 Drumstick | 1420 | 70 | 132 |
| **Extra Crispy Tenders,** 3 pieces | 1080 | 47 | 124 |
| **Grilled Chicken,** 1 Breast, 1 D'stick | 910 | 34 | 110 |

## KFC® cont... (Aug '16)

| KFC Famous Bowls & Pot Pie: | C | F | Cb |
|---|---|---|---|
| **Famous Bowl:** Snack Size, 7 oz | 280 | 13 | 29 |
| Large | 730 | 34 | 83 |
| **Chicken Pot Pie,** 14 oz | 790 | 46 | 66 |
| ***Sandwiches:*** *With Sauce* | | | |
| Chicken Littles | 320 | 19 | 25 |
| Colonal's Original | 500 | 23 | 47 |
| Crispy Twister | 650 | 35 | 54 |
| Doublicious | 570 | 29 | 47 |
| Honey BBQ | 370 | 3.5 | 60 |
| ***Salads:*** *Without Dressing or Croutons* | | | |
| Caesar, Side | 40 | 2 | 2 |
| Crispy Chicken BLT | 370 | 19 | 23 |
| Crispy Chicken Caesar | 350 | 19 | 21 |
| House Side Salad | 15 | 0 | 3 |
| ***Dressings & Add-Ins:*** | | | |
| Creamy Parmesan Caesar, 2 oz | 260 | 26 | 4 |
| Light Italian, 1 oz | 15 | 0.5 | 2 |
| Original Ranch Fat Free, 1.5 oz | 35 | 0 | 8 |
| Croutons, Parm. Garlic, 1 pouch | 60 | 3 | 8 |
| ***Homestyle Sides:*** *Per Single Portion* | | | |
| BBQ Baked Beans, 4.5 oz | 240 | 1.5 | 43 |
| Biscuit, 2 oz | 180 | 9 | 22 |
| Coleslaw, 4.2 oz | 170 | 12 | 14 |
| Corn on the Cob, 2.5 oz | 70 | 0.5 | 16 |
| Cornbread Muffin, 2 oz | 210 | 9 | 28 |
| Macaroni & Cheese, 4.8 oz | 170 | 6 | 22 |
| Mashed Potatoes, with Gravy, 5 oz | 120 | 4 | 19 |
| Potato Wedges, 3.8 oz | 270 | 13 | 34 |
| Sweet Kernel Corn | 100 | 0.5 | 21 |
| ***Homestyle Sides:*** *Per Family Portion* | | | |
| Baked Beans | 790 | 5 | 142 |
| Coleslaw | 630 | 45 | 53 |
| Green Beans | 90 | 0.5 | 17 |
| Macaroni & Cheese | 560 | 22 | 74 |
| Mashed Potatoes & Gray | 560 | 19 | 88 |
| Potato Wedges | 1120 | 54 | 143 |
| ***Desserts:*** | | | |
| Apple Turnover, 2.9 oz | 230 | 10 | 32 |
| Cafe Valley Choc. Chip cake, 1 slice | 300 | 15 | 39 |
| Oreo Cookies & Creme Pie | 290 | 16 | 34 |
| Reese's Peanut Butter Pie, 2.6 oz | 310 | 19 | 31 |

## Kilwins® ~ *see CalorieKing.com*

## Kolache® ~ *see CalorieKing.com*

Updated Nutrition Data ~ www.CalorieKing.com
Persons with Diabetes ~ See Disclaimer (Page 22)

## Krispy Kreme® (Aug '16)

| Doughnuts: | C | F | Cb |
|---|---|---|---|
| **Original Glazed:** | | | |
| Regular | 190 | 11 | 21 |
| Mini size, 1 | 90 | 5.5 | 10 |
| Apple Fritter | 390 | 20 | 50 |
| **Chocolate Iced:** Cake | 280 | 16 | 32 |
| Custard Filled | 350 | 22 | 35 |
| Glazed | 240 | 12 | 32 |
| with Sprinkles | 250 | 12 | 34 |
| Kreme Filling | 340 | 17 | 42 |
| Cinnamon Apple Filled | 330 | 19 | 36 |
| Cinnamon Bun | 220 | 12 | 27 |
| Cinnamon Sugar | 180 | 11 | 19 |
| **Cruller:** Glazed | 250 | 17 | 23 |
| Chocolate Iced Glazed | 300 | 18 | 34 |
| Double Chocolate Éclair | 340 | 15 | 47 |
| Double Dark Chocolate | 400 | 20 | 49 |
| Dulche De Leche | 310 | 17 | 37 |
| Fun Faces, all varieties | 380 | 23 | 41 |
| **Glazed:** with Kreme Filling | | | |
| Lemon Filled | 340 | 21 | 35 |
| Maple Iced | 230 | 11 | 31 |
| Powdered Cake | 260 | 16 | 26 |
| Powdered with Lemon Kreme | 340 | 19 | 37 |
| Strawberry Iced | 240 | 12 | 32 |
| Strawb. Shortcake Éclair | 330 | 15 | 47 |
| Sugar Doughnut | 180 | 11 | 19 |
| White Iced w/ Chocolate Drizzle | 250 | 11 | 36 |
| **Doughnut Holes:** Glazed Cake (4) | 190 | 10 | 24 |
| Chocolate Cake (4) | 180 | 10 | 21 |
| Original Glazed (5) | 200 | 9 | 27 |
| *Kool Kreme:* | | | |
| Cone, Chocolate | 310 | 9 | 52 |
| Doughnut Sundae, Orig. Glazed | 450 | 17 | 69 |
| *Frozen Coffees:* | | | |
| Mocha, 16 oz | 360 | 11 | 58 |
| Vanilla Latte, 16 oz | 420 | 10 | 74 |
| *Frozen Lemonade,* 16 oz | 330 | 0 | 84 |
| *Hot:* Chocolate, w/ 2% Milk, 12 oz | 390 | 14 | 57 |
| Mocha Latte, w/ 2% Milk, 12 oz | 320 | 9 | 51 |
| *Iced Coffees:* Per 12 fl.oz with 2% Milk | | | |
| Caramel Latte, with Wh. Cream | 310 | 7 | 50 |
| Hazelnut/Vanilla Latte, av. | 200 | 3.5 | 34 |
| Mocha, with Whipped Cream | 290 | 8 | 48 |
| *Skinny Iced Lattes:* With Skim Milk | | | |
| Caramel, 12 fl.oz | 160 | 5 | 26 |
| Vanilla, 12 fl.oz | 90 | 3.5 | 12 |

*For Complete Menu & Data ~ See CalorieKing.com*

## Krystal® (Aug '16)

| Burgers: | C | F | Cb |
|---|---|---|---|
| **Big Angus:** Original | 550 | 35 | 46 |
| Dble, w/ Bacon & Cheese | 850 | 59 | 48 |
| **Krystal:** | | | |
| Famous | 130 | 6 | 20 |
| Double | 290 | 13 | 33 |
| Bacon Cheese | 200 | 11 | 20 |
| Cheese | 160 | 8 | 20 |
| Chik | 300 | 16 | 27 |
| Double Cheese | 350 | 17 | 34 |
| **Pups:** Chili Cheese | 230 | 14 | 16 |
| Corn Pup | 240 | 14 | 22 |
| Plain Pup | 150 | 8 | 15 |
| *Fries:* | | | |
| **French Fries:** Small | 180 | 7 | 27 |
| Medium | 310 | 13 | 46 |
| Large | 380 | 15 | 57 |
| Chili Cheese Fries | 570 | 29 | 62 |
| Ranch Chili Cheese Fries | 760 | 49 | 64 |
| *Salad,* Crispy Chicken, 11 oz | 370 | 21 | 20 |
| *Breakfast Items:* | | | |
| **Biscuits:** Chik | 400 | 18 | 43 |
| Bacon, Egg & Cheese | 440 | 24 | 34 |
| Sausage, Egg & Cheese | 520 | 35 | 34 |
| Grits, with Margarine | 160 | 2 | 33 |
| **Sandwiches:** Krystal Sunriser | 200 | 11 | 16 |
| Bacon on Toast | 220 | 10 | 24 |
| Sausage on Toast | 300 | 20 | 24 |
| *Scramblers:* | | | |
| Original: with Bacon | 330 | 16 | 27 |
| with Sausage | 420 | 26 | 27 |
| Low-Carb Scrambler, | | | |
| with Sausage | 620 | 52 | 3 |
| *Dessert,* Apple Turnover | 220 | 8 | 34 |
| *Coca-Cola:* With ¼ Cup Ice | | | |
| Small, 16 oz | 120 | 0 | 30 |
| Medium, 21 oz | 160 | 0 | 40 |
| Large, 32 oz | 240 | 0 | 60 |
| *Milkquakes:* | | | |
| Chocolate | 880 | 50 | 92 |
| Strawberry | 900 | 48 | 105 |
| Vanilla | 850 | 49 | 87 |
| *Iced Tea,* | | | |
| Sweetened, 16 oz | 120 | 0 | 30 |

*For Complete Menu & Data ~ see CalorieKing.com*

# Fast - Foods & *Restaurants*

## LaRosa's Pizzeria® (Aug '16)

*Classic Pizzas:*

| | C | F | Cb |
|---|---|---|---|
| **Hand Tossed:** *Per ⅛ slice of 14" Large Pizza* | | | |
| Chicken Bacon Ranch | 505 | 26 | 44 |
| Double Pepperoni | 420 | 17 | 44 |
| Garlic Chicken | 535 | 31 | 45 |
| Hawaiian | 425 | 16 | 48 |
| Zesty BBQ Chicken | 430 | 15 | 51 |
| **Traditional:** *Per ½ slice of 14" Large Pizza* | | | |
| Chicken Bacon Ranch | 290 | 18 | 18 |
| Double Pepperoni | 230 | 12 | 18 |
| Hawaiian | 235 | 11 | 21 |
| Zesty BBQ Chicken | 240 | 11 | 23 |

*Deluxe Pizzas:*

| | | | |
|---|---|---|---|
| **Hand Tossed:** *Per Slice, ⅛ of 14" Large Pizza* | | | |
| Buddy Deluxe | 495 | 24 | 46 |
| Meat Deluxe | 560 | 28 | 45 |
| Original Deluxe | 490 | 33 | 56 |
| Veggie Deluxe | 360 | 11 | 48 |
| **Pan:** *Per ⅛ Slice, ⅛ of 14" Large Pizza* | | | |
| Buddy Deluxe | 515 | 25 | 48 |
| Meat Deluxe | 580 | 29 | 47 |
| Original Deluxe | 490 | 22 | 46 |
| Veggie Deluxe | 375 | 12 | 50 |

*Calzones:* *Standard Toppings, w/out Dipping Sauce*

| | | | |
|---|---|---|---|
| Baked Buddy | 1060 | 47 | 105 |
| Philly Chicken with 4 Cheese | 810 | 24 | 105 |
| Philly Steak with 4 Cheese | 860 | 31 | 103 |
| Three Meat with 4 Cheese | 1040 | 47 | 102 |

*Pasta Dinner:* *Without Bread, Soup or Salad*

| | | | |
|---|---|---|---|
| Lasagna, with Meat Sauce | 1100 | 66 | 72 |
| **Ravioli:** Cheese, with Spag. Sauce | 750 | 29 | 89 |
| Meat, with Spaghetti Sauce | 730 | 26 | 89 |
| Meat & Cheese, w/ Spag. Sauce | 740 | 27 | 89 |
| **Ziti:** Chicken Alfredo | 1180 | 57 | 121 |
| Sausage Pelucci w/ Spag. Sce | 1040 | 42 | 136 |

*Fresh Salad:* *Regular, w/out Dressing or Breadstick*

| | | | |
|---|---|---|---|
| Antipasto | 390 | 28 | 14 |
| Crispy Chicken | 500 | 27 | 37 |
| Grilled Chicken | 300 | 12 | 16 |
| JoJo's BLT | 160 | 9 | 11 |
| Tossed Salad | 160 | 9 | 12 |
| **Soup:** Baked Onion, w/ crackers | 230 | 10 | 27 |
| Minestrone, with crackers | 140 | 4 | 24 |
| **Salad Dressings:** Bleu Cheese | 280 | 30 | 2 |
| Honey French | 250 | 19 | 18 |
| Italian | 320 | 34 | 4 |

## LaRosa's Pizzeria® cont... (Aug '16)

*Appetizers:* *Without Sauce*

| | C | F | Cb |
|---|---|---|---|
| Garlic Fries | 620 | 32 | 74 |
| Four Taste Sampler | 1630 | 94 | 145 |
| Garlic Bread, 5 pieces | 580 | 12 | 100 |
| Rondo: Pepperoni | 1310 | 75 | 103 |
| Spinach/Cheese, average, 4.5 oz | 1195 | 64 | 103 |
| **Wings, Boneless:** BBQ (5) | 380 | 17 | 36 |
| Diablo (5) | 440 | 25 | 33 |
| Garlic-Romano (5) | 530 | 38 | 26 |

## La Salsa Fresh Mexican® (Aug '16)

*Appetizers:*

| | C | F | Cb |
|---|---|---|---|
| **Salsa & Chips:** Regular, 14.5 oz | 700 | 32 | 87 |
| w/ Guacamole, 14.5 oz | 970 | 55 | 103 |
| Chips (15), 1.4 oz | 200 | 10 | 25 |
| **Nachos:** | | | |
| Black Beans: with Carnitas | 1570 | 83 | 141 |
| with Chicken | 1600 | 83 | 148 |
| with Steak | 1580 | 84 | 142 |
| Pinto Beans: with Carnitas | 1560 | 83 | 139 |
| with Chicken | 1590 | 83 | 146 |
| with Steak | 1565 | 84 | 139 |
| **Burritos:** *Without Chips* | | | |
| **Black Beans & Cheese** | 1100 | 48 | 132 |
| with Carnitas | 1205 | 51 | 132 |
| with Chicken | 1240 | 52 | 139 |
| **Pinto Beans & Cheese** | 1070 | 48 | 115 |
| with Chicken | 1200 | 52 | 122 |
| with Steak | 1175 | 54 | 115 |
| Baja Fish Burrito | 875 | 53 | 58 |
| California Steak w/ Black Beans | 815 | 35 | 89 |
| **Overstuffed Grilled Burrito:** | | | |
| with Carnitas | 1200 | 59 | 108 |
| with Chicken | 1260 | 59 | 110 |
| with Steak | 1290 | 66 | 109 |
| **Grande, Black Beans:** | | | |
| with Carnitas or Chicken, average | 810 | 34 | 92 |
| with Steak | 820 | 35 | 91 |
| **Tacos:** *Without Chips* | | | |
| Baja Fish | 395 | 22 | 29 |
| Baja Shrimp | 320 | 19 | 30 |
| Guadalajara Carnitas | 320 | 15 | 30 |
| Mexico City, Chicken or Steak, av. | 190 | 4 | 27 |
| **Quesadillas:** *Without Chips* | | | |
| **Classic:** Carnitas | 960 | 58 | 57 |
| Chicken | 955 | 57 | 58 |
| Steak | 965 | 59 | 57 |
| **Grande,** Pinto Beans, with choice of meat, average | 1130 | 61 | 90 |
| **Grande,** Black Beans, with choice of meat, average | 1140 | 61 | 91 |

Updated Nutrition Data ~ www.CalorieKing.com
Persons with Diabetes ~ See Disclaimer (Page 22)

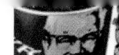

## La Salsa® cont... (Aug '16)

*Favorites: Without Chips* **C** **F** **Cb**

| | C | F | Cb |
|---|---|---|---|
| **Stuffed Fajita Quesadilla:** | | | |
| with Carnitas or Chicken, av. | 860 | 51 | 54 |
| with Shrimp | 800 | 49 | 54 |
| with Steak | 885 | 55 | 53 |
| **Fire Roasted Bowls:** | | | |
| Black Beans: w/ Chicken | 730 | 32 | 74 |
| with Steak | 735 | 34 | 73 |
| without Meat | 630 | 29 | 71 |
| Pinto Beans: w/ Chicken | 730 | 32 | 73 |
| with Steak | 720 | 34 | 70 |
| without Meat | 620 | 29 | 69 |

## Little Caesars® (Aug '16)

*14" Pizza: Per Slice, ⅛ Pizza* **C** **F** **Cb**

| | C | F | Cb |
|---|---|---|---|
| **Optional:** 3 Meat Treat | 330 | 16 | 31 |
| Hula Hawaiian: with Ham | 270 | 9 | 35 |
| with Canadian Bacon | 280 | 9 | 35 |
| Ultimate Supreme | 300 | 13 | 32 |
| Veggie | 270 | 10 | 32 |
| **Hot-N-Ready:** | | | |
| Deep Deep Dish: Cheese | 320 | 11 | 39 |
| Pepperoni | 350 | 14 | 39 |
| Round Pizza: | | | |
| Cheese | 250 | 8 | 31 |
| Pepperoni | 280 | 11 | 31 |
| **Caesar Wings:** *Per Wing* | | | |
| BBQ: Regular | 80 | 5 | 3 |
| Spicy | 70 | 5 | 1 |
| Buffalo, Mild or Hot | 70 | 5 | 0 |
| Garlic Parmesan | 90 | 7 | 1 |
| Lemon Pepper | 90 | 8 | 0 |
| Oven Roasted | 70 | 5 | 0 |
| **Caesar Dips:** *Per 1.5 oz Container* | | | |
| Buffalo Ranch | 230 | 24 | 3 |
| Buttery Garlic, 0.5 oz | 380 | 42 | 0 |
| Cheezy Jalapeno | 210 | 22 | 3 |
| Ranch | 250 | 26 | 3 |
| **Bread:** *Per Piece* | | | |
| Crazy Bread, 1 stick | 100 | 3 | 15 |
| Crazy Sauce, 4 oz | 45 | 0 | 10 |
| Italian Cheese Bread | 140 | 6 | 15 |
| Pepperoni Cheese Bread | 150 | 8 | 13 |

## Lone Star Steakhouse® (Oct '12)

*Appetizers: Per Serving*

| | C | F | Cb |
|---|---|---|---|
| Lone Star Wings, mild, 3.5 oz | 305 | 20 | 5 |
| Spin. & Artichoke Dip, 3.5 oz | 160 | 13 | 4.5 |
| Texas Rose, 3.5 oz | 285 | 19 | 25 |
| *Meals: Without Sides, Toppings & Sauce* | | | |
| Chopped Steak, 9.6 oz | 710 | 52 | 0 |
| NY Strip, 9.6 oz | 525 | 28 | 0 |
| Texas Ribeye, 12.5 oz | 710 | 40 | 5.5 |
| *Ribs Combo:* | | | |
| Baby Back Ribs, with Chicken | 740 | 30 | 46 |
| *Seafood:* | | | |
| Fried Shrimp Entree, 11.7 oz | 865 | 40 | 97 |
| Grilled Shrimp: 3.5 oz | 60 | 2 | 5.5 |
| 11 oz | 190 | 7 | 17 |
| Sweet Bourbon Salmon: 6oz | 240 | 11 | 0 |
| 9 oz | 360 | 16 | 0 |
| *Burgers:* | | | |
| Bubba, 15.7 oz | 1085 | 57 | 67 |
| Swiss & Mushroom, 15.2 oz | 845 | 38 | 53 |
| *Salads: Per Serving, Includes Dressing* | | | |
| Dinner, Caesar, 6.3 oz | 145 | 11 | 8 |
| Grilled Chicken Caesar | 480 | 24 | 19 |
| Lettuce Wedge | 395 | 34 | 10 |
| *Sides: Per Serving* | | | |
| Garlic Mashed Potatoes, ½ cup | 130 | 5 | 19 |
| Steak Fries, 8 oz | 610 | 26 | 86 |
| Texas Seasoned Rice, 8 oz | 100 | 3.5 | 14 |

## Long John Silver's® (June '16)

*Chicken,* **C** **F** **Cb**

| | C | F | Cb |
|---|---|---|---|
| Chicken Tenders, 1 piece 2 oz | 170 | 8 | 11 |
| *Sandwiches & Tacos:* | | | |
| **Baja:** Chicken Taco (1) | 530 | 33 | 40 |
| Fish Taco (1) | 580 | 39 | 41 |
| **Ciabatta:** Chicken Sandwich | 560 | 27 | 52 |
| Fish Sandwich | 490 | 26 | 45 |
| *Seafood:* | | | |
| Baked Cod, 1 piece, 6 oz | 160 | 1 | 1 |
| Battered: Alaskan Pollock, | | | |
| 1 piece, 3.2 oz | 230 | 14 | 14 |
| Cod, 1 piece, 3 oz | 280 | 19 | 6 |
| Shrimp, 3 pieces, 1.5 oz | 130 | 7 | 5 |
| Crab Cake, 1 cake, 2.2 oz | 280 | 15 | 26 |
| **Snack Box:** Breaded Clam Strips | 280 | 16 | 20 |
| Popcorn Shrimp, 3 oz | 330 | 12 | 20 |

*Continued Next Page....*

## Long John's® cont... (Aug '16)
### Sauces & Condiments:

| | | | |
|---|---|---|---|
| **Dipping Sauces:** BBQ, 1 oz | **40** | 0 | 10 |
| Cocktail, 1 oz | **25** | 0 | 6 |
| Honey Mustard, 1 oz | **100** | 6 | 12 |
| Ketchup, 1 pouch, 1 oz | **30** | 0 | 8 |
| Louisiana Hot Sauce, 1 tsp | **0** | 0 | 0 |
| Malt Vinegar, 0.5 oz | **0** | 0 | 0 |
| Ranch, 1 oz | **160** | 17 | 2 |
| Sweet Thai Chili, 1 oz | **60** | 0 | 14 |
| Tartar, 0.5 oz packet | **40** | 4 | 2 |

### Sides:

| | | | |
|---|---|---|---|
| Breaded Mozzarella Sticks (3) | **170** | 10 | 12 |
| Broccoli Cheese Soup, 1 bowl, 7.5 oz | **220** | 18 | 8 |
| Clam Chowder, 1 bowl | **230** | 16 | 16 |
| Cole Slaw, 4 oz | **200** | 15 | 15 |
| Corn Cobbette w/ Butter Oil, 3.5 oz | **150** | 10 | 14 |
| Crumblies, 1 oz | **150** | 13 | 8 |
| Fries, 3.7oz | **350** | 17 | 44 |
| Hushpuppy, 2 pups, 1.5 oz | **160** | 13 | 18 |
| Jalapeno Cheddar Bites (5), 1 oz | **240** | 16 | 18 |
| Rice, 5 oz | **180** | 1 | 37 |

*For Complete Menu & Data ~ see CalorieKing.com*

## Macaroni Grill® (Aug '16)
### Tappas & Antipasti:
*Per Whole Appetizer as Served*

| | C | F | Cb |
|---|---|---|---|
| Calamari Fritti | **760** | 55 | 33 |
| Goat Cheese Peppadew Peppers | **350** | 11 | 56 |
| Loaded Fries | **1020** | 74 | 68 |
| Mac & Cheese Bites w/ Truffle Dip | **920** | 70 | 44 |
| Spicy Ricotta Meatballs | **490** | 35 | 12 |

### Meals: with Menu Set Sides

| | | | |
|---|---|---|---|
| **Carne:** Cremini Pork Shank | **1800** | 124 | 43 |
| Grilled Lamb Chops | **790** | 63 | 19 |
| Rosemary Ribeye | **1430** | 120 | 18 |
| **Chicken:** Caprese | **720** | 34 | 40 |
| Marsala | **790** | 32 | 61 |
| Scallopine | **1110** | 74 | 51 |
| Under a Brick | **1590** | 145 | 20 |
| **Classics:** Eggplant Parmesan | **1340** | 90 | 103 |
| Fettuccine Alfredo | **1040** | 59 | 86 |
| Lasagne Bolognese | **1110** | 67 | 69 |
| Mom's Ricotta Meatballs: | | | |
| with Bolognese | **1130** | 62 | 83 |
| with Pomodoro | **970** | 51 | 79 |

## Macaroni Grill® cont... (Aug '16)
### Meals (Cont): Per Whole Entree

| | | | |
|---|---|---|---|
| **Pasta:** Butternut Asiago tortellaci | **980** | 66 | 63 |
| Carmela's Chicken | **1030** | 60 | 82 |
| Lobster Ravioli | **600** | 35 | 36 |
| Mama's Trio, | | | |
| with Cannelloni | **2040** | 127 | 123 |
| Mushroom Ravioli | **930** | 66 | 53 |
| Penne Rustica | **950** | 45 | 79 |
| Shrimp Scampi | **1180** | 88 | 56 |
| **Pesce:** Grilled Salmon | **1030** | 66 | 53 |
| Parmesan-Crusted Sole | **1330** | 94 | 94 |

### Artisan Pizzas: Per Whole Meal, as Served

| | | | |
|---|---|---|---|
| Cheese | **1170** | 41 | 146 |
| Farmhouse | **1360** | 59 | 146 |
| Margherita | **1270** | 51 | 147 |
| Pepperoni | **1360** | 57 | 146 |

| | | | |
|---|---|---|---|
| **Kids:** Chkn Tenders w/ Broccolini | **860** | 45 | 67 |
| Macaroni & Cheese | **540** | 31 | 44 |
| Pepperoni Pizza | **630** | 25 | 72 |
| Spaghetti & Meatballs, | | | |
| with Pomodoro Sauce | **460** | 21 | 45 |

### Salads: Includes Dressing

| | | | |
|---|---|---|---|
| Bibb & Blue, entrée | **520** | 42 | 17 |
| Caesar, with Chicken, entrée | **650** | 41 | 16 |
| Steak & Greens | **950** | 71 | 32 |
| **Side:** Florentine | **300** | 22 | 22 |
| Fresh Green | **190** | 16 | 11 |

### Dessert: Gelato, Vanilla

| | | | |
|---|---|---|---|
| **Dessert:** Gelato, Vanilla | **310** | 13 | 42 |
| Homemade Choc. Cake | **940** | 58 | 101 |
| Lemon Passion | **740** | 45 | 77 |
| New York Style Cheesecake | **690** | 41 | 70 |
| Tiramisu | **600** | 39 | 54 |

## Manhattan Bagel® (Aug '16)
### Bagels: Per Bagel

| | C | F | Cb |
|---|---|---|---|
| Blueberry, 3.8 oz | **300** | 1 | 65 |
| Chocolate Chip, 3.8 oz | **290** | 2.5 | 58 |
| Cinnamon Raisin, 4 oz | **330** | 1 | 70 |
| Egg; Jalapeno Cheddar, av., 4 oz | **320** | 2 | 67 |
| Everything; Poppy, av 4.3 oz | **335** | 3 | 68 |
| Pumpernickel, 3.5 oz | **240** | 1.5 | 53 |
| Salt, 4.3 oz | **320** | 1 | 68 |
| **Cream Cheese:** Plain, 1.3 oz | **120** | 12 | 2 |
| Scallion, 1.3 oz | **120** | 11 | 5 |

*Continued Next Page...*

Updated Nutrition Data ~ www.CalorieKing.com
Persons with Diabetes ~ See Disclaimer (Page 22)

## Manhattan Bagel® cont... (Aug '16)

*Breakfast:* On Plain Bagel

| | | | |
|---|---|---|---|
| Egg & Cheese | 480 | 13 | 69 |
| Egg Bacon & Cheese | 620 | 25 | 70 |
| Egg, Pork Roll & Cheese | 710 | 31 | 71 |
| Omelet Wrap, Egg, Cheese & Ham | 640 | 29 | 54 |

*Deli Sandwich:*

| | | | |
|---|---|---|---|
| BLT on Multigrain Bread | 500 | 25 | 48 |
| Turkey & Cheddar | 470 | 16 | 58 |
| White Albacore Tuna Wrap | 610 | 34 | 52 |
| *Signature Lunch:* Bronx Bomber | 430 | 14 | 49 |
| Chelsea Chicken | 760 | 31 | 75 |
| Village Veggie Wrap | 470 | 21 | 62 |

*Salad:* Without Dressing

| | | | |
|---|---|---|---|
| Garden Market, 10 oz | 350 | 26 | 25 |
| NY Deli Chef, 14 oz | 690 | 49 | 25 |

## Marie Callender's® (Aug '16)

*Appetizers:* Per Serving — C F Cb

| | | | |
|---|---|---|---|
| Crispy Chicken Tenders, 12.9 oz | 870 | 47 | 72 |
| Crispy Green Beans, 10.5 oz | 810 | 52 | 75 |
| Mozzarella Sticks, 8.6 oz | 690 | 42 | 46 |

*Burgers and Sandwiches:* With Fries

| | | | |
|---|---|---|---|
| Original Burger | 1290 | 87 | 84 |
| Albacore Tuna Melt | 1430 | 92 | 99 |
| French Dip Supreme | 1110 | 53 | 105 |
| Roasted Turkey Croissant Club | 1450 | 97 | 95 |

*Main Meals:* Per Complete Meal as Served

**Comfort Classics:**

| | | | |
|---|---|---|---|
| Artichoke & Mushroom Chicken | 1010 | 71 | 29 |
| Home-Style Meatloaf Dinner | 650 | 38 | 33 |

**From The Grill:**

| | | | |
|---|---|---|---|
| Skewer of Shrimp | 90 | 1 | 0 |
| St. Louis BBQ Ribs Skewer | 800 | 4 | 39 |

**Pasta Perfecto:** Includes Garlic Bread

| | | | |
|---|---|---|---|
| Chicken & Broccoli Fettuccini | 1230 | 66 | 97 |
| Double Shrimp Pasta | 1300 | 7 | 99 |
| **Pies,** Chicken Pot Pie, w/out sides | 1140 | 79 | 70 |

*Salads:* Includes Dressing

| | | | |
|---|---|---|---|
| Calif. Waldorf Chicken with Mango | 740 | 40 | 73 |
| Crunchy BBQ Chicken | 1060 | 56 | 90 |
| Traditional Caesar, with Chicken | 700 | 43 | 28 |

*Sides:* Cornbread,

| | | | |
|---|---|---|---|
| with Honey Butter, 3 oz | 340 | 21 | 33 |
| French Fries, 4 oz | 380 | 20 | 45 |
| Loaded Mashed Potatoes, 6.2 oz | 340 | 23 | 23 |
| Macaroni & Cheese, 6.4 oz | 230 | 9 | 26 |

*Soups:* Per Bowl

| | | | |
|---|---|---|---|
| Chicken Tortilla | 230 | 10 | 26 |
| Clam Chowder | 270 | 13 | 22 |
| Hearty Vegetable | 90 | 3 | 13 |
| Split Pea & Ham | 220 | 13 | 17 |

## Marie Callender's® cont... (Aug '16)

*Breakfast:* As Served — C F Cb

**Griddle Greats:**

| | | | |
|---|---|---|---|
| Belgian Waffles | 600 | 19 | 99 |
| Buttermilk Pancakes (3) | 670 | 28 | 92 |
| Old Fashioned French Toast | 830 | 31 | 123 |

**Eggs:** Marie's Magnificent Six,

| | | | |
|---|---|---|---|
| with Bacon | 750 | 36 | 80 |
| with Sausage | 910 | 52 | 81 |

**Eggs Benedict:**

| | | | |
|---|---|---|---|
| California | 1210 | 67 | 126 |
| Traditional | 1060 | 54 | 110 |
| **Omelettes:** BTA | 1610 | 84 | 161 |
| Oh My | 1710 | 88 | 156 |
| Spanish | 1550 | 78 | 166 |
| **Quiche:** Bacon, 1 slice | 990 | 79 | 45 |
| Ham, 1 slice | 1030 | 83 | 39 |
| **Smashers:** Country | 1320 | 82 | 90 |
| Tex-Mex | 1180 | 71 | 99 |

*Desserts:* Per Slice Unless Indicated

| | | | |
|---|---|---|---|
| **Pies:** Apple | 630 | 39 | 66 |
| Banana Cream, with Meringue | 510 | 24 | 66 |
| Chocolate Cream, with Meringue | 570 | 26 | 77 |
| Coconut Cream with Meringue | 590 | 29 | 75 |
| Razzleberry | 650 | 39 | 71 |

*For Complete Nutritional Data ~ see CalorieKing.com*

## Max & Erma's® (June '16)

*Shareables:* As Served — C F Cb

| | | | |
|---|---|---|---|
| **Black Bean Roll-Ups:** Original | 680 | 31 | 90 |
| Crispy | 890 | 54 | 90 |
| Hand Breaded Buffalo Tenders | 1320 | 99 | 49 |
| Potato Skin, Erma | 640 | 51 | 27 |

*Burgers:* Without Sides

| | | | |
|---|---|---|---|
| Cheeseburger, 6 oz | 790 | 51 | 47 |
| Cola BBQ Bacon, 10 oz | 1200 | 70 | 71 |
| Garbage, 6 oz | 1260 | 92 | 53 |
| Windy City Brat Burger | 970 | 59 | 68 |

*Salads:* Entrée Size, w/ Dressing, w/out Breadstick

| | | | |
|---|---|---|---|
| Apple Harvest | 1180 | 77 | 64 |
| Grilled Chicken Santa Fe | 1090 | 73 | 54 |
| Sthrn Fried Chicken | 1260 | 81 | 78 |
| *Sides:* Baked Potato | 190 | 2.5 | 38 |
| French Fries, 5 oz | 460 | 28 | 47 |
| Fresh Fruit Salad | 120 | 0 | 31 |
| Herb Rice | 240 | 2.5 | 49 |
| Seasoned Vegetables | 100 | 9 | 4 |

*Dessert:*

| | | | |
|---|---|---|---|
| Banana Cream Pie | 890 | 69 | 68 |
| Chocolate Cake Ala Mode | 1610 | 86 | 211 |

*For Complete Menu & Data ~ See CalorieKing.com*

## McAlister's Deli® (Aug '16)

*Sandwiches: Per Whole Sandwich*

| | C | F | Cb |
|---|---|---|---|
| **Classic:** Grilled Chicken | 620 | 32 | 50 |
| Harvest Chicken Salad | 730 | 48 | 55 |
| The Italian | 760 | 39 | 49 |
| Tuna Salad | 510 | 22 | 49 |
| Veggie Pita | 590 | 41 | 46 |
| **Club:** Black Angus | 830 | 40 | 76 |
| Grilled Chicken | 780 | 33 | 80 |
| McAlister's | 800 | 36 | 80 |
| **Grilled:** Four Cheese Griller | 790 | 43 | 65 |
| Smoky Pepper Jack Turkey | 800 | 38 | 72 |
| Sweet Chipotle Chicken | 650 | 19 | 76 |
| **Hot Sandwiches:** Ham Melt | 590 | 25 | 44 |
| California Turkey Reuben | 1000 | 51 | 82 |
| French Dip | 540 | 20 | 42 |
| Reuben | 950 | 46 | 77 |
| Roast Beef Melt | 580 | 24 | 42 |

### Mellow Mushroom® (Sept '16)

| | C | F | Cb |
|---|---|---|---|
| **Burgers:** Carnie Burger | 1030 | 64 | 57 |
| Herb Veggie Burger | 860 | 45 | 89 |
| **Calzones:** Chkn & Cheese | 1200 | 33 | 151 |
| Steak & Cheese | 1280 | 40 | 151 |
| **Hoagies, Whole:** BLT | 1340 | 92 | 64 |
| Jerk | 710 | 24 | 80 |
| Meatball | 600 | 20 | 66 |
| Mushroom Club | 1250 | 73 | 68 |
| Spiked Sausage | 1290 | 68 | 83 |
| Steak & Cheese | 1020 | 61 | 60 |
| **Munchies:** Garlic Bread | 510 | 25 | 55 |
| Magic Mushroom Soup | 350 | 24 | 15 |
| Meatball Trio | 590 | 38 | 21 |
| Roasted Red Potatoes | 120 | 3 | 22 |
| Spinach & Artichoke Dip, w/o bread | 500 | 38 | 14 |
| Stuffed Portobello | 300 | 19 | 14 |
| Wings: BBQ (5) | 330 | 18 | 15 |
| Jerk (5) | 280 | 17 | 1 |

*Pizzas: Per Medium Slice*

| | C | F | Cb |
|---|---|---|---|
| **Bayou Bleu; Holy Shiake Pie,** av. | 460 | 22 | 45 |
| **Buffalo Chkn; Mighty Meaty,** av | 490 | 21 | 46 |
| **Funky Q Chicken** | 450 | 16 | 50 |
| **Kosmic Karma; Mega-Veggie,** av. | 400 | 14 | 48 |

*Salads: Per Regular Size Without Dressing*

| | C | F | Cb |
|---|---|---|---|
| **Caesar,** with Parmean, w/out meat | 410 | 28 | 25 |
| **Greek,** with Feta, w/out meat | 250 | 15 | 17 |
| **Cookies:** Choc Chunk | 600 | 29 | 83 |
| Oatmeal Raisin | 480 | 17 | 75 |
| Peanut Butter | 580 | 32 | 65 |
| **Cookie Sundaes:** Choc. Chip | 480 | 26 | 58 |
| Oatmeal Raisin | 420 | 20 | 54 |
| Peanut Butter | 470 | 27 | 50 |

*Extra Menu Items ~ See CalorieKing.com*

## McDonald's® (Sept '16)

*Beef Burgers/Sandwiches::*

| | C | F | Cb |
|---|---|---|---|
| **Big Mac Burger** | 540 | 28 | 46 |
| **Cheeseburger** | 300 | 12 | 33 |
| **Double Cheeseburger** | 440 | 22 | 35 |
| **Hamburger** | 250 | 8 | 32 |
| **McDouble** | 390 | 18 | 34 |
| **McRib** | 480 | 22 | 45 |
| **Quarter Pounder:** with Cheese | 540 | 27 | 42 |
| Deluxe | 600 | 33 | 44 |
| Double, with Cheese | 780 | 45 | 43 |

*Chicken & Fish Sandwiches:*

| | C | F | Cb |
|---|---|---|---|
| **Artisan Grilled Chicken** | 360 | 6 | 43 |
| **Buttermilk Crispy Chicken Deluxe** | 580 | 24 | 62 |
| **Filet-O-Fish** | 390 | 19 | 39 |
| **Mac Snack Wrap** | 340 | 20 | 26 |
| **McChicken** | 370 | 17 | 40 |

*Chicken McNuggets:*

| | C | F | Cb |
|---|---|---|---|
| 4 pieces | 180 | 11 | 11 |
| 6 pieces | 270 | 16 | 16 |
| 10 pieces | 440 | 27 | 26 |
| 20 pieces | 890 | 53 | 49 |
| **Sauces:** Chipotle BBQ, 1 oz | 50 | 0 | 11 |
| Creamy Ranch, 0.8 oz | 110 | 12 | 1 |
| Spicy Buffalo, 0.8 oz | 35 | 3 | 1 |
| Sweet 'N Sour; Tangy BBQ, 1 oz | 50 | 0 | 12 |
| **French Fries:** Kids, 1.3 oz | 110 | 5 | 15 |
| Small, 2.6 oz | 230 | 11 | 29 |
| Medium, 3.9 oz | 340 | 16 | 44 |
| Large, 5.9 oz | 510 | 24 | 66 |
| Ketchup, packet | 10 | 0 | 2 |

*Breakfast:*

| | C | F | Cb |
|---|---|---|---|
| **Big Breakfast:** with Regular Biscuit | 740 | 48 | 50 |
| with Hotcakes | 1050 | 56 | 105 |
| **Biscuits:** *Regular* | | | |
| Bacon, Egg & Cheese | 450 | 26 | 36 |
| Sausage Biscuit | 440 | 30 | 33 |
| Sausage with Egg | 520 | 35 | 35 |
| Steak, Egg & Cheese | 530 | 32 | 37 |
| Burrito, Sausage | 300 | 16 | 26 |
| **Fruit 'N Yogurt Parfait** | 150 | 2 | 30 |
| **Fruit & Maple Oatmeal:** | | | |
| with Brown Sugar | 290 | 4 | 58 |
| without Brown Sugar | 260 | 4 | 49 |
| **Hash Browns,** (1), 2 oz | 150 | 9 | 16 |
| **Hotcakes:** Plain (3) | 320 | 7 | 54 |
| with 1 Pat Margarine & Syrup | 540 | 12 | 99 |
| with Sausage | 510 | 25 | 55 |

## McDonald's® cont... (Sept '16)

### Breakfast (Cont):

| | C | F | Cb |
|---|---|---|---|
| **McMuffins:** Egg | 300 | 12 | 29 |
| Egg White Delight | 250 | 8 | 29 |
| Sausage | 400 | 25 | 28 |
| Sausage with Egg | 470 | 30 | 29 |
| **McGriddles:** Bacon, Egg & Cheese | 450 | 21 | 48 |
| Sausage | 440 | 25 | 44 |
| Sausage, Egg & Cheese | 570 | 34 | 47 |
| **McMuffins:** Egg | 300 | 12 | 29 |
| Egg White Delight | 250 | 8 | 29 |
| Sausage | 400 | 25 | 28 |
| Sausage with Egg | 470 | 30 | 29 |

### Happy Meals:

| | C | F | Cb |
|---|---|---|---|
| **Chicken McNuggets (4):** | | | |
| +Apple Slices + 1% low fat Milk | 295 | 13 | 27 |
| +Apple Slices + fat free Choc Milk | 325 | 11 | 38 |
| + Go-Gurt Strawb Yog. & Apple Jce | 310 | 12 | 40 |
| **Hamburger:** | | | |
| +Apple Slices + 1% low fat Milk | 365 | 9 | 28 |
| +Apple Slices +fat free Choc Milk | 395 | 8 | 39 |
| + Go-Gurt Strawb Yog. & Apple Jce | 380 | 9 | 41 |
| **Cheeseburger:** | | | |
| +Apple Slices + 1% low fat Milk | 415 | 15 | 49 |
| + Apple Slices & Fat-Free Choc Milk | 445 | 12 | 60 |
| + Go-Gurt Strawb Yog. & Apple Jce | 430 | 13 | 62 |

### Mighty Kid's Meal:

| | C | F | Cb |
|---|---|---|---|
| **Chicken McNuggets (6):** | | | |
| + Apple Slices+ Fat Free Choc Milk | 415 | 16 | 43 |
| + Go-Gurt & Apple Juice | 400 | 17 | 45 |

### Salads: Without Dressing

| | C | F | Cb |
|---|---|---|---|
| **Bacon Ranch:** Grilled Chicken | 320 | 14 | 9 |
| Buttermilk Crispy Chicken | 490 | 29 | 28 |
| **Southwest:** Grilled Chicken | 350 | 12 | 27 |
| B'milk Crispy Chicken | 520 | 25 | 46 |
| **Side Salad** | 15 | 0 | 3 |

### Salad Dressings: Per Package

| | C | F | Cb |
|---|---|---|---|
| **Newman's Own:** Ranch, 2 fl.oz | 200 | 17 | 11 |
| **Low-Fat:** Balsamic Vinaig., 1.5 fl.oz | 35 | 1.5 | 3 |
| Family Recipe Italian, 1.5 fl.oz | 50 | 1.5 | 7 |
| **Snacks:** Apple Slices | 15 | 0 | 4 |
| Mozzarella Sticks (3), w/ Mar. Sce | 200 | 10 | 18 |
| Yoplait Go-Gurt, Strawberry, 1 tube | 50 | 0.5 | 9 |

### Desserts & Shakes:

| | C | F | Cb |
|---|---|---|---|
| **Baked Apple Pie,** 2.6 oz | 230 | 10 | 32 |
| **Cookies:** Choc. Chip Cookie (1) | 160 | 8 | 21 |
| Oatmeal Raisin (1), 1 oz | 150 | 6 | 22 |

## McDonald's® cont... (Sept '16)

### Desserts & Shakes (Cont):

| | C | F | Cb |
|---|---|---|---|
| **Pie,** Strawberry & Creme | 310 | 17 | 36 |
| **McFlurry:** M&M Candies, 12 fl.oz | 650 | 23 | 96 |
| Oreo Cookies, 12 fl.oz cup | 520 | 17 | 80 |
| **Soft Serve:** Kiddie Cone | 45 | 1.5 | 7 |
| Vanilla Cone | 170 | 4.5 | 27 |
| **Sundaes:** | | | |
| Hot Caramel, 6.4 oz | 340 | 8 | 60 |
| Hot Fudge, 6.3 oz | 330 | 9 | 53 |
| Strawberry, 6.3 oz | 280 | 6 | 49 |
| **Shakes:** Chocolate; Strawberry, average: | | | |
| 12 fl.oz cup | 530 | 16 | 86 |
| 16 fl.oz cup | 635 | 18 | 103 |
| 22 fl.oz cup | 850 | 23 | 141 |
| Vanilla: 12 fl.oz cup | 510 | 15 | 83 |
| 16 fl.oz cup | 610 | 18 | 100 |
| 22 fl.oz cup | 820 | 23 | 135 |
| **Smoothies, all flavors:** | | | |
| Small, 12 fl oz cup | 200 | 0.5 | 45 |
| Medium, 16 fl oz cup | 250 | 1 | 56 |
| Large, 22 fl oz cup | 340 | 1 | 77 |
| **Milk:** 1% Low-Fat, 8 fl.oz cup | 100 | 2.5 | 12 |
| Fat-Free Chocolate Milk, 8 fl.oz | 130 | 0 | 23 |
| **Juice:** Apple, 6 fl.oz box | 80 | 0 | 21 |
| Orange: Small, 12 fl.oz | 150 | 0 | 34 |
| Medium, 16 fl.oz cup | 190 | 0 | 44 |
| Large, 22 fl.oz cup | 280 | 0 | 65 |
| **Frappe,** Oreo, small, 12 fl.oz | 420 | 17 | 60 |

### Soda: With Ice, approximately 30%

| | C | F | Cb |
|---|---|---|---|
| **Coca-Cola or Sprite** | | | |
| Extra Small, 12 fl.oz cup | 100 | 0 | 29 |
| Small, 16 fl.oz cup | 140 | 0 | 38 |
| Medium, 21 fl.oz cup | 205 | 0 | 55 |
| Large, 30 fl.oz cup | 280 | 0 | 76 |
| **Diet Coke** | 0 | 0 | 0 |
| **Hi-C Orange Lavaburst:** | | | |
| Extra Small, 12 fl.oz cup | 110 | 0 | 31 |
| Small, 16 fl.oz cup | 160 | 0 | 43 |
| Medium, 21 fl.oz cup | 230 | 0 | 61 |
| Large, 30 fl.oz cup | 310 | 0 | 84 |
| **Powerade,** Mountain Berry Blast: | | | |
| Extra Small, 12 fl.oz cup | 60 | 0 | 15 |
| Small, 16 fl.oz cup | 80 | 0 | 21 |
| Medium, 21 fl.oz cup | 120 | 0 | 30 |
| Large, 30 fl.oz cup | 160 | 0 | 42 |
| **Iced Tea,** medium, 21 fl.oz cup | 0 | 0 | 0 |
| **Sweet Tea,** small, 16 fl oz cup | 150 | 0 | 36 |

*McCafe Coffees ~ Next Page*

## McDonald's® cont... (Sept '16)
*McCafe:*

| | C | F | Cb |
|---|---|---|---|
| **Hot Chocolate:** *With Whipped Cream & Toppings* | | | |
| Whole Milk: Small, 12 fl oz | 360 | 13 | 50 |
| Medium, 16 fl oz cup | 440 | 16 | 61 |
| Large, 20 fl oz cup | 540 | 20 | 73 |
| Nonfat Milk: Small, 12 fl oz | 280 | 3.5 | 50 |
| Medium, 16 fl oz cup | 340 | 3.5 | 61 |
| **Hot White Choc.:** *With Whipped Cream & Toppings* | | | |
| Whole Milk: | | | |
| Small, 12 fl oz | 350 | 13 | 48 |
| Medium, 16 fl oz cup | 420 | 15 | 59 |
| Large, 20 fl.oz cup | 520 | 19 | 71 |
| *Iced Coffee:* | | | |
| **Regular:** *With Whole Milk, Liquid Sugar & Light Cream* | | | |
| Small, 16 fl.oz cup | 130 | 4 | 23 |
| Medium, 22 fl.oz cup | 170 | 5 | 30 |
| **Mocha:** *With Whole Milk, Whipped Cream & Toppings* | | | |
| Small, 16 fl.oz cup | 290 | 11 | 40 |
| Large, 30 fl.oz cup | 470 | 16 | 69 |

## Mimi's Cafe® (Aug '16)
*Breakfast:*

| | C | F | Cb |
|---|---|---|---|
| **Benedicts:** *With Roasted Potatoes* | | | |
| Original | 880 | 56 | 51 |
| Smoked Salmon | 810 | 52 | 52 |
| **Omelets:** *With Roasted Potatoes Unless Indicated* | | | |
| Andouille Sausage & Red Pepper | 760 | 51 | 31 |
| Bacon Avocado | 930 | 67 | 28 |
| Egg White & Veggie, with Fruit | 290 | 8 | 28 |
| Hickory-Smoked Ham & Cheese | 680 | 48 | 25 |
| **Griddle Cakes:** *Includes Mixed Fruit* | | | |
| Brioche French Toast | 580 | 17 | 85 |
| Cinnamon Roll French Toast | 810 | 31 | 113 |
| Orange Crème French Toast | 1160 | 42 | 164 |
| **Appetizers:** | | | |
| Baked Brie To Share | 440 | 17 | 56 |
| Calamari | 350 | 9 | 32 |
| Warm Spinach Artich. Dip, 15 oz | 700 | 40 | 64 |
| *Lunch & Dinner: Without Side Choices* | | | |
| **Burgers:** Bacon Avoc. Sourdough | 1240 | 87 | 41 |
| Brioche Cheeseburger | 820 | 45 | 51 |
| Hickory Bacon Cheddar | 1250 | 67 | 90 |
| **Craft Sandwiches:** | | | |
| Chicken Cordon Bleu | 1100 | 49 | 92 |
| West Coast Reuben | 1190 | 70 | 76 |
| **Entrees:** | | | |
| Chicken Pot Pie | 860 | 56 | 60 |
| French Pot Roast | 510 | 32 | 22 |
| Quiche Lorraine | 420 | 28 | 16 |
| Roasted Chicken Crepes | 360 | 27 | 12 |
| *Sides:* Broccoli; Green Beans, av. | 125 | 9 | 6 |
| Mashed Potatoes | 130 | 4 | 21 |

## Mr. Goodcents® (Aug '16)
*Cold Subs:*

| | C | F | Cb |
|---|---|---|---|
| *Per 8" Wheat Bread Sub with Standard Toppings* | | | |
| Centsable | 450 | 18 | 56 |
| Italian Sub | 635 | 37 | 52 |
| Goodcents Original | 515 | 25 | 54 |
| Oven Roasted Chicken Breast | 340 | 6 | 52 |
| Penny Club | 350 | 6 | 55 |
| Pepperoni | 690 | 43 | 52 |
| Tuna Salad | 475 | 20 | 59 |
| **Toasted Sub:** *Per 8" Wheat Bread Sub with Standard Toppings* | | | |
| Chicken Bacon Ranch, w/ Cheddar | 690 | 27 | 58 |
| Meatball with Mozzarella | 730 | 32 | 70 |
| *Pasta:* | | | |
| with Alfredo Sauce | 740 | 35 | 91 |
| Chicken Alfredo | 930 | 38 | 103 |
| Chicken Parmesan | 780 | 20 | 107 |
| with Marinara Sauce & Meatballs | 860 | 29 | 114 |
| *Garlic Bread,* 1 piece, 2 4 oz | 260 | 15 | 28 |
| *Soup: Per Bowl* | | | |
| Broccoli Cheese | 855 | 60 | 34 |
| Chicken Homestyle Noodle | 295 | 8 | 42 |
| Potato with Bacon | 890 | 59 | 76 |

## Mr. Hero® (Aug '16)
*7" Subs & Burgers:*

| | C | F | Cb |
|---|---|---|---|
| **Burgers:** Cheeseburger | 770 | 54 | 44 |
| Hamburger | 690 | 48 | 44 |
| Romanburger | 860 | 62 | 45 |
| **Chicken Subs:** | | | |
| Bistro Chicken | 560 | 26 | 42 |
| Grilled Chicken Philly | 500 | 21 | 44 |
| Tuscan Chicken | 890 | 52 | 67 |
| **Deli Subs:** *Per 7" Sub with Menu Board Toppings* | | | |
| Italiano | 570 | 27 | 54 |
| Original Italian | 530 | 27 | 50 |
| Tuna 'N Cheese | 670 | 53 | 45 |
| Turkey | 330 | 2.5 | 49 |
| **Steak Subs:** | | | |
| Hot Buttered Cheesesteak Deluxe | 660 | 42 | 41 |
| Sicilian Parm | 570 | 31 | 41 |
| Zesty Bacon & Swiss | 510 | 25 | 43 |
| **Pitas:** Chicken | 450 | 13 | 45 |
| Gyro | 580 | 31 | 50 |
| *Sides:* Per Regular Size | | | |
| Mozzarella Sticks | 525 | 34 | 36 |
| Onion Petals | 545 | 36 | 52 |
| **Fries:** Potato Waffle | 360 | 27 | 29 |
| Zesty Fries | 420 | 34 | 30 |
| **Desserts:** Oreo Cheesecake | 270 | 18 | 24 |
| Snickers Cheesecake | 270 | 18 | 23 |
| Strawb. Swirl Cheesecake | 250 | 17 | 21 |

Updated Nutrition Data ~ www.CalorieKing.com
Persons with Diabetes ~ See Disclaimer (Page 22)

## Mrs Fields Cookies® (June'16)

| Brownies: Per 2.15 oz Brownie | C | F | Cb |
|---|---|---|---|
| Butterscotch Blondie | 260 | 10 | 38 |
| Double Fudge; Pecan Fudge, av. | 265 | 14 | 33 |
| Special Walnut Fudge & Blondie | 260 | 13 | 35 |
| Toffee Fudge; Walnut Fudge, av. | 265 | 14 | 33 |
| **Brownie Bites:** | | | |
| Double Fudge (3) | 200 | 10 | 27 |
| Toffee Fudge (3) | 200 | 11 | 26 |
| **Coffee Cake,** | | | |
| Chocolate Chip, small, 2.35 oz | 240 | 11 | 30 |
| **Cookies:** | | | |
| Bite Size Nibblers: Cinn. Sugar (3) | 180 | 8 | 25 |
| Peanut Butter (3) | 170 | 9 | 19 |
| Semi-Sweet Chocolate (3) | 170 | 8 | 23 |
| Triple Chocolate (3) | 160 | 8 | 22 |
| White Chunk Macadamia (3) | 180 | 9 | 22 |
| Butter (1) | 200 | 8 | 29 |
| Cut Out (1) | 280 | 11 | 44 |
| Debra's Special (1) | 200 | 9 | 27 |
| Oatmeal, Raisins and Walnuts (1) | 200 | 9 | 27 |
| Peanut Butter (1) | 200 | 12 | 24 |
| Semi-Sweet: Chocolate (1) | 210 | 10 | 29 |
| with Walnuts (1) | 220 | 11 | 28 |
| Triple Chocolate (1) | 210 | 10 | 28 |
| White Chunk Macadamia (1) | 230 | 12 | 28 |
| **Muffins:** Per 2 oz | | | |
| Blueberry | 190 | 9 | 24 |
| Chocolate Chip | 200 | 10 | 26 |

*For Complete Nutritional Data ~ See CalorieKing.com*

## My Favorite Muffin® (Aug '16)

| Jumbo Muffins: Per 5.8 oz | C | F | Cb |
|---|---|---|---|
| **Regular:** Blueberry | 505 | 24 | 66 |
| Choc. Chip; Cinn Swirl Cheesecake | 635 | 33 | 82 |
| Deep Dish Apple Pie | 530 | 24 | 75 |
| Pumpkin Spice | 545 | 24 | 78 |
| **Fat Free:** Blueberry | 325 | 0 | 78 |
| Chocolate Marble | 375 | 0 | 87 |
| Cinnamon Bun | 505 | 0 | 126 |

## Nathan's Famous® (Aug '16)

| Burgers: | C | F | Cb |
|---|---|---|---|
| Bacon Cheeseburger, 5 oz | 850 | 47 | 45 |
| Double Beefburger, 10 oz | 1050 | 73 | 45 |
| Hamburger, 5 oz | 640 | 38 | 45 |
| Super Cheeseburger, 5 oz | 980 | 58 | 51 |
| **Nathan's Famous Hot Dogs:** With Natural Casings | | | |
| Original, 3.5 oz | 280 | 18 | 24 |
| Cheese Dog, 4.5 oz | 320 | 20 | 27 |
| Chili Dog, 5.5 oz | 400 | 27 | 30 |
| Chili Cheese, 6.5 oz | 440 | 30 | 33 |
| **Corn Dog,** on a stick, 3.2 oz | 380 | 21 | 36 |

## Nathan's Famous® cont... (Aug'16)

| Chicken: | C | F | Cb |
|---|---|---|---|
| Chicken Tenders, Krispy, | | | |
| 3 pieces, 6.3 oz | 520 | 31 | 32 |
| Grilled: Chicken Sandwich, 8.2 oz | 480 | 21 | 43 |
| Chicken Caesar Wrap, 12 oz | 690 | 30 | 64 |
| Krispy: Chkn Club S'wich, 10 .3oz | 850 | 53 | 60 |
| Chicken Caesar Wrap, 12.7 oz | 890 | 48 | 78 |
| **Fries:** | | | |
| **French:** Regular, 7.5 oz | 540 | 39 | 43 |
| Large, 11.5 oz | 830 | 60 | 66 |
| Family, 15.5 oz | 1120 | 80 | 89 |
| **Cheese:** Regular, 9 oz | 600 | 42 | 48 |
| Large, 13.5 oz | 910 | 64 | 72 |
| **Philly Cheesesteak,** 12.8 oz | 660 | 32 | 47 |

## New York Fries® ~ See CalorieKing.com

## Ninety Nine (Aug '16)

| Standout Starters: As Served | C | F | Cb |
|---|---|---|---|
| Boneless Wings & Skins Sampler | 1890 | 125 | 107 |
| Fried Mozzarella | 770 | 45 | 57 |
| Outrageous Potato Skins | 1470 | 101 | 84 |
| **Burgers:** Without Sides | | | |
| Bacon & Cheese Steakburger | 900 | 58 | 48 |
| BBQ BLT Crunch Burger | 1260 | 76 | 89 |
| Vermont Cheddar Burger | 1040 | 69 | 54 |
| West Coast Turkey Burger | 800 | 48 | 42 |
| **Sandwiches:** Without Sides | | | |
| Honey BBQ Chicken Wrap | 850 | 33 | 100 |
| Triple-Decker Turkey Club | 700 | 31 | 58 |
| **Meals:** Served with Menu Set Sides Unless Indicated | | | |
| Fish & Chips | 1570 | 105 | 107 |
| Macadamia Crusted Chicken | 1240 | 82 | 92 |
| New England Shoreline Combo | 1890 | 126 | 132 |
| Original Crispy Chicken Tenders | 1750 | 112 | 128 |
| Prime Rib: 12 oz, without sides | 670 | 39 | 3 |
| 18 oz, without sides | 940 | 53 | 3 |
| Smthrd Sirloin Tips, w/o sides, 24 oz | 1050 | 62 | 18 |
| **Salads:** As Served | | | |
| Big Kahuna | 810 | 37 | 86 |
| Chicken Caesar | 730 | 42 | 52 |
| Grilled Chicken Kabob | 770 | 48 | 44 |
| **Sides:** | | | |
| Baked Potato with Sour Cream | 310 | 8 | 52 |
| Double Bleu Iceberg Wedge | 460 | 42 | 11 |
| French Fries | 1040 | 64 | 107 |
| Honey Butter Bisc., w/ Honey Butter | 230 | 11 | 29 |
| Pasta: with Butter | 740 | 28 | 104 |
| with Marinara | 660 | 10 | 124 |
| Perfect Coleslaw | 150 | 12 | 10 |
| Russet Mashed Potatoes | 260 | 11 | 36 |
| **Dessert,** | | | |
| Towering Midnight Fudge Cake | 790 | 40 | 96 |

## Noodles & Company® (Aug '16)

*Noodles & Pasta: Regular Size*

| | C | F | Cb |
|---|---|---|---|
| Buttered Noodles | 870 | 39 | 113 |
| Bangkok Curry | 550 | 23 | 76 |
| Indonesian Peanut Sauté | 890 | 26 | 146 |
| Japanese Pan Noodles | 710 | 22 | 112 |
| Mushroom Stroganoff | 980 | 54 | 105 |
| Pad Thai | 1100 | 44 | 153 |
| Penne Rosa w. Parmesan | 680 | 24 | 91 |
| Spaghetti & Meatballs | 990 | 50 | 98 |
| Steak Stroganoff | 1150 | 62 | 107 |
| Wisconsin Mac & Cheese | 1100 | 47 | 128 |

*Sandwiches:* BBQ Pork

| | C | F | Cb |
|---|---|---|---|
| BBQ Pork | 560 | 6 | 69 |
| Spicy Chicken Caesar | 530 | 32 | 41 |
| The Med | 350 | 13 | 38 |
| The Veggie Med | 310 | 12 | 41 |
| Wisconsin Cheesesteak on Petite Baguette | 580 | 25 | 52 |

*Salads: Per Regular Size*

| | C | F | Cb |
|---|---|---|---|
| Chinese Chicken Chop Salad | 490 | 28 | 39 |
| Grilled Chicken Caesar | 420 | 27 | 118 |
| Spinach & Fruit Salad | 610 | 37 | 55 |
| The Med with Chicken | 410 | 15 | 43 |

*Soups: Per Regular Size*

| | C | F | Cb |
|---|---|---|---|
| Chicken Noodle | 320 | 9 | 41 |
| Thai Curry | 510 | 19 | 69 |
| Tomato Basil Bisque | 430 | 28 | 37 |

*Extras:* Cheesy Garlic Bread (3)

| | C | F | Cb |
|---|---|---|---|
| Cheesy Garlic Bread (3) | 330 | 18 | 31 |
| Cucumber Tomato Salad | 80 | 0 | 10 |
| Margherita Flatbread | 340 | 15 | 37 |
| Potsticker (6), without sauce | 380 | 8 | 56 |

## Nothing But Noodles® (Apr '16)

*Noodle Bowls:*

| | C | F | Cb |
|---|---|---|---|
| **American:** Beef Stroganoff | 510 | 31 | 33 |
| Buttery Noodles | 650 | 44 | 46 |
| Santa Fe Pasta | 705 | 54 | 40 |
| Southwest Chipotle | 715 | 58 | 41 |
| Spicy Cajun Pasta | 660 | 50 | 44 |
| **Asian:** Pad Thai Noodles | 600 | 10 | 118 |
| Sesame Lo Mein | 410 | 11 | 64 |
| Spicy Japanese Noodles | 420 | 8 | 74 |
| Thai Peanut | 570 | 20 | 89 |
| **Italian:** Basil Pesto | 575 | 42 | 36 |
| Cappelini Primavera | 500 | 28 | 36 |
| Fettuccini Alfredo | 725 | 56 | 36 |
| Margherita Pasta | 475 | 31 | 36 |
| Marinara Pasta | 485 | 11 | 77 |
| Three-Cheese Macaroni | 445 | 21 | 45 |

*For Complete Menu & Data ~ see CalorieKing.com*

## O'Charley's® (Aug '16)

*Appetizers: As Served*

| | C | F | Cb |
|---|---|---|---|
| Bacon & Cheese Quesadilla | 870 | 59 | 50 |
| Chicken Tenders, Chipotle | 1160 | 40 | 107 |
| Spicy Jack Cheese Wedges (7) | 720 | 48 | 44 |
| Top Shelf Combo Platter | 1880 | 132 | 74 |

*Chicken & Pasta: Without Sides Unless Indicated*

| | C | F | Cb |
|---|---|---|---|
| Bruschetta Chicken | 340 | 10 | 14 |
| Chicken Tender, Buffalo | 1070 | 64 | 31 |
| Prime Rib Pasta | 1400 | 94 | 80 |
| Shrimp Scampi Pasta | 950 | 43 | 104 |

*Classic Combos: Without Sides*

| | C | F | Cb |
|---|---|---|---|
| Panko-Crusted Shrimp, with Battered Cod | 1060 | 58 | 69 |
| Steak & Chicken Tenders, 6 oz | 1030 | 67 | 26 |
| Steak & Grilled Atl. Salmon, 9 oz | 890 | 56 | 3 |
| Steak & Panko-Crstd Shrimp, 9 oz | 780 | 42 | 41 |
| Steak & Savannah Crab Cake | 910 | 67 | 26 |

*Hand-Crushed Burgers: Without Sides*

| | C | F | Cb |
|---|---|---|---|
| Better Cheddar Bacon | 1000 | 68 | 49 |
| Pretzel Burger | 1260 | 86 | 68 |
| Southwest Blackbean | 760 | 38 | 77 |
| Wild West Burger | 1290 | 94 | 64 |

*Ribs: Without Sides*

O'Charley's: Baby Back Ribs:

| | C | F | Cb |
|---|---|---|---|
| Full Rack | 1460 | 85 | 96 |
| Half Rack | 730 | 43 | 48 |
| **Slow Roasted Prime Rib:** 8oz | 830 | 70 | 3 |
| 16 oz | 1460 | 120 | 3 |

*Seafood! Favorites: Without Sides*

| | C | F | Cb |
|---|---|---|---|
| Grilled Atlantic Salmon, 9 oz | 500 | 31 | 2 |
| Hand Battered: Fish & Chips Entrée | 1460 | 91 | 85 |
| Fish & Shrimp | 1810 | 127 | 106 |
| Panko Crusted Fried Shrimp Dinner | 560 | 24 | 56 |

*Sides:* Baked Potato

| | C | F | Cb |
|---|---|---|---|
| Baked Potato | 200 | 1 | 50 |
| Broccoli | 110 | 8 | 6 |
| French Fries | 400 | 24 | 40 |
| Loaded Baked Potato | 490 | 27 | 53 |
| Sweet Potato Fries | 280 | 19 | 27 |

*Salads: Per Full Salad, with Dressing Unless Indicated*

| | C | F | Cb |
|---|---|---|---|
| California Chicken, w/out Dressing | 980 | 63 | 68 |
| Classic Cobb | 1130 | 92 | 35 |
| Southern Fried Chicken Salad | 1620 | 114 | 50 |
| Southern Pecan Chicken Tender | 1600 | 114 | 89 |

*Signature Soup: Per Bowl*

| | C | F | Cb |
|---|---|---|---|
| Chicken Harvest | 210 | 13 | 20 |
| Chicken Tortilla | 190 | 7 | 20 |

*Desserts:*

| | C | F | Cb |
|---|---|---|---|
| Double-Crust Peach Pie, 1 slice | 570 | 35 | 64 |
| Ooey Gooey Caramel Pie, 1 slice | 640 | 39 | 76 |

*For Complete Menu & Data ~ see CalorieKing.com*

# Olive Garden® (Aug '16)

| | C | F | Cb |
|---|---|---|---|
| *Appetizers:* | | | |
| Bruschetta Caprese | 540 | 30 | 43 |
| Classic Calamari | 870 | 56 | 67 |
| Sauce: Marinara | 45 | 2.5 | 6 |
| Parmesan-Peppercorn | 250 | 25 | 3 |
| Spicy Shrimp Scampi Fritta | 560 | 37 | 34 |
| Stuffed Mushrooms | 380 | 30 | 13 |
| *Entrées:* | | | |
| **Lighter Lunch:** | | | |
| Citrus Chicken Sorrento | 410 | 16 | 35 |
| Garlic Rosemary Chicken | 400 | 16 | 29 |
| Ravioli di Portobello | 570 | 31 | 52 |
| Grilled Chicken Caesar Salad | 390 | 20 | 11 |
| **Dinner:** | | | |
| Eggplant Parmigiana | 1060 | 52 | 86 |
| Fettuccini Alfredo | 1090 | 68 | 92 |
| Five Cheese Ziti al Forno | 1220 | 71 | 103 |
| Lasagna Classico | 960 | 58 | 54 |
| Ravioli di Portobello | 820 | 46 | 73 |
| Sausage Stuffed Giant Rigatoni | 1020 | 60 | 58 |
| Tour of Italy | 1520 | 96 | 92 |
| *Desserts:* | | | |
| Chocolate Hazelnut Mousse Cake | 480 | 36 | 38 |
| Salted Caramel tiramisu | 330 | 12 | 48 |
| Vanilla Panna Cotta & Raspb. Sce | 300 | 16 | 17 |

# Old Spaghetti Factory® (Aug '16)

| | C | F | Cb |
|---|---|---|---|
| *Appetizers: As Served* | | | |
| Shrimp, Spinach & Artichoke Dip | 590 | 40 | 39 |
| Sicilian Garlic Cheese Bread | 1220 | 78 | 97 |
| *Entrées, Lunch/Dinner:* | | | |
| **Classics:** | | | |
| Spaghetti: with Clam Sauce, 15 oz | 810 | 31 | 107 |
| with Marina Sauce, 15 oz | 560 | 5 | 108 |
| with Meat Sauce, 15 oz | 650 | 11 | 108 |
| with Sicilian Meatballs, 21 oz | 1040 | 36 | 115 |
| **Factory Favorites:** | | | |
| Chicken Parmigiana, 18 oz | 750 | 29 | 70 |
| Spinach & Cheese Ravioli, 11 oz | 470 | 16 | 63 |
| Spinach Tortellini w/ Alfredo Sce | 940 | 56 | 86 |
| **Managers Favorites:** | | | |
| Marinara: Clam, 15 oz | 490 | 15 | 74 |
| Meat, 15 oz | 420 | 6 | 74 |
| Mushroom, 16.5 oz | 460 | 11 | 76 |
| *Signature Selection:* | | | |
| Crab Ravioli, 11 oz | 810 | 45 | 73 |
| Garlic Mizithra, 16.9 oz | 1360 | 85 | 102 |
| Sausage Ravioli | 840 | 56 | 60 |

# On the Border® (Aug '16)

| | C | F | Cb |
|---|---|---|---|
| *Appetizers: As Served* | | | |
| Border Sampler | 1940 | 131 | 102 |
| Fajita Quesadillas: Chicken | 1190 | 83 | 60 |
| Steak | 1230 | 88 | 58 |
| *Burritos: Includes Rice, without Beans & Sauce* | | | |
| Classic Chicken Tinga | 920 | 35 | 96 |
| Classic Shredded Beef | 970 | 40 | 96 |
| *Chimichangas: Includes Rice, without Beans & Sauce* | | | |
| Chicken Tinga | 1340 | 78 | 109 |
| Ground Beef | 1500 | 95 | 111 |
| *Enchiladas: With Rice, without Beans* | | | |
| Hatch Chili Chicken | 810 | 31 | 99 |
| La Bandera | 900 | 40 | 98 |
| Suizas | 990 | 44 | 103 |
| *Fajita Grill: Without Rice, Beans, Tortillas or Condiments* | | | |
| Monterey Ranch Chicken | 690 | 46 | 10 |
| The Ultimate | 1150 | 95 | 25 |
| *Fresh Grill:* Queso Chicken | 810 | 39 | 64 |
| Jalapeno- BBQ Salmon | 640 | 25 | 55 |
| *Salads: Without Dressing* | | | |
| House Salad | 160 | 6 | 25 |
| **Grande Taco Salad:** Chkn Tinga | 750 | 40 | 68 |
| with Ground Beef | 850 | 51 | 69 |
| *Soup:* Chicken Tortilla, 1 cup | 300 | 14 | 26 |
| 1 Bowl | 470 | 17 | 51 |
| *Sides:* Black Beans | 170 | 1.5 | 29 |
| Corn Tortillas (3) | 130 | 2.5 | 33 |
| Mexican Rice | 280 | 4.5 | 54 |
| Flour Tortillas (3) | 360 | 11 | 55 |
| Refried Beans | 150 | 8 | 25 |
| *Dressings: Per Serving* | | | |
| Ranch Dressing | 230 | 24 | 2 |
| Smoked Jalapeno Vinaigrette | 250 | 24 | 8 |

*For Complete Nutritional Data ~ see CalorieKing.com*

# Orange Julius® (Aug '16)

| | C | F | Cb |
|---|---|---|---|
| *Julius Originals: Per Medium Size* | | | |
| Berry Pomegranate | 430 | 0 | 108 |
| Mango Pineapple | 450 | 0 | 114 |
| OrangeBerry | 330 | 0 | 82 |
| Strawberry Banana | 530 | 8 | 114 |
| *Premium Fruit Smoothies: Per Medium Size* | | | |
| Berry Pomegranate | 380 | 0 | 91 |
| Pina Colada | 340 | 0 | 80 |
| Strawberry | 300 | 0.5 | 71 |
| *Light Smoothies: Per Medium Size* | | | |
| Orange | 170 | 0 | 41 |
| Strawberry | 200 | 0 | 50 |
| Tripleberry | 210 | 0 | 55 |
| *Boost,* Banana, Small drink | 30 | 0 | 7 |

## Outback Steakhouse® (Aug '16)

*Aussie-Tizers:* Per Whole Dish, with Selected Dressing/Sauce

| | C | F | Cb |
|---|---|---|---|
| Alice Springs Chicken Quesadillas | 1600 | 95 | 90 |
| Aussie Cheese Fries: Small | 1155 | 85 | 63 |
|   Regular | 1755 | 122 | 111 |
| Bloomin' Onion | 1955 | 155 | 123 |
| Coconut Shrimp | 635 | 35 | 60 |
| Wings | 1165 | 100 | 11 |

*Forkless Features:* wWhout Sides

| | C | F | Cb |
|---|---|---|---|
| Aussie Chicken Tacos | 1040 | 58 | 55 |
| Cripsy Chicken Sandwich | 775 | 41 | 68 |
| Double Burger | 930 | 61 | 44 |
| Outback Burger, without Cheese | 625 | 38 | 33 |
| Prime Rib Sandwich | 855 | 46 | 72 |
| Ribeye Melt | 1030 | 51 | 71 |
| The Bloomin' Burger | 1075 | 77 | 48 |
| Wood Grilled, California Chicken Sandwich | 590 | 27 | 43 |

*Chicken, Ribs, Chops:* Without sides

| | C | F | Cb |
|---|---|---|---|
| Alice Springs Chicken | 750 | 44 | 15 |
| Baby Back Ribs | 880 | 57 | 22 |
| Chicken Tender Platter | 1015 | 68 | 58 |
| Grilled Chicken On The Barbie | 200 | 2 | 11 |
| New Zealand Lamb Chops | 595 | 39 | 1 |
| Parmesan-Herb Crusted Chicken | 510 | 22 | 13 |
| Pork Porterhouse | 515 | 26 | 0 |
| Ribs & Chicken On The Barbie | 500 | 23 | 13 |

*Signature Outback Classic Cuts:* Without Sides

| | C | F | Cb |
|---|---|---|---|
| New York Strip, 14 oz | 615 | 26 | 0 |
| Outback: 6 oz Sirloin | 255 | 13 | 0 |
|   9 oz Sirloin | 380 | 19 | 0 |
|   12 oz Sirloin | 510 | 25 | 0 |
| Victoria's Filet Mignon, 6 oz | 220 | 9 | 0 |

*Steaks Bold Creations:* Without Sides

| | C | F | Cb |
|---|---|---|---|
| Sirloin: 9 oz, with Coconut Shrimp | 745 | 36 | 41 |
|   12 oz, with Coconut Shrimp | 870 | 43 | 41 |
|   9 oz, with Grilled Shrimp | 385 | 21 | 4 |
|   12 oz, with Grilled Shrimp | 555 | 30 | 4 |

*Steak Toppings:*

| | C | F | Cb |
|---|---|---|---|
| Blue Cheese Crumbles | 105 | 9 | 0 |
| Bloom Petals | 100 | 7 | 7 |

## Outback Steakhouse® cont... (Aug '16)

*Straight From The Sea:* without Sides

| | C | F | Cb |
|---|---|---|---|
| Firecracker Salmon | 480 | 25 | 25 |
| Hearts of Gold Mahi | 390 | 17 | 8 |
| Simply Grilled Mahi | 225 | 4 | 1 |
| Tilapia, with Pure Lump Crab Meat | 465 | 22 | 10 |

*Surf Add-Ons:*

| | C | F | Cb |
|---|---|---|---|
| Coconut Shrimp | 365 | 17 | 41 |
| Grilled Shrimp | 170 | 11 | 4 |

*Under 600 Calories:* Per Total Meal

| | C | F | Cb |
|---|---|---|---|
| Ahi Sesame Salad, full | 250 | 8 | 15 |
| Crab & Avocado Stack | 580 | 37 | 43 |
| Perfectly Gr. Salmon, w/ Veggies | 535 | 35 | 17 |

*Salads:* Without Dressing

| | C | F | Cb |
|---|---|---|---|
| Blue Cheese Pecan Chopped | 340 | 17 | 39 |
| Blue Cheese Wedge Salad | 340 | 17 | 39 |
| Caesar Side Salad | 95 | 5 | 11 |
| Sesame Salad | 250 | 8 | 15 |
| *Soup,* Clam Chowder, 1 Bowl | 700 | 45 | 46 |

*Sides:* As Per Menu Description

| | C | F | Cb |
|---|---|---|---|
| Aussie Fries | 320 | 16 | 40 |
| Blue Cheese Pecan Chopped Salad | 325 | 15 | 37 |
| Broccoli & Cheese | 380 | 30 | 14 |
| Classic Blue Cheese Wedge Salad | 110 | 6 | 58 |
| Fresh Seasonal Mixed Veggies | 150 | 9 | 15 |
| Garlic Mashed Potatoes | 275 | 15 | 30 |
| Loaded Mashed Potatoes | 350 | 19 | 33 |
| Sweet Potato, w/ Butter & Sugar | 290 | 2 | 63 |

*Desserts:* Per Whole Dish

| | C | F | Cb |
|---|---|---|---|
| Chocolate Thunder | 1560 | 106 | 138 |
| NY Style Cheesecake | 1410 | 96 | 120 |
| Triple Layer Carrot Cake | 1285 | 68 | 174 |

*Mini Milkshakes,*

| | C | F | Cb |
|---|---|---|---|
| Chocolate | 600 | 38 | 58 |

For Complete Menu & Data ~ see CalorieKing.com

## Panda Express® (Aug '16)

*Appetizers:*

| | C | F | Cb |
|---|---|---|---|
| Chicken Egg Roll (1), 2.75 oz | 200 | 10 | 20 |
| Chicken Potsticker (3), 3.3 oz | 160 | 6 | 20 |
| Cream Cheese Rangoon (3), 2.4 oz | 190 | 8 | 24 |
| Crispy Shrimp (3), 1.8 oz | 130 | 6 | 13 |
| Veggie Spring Rolls (2), 3.4 oz | 190 | 8 | 27 |

*Continued Next Page...*

## Panda Express® cont... (Aug '16)

*Entrées:*

| | C | F | Cb |
|---|---|---|---|
| **Beef:** Beijing Beef, 5.6 oz | 470 | 26 | 46 |
| Broccoli Beef, 5.4 oz | 150 | 7 | 13 |
| Shanghai Angus Beef, 5.4 oz | 310 | 19 | 16 |
| **Chicken Breast:** | | | |
| String Bean, 5.6 oz | 190 | 9 | 13 |
| Sweet & Sour, 5.8 oz | 300 | 12 | 40 |
| SweetFire, 5.8 oz | 380 | 15 | 47 |
| **Shrimp:** Crispy Shrimp (6), 3.5 oz | 260 | 13 | 26 |
| Honey Walnut Shrimp, 3.7 oz | 360 | 23 | 35 |

*Sides: Per Serving*

| | C | F | Cb |
|---|---|---|---|
| Chow Mein, 9.4 oz | 510 | 22 | 65 |
| Fried Rice, 9.3 oz | 520 | 16 | 85 |
| Steamed White Rice, 8.1 oz | 380 | 0 | 87 |

## Panera Bread® (Aug '16)

*Bagels:*

| | C | F | Cb |
|---|---|---|---|
| Asiago Cheese | 330 | 6 | 55 |
| Cinnamon Crunch | 430 | 7 | 81 |

*Breakfast Sandwiches, Grilled:*

| | C | F | Cb |
|---|---|---|---|
| Bacon, Egg & Cheese on Ciabatta | 520 | 25 | 44 |
| Sausage, Egg & Cheese on Ciabatta | 560 | 29 | 44 |
| Steak & Egg on Everthing Bagel | 540 | 18 | 59 |

*Sandwiches: Per Full Sandwich*

| | C | F | Cb |
|---|---|---|---|
| Bacon Turkey Bravo on Tomato Basil | 780 | 26 | 83 |
| Medit. Veggie on Tomato Basil | 560 | 12 | 94 |
| Napa Almond Chicken Salad, on Sesame Semolina | 700 | 26 | 90 |
| Sierra Turkey, on Asiago Cheese Foccacia | 730 | 26 | 81 |
| Smoked Turkey Breast on Country | 440 | 3.5 | 68 |
| Smoked Ham & Swiss on Rye | 610 | 18 | 67 |
| Flatbread: BBQ Chicken (1) | 370 | 16 | 40 |
| Tomato Mozzarella (1) | 340 | 18 | 34 |

*Paninis: Per Full Panini*

| | C | F | Cb |
|---|---|---|---|
| Frontega Chicken on Focaccia | 750 | 24 | 85 |
| Roasted Turkey & Caramelized Kale | 590 | 22 | 58 |
| **Pasta:** Chkn Tortellini Alfredo, 2 cups | 740 | 39 | 68 |
| Mac & Cheese, small | 490 | 30 | 38 |
| Tortellini Alfredo, 2 cups | 680 | 38 | 65 |

*Salads: Full Size, with Dressing, without Bread*

| | C | F | Cb |
|---|---|---|---|
| BBQ Chicken | 450 | 20 | 37 |
| Chicken Caesar | 420 | 25 | 16 |
| Chinese Citrus Cashew & Chicken | 540 | 27 | 45 |
| Greek | 400 | 36 | 13 |
| Strawberry Poppyseed with Chkn | 340 | 13 | 31 |

## Panera Bread® cont... (Aug '16)

*Soups: Per Bowl, w/o Bread*

| | C | F | Cb |
|---|---|---|---|
| Baked Potato | 330 | 20 | 33 |
| Broccoli Cheddar | 350 | 23 | 22 |
| Cream of Chicken & Wild Rice | 260 | 16 | 27 |
| New England Clam Chowder | 520 | 42 | 29 |
| Vegetarian Creamy Tomato | 310 | 20 | 31 |
| **Cake:** Cinn. Crumb Coffee, 1 slice | 470 | 25 | 53 |
| Strawberry Rhubarb Mini Cake | 250 | 7 | 45 |
| **Cookies:** Flip Flop (1) | 430 | 21 | 58 |
| Oatmeal Raisin, 3.3 oz | 400 | 14 | 62 |

*Pastries & Sweets:*

| | C | F | Cb |
|---|---|---|---|
| Bear Claw, 4.5 oz | 570 | 28 | 69 |
| Cobblestone, 7 oz | 560 | 12 | 103 |
| Pecan Roll (1) | 740 | 39 | 89 |
| **Muffins:** Apple Crunch, 5 oz | 450 | 12 | 80 |
| Chocolate Chip Muffie | 320 | 14 | 46 |
| Pumpkin | 580 | 22 | 90 |

## Papa Gino's® (Aug '16)

*Appetizers: Per Small Serving*

| | C | F | Cb |
|---|---|---|---|
| BBQ Chicken Tender (2), 5.2 oz | 360 | 18 | 33 |
| Buffalo Chicken Tender (2), 5.4 oz | 390 | 25 | 22 |
| Cheese Breadsticks, 4.23 oz | 260 | 8 | 35 |
| Chicken Tender (2), 4.4 oz | 350 | 20 | 24 |
| **Burgers:** Cheeseburger, 6.7 oz | 570 | 32 | 37 |
| Classic Double, 12.8 oz | 1040 | 67 | 43 |
| Hamburger, 6.3 oz | 520 | 28 | 36 |
| **French Fries,** small, 5 oz | 230 | 10 | 33 |

*Pastas: r*

| | C | F | Cb |
|---|---|---|---|
| Mac & Cheese, 17.8 oz | 1040 | 60 | 87 |
| Ravioli, 12.4 oz | 560 | 21 | 67 |
| Spaghetti & Meatballs, 19.8 oz | 780 | 28 | 109 |

*Pizzas:*

**Thin Crust:** *Per slice, ⅛ of Large Pizza*

| | C | F | Cb |
|---|---|---|---|
| Boss BBQ Chicken | 320 | 12 | 38 |
| Cheese | 230 | 7 | 32 |
| Meat Combo | 330 | 16 | 32 |
| PapRoni | 340 | 16 | 32 |
| Pepperoni | 280 | 11 | 32 |
| Super Veggie | 250 | 8 | 35 |
| Works | 330 | 14 | 34 |

*Subs: Per Small Sub*

| | C | F | Cb |
|---|---|---|---|
| BLT | 690 | 35 | 67 |
| Italian | 590 | 24 | 64 |
| Meatball Parmesan | 790 | 38 | 79 |
| Steak & Cheese | 710 | 33 | 63 |
| Super Steak | 750 | 33 | 72 |
| Tuna | 730 | 39 | 64 |
| Turkey Club | 600 | 22 | 67 |

## Papa John's® (Aug '16)

**Pizzas:**

| | C | F | Cb |
|---|---|---|---|
| **Original Crust (14"):** *Per ⅛ of Large 14" Pizza* | | | |
| Chicken Margherita | 320 | 11 | 39 |
| Double Bacon 6 Cheese | 350 | 14 | 38 |
| Greek | 360 | 14 | 39 |
| Philly Cheesesteak | 360 | 17 | 38 |
| Spicy Italian, 5.25 oz | 380 | 18 | 38 |
| Spinach Alfredo, 4 oz | 280 | 10 | 36 |
| The Meats, 3.8 oz | 380 | 17 | 39 |
| The Works, 5.5 oz | 360 | 14 | 39 |
| **Thin Crust (14"):** *Per ⅛ of Large 14" Pizza* | | | |
| Chicken Margherita | 250 | 12 | 21 |
| Double Bacon 6 Cheese | 290 | 16 | 22 |
| Greek | 280 | 16 | 21 |
| Philly Cheesesteak | 290 | 18 | 20 |
| Spicy Italian, 4 oz | 310 | 20 | 21 |
| Spinach Alfredo, 2.8 oz | 210 | 11 | 18 |
| The Meats, 3.8 oz | 300 | 19 | 21 |
| The Works, 4.3 oz | 290 | 15 | 21 |

**Wings:** *Without Dipping Sauce*

| | C | F | Cb |
|---|---|---|---|
| BBQ, 2 wings, 3 oz | 220 | 14 | 5 |
| Spicy Buffalo, 2 wings, 3 oz | 210 | 14 | 2 |

**Dipping Sauces:** *Per 1 oz Container*

| | C | F | Cb |
|---|---|---|---|
| Barbeque | 45 | 0 | 11 |
| Blue Cheese | 160 | 16 | 1 |
| Buffalo | 15 | 0.5 | 2 |
| Ranch | 100 | 10 | 1 |

**Sides:**

| | C | F | Cb |
|---|---|---|---|
| Breadsticks (2) | 300 | 4.5 | 55 |
| Cheesesticks (4) | 460 | 20 | 51 |
| Papa's Chicken Poppers (5) | 180 | 7 | 15 |

## Papa Murphy's® (Aug '16)

**Pizzas:**

| | C | F | Cb |
|---|---|---|---|
| **Original Crust:** *Per ½ of Family Size Pizza* | | | |
| BBQ Chicken | 350 | 13 | 37 |
| Chicken Garlic | 340 | 15 | 30 |
| Cowboy | 370 | 19 | 32 |
| Gourmet Vegetarian | 320 | 16 | 32 |
| Murphy's Combo | 350 | 18 | 33 |
| Papa's Favorite | 350 | 17 | 33 |
| Pepperoni | 300 | 14 | 31 |
| Rancher | 320 | 14 | 32 |
| Spicy Fennel Sausage | 350 | 16 | 35 |
| Taco Granee, Chicken | 320 | 12 | 34 |
| Thai Chicken | 350 | 12 | 40 |
| **Stuffed Pizzas:** *Per 1⁄16 of Family Size Pizza* | | | |
| 5 Meat | 460 | 18 | 52 |
| Big Murphy | 450 | 18 | 53 |
| Chicago Style | 450 | 18 | 52 |
| Chicken and Bacon | 450 | 17 | 51 |

## Papa Murphy's® cont... (Aug '16)

**Pizzas (Cont):**

| | C | F | Cb |
|---|---|---|---|
| **Thin Crust:** *Per ⅛ of Large Pizza* | | | |
| All Meat | 230 | 13 | 18 |
| Hawaiian | 180 | 7 | 20 |
| Murphy's Combo | 240 | 13 | 19 |
| Pepperoni | 220 | 12 | 18 |
| Rancher | 210 | 10 | 19 |

**Salads:** *Per Whole Salad, w/out Dressing or Croutons*

| | C | F | Cb |
|---|---|---|---|
| Club, 13 oz | 290 | 17 | 12 |
| Garden, 14.5 oz | 190 | 11 | 15 |
| Italian, 13 oz | 260 | 19 | 13 |

## Pei Wei Asian Diner (Aug '16)

**Perfect Additions:** *Without Sauce*

| | C | F | Cb |
|---|---|---|---|
| Crab Wontons (4) | 340 | 20 | 26 |
| Crispy Potstickers (4) | 300 | 16 | 25 |
| Traditional Edamame, small | 160 | 7 | 10 |
| Vegetable Spring Rolls (4) | 460 | 20 | 52 |
| **Sauces:** Potsticker, 2 oz | 35 | 1.5 | 3 |
| Sweet Chile, 2 oz | 140 | 0 | 34 |
| Thai Peanut Dipping Sauce, 2 oz | 230 | 15 | 20 |

**Lettuce Wraps:** *With Sauce*

| | C | F | Cb |
|---|---|---|---|
| Thai Chicken | 540 | 30 | 31 |
| Traditional Chicken | 720 | 36 | 66 |
| Sauce, 2 oz | 70 | 3.5 | 4 |

**Wok Fresh Classic Entrées:** *Per Small Serving without Sides*

| | C | F | Cb |
|---|---|---|---|
| Honey Seared: with Chicken | 720 | 30 | 83 |
| with Shrimp | 660 | 28 | 80 |
| with Steak | 730 | 31 | 83 |
| Reglar: | | | |
| with Chicken | 1030 | 44 | 112 |
| with shrimp | 980 | 46 | 109 |
| with Steak | 1020 | 45 | 110 |
| **Pei Wei Spicy:** | | | |
| with Chicken | 600 | 21 | 80 |
| with Steak | 780 | 30 | 111 |
| **Sweet & Sour:** | | | |
| with Chicken | 480 | 19 | 59 |
| with Shrimp | 430 | 18 | 56 |
| with Steak | 490 | 20 | 59 |

**Wok Classics Noodle Bowls:** *Small, includes Noodles*

| | C | F | Cb |
|---|---|---|---|
| Lo Mein Chicken | 760 | 26 | 92 |
| Lo Mein Shrimp | 640 | 21 | 90 |
| Lo Mein Steak | 700 | 24 | 91 |
| Pad Thai Vegetables & Tofu | 1230 | 33 | 167 |
| **Add Ons:** Egg Noodles, regular | 450 | 8 | 79 |
| Fried Rice, regular | 630 | 20 | 93 |
| White Rice, 8 oz | 290 | 0 | 65 |

## Pepe's Mexican® ~ see CalorieKing.com

Updated Nutrition Data ~ www.CalorieKing.com
Persons with Diabetes ~ See Disclaimer (Page 22)

## Perkins® (Aug '16)

*Breakfast:* With all components  **C**  **F**  **Cb**

| | C | F | Cb |
|---|---|---|---|
| **Classic:** Eggs Benedict | 1220 | 54 | 148 |
| Country Fried Steak & Eggs | 1100 | 60 | 93 |
| Eggs & Bacon | 670 | 40 | 48 |
| Steak Medallions & Eggs | 910 | 44 | 60 |
| **Griddle Greats:** | | | |
| Belgian Waffle | 470 | 23 | 57 |
| Belgian Waffle Platter, with Bacon | 680 | 42 | 53 |
| Blueb. Pancakes (3), w/- Syrup | 700 | 26 | 106 |
| Brioche French Toast Platter, with Bacon, 2 slices toast | 700 | 35 | 66 |
| Cinn. Roll French Toast Platter | 870 | 51 | 71 |
| Ooh-la-la French Toast & Bacon | 720 | 39 | 54 |
| Potato Pancakes (3) | 990 | 43 | 130 |
| The Buttermilk Five | 780 | 35 | 101 |
| The Buttermilk Pancake, Short Stack | 510 | 25 | 61 |
| **Pancake Syrup,** 2 oz | 140 | 0 | 35 |
| **Omelets:** *Without Optional Sides* | | | |
| Everything | 550 | 40 | 14 |
| Farmers | 660 | 54 | 8 |
| Granny's Country, without hashbrowns | 510 | 38 | 11 |
| **Hearty Extras:** | | | |
| Breakfast Potatoes, 5 oz | 250 | 12 | 32 |
| English Muffin, w/ butter, 2.7 oz | 230 | 11 | 28 |
| Fresh Cut Fruit, 4 oz | 70 | 0 | 19 |
| Hash Browns, 4 oz | 490 | 13 | 87 |
| Oatmeal, w/ 2% Milk & Br. Sugar | 330 | 6 | 60 |
| Sausage Links (4) | 460 | 44 | 2 |
| **Burgers:** *With Standard Toppings w/out Fruit Cup* | | | |
| BBQ Bacon Supreme | 1070 | 62 | 76 |
| Classic Burger | 710 | 42 | 44 |
| Classic Cheeseburger | 870 | 56 | 45 |
| The Beef Tangler | 1040 | 69 | 56 |
| **Melt:** *With Standard Toppings, without Fruit Cup* | | | |
| Chicken Strips, on Sourdough | 1290 | 80 | 88 |
| Patty Melt | 1170 | 80 | 60 |
| **Sandwiches:** *With Standard Toppings, w/o Fruit Cup* | | | |
| BLT, half | 320 | 22 | 20C |
| Classic Chicken Breast | 670 | 33 | 45 |
| Roast Turkey | 490 | 17 | 45 |
| Ultimate Club | 950 | 55 | 63 |

## Perkins® cont... (Aug '16)

*Lunch & Dinners:*  **C**  **F**  **Cb**

**Fork Worthy Entrées:** With Menu Set Sides Unless Indicated

| | C | F | Cb |
|---|---|---|---|
| Chicken Pot Pie, without sides | 1380 | 92 | 84 |
| Chicken Strips Dinner | 940 | 52 | 68 |
| Country Fried Steak Dinner | 710 | 41 | 55 |
| Fish 'n Chips, with Tartaire Sce, without sides | 1370 | 87 | 107 |
| Grilled Pork Chops | 920 | 48 | 58 |
| Grilled Salmon | 430 | 29 | 2 |
| Steak Medallions & Mushrooms | 620 | 37 | 16 |
| Turkey & Dressing, w/- Cranb Sce | 670 | 29 | 59 |
| *Sides:* | | | |
| Baked Potato, Loaded | 620 | 20 | 42 |
| Buttered Corn | 150 | 8 | 17 |
| French Fries, 7 oz | 570 | 36 | 56 |
| Green Beans & Bacon, 4 oz | 45 | 2.5 | 4 |
| Macaroni & Five Cheese, 5.2 oz | 300 | 16 | 26 |
| Mashed Potatoes, 4 oz | 120 | 3.5 | 19 |
| Add Brown Gravy, 2 oz | 50 | 4 | 3 |
| Sauteed Spinach, 4 oz | 70 | 3.5 | 4 |
| Side Salad with Croutons, and Ranch Dressing, 6.5 oz | 300 | 25 | 15 |
| Vegetable Medley, 4 oz | 110 | 8 | 6 |
| *Soups:* Per Bowl, Includes Crackers | | | |
| Homestyle Chicken Noodle | 260 | 6 | 37 |
| Tomato Basil | 460 | 26 | 46 |
| *Salads:* Includes Dinner Roll & Dressing | | | |
| Honey Mustard Chicken Crunch with Honey Mustard Dressing | 1030 | 67 | 66 |
| *Dessert:* | | | |
| **Muffins:** *Includes Whipped Butter Blend* | | | |
| Apple Cinnamon | 570 | 31 | 66 |
| Banana Nut | 700 | 40 | 78 |
| Blueberry | 600 | 31 | 72 |
| *Pies:* Per Slice | | | |
| Caramel Apple, 7.2 oz | 500 | 22 | 68 |
| Cherry | 580 | 27 | 75 |
| Lem. Meringue, 7 oz | 500 | 17 | 80 |
| Southern Pecan, 5.5 oz | 670 | 33 | 86 |
| Wildberry, no sugar added, 7 oz | 470 | 27 | 50 |

## Peter Piper Pizza® (Aug '16)

| Appetizers: | C | F | Cb |
|---|---|---|---|
| **Boneless Wings:** *Per 10 oz Serving* | | | |
| Mild Buffalo | 1010 | 67 | 56 |
| Sweet BBQ | 1130 | 58 | 110 |
| Cheddar Bacon Roll (1) | 350 | 18 | 34 |
| Garlic Cheese Bread, 3.25 oz | 390 | 17 | 45 |
| Handmade Breadsticks, with Marinara Sauce (6) | 1000 | 9 | 198 |

| Dipping Sauces: | | | |
|---|---|---|---|
| BBQ | 240 | 0 | 60 |
| Buffalo | 120 | 9 | 6 |
| Ranch | 320 | 36 | 2 |
| Sweet Chili | 200 | 0 | 46 |
| Xtra Hot Buffalo | 90 | 6 | 5 |

| Signature Pizzas: | | | |
|---|---|---|---|
| **Original Crust:** *Per ⅛ of Large 14" Pizza* | | | |
| 5 Meat Supreme | 390 | 18 | 39 |
| Buffalo Ranch | 400 | 20 | 37 |
| California Veggie | 290 | 9 | 41 |
| Cheddar & Bacon | 540 | 28 | 45 |
| Cheese | 310 | 11 | 39 |
| Chicago Classic | 330 | 12 | 40 |
| Double Pepperoni Parmesan | 310 | 15 | 27 |
| Extreme Pepperoni | 260 | 13 | 26 |
| New York 3 Cheese w/ Pepperoni | 480 | 25 | 40 |
| Pizza Mexicana | 390 | 18 | 39 |
| The Werx | 340 | 14 | 40 |
| **Original Crust:** *Per ½12 of Extra Large 16" Pizza* | | | |
| 5 Meat Supreme | 340 | 16 | 34 |
| Buffalo Ranch | 340 | 17 | 32 |
| California Veggie | 250 | 7 | 36 |
| Cheddar & Bacon | 480 | 25 | 39 |
| Cheese | 270 | 9 | 33 |
| Chicago Classic | 290 | 11 | 35 |
| Double Pepperoni Parmesan | 400 | 19 | 35 |
| Extreme Pepperoni | 340 | 16 | 34 |
| New York 3 Cheese w/ Pepperoni | 410 | 21 | 34 |
| Pizza Mexicana | 340 | 15 | 34 |
| The Werx | 290 | 11 | 35 |

| Salads: *without Dressing* | | | |
|---|---|---|---|
| Apple Harvest with Walnuts | 270 | 16 | 27 |
| Caesar, small | 320 | 14 | 35 |
| Chopped House, small | 210 | 6 | 35 |
| Mandarin Cranberry, small | 150 | 6 | 26 |

| Dessert: | | | |
|---|---|---|---|
| Cinnamon Crunch, 3 pieces | 380 | 9 | 69 |
| Vanilla Soft Serve: Cone | 200 | 6 | 35 |
| Cup | 180 | 6 | 31 |

## P.F. Chang's® (Aug '16)

| Small Plates: *Per Whole Dish* | C | F | Cb |
|---|---|---|---|
| Chicken Satay | 420 | 22 | 21 |
| Chang's BBQ Spare Ribs | 1210 | 64 | 62 |
| Chang's Vegetarian Lettuce Wraps | 470 | 21 | 39 |
| Crispy Green Beans, small | 690 | 58 | 37 |
| Dynamite Shrimp | 490 | 39 | 26 |
| Kale & Quinoa Dip | 280 | 6 | 43 |
| Jicama Lobster & Shrimp | 380 | 30 | 13 |
| Northern Style spare Ribs | 1130 | 63 | 41 |
| Orange Ginger Edamame | 420 | 19 | 33 |

| Entrées: | | | |
|---|---|---|---|
| **Beef:** *Per Whole Meal, without Rice* | | | |
| A La Sichuan | 810 | 35 | 77 |
| Beef with Broccoli | 710 | 37 | 45 |
| Mongolian | 790 | 45 | 37 |
| Orange Peel Beef | 820 | 37 | 77 |
| Shaking | 770 | 47 | 44 |
| **Chicken:** *Per Whole Dish, without Rice* | | | |
| Almond Cashew | 730 | 29 | 57 |
| Cantonese-Style Lemon | 1190 | 43 | 133 |
| Chang's Spicy | 960 | 35 | 102 |
| Crispy Honey Chicken | 1200 | 48 | 130 |
| Korean BBQ Chicken Stir-Fry | 910 | 46 | 73 |
| Kung Pao | 1090 | 64 | 58 |
| Sesame Chicken | 990 | 36 | 102 |
| **Pork,** Sweeet & Sour | 740 | 24 | 104 |
| **Seafood:** *Per Whole Meal, without Rice* | | | |
| Asian Grilled Salmon | 600 | 35 | 15 |
| Chang's Lobster & Shrimp Rice | 1030 | 48 | 98 |
| Crispy Honey Shrimp | 1040 | 41 | 131 |
| Hunan-Style Hot Fish | 650 | 28 | 51 |
| Oolong Chilean Sea Bass | 630 | 37 | 36 |
| Orange Peel Shrimp | 820 | 37 | 77 |
| Salt & Pepp. Prawns | 650 | 32 | 45 |
| Sauce, 2 oz | 70 | 1.5 | 13 |
| Walnut Shrimp with Melon | 1420 | 113 | 69 |

| Happy Hour: | | | |
|---|---|---|---|
| California Roll | 350 | 9 | 52 |
| Chang's Chicken Lettuce Wraps | 580 | 29 | 48 |
| Jicama Kung Pao Chicken Tacos | 370 | 24 | 17 |
| Jicama Pork Tacos | 320 | 19 | 23 |
| Spicy Tuna Roll | 280 | 3 | 43 |

*Continued Next Page...*

**226**

## P.F. Chang's® cont... (Aug '16)

*Entrées Cont:*

| | C | F | Cb |
|---|---|---|---|
| **Vegetarian Plates:** *without Rice* | | | |
| Buddha's Feast, steamed | 250 | 4 | 32 |
| Coconut Curry Vegetables | 1270 | 90 | 73 |
| Ma Po Tofu | 950 | 62 | 61 |
| Stir-Fried Eggplant | 480 | 23 | 65 |
| **Noodles & Rice:** Fried Rice w/ Beef | 960 | 17 | 156 |
| Garlic Noodles | 760 | 11 | 147 |
| Lo Mein Pork | 790 | 25 | 107 |
| Pad Thai Combo | 1090 | 23 | 159 |
| Singapore Street Noodles | 920 | 24 | 130 |
| **Sides:** *Per Small Dish* | | | |
| Brown Rice, 6 oz | 190 | 0 | 40 |
| Sichuan-Style Asparagus, small | 70 | 4 | 8 |
| Shanghai Cucumbers | 70 | 3 | 7 |
| Spinach with Garlic | 120 | 8 | 8 |
| White Rice, 6 oz | 220 | 0 | 49 |
| **Salad:** Crisp Salad with Seared Ahi | 690 | 53 | 30 |
| Lemongrass Chicken Salad | 660 | 40 | 55 |
| Waldorf Salad | 630 | 51 | 36 |
| Waldorf Salad with Chicken | 740 | 54 | 37 |
| **Dessert:** Apple Chai Cobbler, small | 310 | 10 | 54 |
| Banana Sprimg Rolls | 1030 | 42 | 152 |
| Berry Ginger Shortcake, small | 500 | 38 | 37 |
| New York Style Cheese Cake | 890 | 57 | 82 |
| The Great Wall of Chocolate | 1490 | 72 | 209 |

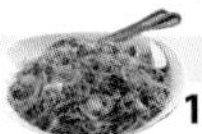

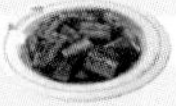

## Pita Pit® ~ *See CalorieKing.com*

## Pizza Hut® (Aug '16)

| | C | F | Cb |
|---|---|---|---|
| **Hand-Tossed Style:** *Per ⅛ of Medium 12" Pizza* | | | |
| Cheese | 210 | 8 | 25 |
| Chicken-Bacon Parmesan | 230 | 9 | 25 |
| Meat Lover's | 280 | 15 | 25 |
| Pepperoni | 220 | 9 | 25 |
| Pepperoni Lover's | 270 | 13 | 25 |
| Primo Meats | 280 | 14 | 25 |
| Supreme | 240 | 10 | 26 |
| Ultimate Cheese Lover's | 230 | 10 | 25 |
| Veggie Lover's | 190 | 7 | 26 |
| **Original Pan:** *Per ⅛ of Medium 12" Pizza* | | | |
| Cheese | 240 | 10 | 27 |
| Meat Lover's | 310 | 17 | 27 |
| Pepperoni | 260 | 12 | 27 |
| Pepperoni Lover's | 300 | 16 | 28 |
| Premium Garden Veggie | 230 | 9 | 29 |
| Supreme | 260 | 12 | 28 |
| Ultimate Cheese Lover's | 260 | 13 | 27 |
| Veggie Lover's | 220 | 9 | 28 |

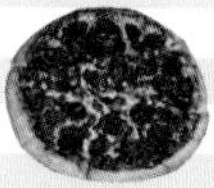

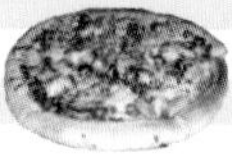

## Pizza Hut® cont... (Aug '16)

| | C | F | Cb |
|---|---|---|---|
| **Personal Pan:** *Per ¼ Slice of Pizza* | | | |
| BBQ Bacon Cheeseburger | 190 | 9 | 19 |
| Meat Lover's | 210 | 12 | 17 |
| Pepperoni | 160 | 7 | 17 |
| Pepperoni Lover's | 180 | 9 | 17 |
| Primo Meats | 210 | 12 | 17 |
| Supreme | 180 | 9 | 17 |
| Ultimate Cheese Lover's | 170 | 8 | 17 |
| Veggie Lover's | 140 | 5 | 17 |
| **Regional Large Original Stuffed:** *Per ⅛ Large 14" Pizza* | | | |
| BBQ Beef | 380 | 17 | 39 |
| Chicken Supreme | 310 | 12 | 35 |
| Fiesta Taco Beef | 380 | 18 | 39 |
| Hawaiian Luau | 320 | 13 | 36 |
| Italian Trio | 360 | 18 | 35 |
| Super Supreme | 420 | 23 | 36 |
| Triple Meat Italiano | 370 | 18 | 35 |
| **Thin 'n Crispy:** *Per ⅛ of Medium 12" Pizza* | | | |
| Cheese | 180 | 7 | 22 |
| Chicken-Bacon Parmesan | 220 | 10 | 21 |
| Five Pepper Pepperoni | 190 | 7 | 23 |
| Meat Lover's | 260 | 14 | 22 |
| Pepperoni | 200 | 9 | 21 |
| Pepperoni Lover's | 250 | 13 | 22 |
| Supreme | 210 | 9 | 23 |
| Ultimate Cheese Lover's | 210 | 10 | 21 |
| Veggie Lover's | 170 | 6 | 23 |
| **Skinny Slice:** *Per ⅛ of Medium 12" Pizza* | | | |
| BBQ Bacon Cheeseburger | 270 | 11 | 32 |
| Bacon Spinach Alfredo | 230 | 10 | 26 |
| Italian Meatball | 220 | 8 | 27 |
| Supreme | 240 | 11 | 26 |
| **Pastas, Tuscani:** *Per ½ Pan* | | | |
| Creamy Chicken Alfredo | 510 | 26 | 47 |
| Meaty Marinara | 450 | 19 | 48 |
| **Sides:** Baked Wings (1), av. | 50 | 3.5 | 0.5 |
| Breadstick (1), without sauce | 140 | 4.5 | 19 |
| Garlic Bread, 1 piece | 140 | 8 | 15 |
| **Desserts:** Hot Cinnamon Apple Pie | 170 | 9 | 22 |
| Hershey's: Hot Choc. Brownie | 290 | 11 | 45 |
| Tstd S'mores Cookie, 1 slice | 240 | 10 | 33 |
| Ultimate Choc Chip Cookie (1) | 190 | 9 | 26 |

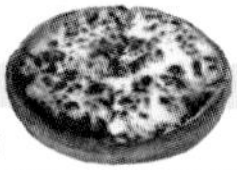

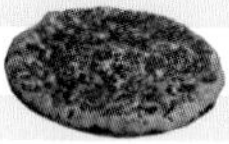

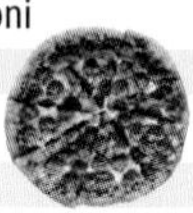

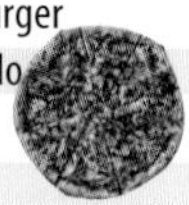

## Pizza Ranch® (Aug '16)

*Figures based on West Coast Outlets* **C** **F** **Cb**

*Pizza:*
**Breakfast,** average all varieties,

| | C | F | Cb |
|---|---|---|---|
| ⅛ of medium carry out pizza | 315 | 13 | 35 |

**Original Crust:** *Per ⅒ Slice of Medium Buffet Pizza*

| | C | F | Cb |
|---|---|---|---|
| Bacon Cheeseburger | 240 | 9 | 29 |
| BLT | 280 | 14 | 29 |
| Bronco | 250 | 10 | 29 |
| Buffalo Chicken | 240 | 9 | 28 |
| California Chicken | 260 | 11 | 28 |
| Chicken Bacon Ranch | 270 | 12 | 28 |
| Chicken Broccoli Alfredo | 230 | 8 | 28 |
| Garlic Cheese | 240 | 11 | 27 |
| Italian Sausage | 230 | 8 | 29 |
| Pepperoni | 240 | 9 | 29 |
| Prairie (Veggie) | 220 | 7 | 30 |
| Roundup | 240 | 9 | 30 |
| Stampede | 250 | 9 | 30 |
| Sweet Swine | 220 | 6 | 30 |
| Texan Taco | 270 | 9 | 37 |

**Thin Crust:** *Per ⅛ Slice of Medium Carry Out Pizza*

| | C | F | Cb |
|---|---|---|---|
| BBQ Chicken | 180 | 7 | 16 |
| Beef | 170 | 7 | 14 |
| BLT | 250 | 16 | 14 |
| Cheese | 190 | 9 | 14 |

*For Complete Menu & Data ~ see CalorieKing.com*

## Pollo Tropical® ~ *See CalorieKing.com*

## Popeye's® (Aug '16)

**Chicken Pieces:** *Mild & Spicy with Skin* **C** **F** **Cb**

| | C | F | Cb |
|---|---|---|---|
| Breast, average | 430 | 27 | 14 |
| Leg, average | 165 | 10 | 5 |
| Thigh, average | 270 | 20 | 8 |
| Wing | 210 | 14 | 8 |
| *Nuggets:* 4 pieces, 1.8 oz | 150 | 9 | 10 |
| 6 Pieces 2.7 oz | 230 | 14 | 14 |
| *Tenders:* Mild, 3 pieces, 4.5 oz | 340 | 14 | 26 |
| Spicy, 3 pieces, 4.5 oz | 310 | 15 | 16 |

*Sandwiches & Wraps: Each*

| | C | F | Cb |
|---|---|---|---|
| Blackened BBQ Chicken Po'Boy | 340 | 7 | 49 |
| Chicken & Sausage Jambalaya | 220 | 11 | 20 |
| Chicken Po'Boy | 660 | 34 | 61 |
| Loaded Chicken Wrap | 310 | 13 | 33 |
| Shrimp Po' Boy | 690 | 42 | 66 |
| *Seafood:* Catfish Fillets, 5 oz | 460 | 29 | 27 |
| Butterfly Shrimp (8) | 290 | 17 | 21 |
| Popcorn Shrimp, 3 oz | 330 | 9 | 28 |

## Popeye's®... cont (Aug '16)

*Sides:* **C** **F** **Cb**

| | C | F | Cb |
|---|---|---|---|
| Biscuit, 2 oz | 260 | 15 | 26 |
| Cajun Fries, regular, 3 oz | 260 | 14 | 30 |
| Cajun Rice, regular, 4.3 oz | 170 | 5 | 25 |
| Cole Slaw, regular, 4.9 oz | 220 | 15 | 19 |
| Corn on the Cob (1), 7.8 oz | 190 | 2 | 37 |
| Mashed Potatoes, regular, 5 oz | 110 | 4 | 18 |
| Onion Rings (12) | 560 | 38 | 50 |
| Red Beans & Rice, regular, 5.2 oz | 230 | 14 | 23 |

*Breakfast:*
**Biscuits:** Bacon

| | C | F | Cb |
|---|---|---|---|
| Bacon | 400 | 25 | 37 |
| Chicken | 490 | 26 | 47 |
| Egg | 510 | 29 | 41 |
| Egg & Sausage | 690 | 45 | 43 |
| Sausage | 540 | 36 | 41 |
| Sausage & Gravy | 510 | 33 | 42 |
| Grits | 370 | 5 | 80 |
| Hashbrowns | 360 | 20 | 41 |

*Desserts:*

| | C | F | Cb |
|---|---|---|---|
| Hot Sweet Potato Pie 3.4 oz | 350 | 19 | 41 |
| Mardi Gras Cheesecake, 3 oz | 310 | 19 | 32 |
| Mississippi Mud Pie, 3 oz | 280 | 7 | 51 |
| Sliced Pecan Pie, 3.4 oz | 410 | 21 | 52 |

## Port of Subs® (Aug '16)

*Figures Based on West Coast Outlets* **C** **F** **Cb**
*Cold Submarine S'wiches: Per 5" Sub with Cheese,
Lettuce, Tomato Vinegar, Oil, Salt & Oregano*

| | C | F | Cb |
|---|---|---|---|
| #1 Ham, Salami, Capicolla Pepperoni, Provolone | 475 | 22 | 43 |
| #2 Ham & Turkey, Provolone | 400 | 13 | 42 |
| #3 Salami & Turkey, Provolone | 440 | 18 | 43 |
| #4 Ham, Salami, Provolone | 425 | 18 | 42 |
| #5 Smoked Ham, Turkey, Cheddar | 405 | 14 | 43 |
| #6 Vegetarian, 3 Chse | 430 | 20 | 44 |
| #7 Roast Beef, Prov. | 400 | 14 | 42 |
| #8 Turkey, Provolone | 415 | 13 | 45 |
| #10 Rstd Chicken Breast, Provolone | 390 | 12 | 42 |
| #11 Ham, American Cheese | 470 | 22 | 44 |
| #12 Salami, Provolone | 435 | 20 | 42 |
| #13 Peppered Pastrami Turkey, Swiss | 410 | 15 | 43 |
| #15 Salami, Pepperoni, Provolone | 445 | 22 | 42 |
| #16 Chicken, Pepperoni, Pepper Jack | 350 | 14 | 41 |
| #17 Tuna, Provolone | 490 | 25 | 43 |
| #18 Roast Beef,Turkey, Provolone | 410 | 14 | 43 |

*Continued Next Page...*

**Updated Nutrition Data ~ www.CalorieKing.com
Persons with Diabetes ~ See Disclaimer (Page 22)**

## Port of Subs® ... cont (June'16)

*Figures Based on West Coast Outlets* **C** **F** **Cb**

*Wraps: With 12" Flour Tortilla, Cheese, Lettuce, Tomato, Onion, Vinegar, Oil, Salt & Oregano*

| | C | F | Cb |
|---|---|---|---|
| #2 Ham, Turkey, Provolone | 590 | 24 | 57 |
| # 8 Turkey Provolone | 610 | 24 | 60 |
| #11 Ham, with American Cheese | 740 | 38 | 60 |

*Fresh Salads: With Lettuce, Tomato & Onion, w/o Dressing*

| | C | F | Cb |
|---|---|---|---|
| Caesar: with Parmesan, 6 oz | 35 | 0 | 7 |
| Garden, 10 oz | 65 | 2 | 10 |
| Grilled Chicken, 10 oz | 235 | 4 | 11 |

*Salad Dressings:*

| | C | F | Cb |
|---|---|---|---|
| Blue Cheese, 1.5 oz | 220 | 23 | 2 |
| Ranch, 1.5 oz | 260 | 28 | 2 |
| Fat Free Ranch, 1.5 oz | 50 | 0 | 13 |

*Sides: Per Regular, 8 oz*

| | C | F | Cb |
|---|---|---|---|
| Caesar Bow Tie Pasta Salad, 8 oz | 355 | 18 | 37 |
| Potato Salad | 325 | 13 | 52 |

*Desserts:*

| | C | F | Cb |
|---|---|---|---|
| Brownie, 2.3 oz | 280 | 6 | 50 |
| Chocolate Chunk Cookie, 4 oz | 500 | 22 | 70 |
| Oatmeal Raisin Cookie, 4 oz | 460 | 20 | 68 |

*Fountain Beverages: Without Ice*

| | C | F | Cb |
|---|---|---|---|
| Coca Cola: 22 oz | 270 | 0 | 74 |
| 32 oz | 395 | 0 | 108 |
| Barq's Root Beer: 22 oz | 305 | 0 | 83 |
| 32 oz | 445 | 0 | 120 |
| Cherry Coke: 22 oz | 285 | 0 | 77 |
| 32 oz | 415 | 0 | 112 |

*Smoothies:*

| | C | F | Cb |
|---|---|---|---|
| Strawb. Bomb, 8 oz | 250 | 0 | 63 |
| Mand. Orange Passion Fruit, 8 oz | 240 | 1 | 59 |
| Average other flavors, 8 oz | 220 | 1 | 53 |

## Pret A Manger® (Aug'16)

*Baguettes:* **C** **F** **Cb**

| | C | F | Cb |
|---|---|---|---|
| Chicken Mozzarella,11 oz | 690 | 19 | 88 |
| Pret's Tuna & Cucumber, 11 oz | 710 | 28 | 84 |
| Roast Beef & Horseradish, 8.4 oz | 580 | 25 | 63 |

*Hot Food: Per Pack*

| | C | F | Cb |
|---|---|---|---|
| Baguettes: Southern BBQ Chicken | 680 | 12 | 95 |
| Turkey, Ham & Wisconsin Chedd | 660 | 28 | 63 |
| Burrito, Chicken | 660 | 24 | 72 |
| Spinach Tomato Mac & Cheese | 420 | 21 | 41 |
| Wrap, Falafel & Red Pepper | 580 | 25 | 69 |

## Pret A Manger® ... cont (Aug '16)

*Sandwiches:* **C** **F** **Cb**

| | C | F | Cb |
|---|---|---|---|
| Balsmc Chicken & Avocado, 8.5 oz | 480 | 25 | 40 |
| California Club, 9.4 oz | 390 | 17 | 39 |
| Chicken & Bacon, 7.9 oz | 480 | 27 | 35 |
| Classic Cheddar & Tomato. 7 oz | 430 | 25 | 35 |
| Pret's Tuna Salad, 8.7 oz | 460 | 29 | 32 |
| Turkey & Wisconsin Cheddar, 8.5 oz | 500 | 22 | 46 |

*Soups: Per Large Serve*

| | C | F | Cb |
|---|---|---|---|
| Carrot Ginger | 210 | 8 | 33 |
| Crmy Chicken & Veggie | 350 | 16 | 37 |
| Gazpacho, 8.5 oz | 90 | 5 | 9 |
| Moroccan Lentil | 380 | 17 | 45 |
| Tomato Feta, 12.6 oz | 230 | 14 | 23 |

*Salads: Without Dressing*

| | C | F | Cb |
|---|---|---|---|
| Chef, 11.8 oz | 280 | 15 | 14 |
| Chicken Avoc., 9.3 oz | 370 | 21 | 18 |
| Falafel Mezze, 13.5 oz | 330 | 14 | 36 |
| Kale Chicken Caesar, 10 oz | 400 | 14 | 18 |
| Maine Lobster, 7 oz | 140 | 7 | 7 |

*Dressings:*

| | C | F | Cb |
|---|---|---|---|
| Balsamic Vinaigrette | 140 | 15 | 2 |
| Caesar | 170 | 17 | 3 |
| Lemon Shallot Vinaigrette | 100 | 10 | 2 |
| Skinny Honey Dijon Vinaigrette | 50 | 0 | 10 |

*Bakery: Per Pack*

| | C | F | Cb |
|---|---|---|---|
| Croissants: Almond | 410 | 23 | 41 |
| Pain au Chocolate | 300 | 15 | 34 |
| Cookies: Carrot Cake, 2.5 oz | 270 | 14 | 35 |
| Chocolate Chunk, 2.5 oz | 320 | 15 | 41 |
| Harvest, 2.5 oz | 280 | 12 | 40 |
| Muffin, Blueberry, 4.5 oz | 420 | 16 | 63 |
| Yogurt Pots: Banana & Honey | 400 | 14 | 53 |
| Blueberry & Granola | 290 | 11 | 31 |

## Pretzelmaker® (Aug'16)

*Pretzels: Per Serving* **C** **F** **Cb**

| | C | F | Cb |
|---|---|---|---|
| Bites: Plain, salted, large, 3.5 oz | 250 | 1 | 52 |
| Cinnamon Sugar, 3.8 oz | 330 | 4 | 65 |
| Whole: Caramel Crunch, 4.2 oz | 300 | 4 | 58 |
| Cinnamon Sugar, 3.9 oz | 330 | 4 | 65 |
| Garlic; Salted, average, 4.2 oz | 310 | 4 | 60 |
| Iced Cinnamon Swirl, 3.9 oz | 330 | 4 | 65 |
| Ranch, 4.2 oz | 320 | 4.5 | 60 |
| Pretzel Dogs: Mini (6) | 300 | 19 | 23 |
| Jalapeno (1), 6.4 oz | 410 | 19 | 32 |

*Continued Next Page...*

## Pretzelmaker® cont... (Aug '16)

*Sauces:* Per Single Portion

| | C | F | Cb |
|---|---|---|---|
| Caramel | 140 | 0 | 35 |
| Cheddar Cheese | 80 | 5 | 4 |
| Cream Cheese | 200 | 20 | 2 |
| Honey Mustard | 80 | 0 | 20 |
| Icing | 180 | 0 | 45 |
| Ketchup | 20 | 0 | 4 |
| Mustard | 10 | 0 | 1 |
| Nacho Cheese | 80 | 5 | 4 |
| Pizza | 20 | 0.5 | 6 |

*Beverages:* Per 20 fl.oz Unless Indicated

**Blended Drinks:**

| | | C | F | Cb |
|---|---|---|---|---|
| Cool Cappuccino | | 640 | 21 | 107 |
| Lemon Twist | | 540 | 16 | 99 |
| Mango Madness | | 520 | 16 | 89 |
| Mocha Mania | | 620 | 20 | 106 |
| Power Pomegranate | | 490 | 16 | 86 |
| Strawberry Bananza | | 650 | 20 | 115 |
| **Lemonade:** Original, 20oz | | 230 | 0 | 59 |
| Strawberry; Raspberry, 20 oz | | 290 | 0 | 74 |

## Qdoba® (Apr '16)

| | C | F | Cb |
|---|---|---|---|

*Please Note: Nutritional Information is based on a single serving of each menu ingredient listed.*

*Burritos:* Each with 12.5" Flour Tortilla, Cilantro-Lime Rice, Black Beans, Salsa Verde, Lite Sour Cream, Lettuce and Shredded Cheese

| | C | F | Cb |
|---|---|---|---|
| Grilled Chicken | 1035 | 37 | 124 |
| Pulled Pork | 1025 | 34 | 130 |
| Seasoned Ground Beef | 1055 | 40 | 124 |

*Burritos:* With 12.5" Flour Tortilla, 3-Cheese Queso, Pinto Beans, Roasted Chili Corn Salsa, Guacamole & Lite Sour Cream

| | C | F | Cb |
|---|---|---|---|
| Grilled Chicken | 920 | 40 | 101 |
| Grilled Steak | 930 | 41 | 99 |
| Pulled Pork | 910 | 37 | 107 |
| Seasoned Ground Beef | 940 | 43 | 101 |

*Grilled Quesadillas:* With 12.5" Flour Tortilla, Shredded Cheese, Pico de Gallo and Fajita Vegetables

| | C | F | Cb |
|---|---|---|---|
| Grilled Chicken | 685 | 30 | 64 |
| Shredded Beef | 705 | 29 | 66 |

*3-Cheese Nachos:* Per Serving, with Tortilla Chips, 3-Cheese Queso, Salsa Roja, Guacamole & Sour Cream

| | C | F | Cb |
|---|---|---|---|
| Grilled Chicken | 1020 | 57 | 95 |
| Pulled Pork | 1010 | 54 | 101 |

## Qdoba® cont... (Apr '16)

*Knock Out Tacos:* Set Ingredients

| | C | F | Cb |
|---|---|---|---|
| Bohemian Veg | 230 | 9 | 28 |
| Drunken Yardbird | 220 | 8 | 25 |
| Mad Rancher | 230 | 10 | 21 |
| Two Timer | 290 | 13 | 28 |
| Triple Threat | 250 | 12 | 17 |
| The Gladiator | 280 | 17 | 16 |

*Taco Salads:* With Crunchy Flour Tortilla Bowl, Black Beans, Lettuce, Shredded Cheese, Brown Rice, Sour Cream, Guacamole & Cilantro Lime Dressing

| | C | F | Cb |
|---|---|---|---|
| Grilled Chicken | 1270 | 66 | 116 |
| Pulled Pork | 1260 | 63 | 122 |
| Seasoned Ground Beef | 1290 | 69 | 116 |

*Chips & Dip:* Includes Tortilla Chips

| | C | F | Cb |
|---|---|---|---|
| 3- Cheese Queso | 940 | 57 | 87 |
| 3-Cheese Queso, Guac. & Salsa Roja | 955 | 56 | 98 |

*Breakfast Burritos:* With Flour Tortilla

*Chorizo, Egg & Potato:*

| | C | F | Cb |
|---|---|---|---|
| with 3-Cheese Queso Sauce | 750 | 37 | 74 |
| with Shred. Chse & Salsa Roja | 850 | 45 | 76 |

## Quiznos Subs® (Aug '16)

*Subs:* Per 8" Regular Japaleno Cheddar Sub, with Standard Menu Toppings Unless Indicated

**All Natural Chicken:**

| | C | F | Cb |
|---|---|---|---|
| Baja | 800 | 37 | 65 |
| Carbonara | 880 | 46 | 63 |
| Honey Mustard | 850 | 41 | 69 |
| Mesquite | 800 | 38 | 62 |
| Pesto Caesar on Rosemary Parm | 740 | 33 | 61 |

**Steak:**

| | C | F | Cb |
|---|---|---|---|
| Black Angus Steak | | | |
| On Rosemary Parmesan | 770 | 29 | 76 |
| Chipotle Steak & Cheddar | 830 | 46 | 62 |
| Peppercorn Steak | 830 | 44 | 64 |
| Steak, Bacon & Swiss | 840 | 40 | 65 |

**Deli Classic:**

| | C | F | Cb |
|---|---|---|---|
| Classic Italian | 900 | 53 | 67 |
| Honey Bacon Club | 850 | 40 | 80 |
| Italian Meatball | 1110 | 59 | 86 |
| Spicy Monterey | 610 | 21 | 72 |
| The Traditional | 710 | 33 | 66 |
| Tuna | 760 | 37 | 67 |
| Veggie Guacamole | 760 | 43 | 68 |

*Grilled Flatbreads:* Per Menu Board Toppings

| | C | F | Cb |
|---|---|---|---|
| Basil Pesto Turkey | 380 | 18 | 31 |
| Classic Italian | 480 | 29 | 34 |
| Honey Mustard Chkn | 480 | 25 | 35 |
| Turkey Bacon Guacamole | 490 | 28 | 35 |

*Continued Next Page...*

Updated Nutrition Data ~ www.CalorieKing.com
Persons with Diabetes ~ See Disclaimer (Page 22)

## Quiznos Subs® cont... (Aug '16)

| | C | F | Cb |
|---|---|---|---|
| **Salads:** Per Full, without Dressing | | | |
| Apple Harvest Chicken | 390 | 16 | 41 |
| Honey Mustard Chicken | 290 | 14 | 7 |
| Peppercorn Caesar | 190 | 5 | 7 |
| **Savory Soups:** Per Regular Bowl, with 2 Crackers | | | |
| Broccoli Cheese | 180 | 9 | 17 |
| Chicken Noodle | 140 | 4.5 | 19 |
| **Breakfast:** | | | |
| **Subs:** Bacon, Egg & Cheddar | 470 | 24 | 38 |
| Ham, Egg & Cheddar | 360 | 13 | 39 |
| Sausage, Egg & Cheddar | 490 | 28 | 39 |
| **Desserts:** | | | |
| Chocolate Chunk Cookie | 390 | 19 | 54 |
| Chocolate Brownie | 310 | 16 | 40 |
| Cinnamon Sugar Cookie | 400 | 17 | 58 |
| Oatmeal Raisin Cookie | 360 | 12 | 58 |

## Rally's/Checkers® (Aug '16)

| | C | F | Cb |
|---|---|---|---|
| **Burgers/Sandwiches:** | | | |
| Baconzilla | 810 | 52 | 40 |
| Big Buford | 660 | 3 | 39 |
| Cheese Champ | 430 | 21 | 39 |
| Cheese Double | 480 | 25 | 38 |
| Rallyburger | 320 | 12 | 39 |
| **Classic Wings:** Buffalo, 5 pieces | 360 | 23 | 3 |
| Honey BBQ, 5 pieces | 430 | 23 | 19 |
| Garlic Parmesan, 5 pieces | 510 | 40 | 3 |
| **Fries:** | | | |
| Fries, medium | 500 | 24 | 63 |
| Chili Cheese | 590 | 30 | 72 |
| Fully Loaded | 640 | 44 | 51 |

## Ranch One® (Aug '16)

| | C | F | Cb |
|---|---|---|---|
| **Sandwiches:** | | | |
| Chicken & Cheese | 390 | 12 | 40 |
| Chkn Philly, 9.3 oz | 410 | 13 | 40 |
| Grilled Classic Chicken, 9.4 oz | 680 | 47 | 37 |
| Original Crispy Chicken, 11.5 oz | 870 | 56 | 72 |
| **Other Favorites:** | | | |
| Chicken Fajita, 10 oz | 540 | 24 | 53 |
| Chicken Platter, with Rice, 11.9 oz | 270 | 6 | 28 |
| Popcorn Chicken: Small, 5.5 oz | 310 | 10 | 30 |
| Large, 7.5 oz | 420 | 14 | 40 |
| Kids, 2 oz | 120 | 4 | 11 |
| **Salads:** Completed | | | |
| Grilled Chicken Caesar, 13.3 oz | 430 | 30 | 14 |
| Southwest Chicken, 17.5 oz | 680 | 43 | 44 |
| **Fries:** Medium, 5.8 oz | 380 | 19 | 43 |
| Kids, 4.3 oz | 280 | 14 | 31 |
| **Cheese:** Medium, 7.3 oz | 490 | 27 | 46 |
| Large, 11 oz | 760 | 44 | 66 |

## Red Hot & Blue® (Aug '16)

| | C | F | Cb |
|---|---|---|---|
| **Entrées:** Per Serving | | | |
| **Delta Double:** | | | |
| with Memphis Chicken | 900 | 54 | 12 |
| with Pulled Pork | 795 | 60 | 9 |
| Five Meat Treat | 935 | 63 | 15 |
| **Ribs, Half Slab:** Dry | 935 | 72 | 14 |
| Sweet | 950 | 71 | 22 |
| **Sandwiches:** Regular, without Sides | | | |
| Beef Brisket | 390 | 15 | 37 |
| Carolina Chopped Pork | 360 | 14 | 34 |
| Pulled Pork | 370 | 15 | 37 |
| **Salads:** Without Dressing | | | |
| Grilled Chicken Caesar Salad | 770 | 46 | 47 |
| Pulled Chicken Salad | 295 | 8 | 14 |
| Smokehouse Salad | 670 | 36 | 36 |
| Southern Fried Chicken Salad | 710 | 31 | 60 |
| **Soup,** Memphis Corn Chowder, 1 bowl | 270 | 12 | 23 |
| **Sides:** | | | |
| BBQ Beans | 255 | 2 | 48 |
| Mashed Potatoes with Gravy | 310 | 14 | 44 |
| Memphis Fries, 6 oz | 345 | 19 | 38 |
| Potato Salad | 405 | 28 | 33 |

## Red Lobster® (Aug '16)

| | C | F | Cb |
|---|---|---|---|
| **Seaside Starters:** | | | |
| Crispy Calamari & Vegetables | 1830 | 127 | 138 |
| Crispy Shrimp Lettuce Wraps | 620 | 18 | 93 |
| Lobster, Artich. & Seafood Dip | 1040 | 57 | 102 |
| Lobster & Langostino Pizza | 710 | 35 | 55 |
| Mozzarella Cheesesticks | 810 | 44 | 67 |
| Parrot Isle Jumbo Cocktail Shrimp | 610 | 39 | 52 |
| Seafood-Stuffed Mushrooms | 450 | 28 | 20 |
| Signature Shrimp Cocktail | 130 | 0 | 11 |
| Sweet Chili Shrimp | 1140 | 79 | 80 |
| **Lunch Entrées:** Includes Menu Set Sides, without Condiments or Dipping Sauces | | | |
| Cajun Chicken Linguini Alfredo, lunch | 720 | 34 | 56 |
| Crab Linguine Alfredo, lunch | 910 | 57 | 59 |
| Crunchy Popcorn Shrimp | 420 | 18 | 49 |
| Hand Battered Fish & Chips | 970 | 54 | 80 |
| Sailor's Platter | 480 | 19 | 18 |
| Shrimp Linguine Alfredo, lunch | 590 | 30 | 54 |
| Wild Caught Flounder/Sole, Fried | 520 | 36 | 21 |

Continued Next Page...

## Red Lobster® cont... (Aug '16)

*Dinner Entrées: Includes Menu Set Sides, without Condiments or Dipping Sauces.*

| | C | F | Cb |
|---|---|---|---|
| **Fish:** Hand Battered Fish & Chips | 970 | 54 | 80 |
| Parmesan-Crusted Tilapia | 660 | 37 | 20 |
| **Walleye:** Golden-Fried | 590 | 29 | 12 |
| Batter Fried | 1170 | 73 | 51 |
| **Live Main Lobster:** | | | |
| Roasted and Stuffed | 630 | 13 | 61 |
| Steamed | 730 | 38 | 40 |
| **Lighthouse/Fresh Fish Menu:** | | | |
| Garlic-Grilled Shrimp | 390 | 16 | 34 |
| Maple-Glazed Chicken | 370 | 5 | 53 |
| Wood-Grilled Peppercorn Sirloin & Shrimp | 520 | 18 | 36 |
| Parrot Isle Jumbo Coconut Shrimp | 960 | 61 | 78 |
| Rock Lobster Tail | 700 | 42 | 35 |
| Shrimp Linguini Alfredo, full | 1160 | 58 | 108 |
| Walt's Favorite Shrimp | 620 | 28 | 68 |
| **Soup:** *Per Cup* | | | |
| Creamy Potato & Bacon | 250 | 18 | 19 |
| Lobster & Langostino Bisque | 290 | 23 | 15 |
| New England Clam Chowder | 200 | 15 | 11 |
| **Side Dishes:** | | | |
| Baked Potato, Plain | 210 | 2 | 45 |
| Cheddar Bay Biscuit | 160 | 10 | 16 |
| Coleslaw | 260 | 20 | 17 |
| Creamy Lobster Mashed Potatoes | 370 | 24 | 28 |
| French Fries | 430 | 17 | 62 |
| Garden Salad, without dressing | 70 | 1.5 | 13 |
| Wild Rice Pilaf | 130 | 2.5 | 25 |
| **Salads:** *Includes Dressing* | | | |
| Caesar Salad: with Grilled Chicken | 640 | 48 | 19 |
| with Grilled Shrimp | 580 | 46 | 18 |
| **Sauces:** *Per Dinner Menu* | | | |
| 100% Pure Melted Butter | 300 | 33 | 0 |
| Cocktail Sauce | 45 | 0 | 11 |
| Honey Mustard Dipping Sauce | 190 | 17 | 8 |
| Marinara | 35 | 2 | 4 |
| **Desserts:** | | | |
| Chocolate Wave | 1100 | 62 | 133 |
| Key Lime Pie | 430 | 19 | 64 |
| New York-Style Cheesecake with Strawberries | 590 | 41 | 48 |
| Warm Apple Crostada | 650 | 32 | 82 |
| Warm Chocolate Chip Lava Cookie | 920 | 42 | 126 |

*For Complete Nutritional Data ~ see CalorieKing.com*

## Red Robin® (Aug '16)

*Nutritional Information varies between restaurants. Please refer to Red Robin's website for further information*

| *Appetizers:* | C | F | Cb |
|---|---|---|---|
| Chili Chili Con Queso | 650 | 34 | 51 |
| Creamy Artichoke & Spinach Dip | 685 | 41 | 52 |
| Guacamole, Salsa & Chips | 430 | 22 | 43 |
| Red's Tavern Fries | 1355 | 87 | 107 |
| Towering Onion Rings, w/ Ranch Dressing & Mayo | 1935 | 125 | 173 |
| Warm Pretzel Bites, w/ Beer Chse | 635 | 19 | 96 |
| *Jump Starters:* | | | |
| Jalepeno Coins, fried, w/out Dress. | 490 | 33 | 45 |
| Swt Potato Fries, w/out Dressing | 285 | 15 | 35 |
| Zucchini, Breaded & Fried, without Dressing | 215 | 15 | 17 |
| *Entrées:* *With Standard Menu Components* | | | |
| Arctic Cod Fish & Chips | 1050 | 65 | 74 |
| Clucks & Fries | 1320 | 78 | 102 |
| Ensenada Chicken Platter, 1 piece | 215 | 9 | 11 |
| Prime Rib Dip | 765 | 29 | 76 |
| Red's Nantucket Seafood Scatter | 1205 | 72 | 92 |
| *Finest Burgers:* Black & Bleu | 1115 | 69 | 65 |
| DGB | 1165 | 81 | 50 |
| Smoke & Pepper | 1030 | 51 | 74 |
| Southern Charm | 1220 | 61 | 98 |
| *Gourmet Burgers:* | | | |
| A.1. Peppercorn | 1365 | 82 | 93 |
| All American Patty Melt | 1175 | 80 | 72 |
| Bleu Ribbon | 1360 | 84 | 97 |
| Burnin' Love | 895 | 53 | 60 |
| Chili Chili Cheeseburger | 915 | 49 | 61 |
| Garden Burger | 550 | 23 | 72 |
| Guacamole Bacon | 990 | 61 | 50 |
| Keep It Simple | 625 | 33 | 47 |
| Prime Chophouse | 1385 | 83 | 105 |
| Red Robin Gourmet Cheeseburger | 835 | 51 | 48 |
| Royal Red Robin | 1205 | 83 | 47 |
| Sauteed Mushroom | 840 | 49 | 52 |
| Whiskey River BBQ | 1390 | 89 | 94 |
| *Sandwiches & Wraps:* | | | |
| BLTA Croissant | 695 | 39 | 45 |
| Caesars Chkn Wrap | 765 | 42 | 54 |
| Whiskey River BBQ Chicken Wrap | 995 | 54 | 68 |

*Continued Next Page... ...*

**Updated Nutrition Data ~ www.CalorieKing.com**
**Persons with Diabetes ~ See Disclaimer (Page 22)**

# Red Robin® cont... (Aug '16)

| Soups: | C | F | Cb |
|---|---|---|---|
| **Chicken Tortilla:** *Includes Tortilla Strips* | | | |
| 1 Cup | 205 | 11 | 17 |
| 1 Bowl | 410 | 20 | 35 |
| **Clam Chowder:** *Includes Croutons* | | | |
| 1 Cup | 250 | 16 | 19 |
| 1 Bowl | 470 | 31 | 34 |
| **French Onion:** *Includes Baguette, Au Jus & Croutons* | | | |
| 1 Cup | 200 | 13 | 13 |
| 1 Bowl | 465 | 25 | 40 |
| **Salads:** *wWthout Bread or Dressing* | | | |
| Avo-Cobb-O | 500 | 28 | 20 |
| Crispy Chicken Tender | 875 | 49 | 53 |
| Insane Romain | 510 | 25 | 50 |
| Spicy Sombrero | 620 | 40 | 32 |
| Whiskey Rio BBQ Chicken | 295 | 10 | 28 |
| **Desserts:** | | | |
| Gooey Chocolate Brownie Cake | 795 | 28 | 132 |
| Mountain High Mudd Pie | 1390 | 59 | 194 |
| **Milkshakes:** | | | |
| **Classic:** Banana | 530 | 21 | 77 |
| Chocolate | 535 | 21 | 77 |
| **Smoothie:** Groovy | 340 | 2 | 81 |
| Hawaiian Heart Throb | 375 | 2 | 91 |

# Roly Poly® (Aug '16)

| Wraps: | C | F | Cb |
|---|---|---|---|
| *Per 6" White Tortilla Unless Indicated* | | | |
| **Chicken:** Basil Cashew Chicken | 300 | 10 | 30 |
| Catalina Chicken | 315 | 11 | 28 |
| Chicken Caesar | 310 | 11 | 30 |
| Chicken Fajita | 315 | 9 | 28 |
| Cobb Salad | 255 | 12 | 27 |
| Oriental Chicken | 230 | 4 | 29 |
| Santa Fe Chicken | 305 | 11 | 28 |
| **Ham & Smoked Pork:** | | | |
| Italian Classic | 335 | 12 | 32 |
| Key West Cuban Mix | 330 | 9 | 44 |
| Peachtree Melt | 310 | 11 | 27 |
| Pork Melt | 310 | 11 | 26 |
| Porky's Nightmare | 320 | 12 | 28 |
| **Tuna:** Classic Tuna Melt | 340 | 17 | 26 |
| Popeyes Tuna on Wheat | 305 | 10 | 31 |
| Texas Tuna | 310 | 12 | 30 |
| Thai Hot Tuna | 290 | 11 | 30 |
| **Turkey:** California | 330 | 12 | 30 |
| Tuscan | 220 | 2 | 31 |

# Round Table Pizza® (Aug '16)

| Appetizers: | C | F | Cb |
|---|---|---|---|
| Boneless Wings: | | | |
| with BBQ Sauce, 8 pieces | 565 | 14 | 73 |
| with Buffalo Sauce, av., 8 pcs | 440 | 14 | 41 |
| Garlic Bread: 1 piece | 70 | 3.5 | 9 |
| with Cheese, 1 piece | 100 | 6 | 9 |
| Garlic Parmesan Twists, 1 twist | 170 | 5 | 26 |
| **Pizzas:** *Per ½ of Large 14" Pizza* | | | |
| **Original Crust:** Cheese | 230 | 9 | 25 |
| Chicken & Garlic Gourmet | 250 | 11 | 25 |
| Gourmet Veggie | 240 | 10 | 27 |
| Guinevere's Garden Delight | 220 | 8 | 26 |
| Hawaiian | 220 | 8 | 27 |
| Italian Garlic Supreme | 270 | 14 | 25 |
| King Arthur Supreme | 270 | 13 | 26 |
| Maui Zaui, with Polynesian Sce | 260 | 10 | 29 |
| Montague's All Meat Marvel | 290 | 15 | 25 |
| Smokehouse Combo, Chicken | 290 | 14 | 26 |
| Triple Play Pepperoni | 250 | 12 | 24 |
| **Pan Crust:** Cheese | 300 | 11 | 38 |
| Chicken & Garlic Gourmet | 340 | 13 | 39 |
| Gourmet Veggie | 320 | 12 | 41 |
| Guinevere's Garden Delight | 300 | 10 | 39 |
| Hawaiian | 300 | 10 | 40 |
| Italian Garlic Supreme | 360 | 16 | 39 |
| King Arthur Supreme | 340 | 14 | 39 |
| Maui Zaui w/ Polynesian Sauce | 340 | 12 | 43 |
| Montague's All Meat Marvel | 350 | 15 | 37 |
| Smokehouse Combo, Chicken | 370 | 16 | 40 |
| Triple Play Pepperoni | 330 | 14 | 36 |
| **Skinny Crust:** Cheese | 190 | 9 | 18 |
| Chicken & Garlic Gourmet | 220 | 11 | 18 |
| Gourmet Veggie | 200 | 10 | 20 |
| Guinevere's Garden Delight | 180 | 8 | 19 |
| Hawaiian | 190 | 8 | 20 |
| Italian Garlic Supreme | 240 | 14 | 18 |
| King Arthur Supreme | 240 | 13 | 19 |
| Maui Zaui w/ Polynesian Sauce | 220 | 10 | 22 |
| Montague's All Meat Marvel | 260 | 15 | 18 |
| Smokehouse Combo, Chicken | 250 | 14 | 20 |
| Triple Play Pepperoni | 220 | 12 | 17 |
| **Sandwiches:** | | | |
| Chicken Club | 800 | 43 | 59 |
| Ham Club | 740 | 40 | 60 |
| RT Veggie | 630 | 32 | 65 |
| Turkey Club | 720 | 38 | 59 |
| Turkey Sante-Fe | 730 | 40 | 57 |

*For Complete Nutritional Data ~ see CalorieKing.com*

## Rubio's Mexican Grill® (Aug '16)

*Burritos:* Each with Flour Tortilla, without Chips

| Beef: | C | F | Cb |
|---|---|---|---|
| Baja Grilled, with Steak | 690 | 33 | 56 |
| Especial, w/ Steak | 950 | 38 | 113 |
| **Chicken:** | | | |
| Baja Grilled, w/ Chkn | 640 | 28 | 59 |
| Especial, with Chicken | 860 | 31 | 106 |
| **Seafood:** Beer Battered Fish | 910 | 57 | 77 |
| Blackened Atlantic Salmon | 820 | 42 | 80 |
| Classic Grilled Shrimp | 730 | 35 | 74 |
| Grilled Pacific Mahi Mahi | 770 | 35 | 77 |
| **Veggies & More:** Bean & Cheese | 760 | 34 | 79 |
| Especial with Veggies | 870 | 36 | 120 |

*Enchiladas:* With Black Beans & Citrus Rice

| | | | |
|---|---|---|---|
| Two Cheese, with Fire-Rstd Sauce | 1090 | 63 | 89 |
| Two Chicken, with Fire-Rstd Sauce | 1070 | 56 | 91 |
| Two Shrimp, with Verde Sauce | 1050 | 59 | 94 |

*Tacos:* Each, with Corn Tortilla

| **Grilled Gourmet:** Chicken | 330 | 19 | 22 |
|---|---|---|---|
| Steak | 340 | 20 | 21 |
| **Seafood, Blackened:** | | | |
| Atlantic Salmon | 220 | 10 | 22 |
| Pacific Mahi Mahi | 220 | 10 | 22 |
| **Seafood, Grilled:** | | | |
| Atlantic Salmon | 270 | 13 | 23 |
| Pacific Mahi Mahi | 240 | 10 | 23 |
| Regal Springs Tilapia | 260 | 11 | 20 |

*Sides:*

| **Black Beans:** Regular, 4 oz | 140 | 2 | 25 |
|---|---|---|---|
| Large, 9.4 oz | 320 | 3 | 58 |
| **Chips:** Regular, 1.8 oz | 210 | 3 | 43 |
| Large, 4 oz | 460 | 5 | 96 |
| **Citrus Rice:** Regular, 2.3 oz | 110 | 2 | 22 |
| Large, 6 oz | 300 | 5 | 59 |
| **Mexican Rice:** Regular, 2.3 oz | 100 | 2 | 20 |
| Large, 6 oz | 270 | 4 | 53 |
| **No Fried Pinto Beans:** Reg., 4 oz | 130 | 2 | 21 |
| Large, 10.9 oz | 330 | 3 | 56 |

*Salad & Bowls:* Entrée Size, Includes Dressing

| **Chipotle Ranch:** W/- Grilled Chkn | 500 | 36 | 22 |
|---|---|---|---|
| with Grilled Mahi Mahi | 510 | 37 | 19 |
| with Grilled Tilapia | 550 | 39 | 19 |

*Salsas:* Per 1 oz

| Mango, Picante, Tomatillo, average | 20 | 0.5 | 3 |
|---|---|---|---|
| Other Varieties | 10 | 0 | 2 |

## Ruby Tuesday® (Aug '16)

*Shareables:* Per Serve, w/out Sauce

| | C | F | Cb |
|---|---|---|---|
| BBQ Chicken Flatbread | 105 | 5 | 10 |
| Cheese Fries | 270 | 19 | 22 |
| Fire Wings | 195 | 12 | 4 |
| Fried Mozzarella | 145 | 8 | 11 |
| Shrimp Fondu, with chips | 300 | 18 | 25 |
| Spinach Artichoke Dip, with chips | 285 | 18 | 25 |
| Thai Spring Rolls | 130 | 6 | 14 |

*Burgers/Sandwiches:* With Fries

| Avocado Turkey Burger | 1190 | 67 | 90 |
|---|---|---|---|
| Buffalo Chicken | 1120 | 54 | 106 |
| Chicken BLT | 1060 | 56 | 89 |
| **Half Pounders:** Ruby's Classic Bgr | 1060 | 56 | 89 |
| Smokehouse Burger | 1370 | 73 | 115 |
| Triple Prime: Original Burger | 1060 | 56 | 89 |
| Bacon Cheddar Burger | 1210 | 68 | 89 |
| Cheddar Burger | 1115 | 60 | 90 |

*Fit & Trim Choices:* Without Sides

| Chicken Bella | 425 | 20 | 19 |
|---|---|---|---|
| Grilled Salmon | 425 | 27 | 9 |
| Hickory Bourbon: | | | |
| Chicken | 345 | 10 | 27 |
| Salmon | 485 | 18 | 16 |
| Top Sirloin | 425 | 22 | 12 |
| **Sides:** Green Beans | 70 | 4 | 5 |
| Grilled Zucchini | 40 | 2 | 4 |
| Roasted Spaghetti Squash | 55 | 3 | 6 |
| Steamed Broccoli | 50 | 2 | 7 |

*Fresh All Natural Chicken:* Without Sides

| Chicken Bella | 330 | 15 | 9 |
|---|---|---|---|
| Chicken Fresco | 355 | 20 | 12 |
| Double Decker Chicken | 675 | 31 | 14 |
| Smoky Mountain Chicken | 500 | 25 | 18 |

*Petite Plates:* With Mashed Potatoes & Steamed Broccoli

| Blackened Tilapia | 285 | 12 | 23 |
|---|---|---|---|
| Parmesan Shrimp Pasta | 625 | 30 | 58 |
| Sliced Sirloin | 380 | 20 | 23 |

*Ribs & Chops:* With Fries

| BBQ Baby-Back Ribs, Half-Rack with Fries | 470 | 24 | 21 |
|---|---|---|---|
| Hickory Bourbon-Glazed Pork Chops | 885 | 42 | 57 |

*Seafood:* Without Sides

| Grilled Salmon | 330 | 22 | 0 |
|---|---|---|---|
| Herb-Crusted Tilapia | 400 | 24 | 11 |
| Jumbo Skewered Shrimp | 275 | 15 | 0 |
| New Orleans Seafood | 315 | 14 | 6 |

*Continued Next Page...*

Updated Nutrition Data ~ www.CalorieKing.com
Persons with Diabetes ~ See Disclaimer (Page 22)

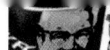
## Ruby Tuesday® cont... (Aug '16)

| *Pasta & More:* | **C** | **F** | **Cb** |
|---|---|---|---|
| Cajun Jambalaya | 1525 | 102 | 85 |
| Chicken & Broccoli | 1415 | 86 | 101 |
| Grilled Chicken Sonora | 1315 | 53 | 126 |
| Parmesan Chicken | 1285 | 63 | 105 |
| Parmesan Shrimp | 995 | 46 | 96 |

| *Steaks: Without Sides* | | | |
|---|---|---|---|
| Asiago Peppercorn Strip | 585 | 37 | 7 |
| Bella Mushroom Sirloin | 385 | 19 | 7 |
| Cajun Rib Eye | 780 | 60 | 6 |
| New York Strip | 520 | 36 | 0 |
| Rib Eye | 700 | 53 | 0 |

| *Salads: Without Dressing* | | | |
|---|---|---|---|
| Carolina Chicken | 1100 | 83 | 67 |
| Fried Chicken Caesar | 1055 | 76 | 49 |
| Grilled Chicken | 705 | 53 | 43 |
| Grilled Salmon Caesar | 935 | 75 | 31 |

| *Dressing: Per 1 oz* | | | |
|---|---|---|---|
| Balsamic Vinaigrette | 40 | 2 | 5 |
| Blue Cheese | 180 | 19 | 1 |
| Caesar | 190 | 20 | 1 |
| French | 120 | 11 | 6 |
| Honey Mustard; Thsnd Island, av. | 85 | 8 | 5 |
| Italian | 130 | 14 | 1 |
| Ranch | 90 | 9 | 1 |

| *Fresh Sides:* | | | |
|---|---|---|---|
| Baked Mac 'n Cheese | 430 | 28 | 27 |
| Baked Potato: Plain | 250 | 3 | 51 |
| Loaded | 595 | 33 | 53 |
| French Fries | 480 | 24 | 54 |
| Garlic Cheese Biscuit | 100 | 6 | 12 |
| Mashed Potatoes | 265 | 15 | 29 |
| Onion Rings | 340 | 19 | 37 |
| Rice Pilaf | 190 | 1 | 40 |
| Sweet Potato Fries | 445 | 24 | 56 |

| *Kid's Menu: Includes Fries* | | | |
|---|---|---|---|
| Chicken Breast | 430 | 17 | 29 |
| Chicken Tenders | 570 | 27 | 45 |
| Cheese Pizza | 470 | 14 | 61 |
| Corn Dogs | 620 | 38 | 57 |

| *Desserts:* | | | |
|---|---|---|---|
| Blondie | 1110 | 52 | 150 |
| Chocolate Goblet Sundae | 865 | 52 | 97 |
| New York Cheesecake | 785 | 60 | 96 |
| White Choc. Cherry Cheesecake | 675 | 44 | 65 |

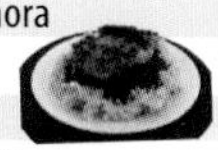

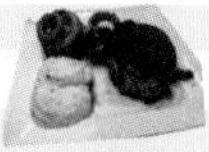

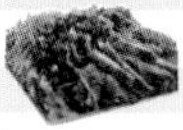

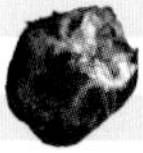

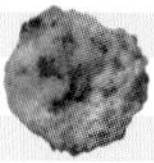

*For Complete Menu ~ see CalorieKing.com*

## Runza® (Aug '16)

| *Burgers:* | **C** | **F** | **Cb** |
|---|---|---|---|
| ¼ lb BBQ Bacon & Swiss | 530 | 32 | 26 |
| ¼ lb Bacon Cheeseburger | 510 | 31 | 26 |
| ¼ lb French Onion | 490 | 29 | 26 |
| ¼ lb Legend Supreme | 520 | 32 | 26 |
| ¼ lb Spicy Jack | 570 | 38 | 23 |
| ¼ lb Swiss Mushroom | 480 | 29 | 24 |
| Runza Way: ¼ lb Cheeseburger | 420 | 22 | 28 |
| ¼ lb Hamburger | 370 | 18 | 26 |
| ½ lb Double Cheeseburger | 670 | 39 | 30 |
| ½ lb Double Hamburger | 570 | 31 | 26 |

| *Runza Sandwiches:* | | | |
|---|---|---|---|
| BBQ Bacon Runza | 730 | 34 | 72 |
| BLT Runza | 745 | 40 | 68 |
| Cheese Runza | 580 | 24 | 69 |
| Cheesesburger Runza | 590 | 24 | 72 |
| Spicy Jack Runza | 750 | 41 | 69 |

| *Sides:* | | | |
|---|---|---|---|
| French Fries: Small | 220 | 11 | 29 |
| Medium | 320 | 15 | 41 |
| Large | 460 | 23 | 60 |
| Frings: Medium | 330 | 18 | 39 |
| Large | 470 | 25 | 55 |
| Onion Rings: Medium | 320 | 19 | 35 |
| Large | 550 | 31 | 58 |

| *Salads:* | | | |
|---|---|---|---|
| Asian Grilled Chicken w/ dressing | 360 | 7 | 48 |
| Southwest Chicken Salad w/ Salsa | 330 | 16 | 31 |
| Sweet Berry Chicken w/o dressing | 370 | 19 | 21 |

| *Dressings:* Honey Mustard | 200 | 18 | 9 |
|---|---|---|---|
| Ranch | 180 | 18 | 3 |

| *Soups: Per Bowl* | | | |
|---|---|---|---|
| Boston Clam Chowder | 280 | 15 | 29 |
| Broccoli Cheese | 240 | 16 | 20 |
| Chicken Tortilla | 150 | 6 | 16 |
| Homemade Chili | 320 | 15 | 23 |
| Wisconsin Cheese | 340 | 23 | 29 |

| *Kids:* | | | |
|---|---|---|---|
| Junior: Cheeseburger, plain | 250 | 13 | 18 |
| Hamburger, plain | 200 | 9 | 16 |
| Swiss Cheese Mushroom Burger | 300 | 17 | 17 |
| **Runza Way:** Cheeseburger | 270 | 13 | 22 |
| Hamburger | 220 | 9 | 20 |

| *Desserts:* | | | |
|---|---|---|---|
| Ice Cream Cones, all flavors | 260 | 7 | 40 |
| Ice Cream Dish, all flavors | 230 | 7 | 34 |
| Sundaes: Caramel; Chocolate | 300 | 7 | 51 |
| Turtle | 360 | 13 | 53 |

| *Shakes: Per Regular, 16 oz* | | | |
|---|---|---|---|
| Cappucc.; Choc., Strawb., average | 485 | 12 | 80 |
| Vanilla | 430 | 12 | 66 |

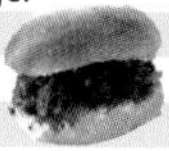

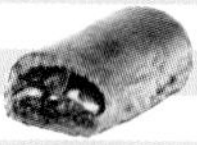

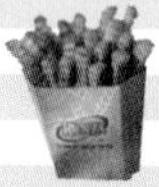

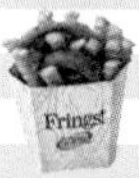

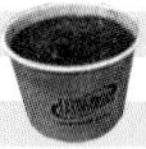

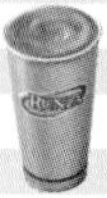

## Ryan's Grill Buffet & Bakery® (Aug '16)

*Entrées: Without Sides*

| | C | F | Cb |
|---|---|---|---|
| **Beef:** BBQ'd, 4 oz | 140 | 5 | 16 |
| Country Fried Steak, w/ gravy, 2.6 oz | 220 | 13 | 16 |
| Meatloaf, 3 oz | 180 | 11 | 7 |
| Perfect Pot Roast, 4.9 oz | 160 | 7 | 9 |
| Salisbury Steak, 3.5 oz | 150 | 9 | 8 |
| **Chicken:** | | | |
| Breasts: Country BBQ, 5.8 oz | 310 | 16 | 6 |
| Rotisserie, 5.3 oz | 310 | 17 | 1 |
| Chicken & Dumplings, 5 oz | 160 | 5 | 17 |
| New Orleans Bourbon Street, 3 oz | 180 | 8 | 9 |
| Orange Chicken, 3 oz | 340 | 22 | 26 |
| **Fish/Seafood:** Baked Fish, 2 oz | 90 | 4.5 | 0 |
| Butter Crumb Alaskan Pollock, 1.8 oz | 110 | 5 | 2 |
| Butterfly Shrimp (6), 2.3 oz | 210 | 9 | 24 |
| Carved Salmon Filet, 3 oz | 190 | 11 | 0 |
| Clam Strips, 3 oz | 320 | 20 | 28 |
| Fried: Fish, 3 pieces, 3 oz | 240 | 12 | 27 |
| Shrimp (22), 3 oz | 240 | 12 | 24 |
| Wood Seared Salmon, 1 pce, 3 oz | 220 | 16 | 0 |
| **Pasta/Spaghetti:** *Per 5 oz Serving* | | | |
| Country Pasta Gratine | 160 | 4 | 24 |
| Creamy Penne Carbonara | 260 | 17 | 17 |
| Fire Grilled Chicken Alfredo | 220 | 14 | 14 |
| Grilled Italian Sausage Penne | 180 | 11 | 14 |
| **Pork:** | | | |
| Carved: Grilled Loin, 3 oz | 140 | 10 | 0 |
| Ham, 3 oz | 100 | 5 | 0 |
| Honey Glazed Baked, 1 sl, 3 oz | 120 | 5 | 1 |
| Ribs, BBQ/County-Style (3), 3.5 oz | 420 | 27 | 15 |
| Steak: Grilled, 2 oz | 140 | 9 | 0 |
| BBQ, grilled, 2 oz | 150 | 9 | 3 |
| **Salads:** *Without Dressing* | | | |
| Asian Chopped, 3.5 oz | 90 | 4 | 13 |
| Caesar, 1 cup, 2.5 oz | 70 | 6 | 4 |
| Greek, 2.6 oz | 120 | 8 | 10 |
| Seafood, 4.2 oz | 310 | 26 | 15 |

## Ryan's Grill Buffet & Bakery®..cont. (Aug '16)

*Sides:*

| | C | F | Cb |
|---|---|---|---|
| Baked Potato, plain, 4.3 oz | 150 | 0 | 36 |
| BBQ Baked Beans, 3 oz | 130 | 3 | 26 |
| Cauliflower Au Gratin, 3 oz | 50 | 2 | 8 |
| French Fries, 2 oz | 170 | 9 | 23 |
| Fried Okra, 3 oz | 220 | 12 | 28 |
| Mashed Potatoes, 4 oz | 70 | 0.5 | 13 |
| **Desserts:** Cheesecake, plain,1 sl. | 230 | 12 | 28 |
| Key Lime Pie, scratch, 1 sl., 2.5 oz | 220 | 9 | 31 |
| Lemon Meringue Pie, 2.3 oz | 130 | 4.5 | 23 |

## 7-Eleven® (Aug '16)

*7-Select Burritos:*

| | C | F | Cb |
|---|---|---|---|
| Bean and Cheese: 5 oz | 320 | 10 | 47 |
| 10 oz | 640 | 21 | 94 |
| Beef & Bean/ Beef, Bean & Chili: | | | |
| 5 oz | 360 | 16 | 44 |
| 10 oz | 720 | 31 | 89 |
| Red Hot Beef: 5 oz | 340 | 15 | 41 |
| 10 oz | 670 | 30 | 83 |
| **Breakfast Sandwiches:** | | | |
| Biscuits, Sausage, 3.3 oz | 330 | 22 | 28 |
| Croissant, Egg, Cheese & Ssg, 4.8 oz | 410 | 30 | 20 |
| Eng. Muffin, Egg, Chse & Ssg, 5 oz | 390 | 25 | 24 |
| **Chicken:** | | | |
| **Dippers:** 1 piece, 0.85 oz | 70 | 3.5 | 4 |
| 6 pieces, 5.1 oz | 400 | 20 | 22 |
| Tenders (1), 3.3 oz | 160 | 5 | 11 |
| Wing (1), 1.2 oz | 80 | 4.5 | 3 |
| **Salads:** | | | |
| BLT Salad, 8 oz | 270 | 18 | 12 |
| Chicken Caesar Salad, 7.5 oz | 390 | 28 | 17 |
| Side, 5 oz | 30 | 0 | 7 |
| **Sandwiches/Melts:** | | | |
| Chicken, Bacon Ranch Melt, 7.4 oz | 560 | 22 | 56 |
| Chicken Salad Sandwich, 6.2 oz | 400 | 14 | 44 |
| Go!Smart Turkey Sandwich | 300 | 2.5 | 48 |
| Italian Melt, 7.8 oz | 610 | 39 | 38 |
| Southwest Turkey Sandwich, 8 oz | 560 | 28 | 48 |
| Steak & Cheese Melt, 7.8 oz | 680 | 35 | 57 |
| **Sides:** Hash Browns (1), 2 oz | 100 | 5 | 12 |
| Potato Wedges (6), 0.7 oz | 240 | 4.5 | 27 |
| **Slurpees,** average all flavors: | | | |
| 12 oz cup | 95 | 0 | 26 |
| 22 oz cup | 175 | 0 | 44 |
| 28 oz cup | 220 | 0 | 56 |
| Sugar Free, 12 oz cup | 30 | 0 | 9 |

**Updated Nutrition Data ~ www.CalorieKing.com**
**Persons with Diabetes ~ See Disclaimer (Page 22)**

## Saladworks® (Aug '16)

| Salads: *Without Dressing or Bread* | C | F | Cb |
|---|---|---|---|
| Bently | 290 | 15 | 11 |
| Buffalo Bleu | 350 | 12 | 29 |
| Chicken Caesar | 370 | 15 | 29 |
| Cobb | 370 | 23 | 19 |
| Fire Roasted Cabo | 350 | 17 | 25 |
| Greek | 200 | 11 | 17 |
| Nuevo Nicoise | 360 | 13 | 40 |
| Sophie's Salad | 310 | 13 | 35 |
| *Paninis:* Buffalo Chicken | 870 | 36 | 85 |
| Caprese | 940 | 47 | 94 |
| Turkey Melt | 1020 | 49 | 90 |
| *Sandwiches:* Avocado BLT | 670 | 44 | 60 |
| Loaded Chicken | 330 | 9 | 28 |
| Tuna Salad | 380 | 8 | 57 |
| *Wraps:* Chicken Caesar | 550 | 21 | 63 |
| Madarin Chicken | 530 | 12 | 83 |
| Thai Chicken | 410 | 9 | 70 |

*Extra Menu Items ~ See CalorieKing.com*

## Sandella's® (Aug '16)

| | C | F | Cb |
|---|---|---|---|
| *Grilled Flatbread: With Standard Toppings* | | | |
| Brazilian Bacon | 560 | 17 | 79 |
| Brazilian Chicken | 510 | 10 | 73 |
| Pesto Chicken | 610 | 28 | 56 |
| Spinach & Bacon | 660 | 39 | 52 |
| *Paninis: wWth Standard Toppings* | | | |
| Philly Cheese | 590 | 25 | 55 |
| Spin., Ham & Swiss | 550 | 20 | 61 |
| Tuscan Chicken | 540 | 21 | 55 |
| *Quesadillas: With Standard Toppings* | | | |
| California | 500 | 23 | 53 |
| Mediterranean | 400 | 16 | 53 |
| *Salads: Includes ½ Flatbread* | | | |
| Fiesta, with Light Bals. Vinaigrette | 360 | 8 | 54 |
| Greek, with Light Bals. Vinaigrette | 310 | 15 | 37 |
| *Rice Bowls: Includes Flatbread & Standard Toppings* | | | |
| Black Bean & Rice | 840 | 20 | 130 |
| Chicken Fajita | 750 | 20 | 104 |
| *Wraps: with Standard Toppings* | | | |
| California Turkey | 410 | 10 | 55 |
| Chipotle Chicken | 350 | 7 | 55 |
| Pesto Turkey | 460 | 15 | 54 |
| Sweet & Spicy Chicken | 400 | 7 | 64 |

## Sarku Japan® (Apr'16)

| D'Lite Meals: | C | F | Cb |
|---|---|---|---|
| Rice & Chicken Tempura, 15 oz | 970 | 58 | 81 |
| Rice & Shrimp Tempura, 11 oz | 540 | 21 | 70 |
| Vegetarian, 14 oz | 360 | 0.5 | 79 |
| Vegetarian Soba Noodle, 14 oz | 710 | 24 | 106 |
| *Combos:* | | | |
| **Tempura:** Chicken, 23 oz | 1270 | 78 | 102 |
| Chicken & Shrimp, 20 oz | 980 | 53 | 95 |
| **Teriyaki:** Beef, 19 oz | 690 | 26 | 81 |
| Beef & Shrimp, 21 oz | 630 | 11 | 85 |
| Chicken, 22 oz | 640 | 13 | 90 |
| Chkn & Shrimp, 24 oz | 700 | 14 | 90 |
| Shrimp, 19 oz | 500 | 2.5 | 83 |
| *Sauce,* Teriyaki, 1.5 oz | 45 | 0 | 9 |
| *Sides:* Maki Roll, 2 oz | 140 | 11 | 9 |
| Rice: Steamed, 9 oz | 290 | 0 | 64 |
| Fried, 9 oz | 330 | 4.5 | 62 |
| Tempura Chicken, 1 piece, 2 oz | 230 | 19 | 8 |
| Tempura Shrimp, 1 piece, 0.8 oz | 90 | 7 | 4 |

## Schlotzsky's® (Aug '16)

*Sandwiches: Per Medium Size*

| Angus: | C | F | Cb |
|---|---|---|---|
| Corned Beef Reuben | 890 | 38 | 81 |
| Pastrami Reuben | 900 | 40 | 84 |
| Roast Beef & Cheese | 780 | 30 | 81 |
| Beef Bacon SmokeCheesy | 810 | 43 | 77 |
| Chipotle Chicken | 530 | 9 | 78 |
| Deluxe Original | 980 | 47 | 81 |
| Fiesta Chicken | 810 | 31 | 78 |
| French Dip on Pretzel Bun | 670 | 28 | 59 |
| Fresh Veggie | 500 | 14 | 74 |
| Ham & Cheese Original-Style | 730 | 25 | 81 |
| Smoked Turkey Breast Orig.-Style | 500 | 17 | 53 |
| The Caprese (Vegetarian) | 570 | 27 | 64 |
| The Original | 780 | 34 | 78 |
| The Sicilian | 730 | 44 | 42 |
| The Tuscan | 700 | 42 | 48 |
| Turkey Original | 830 | 33 | 81 |
| Turkey & Guacamole | 520 | 11 | 78 |
| Turkey Bacon Club | 770 | 30 | 81 |

*Large Size Sandwiches ~ Double above Medium figures*

*Other Menu Items ~ Next Page...*

## Schlotzsky's® cont... (Aug '16)

*10" Pizzas: Per Pizza*

| | C | F | Cb |
|---|---|---|---|
| BBQ Chicken & Jalapeno | 920 | 21 | 148 |
| Combination Special | 960 | 38 | 119 |
| Double Cheese | 840 | 27 | 115 |
| Fresh Veggie | 920 | 35 | 118 |
| Grilled Chicken & Pesto | 910 | 29 | 114 |
| Pepperoni & Double Cheese | 980 | 42 | 115 |

*Oven Baked Pasta:*

| | | | |
|---|---|---|---|
| Bayou Chicken | 800 | 41 | 66 |
| Chicken Pesto Carbonara | 930 | 45 | 79 |
| Tomato-Basil Canestrelli | 550 | 19 | 70 |

*Salads: Without Dressing or Breadsticks*

| | | | |
|---|---|---|---|
| Cranberry, Apple, Pecan & Chicken | 640 | 27 | 68 |
| Hearts of Romaine Chicken Caesar | 680 | 17 | 29 |
| Southwest Chicken | 600 | 29 | 44 |
| Turkey Avocado Cobb | 610 | 33 | 42 |

*Dressings: Per 3 oz*

| | | | |
|---|---|---|---|
| Butttermilk Ranch | 320 | 33 | 4 |
| Chunky Blue Cheese | 460 | 49 | 3 |
| Red Wine Vinaigrette | 430 | 43 | 9 |
| Robusto Italian | 280 | 28 | 3 |
| Tuscan Caesar | 430 | 45 | 2 |

*Soup: Per Bowl*

| | | | |
|---|---|---|---|
| Broccoli Cheddar | 185 | 12 | 14 |
| Chicken Enchilada | 315 | 16 | 27 |
| Chicken & Wild Rice | 280 | 14 | 25 |
| Loaded Baked Potato | 385 | 31 | 29 |
| Timberline Chili | 380 | 21 | 27 |
| Tomato Basil Bisque | 320 | 26 | 21 |

*Chips:*

| | | | |
|---|---|---|---|
| Baked: Regular; BBQ, average | 130 | 3 | 25 |
| Other varieties, average | 230 | 14 | 24 |

*Kidz Meals: Without Cookie or Drink*

| | | | |
|---|---|---|---|
| Cheese Pizza | 540 | 17 | 78 |
| Cheese Sandwich | 400 | 14 | 49 |
| Ham Sandwich | 220 | 2 | 40 |
| Pepperoni Pizza | 590 | 22 | 78 |
| Turkey Sandwich | 220 | 1.5 | 40 |

*Desserts:*

| | | | |
|---|---|---|---|
| Brownie (1) | 420 | 24 | 46 |
| Cookies: Per Cookie | | | |
| Chocolate Chip | 160 | 7 | 24 |
| Oatmeal Raisin; Sugar, average | 155 | 5 | 24 |

## Second Cup® ~ *see CalorieKing.com*

## Shakey's® (Aug '16)

*Pizzas: Per Slice, ½ Large Pizza*

| | C | F | Cb |
|---|---|---|---|
| **Cheese:** | | | |
| Pan Crust | 185 | 6 | 26 |
| Thin Crust | 150 | 5.5 | 18 |
| **Firehouse:** Pan Crust | 255 | 12 | 27 |
| Thin Crust | 220 | 12 | 19 |
| **Garden Veggie:** Pan Crust | 185 | 5.5 | 27 |
| Thin Crust | 150 | 5 | 19 |
| **Margherita:** | | | |
| Pan Crust | 175 | 5 | 26 |
| Thin Crust | 135 | 4.5 | 18 |
| **Rustic Garlic Chicken:** Pan Crust | 190 | 5.5 | 26 |
| Thin Crust | 155 | 5.5 | 18 |
| **Shakey's Special:** Pan Crust | 210 | 6.5 | 31 |
| Thin Crust | 195 | 10 | 18 |
| **Texas BBQ Chicken:** Pan Crust | 205 | 5 | 29 |
| Thin Crust | 170 | 5 | 21 |
| **Ultimate Meat:** Pan Crust | 280 | 14 | 26 |
| Thin Crust | 245 | 13 | 18 |
| **Additional Toppings:** Beef | 35 | 3 | 0 |
| Cheese | 15 | 1 | 1 |
| Chicken | 15 | 0.5 | 0 |
| Pepperoni | 25 | 2.5 | 0 |
| Sausage | 45 | 4 | 1 |

*Shareables: Per Serving, Unless Indicated*

| | | | |
|---|---|---|---|
| Chicken Strips (5) | 620 | 31 | 48 |
| Mojo Potatoes (5) | 215 | 11 | 25 |
| Mojo Supreme, serves 4-6 | 1950 | 120 | 160 |
| Shakey's Spicy Wings (6) | 495 | 29 | 27 |

*Shakey's Famous Chicken: Per Piece*

| | | | |
|---|---|---|---|
| **Fried Chicken:** Breast | 475 | 26 | 16 |
| Leg | 170 | 9 | 6 |
| Thigh | 350 | 24 | 10 |
| Wing | 130 | 9 | 4 |

## Shari's® (Aug '16)

*Breakfast:*

| | C | F | Cb |
|---|---|---|---|
| **Favorites:** *Without Options* | | | |
| Breakfast Sampler Platter | 1030 | 72 | 56 |
| Farmhouse Platter | 1150 | 70 | 94 |
| Traditional Eggs Benedict, with Hashbrowns | 810 | 46 | 61 |
| **Fruit Crepes,** Apples; Strawb., av. | 685 | 36 | 79 |
| **Omelettes:** *Without Options* | | | |
| BMP | 850 | 72 | 9 |
| Chicken Fajita | 680 | 52 | 14 |
| Denver; Spring Spinach, average | 580 | 47 | 12 |

*Continued Next Page...*

Updated Nutrition Data ~ www.CalorieKing.com
Persons with Diabetes ~ See Disclaimer (Page 22)

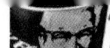

## Shari's® cont... (Aug '16)

### Breakfast (Cont):

| | C | F | Cb |
|---|---|---|---|
| **Pancakes:** | | | |
| Buttermilk, without toppings | 420 | 10 | 73 |
| Potato Pancakes, without meat | 570 | 17 | 96 |
| **Specialties:** *Without Options* | | | |
| Classic Quiche: BMP | 640 | 39 | 57 |
| Lorraine | 680 | 40 | 56 |
| Meat Lover's Skillet | 1140 | 91 | 34 |
| Morning Start Panini | 890 | 56 | 64 |
| T-Bone Steak & Eggs | 1320 | 85 | 31 |
| Ultimate Ctry Fried Steak & Eggs | 1230 | 86 | 73 |
| **Lunch:** | | | |
| **Flame-Grilled Burgers:** *Without Side Choices* | | | |
| Bavarian | 1030 | 47 | 59 |
| Bleu Cheeseburger | 650 | 33 | 46 |
| Cheddar Cheesebuger | 660 | 34 | 46 |
| Hamburger | 600 | 29 | 46 |
| Pepperjack Cheese | 700 | 38 | 46 |
| Srira-Cha-Cha | 730 | 40 | 50 |
| Swiss Cheese Mushroom | 1030 | 72 | 44 |
| Trail Boss | 1030 | 57 | 54 |
| **Flatbread Paninis:** *Without Side Choices* | | | |
| All American | 740 | 33 | 62 |
| Pastrami | 760 | 32 | 58 |
| **Salads:** *Entrée Size* | | | |
| American Chopped, w/o Dress. | 590 | 28 | 39 |
| Northwest Steak | 710 | 31 | 67 |
| Spinach Cobb | 760 | 44 | 46 |
| **Sandwiches:** *Per Whole Sandwich, w/o Side Choices* | | | |
| Crispy Chicken BLT | 940 | 58 | 64 |
| Cuban, on Ciabatta | 600 | 27 | 46 |
| Prime Rib Dip | 540 | 21 | 52 |
| **Dinner:** | | | |
| Alaskan Amber Cod Dinner | 1740 | 134 | 118 |
| Country Fried Steak Dinner | 1340 | 81 | 119 |
| Grilled Chicken Penne Alfredo | 1080 | 54 | 94 |
| Home-style Pot Roast & Veggies | 1410 | 78 | 87 |
| Hot Turkey Sandwich | 840 | 28 | 107 |
| **Meals without Sides, as served:** | | | |
| NY Strip Steak, w ith toppings | 940 | 64 | 33 |
| Sthrn Style Chicken & Waffles | 1430 | 86 | 113 |
| **Steaks:** | | | |
| with Golden Fried Shrimp | 1040 | 50 | 89 |
| with Shrimp Scampi | 930 | 62 | 36 |
| with Shrimp Skewers | 760 | 43 | 35 |
| T-Bone Steak, 16 oz | 1100 | 67 | 35 |

## Shari's® cont... (Aug '16)

### Sides, Lunch/Dinner:

| | C | F | Cb |
|---|---|---|---|
| Baked Potato w/ Butter & Sour Crm | 280 | 13 | 38 |
| Country Vegetables | 120 | 9 | 8 |
| French Fries | 390 | 25 | 40 |
| Red Skins Mashed Potato | 260 | 8 | 40 |
| Rice Pilaf | 90 | 4.5 | 10 |
| Tater Tots | 370 | 26 | 33 |
| **Desserts:** | | | |
| Cheese Cake, 1 slice | 420 | 29 | 37 |
| **Classic Pies:** *Per Slice, as Served* | | | |
| Banana Cream Dream | 410 | 19 | 55 |
| Chocolate Cream Supreme | 540 | 30 | 62 |
| **Gourmet Pies:** *Per Slice, As Served* | | | |
| Caramel Pecan Crunch | 710 | 45 | 71 |
| Peanut Butter Chocolate Silk | 660 | 45 | 60 |
| S'mores Galore | 570 | 31 | 68 |
| Velvet Chocolate Silk | 580 | 38 | 56 |
| World's Greatest Carrot Cake | 330 | 18 | 39 |

## Sheetz® (Aug '16)

### Breakfast Sandwiches:

| | C | F | Cb |
|---|---|---|---|
| Dreamy Bacon Croissant | 390 | 22 | 33 |
| Twisted BLT | 740 | 41 | 62 |
| Walker Breakfast Ranger | 580 | 22 | 68 |
| **Burgerz:** | | | |
| Big Mozz Burger | 610 | 27 | 50 |
| Boss Bacon Burger | 720 | 50 | 26 |
| Cowboy Burger | 650 | 33 | 46 |
| El Gringo Burger | 640 | 33 | 55 |
| Twisted Swiss Burger | 770 | 40 | 60 |
| **Hot Dogz:** | | | |
| BLT | 450 | 27 | 33 |
| Firehouse | 390 | 22 | 35 |
| Junkyard | 340 | 16 | 38 |
| Philly | 340 | 17 | 35 |
| Shmokehouse | 370 | 18 | 37 |
| **Sidez:** | | | |
| Coleslaw | 80 | 3.5 | 12 |
| Crispy Chicken Stripz: 3 pieces | 330 | 11 | 39 |
| 5 pieces | 550 | 18 | 65 |
| Fryz, no sauce, 1 cup | 390 | 13 | 64 |
| Hard Cooked Eggs, 1 order | 70 | 4.5 | 0 |
| Jalapeno Poppers, 1 order | 330 | 18 | 35 |
| Loaded Fryz, plain | 600 | 20 | 97 |
| Mac & Cheese, plain, 1 order | 130 | 6 | 15 |
| Onion Rings, no sauce, 1 cup | 470 | 27 | 52 |
| **Popcorn Chicken, without Sauce:** | | | |
| Regular | 300 | 14 | 28 |
| Large | 610 | 28 | 55 |

*Continued Next Page...*

## Sheetz® cont... (Aug '16)

| Donuts: | C | F | Cb |
|---|---|---|---|
| Apple Fritter | 510 | 30 | 54 |
| Chocolate Cake Donut | 520 | 33 | 54 |
| Cream Filled Glazed Donut | 380 | 20 | 46 |
| Custard Filled Chocolate Iced D'nut | 380 | 19 | 48 |
| Glazed Ring Donut | 340 | 19 | 38 |
| P'nut Butter Filled Choc Iced D'nut | 410 | 23 | 48 |
| Vanilla Cake Donut | 480 | 26 | 57 |
| *Muffin*, Blueberry (1) | 440 | 22 | 56 |

| Beverages: Per 8 fl.oz | C | F | Cb |
|---|---|---|---|
| Brewed Americano, small | 0 | 0 | 0 |
| Cupo'ccino: | | | |
|   C'rml Brownie Cocoa | 200 | 8 | 36 |
|   Creme Brulee | 160 | 5 | 31 |
|   French Vanilla | 150 | 1.5 | 33 |
| Hot Chocolate | 180 | 2 | 40 |

## Sizzler® (Aug '16)

| | C | F | Cb |
|---|---|---|---|
| **Burgers:** *Without Condiments, Dipping Sauce or Optional Accompaniments* | | | |
| Mega Bacon Cheeseburger, ½ lb | 1010 | 61 | 48 |
| Sizzler Burger: ⅓ lb | 620 | 30 | 47 |
|   ½ lb | 760 | 40 | 47 |
| **Hot Entrées:** *Without Condiments, Dipping Sauce or Optional Accompaniments* | | | |
| **Chicken:** Hibachi Chicken, Single | 180 | 4 | 7 |
|   Lemon-Herb Chicken, Single | 170 | 6 | 0 |
|   Malibu Chicken, Single | 360 | 25 | 11 |
| **Pasta:** Fettuccine Alfredo | 995 | 64 | 73 |
|   Cajun Fettuccine Alfredo | 1035 | 64 | 82 |
| **Pork Chop,** Single, w/ Apple Sauce | 420 | 27 | 15 |
| **Ribs:** | | | |
|   Half Rack | 625 | 39 | 37 |
|   Full Rack | 1155 | 79 | 51 |
| **Seafood:** | | | |
| Grilled Salmon with Rice Pilaf | 530 | 20 | 40 |
| Ultimate Shrimp Platter | 1010 | 39 | 103 |
| **Steaks:** Bacon Wrapped Sirloin Filet | 555 | 35 | 5 |
|   Burgundy M'shroom Sirloin Tips, with Rice Pilaf | 870 | 36 | 85 |
|   Chopped Steak, 8 oz | 520 | 30 | 17 |
|   Classic, 8 oz | 395 | 21 | 1 |
|   NY Strip, 12 oz | 810 | 57 | 1 |
|   Combos: Classic Trio | 860 | 47 | 36 |
|     Steak & Hibachi Chicken | 475 | 20 | 7 |
|     Steak & Lobster Tail | 410 | 17 | 2 |
|     Steak & Malibu Chicken | 660 | 41 | 12 |
| **Sandwiches:** | | | |
| Grilled Chicken Club | 645 | 28 | 48 |
| Malibu Chicken | 705 | 37 | 59 |

## Sizzler® cont... (Aug '16)

| Prepared Salads: W/out Dressing | C | F | Cb |
|---|---|---|---|
| Ambrosia Salad, 4 oz | 125 | 4 | 22 |
| Asian Chopped Salad, 4 oz | 30 | 2 | 3 |
| Caesar Salad, 2 oz | 25 | 2 | 1 |
| Carrot Raisin Salad, 4 oz | 100 | 6 | 12 |
| Potato Salad, 4 oz | 325 | 27 | 18 |

| Salad Dressings: Per 1 oz | C | F | Cb |
|---|---|---|---|
| Blue Cheese | 105 | 11 | 1 |
| Honey Mustard | 110 | 8 | 9 |
| Italian | 80 | 8 | 2 |
| Ranch | 115 | 12 | 1 |
| Thousand Island | 95 | 9 | 5 |

| Sides: | C | F | Cb |
|---|---|---|---|
| Baked Potato, plain | 265 | 4 | 51 |
| Broccoli, 5 oz | 50 | 0 | 7 |
| French Fries, 5 oz | 285 | 13 | 42 |
| Rice Pilaf, 5 oz | 225 | 4 | 39 |

*For Complete Menu & Data ~ see CalorieKing.com*

## Skyline Chili® (Aug '16)

| Burritos: | C | F | Cb |
|---|---|---|---|
| Chili Deluxe | 590 | 37 | 34 |
| Original | 600 | 33 | 49 |
| **Coneys:** Cheese | 350 | 23 | 25 |
|   Chili Cheese Sandwich | 290 | 17 | 24 |
|   Chili Sandwich | 180 | 8 | 23 |

| Ways: Per Regular Serving | C | F | Cb |
|---|---|---|---|
| **Chili Spaghetti with Cheese:** | | | |
|   3 Way | 800 | 44 | 50 |
|   4 Way Onion | 820 | 44 | 54 |
|   4 Way Bean | 890 | 44 | 66 |
|   5 Way | 900 | 44 | 70 |
| **Bowls:** Chili | 200 | 12 | 0 |
|   Loaded Chili | 480 | 29 | 21 |
|   Vegetarian Black Beans & Rice | 400 | 15 | 49 |

| Steamed Potatoes: | C | F | Cb |
|---|---|---|---|
| 3-Way Potato | 620 | 26 | 65 |
| Cheddar Potato | 630 | 33 | 65 |
| Sour Cream Potato | 460 | 19 | 66 |

| Salads: Without Dressing | C | F | Cb |
|---|---|---|---|
| Buffalo Chicken | 200 | 10 | 11 |
| Greek | 160 | 9 | 10 |

| Wraps: | C | F | Cb |
|---|---|---|---|
| Buffalo Chicken, w/ Ranch Dress. | 720 | 40 | 59 |
| Classic Chkn w/ Chili Ranch Dress. | 680 | 36 | 56 |
| Greek Chicken, w/ Greek Dressing | 700 | 37 | 58 |

| Sides: | C | F | Cb |
|---|---|---|---|
| Fries: Chili Cheese | 840 | 53 | 61 |
|   French | 430 | 24 | 51 |

## Smoothie King® (Aug '16)

*Fruit Smoothies: Per 20 oz Cup*  **C  F  Cb**
*Figures Include Turbinado. without Turbinado,
deduct 100 calories and 23 carbs.*

**Fitness Blends:**

| | C | F | Cb |
|---|---|---|---|
| High Protein: Almond Mocha | 345 | 9 | 42 |
| Chocolate | 365 | 9 | 42 |
| Peanut Power Plus: | | | |
| Chocolate | 700 | 26 | 98 |
| Strawberry | 680 | 21 | 112 |
| The Activator: Chocolate | 340 | 1 | 67 |
| Strawberry | 495 | 1 | 105 |
| Vanilla | 345 | 1 | 67 |
| The Hulk: Chocolate | 800 | 31 | 108 |
| Strawberry | 965 | 32 | 145 |
| Vanilla | 800 | 32 | 105 |

**Take A Break Blends:**

| | C | F | Cb |
|---|---|---|---|
| Banana Boat | 475 | 4 | 101 |
| Caribbean Way | 395 | 0 | 97 |
| Muscle Punch | 360 | 1 | 84 |
| Pineapple Surf | 460 | 1 | 104 |
| Yogurt D-Lite | 275 | 4 | 46 |
| **Wellness Blends:** Acai Adventure | 435 | 5 | 92 |
| Mangosteen Madness | 380 | 0 | 92 |
| Orange Ka-BAM | 470 | 0 | 117 |

*32 fl.oz Cup: Multiply 20 fl.oz figures by 1.5*
*40 fl.oz Cup: Multiply 20 fl.oz figures by 2*

**Kids Cup Smoothies:** *Per 12 fl.oz Cup*

| | C | F | Cb |
|---|---|---|---|
| Apple Kiwi Bunga | 155 | 0 | 37 |
| Choc-A-Laka | 210 | 4 | 32 |
| Lil' Angel | 210 | 0 | 52 |
| Strawberry Bluegurt Blitz | 175 | 0 | 70 |

## Snappy Tomato (Aug '16)

*Pizza: Per Slice, ⅛ of Large Pizza*  **C  F  Cb**

| | C | F | Cb |
|---|---|---|---|
| Buffalo Grilled Chicken | 250 | 5 | 32 |
| Cheese | 220 | 7 | 30 |
| Hawaiian | 370 | 18 | 33 |
| Pepperoni | 340 | 17 | 31 |
| Ranch | 370 | 21 | 31 |
| Snapperoni | 390 | 22 | 31 |
| Snappy Ultimate | 460 | 26 | 33 |
| Supreme | 340 | 17 | 32 |
| Veggie | 240 | 8 | 33 |

*Snappetizers, Snappy Wings,*

| | C | F | Cb |
|---|---|---|---|
| Plain, without sauce (3), 2.6 oz | 160 | 11 | 0 |

## Sonic Drive-In® (Aug '16)

**Burgers:**  **C  F  Cb**

| | C | F | Cb |
|---|---|---|---|
| **Cheeseburger:** w/ Mayo | 750 | 48 | 44 |
| with Ketchup | 720 | 43 | 47 |
| Double Cheeseburger w/ Mayo | 1170 | 81 | 44 |
| Bacon Cheeseburger | 820 | 54 | 43 |
| Bacon Double Cheeseburger | 1240 | 87 | 44 |
| Jr. Burger | 340 | 17 | 32 |
| Jr. Double Cheeseburger | 520 | 33 | 31 |
| Jr. Deluxe Burger | 360 | 20 | 32 |
| Jr. Deluxe Cheeseburger | 420 | 25 | 32 |
| Toaster, Bacon Cheeseburger | 850 | 50 | 59 |

**Chicken Sandwiches:**

| | C | F | Cb |
|---|---|---|---|
| Classic Crispy Chicken | 580 | 29 | 57 |
| Classic Grilled Chicken | 450 | 17 | 44 |
| Grilled Asiago Caesar Chicken | 530 | 24 | 44 |

**Breakfast:**

| | C | F | Cb |
|---|---|---|---|
| Breakfast Bacon Toaster | 600 | 31 | 52 |
| **Burrito:** Breakfast, with Bacon | 480 | 26 | 39 |
| SuperSonic Breakfast | 580 | 32 | 49 |
| Jr. Breakfast Burrito | 280 | 15 | 23 |
| **CroiSonic Sandwich:** with Bacon | 550 | 37 | 31 |
| with Sausage | 630 | 45 | 31 |
| **Cinnasnacks,** (3) with Frosting | 630 | 33 | 75 |
| **French Toast Sticks,** (4) with Syrup | 590 | 31 | 71 |

**Coneys & Hot Dogs:**

| | C | F | Cb |
|---|---|---|---|
| All American Dog | 380 | 18 | 40 |
| Chili Cheese | 420 | 26 | 30 |
| Footlong, ¼ pound | 830 | 55 | 54 |
| New York Dog | 340 | 19 | 30 |

**Chicken:**

| | C | F | Cb |
|---|---|---|---|
| **Jumbo Popcorn Chicken:** | | | |
| Small | 280 | 16 | 21 |
| Large | 640 | 37 | 47 |
| Super Crunch Chicken Strips (5) | 590 | 26 | 52 |
| **Wraps:** Crispy Chicken | 510 | 22 | 57 |
| Grilled Chicken | 430 | 14 | 42 |

**Sides:**

| | C | F | Cb |
|---|---|---|---|
| **Apple Slices** | 35 | 0 | 9 |
| **Cheese Fries,** medium | 500 | 26 | 53 |
| **Mozzarella Sticks,** medium | 540 | 27 | 52 |
| **Natural Cut Fries:** Small | 250 | 12 | 33 |
| Medium | 290 | 13 | 38 |
| Large | 470 | 22 | 63 |
| **Onion Rings,** Medium | 580 | 29 | 74 |
| **Tater Tots:** *Per Medium* | | | |
| Plain | 360 | 19 | 43 |
| Cheese Tots | 450 | 28 | 43 |

*Continued Next Page…*

## Sonic Drive-In® cont... (Aug '16)

| | C | F | Cb |
|---|---|---|---|
| **Sundaes:** | | | |
| **Ice Cream,** Caramel; Fudge, av. | 520 | 24 | 67 |
| **Molten Cake Sundae,** Fudge | 800 | 34 | 117 |
| **Cones:** | | | |
| Vanilla Cone | 250 | 13 | 31 |
| Waffle Cone, Vanilla | 320 | 15 | 43 |
| **Malts:** *Medium* | | | |
| Caramel | 900 | 42 | 117 |
| Chocolate | 870 | 40 | 116 |
| Fresh Banana | 890 | 41 | 124 |
| Hot Fudge | 920 | 47 | 112 |
| Peanut Butter | 1110 | 73 | 101 |
| **Shakes:** *Small* | | | |
| Banana; Caramel, av. | 615 | 31 | 79 |
| Pineapple; Strawberry, av. | 575 | 31 | 67 |
| **Fruit Slushes, average:** | | | |
| Small | 190 | 0 | 50 |
| Medium | 275 | 0 | 73 |
| **Sonic Blast:** *Small* | | | |
| Butterfingers | 890 | 46 | 107 |
| Reese's | 870 | 41 | 111 |
| Snickers | 800 | 45 | 90 |
| **Sonic Master Blast:** | | | |
| **Triple Choc:** Small | 900 | 47 | 112 |
| Medium | 1370 | 68 | 178 |
| Large | 2000 | 99 | 259 |
| **Limeade:** | | | |
| Small | 140 | 0 | 37 |
| Medium | 170 | 0 | 46 |
| **Iced Tea,** Sweetened, Blackberry, Raspberry, Mango, medium size, average | 180 | 0 | 46 |

*For Complete Nutritional Data ~ see CalorieKing.com*

## Souplantation® (Aug '16)

| | C | F | Cb |
|---|---|---|---|
| **Soups:** *Per Cup* | | | |
| Chesapeake Corn Chdr w/ Bacon | 220 | 11 | 26 |
| Creamy Cauliflower & Cheese | 280 | 21 | 19 |
| Classical Minestrone | 120 | 2 | 20 |
| Cream of Mushroom | 250 | 20 | 14 |
| New Orleans Jambalaya | 210 | 11 | 18 |
| Texas Red Chili | 190 | 7 | 24 |
| Vegetarian Harvest | 130 | 8 | 14 |

## Souplantation® cont... (Aug '16)

| | C | F | Cb |
|---|---|---|---|
| **Hot Pastas:** *Per 1 Cup* | | | |
| Carbonara Pasta, with Bacon | 290 | 10 | 43 |
| Creamy Cilantro Lime Pesto | 470 | 31 | 37 |
| Fettuccine Alfredo | 390 | 18 | 41 |
| Garden Vegetable with Meatballs | 310 | 10 | 44 |
| Macaroni & Cheese | 330 | 14 | 40 |
| Vegetarian Marinara with Basil | 240 | 5 | 39 |
| **Prepared Salads:** *Per ½ Cup* | | | |
| BBQ Potato | 150 | 9 | 17 |
| Carrot Raisin | 80 | 2.5 | 16 |
| Dijon Potato with Garlic Dill Vinegar | 150 | 12 | 9 |
| Lemon Rice with Cashews | 160 | 7 | 23 |
| Thai Chicken Noodle & Peanut Sce | 150 | 8 | 14 |
| **Muffins:** Banana Nut | 150 | 7 | 22 |
| Chocolate Brownie | 180 | 8 | 26 |
| Fruit Medley Bran | 130 | 0.5 | 29 |
| Tangy Lemon | 170 | 6 | 27 |
| **Breads & Focaccia:** *Per Piece* | | | |
| Bruschetta Focaccia | 80 | 3 | 12 |
| Buttermilk Cornbread Muffin | 140 | 5 | 21 |
| Cheesy Garlic Focaccia | 70 | 2.5 | 9 |
| Indian Grain Bread | 200 | 1.5 | 35 |
| Sourdough Bread | 150 | 0.5 | 27 |
| **Desserts:** *Per ½ Cup* | | | |
| Apple Medley | 70 | 0 | 18 |
| Banana Royale | 80 | 0 | 20 |
| Caramel Apple Cobbler | 390 | 12 | 68 |
| Tapioca Pudding | 140 | 2.5 | 24 |
| **Soft Serve:** *Per ½ Cup* | | | |
| Chocolate | 100 | 2 | 20 |
| Vanilla | 100 | 3 | 20 |

*For Complete Nutritional Data ~ see CalorieKing.com*

## Southern Tsunami® (Aug '16)

| | C | F | Cb |
|---|---|---|---|
| **Rolls:** | | | |
| **Hybrid:** *With White Rice* | | | |
| Berry, 6 oz | 260 | 6 | 48 |
| Blueberry: Salmon | 370 | 15 | 51 |
| Shrimp | 340 | 12 | 51 |
| Done Deal, Tuna | 350 | 14 | 45 |
| Happy Mango | 430 | 19 | 60 |
| Jalapeno, Tilapia | 330 | 12 | 51 |
| Mango Shrimp | 370 | 21 | 46 |
| Red Rock Fujisan | 370 | 14 | 49 |
| Spicy Mango Roll, Tuna | 390 | 10 | 65 |
| Ultimate Chili, Salmon | 290 | 11 | 44 |
| **Chef Samplers:** *With White Rice* | | | |
| A, 12 oz | 570 | 17 | 81 |
| F & H, 15.5 oz | 570 | 6 | 95 |

*Continued Next Page... ...*

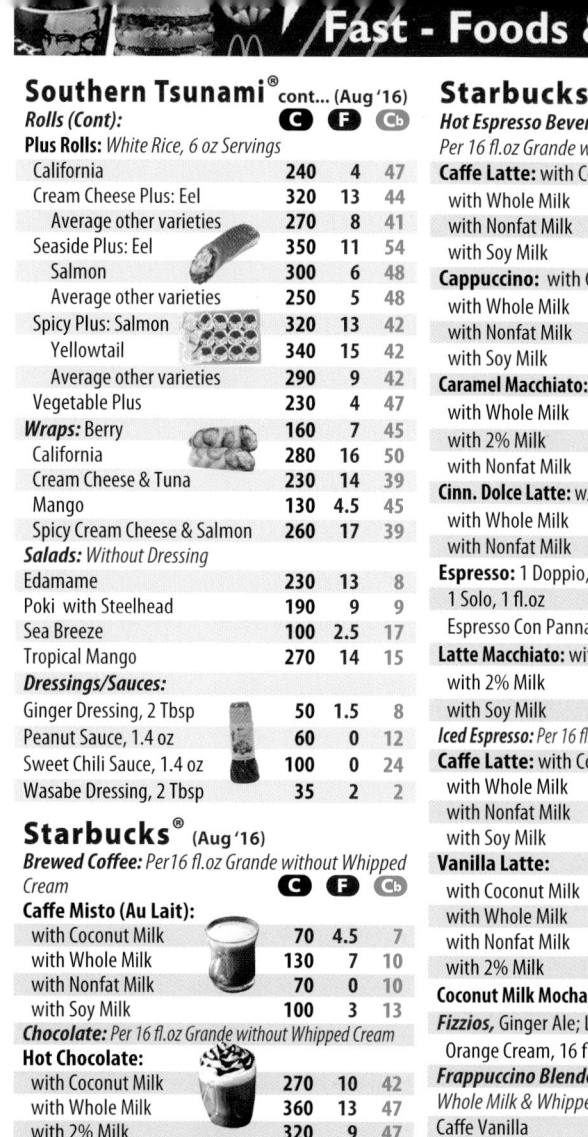

## Southern Tsunami® cont... (Aug '16)

*Rolls (Cont):*

**Plus Rolls:** *White Rice, 6 oz Servings*

| | C | F | Cb |
|---|---|---|---|
| California | 240 | 4 | 47 |
| Cream Cheese Plus: Eel | 320 | 13 | 44 |
| Average other varieties | 270 | 8 | 41 |
| Seaside Plus: Eel | 350 | 11 | 54 |
| Salmon | 300 | 6 | 48 |
| Average other varieties | 250 | 5 | 48 |
| Spicy Plus: Salmon | 320 | 13 | 42 |
| Yellowtail | 340 | 15 | 42 |
| Average other varieties | 290 | 9 | 42 |
| Vegetable Plus | 230 | 4 | 47 |
| *Wraps:* Berry | 160 | 7 | 45 |
| California | 280 | 16 | 50 |
| Cream Cheese & Tuna | 230 | 14 | 39 |
| Mango | 130 | 4.5 | 45 |
| Spicy Cream Cheese & Salmon | 260 | 17 | 39 |

*Salads: Without Dressing*

| | C | F | Cb |
|---|---|---|---|
| Edamame | 230 | 13 | 8 |
| Poki with Steelhead | 190 | 9 | 9 |
| Sea Breeze | 100 | 2.5 | 17 |
| Tropical Mango | 270 | 14 | 15 |

*Dressings/Sauces:*

| | C | F | Cb |
|---|---|---|---|
| Ginger Dressing, 2 Tbsp | 50 | 1.5 | 8 |
| Peanut Sauce, 1.4 oz | 60 | 0 | 12 |
| Sweet Chili Sauce, 1.4 oz | 100 | 0 | 24 |
| Wasabe Dressing, 2 Tbsp | 35 | 2 | 2 |

## Starbucks® (Aug '16)

**Brewed Coffee:** *Per 16 fl.oz Grande without Whipped Cream*

**Caffe Misto (Au Lait):**

| | C | F | Cb |
|---|---|---|---|
| with Coconut Milk | 70 | 4.5 | 7 |
| with Whole Milk | 130 | 7 | 10 |
| with Nonfat Milk | 70 | 0 | 10 |
| with Soy Milk | 100 | 3 | 13 |

**Chocolate:** *Per 16 fl.oz Grande without Whipped Cream*

**Hot Chocolate:**

| | C | F | Cb |
|---|---|---|---|
| with Coconut Milk | 270 | 10 | 42 |
| with Whole Milk | 360 | 13 | 47 |
| with 2% Milk | 320 | 9 | 47 |
| with Soy Milk | 320 | 8 | 51 |

**Peppermint Hot Chocolate:**

| | C | F | Cb |
|---|---|---|---|
| with Whole Milk | 420 | 13 | 65 |
| with 2% Milk | 390 | 9 | 65 |
| with Nonfat Milk | 340 | 2.5 | 65 |
| with Soy Milk | 390 | 7 | 69 |

## Starbucks® cont... (Aug '16)

**Hot Espresso Beverages:**
*Per 16 fl.oz Grande without Whipped Cream*

| | C | F | Cb |
|---|---|---|---|
| **Caffe Latte:** with Coconut Milk | 140 | 8 | 15 |
| with Whole Milk | 220 | 11 | 18 |
| with Nonfat Milk | 130 | 0 | 19 |
| with Soy Milk | 170 | 4.5 | 23 |
| **Cappuccino:** with Coconut Milk | 140 | 8 | 14 |
| with Whole Milk | 140 | 7 | 12 |
| with Nonfat Milk | 80 | 0 | 12 |
| with Soy Milk | 120 | 3.5 | 16 |
| **Caramel Macchiato:** w/ Coconut Mlk | 190 | 8 | 30 |
| with Whole Milk | 270 | 11 | 34 |
| with 2% Milk | 240 | 7 | 34 |
| with Nonfat Milk | 190 | 1 | 35 |
| **Cinn. Dolce Latte:** w/ Coconut Milk | 220 | 7 | 36 |
| with Whole Milk | 300 | 10 | 40 |
| with Nonfat Milk | 210 | 0 | 40 |
| **Espresso:** 1 Doppio, 2 fl.oz | 10 | 0 | 2 |
| 1 Solo, 1 fl.oz | 5 | 0 | 1 |
| Espresso Con Panna, 1 Solo, 1 fl.oz | 30 | 2.5 | 2 |
| **Latte Macchiato:** with Whole Milk | 220 | 11 | 19 |
| with 2% Milk | 190 | 7 | 19 |
| with Soy Milk | 180 | 5 | 23 |

**Iced Espresso:** *Per 16 fl.oz Grande without Whipped Cream*

| | C | F | Cb |
|---|---|---|---|
| **Caffe Latte:** with Coconut Milk | 90 | 5 | 10 |
| with Whole Milk | 150 | 7 | 13 |
| with Nonfat Milk | 90 | 0 | 13 |
| with Soy Milk | 130 | 3.5 | 17 |
| **Vanilla Latte:** | | | |
| with Coconut Milk | 160 | 4.5 | 28 |
| with Whole Milk | 210 | 6 | 30 |
| with Nonfat Milk | 160 | 0 | 31 |
| with 2% Milk | 190 | 4 | 30 |
| **Coconut Milk Mocha Macchiato** | 220 | 10 | 32 |

**Fizzios,** *Ginger Ale; Lemon Ale,*

| | C | F | Cb |
|---|---|---|---|
| Orange Cream, 16 fl oz Grande | 100 | 0 | 26 |

**Frappuccino Blended:** *Cold, Per 16 fl.oz Grande with Whole Milk & Whipped Cream*

| | C | F | Cb |
|---|---|---|---|
| Caffe Vanilla | 430 | 14 | 72 |
| Caramel | 410 | 15 | 66 |
| Cinnamon Dolce | 380 | 14 | 60 |
| Java Chip | 470 | 18 | 72 |
| Mocha | 410 | 15 | 65 |
| White Chocolate Mocha | 440 | 16 | 68 |

*Continued Next Page.... ...*

## Starbucks® cont... (Aug '16)

### Frappuccino Blended Creme: **C** **F** **Cb**

*Per 16 fl.oz Grande with Whole Milk and Whipped Cream*

| | C | F | Cb |
|---|---|---|---|
| Double Chocolaty Chip | 420 | 20 | 57 |
| Green Tea | 430 | 16 | 68 |
| Vanilla Bean Creme | 400 | 16 | 59 |
| **Refreshers:** Cool Lime, 16 oz | 60 | 0 | 15 |
| Valencia Orange, 16 oz | 90 | 0 | 23 |
| Very Berry Hibiscus, 16 oz | 70 | 0 | 18 |

**Smoothies:** *Per 16 fl.oz Grande with 2% Milk, without Whipped Cream*

| | | | |
|---|---|---|---|
| Chocolate | 320 | 5 | 53 |
| Strawberry | 300 | 2 | 60 |

**Teas:** *Per 16 fl.oz Grande, with Whole Milk*

| **Hot Tea Latte:** | | | |
|---|---|---|---|
| Classic Chai Tea | 270 | 7 | 45 |
| Green Tea, sweetened | 280 | 11 | 34 |
| **Iced Tea Latte:** Classic Chai | 260 | 7 | 44 |
| Green Tea | 250 | 10 | 31 |

### Drink Extras:

| | | | |
|---|---|---|---|
| **Caramel Drizzle,** 1 teaspoon | 15 | 0.5 | 2 |
| **Flavored Syrup:** 1 Pump | 20 | 0 | 5 |
| Sugar-Free, 1 Pump | 0 | 0 | 0 |
| **Mocha Syrup,** 1 Pump | 25 | 0.5 | 6 |
| **Sweetened Whipped Cream:** | | | |
| Grande/Venti, cold drinks, average | 110 | 11 | 3 |
| Grande/Venti, hot drinks | 75 | 7 | 3 |

### Breakfast, Hot:

| | | | |
|---|---|---|---|
| Bacon, Gouda & Parmesan Frittata, on Artisan Roll | 350 | 18 | 30 |
| Egg & Cheddar Sandwich | 280 | 13 | 27 |
| Sausage & Cheddar Sandwich | 500 | 28 | 41 |

### Bistro Boxes:

| | | | |
|---|---|---|---|
| Cheese & Fruit | 470 | 28 | 38 |
| Edamame Hummus | 460 | 25 | 47 |
| Protein | 370 | 19 | 37 |
| Thai Style Peanut Chicken Wrap | 450 | 20 | 51 |

### Sandwiches & Paninis:

| | | | |
|---|---|---|---|
| Chicken Artichoke Flatbread S'wich | 510 | 27 | 37 |
| Chicken BLT Salad Sandwich | 470 | 25 | 35 |
| Ham & Swiss Panini | 380 | 11 | 46 |
| Roasted Tomato & Mozz. Panini | 420 | 18 | 47 |
| Turkey & Havarti Sandwich | 460 | 21 | 31 |
| Turkey Pesto Panini | 520 | 21 | 46 |

## Starbucks® cont... (Aug '16)

### Bakery: *Each* **C** **F** **Cb**

| | C | F | Cb |
|---|---|---|---|
| Banana Nut Bread, 4.4 oz | 420 | 22 | 52 |
| Blueberry Muffin, with Yogurt & Honey | 380 | 16 | 53 |
| Butter Croissant | 240 | 12 | 28 |
| Cheese Danish | 320 | 16 | 36 |
| Chewy Chocolate Cookie | 170 | 5 | 30 |
| Chocolate Chip Cookie | 310 | 15 | 42 |
| Cinnamon Morning Bun | 390 | 15 | 58 |
| Classic Coffee Cake | 390 | 16 | 57 |
| Devil's Food Doughnut | 430 | 23 | 53 |
| Iced Lemon Pound Cake | 470 | 20 | 68 |
| Old-Fashioned Glazed Doughnut | 480 | 27 | 56 |

### Yogurt Parfaits:

| | | | |
|---|---|---|---|
| Greek Yog., Cherries & Alm Granola | 280 | 7 | 39 |
| Greek Yogurt, Strawberry | 250 | 7 | 34 |

*Bottled Drinks ~ See Page 37*

## Steak Escape® (Aug '16)

### Sandwiches: *with Menu Board* **C** **F** **Cb**
*Toppings*

| **Regular:** Buffalo Chicken | 820 | 33 | 97 |
|---|---|---|---|
| Cajun Chicken | 660 | 23 | 68 |
| French Onion | 830 | 33 | 75 |
| **Grand:** Chicken | 620 | 19 | 68 |
| Escape | 660 | 19 | 68 |
| Turkey Club | 550 | 14 | 65 |
| Wild West BBQ | 700 | 20 | 75 |

### Wraps: *With Menu Board Toppings*

| | | | |
|---|---|---|---|
| Cajun Chicken | 470 | 17 | 50 |
| **Grand:** Chicken | 490 | 18 | 51 |
| Escape | 520 | 18 | 50 |
| Turkey Club | 440 | 15 | 49 |
| Wild West BBQ | 550 | 19 | 56 |

### Salads:

| **Grilled:** Chicken | 410 | 25 | 14 |
|---|---|---|---|
| Steak | 440 | 24 | 15 |
| Turkey | 360 | 21 | 15 |
| without Meat | 280 | 20 | 13 |
| **Loaded Potatoes:** Bacon & Ranch | 670 | 46 | 51 |
| Cheddar & Bacon | 430 | 17 | 56 |

*For Complete Nutritional Data ~ see CalorieKing.com*

## Steak 'n Shake® (Aug '16)

| The Original Steakburgers: | C | F | Cb |
|---|---|---|---|
| Single, without Cheese | 280 | 11 | 30 |
| **Double:** with Cheese | 440 | 25 | 31 |
| Bacon 'n Cheese | 480 | 28 | 31 |
| Cheesy Cheddar | 480 | 27 | 32 |
| Guacamole | 670 | 44 | 47 |
| Wisconsin Buttery | 700 | 47 | 45 |
| Triple, without cheese | 510 | 30 | 30 |
| *Chili:* 3-Way (1) | 830 | 36 | 94 |
| 5-Way (1) | 1170 | 63 | 99 |
| Deluxe, bowl | 1220 | 74 | 81 |
| *Sandwiches:* | | | |
| Grilled Cheese | 410 | 23 | 37 |
| Grilled Chicken | 370 | 12 | 51 |
| Spicy Chicken | 460 | 18 | 51 |
| *Signature Steak Franks:* | | | |
| Regular | 380 | 27 | 22 |
| Chicago Style | 420 | 27 | 30 |
| Chili Cheese | 620 | 44 | 31 |
| *Salads: Without Dressing* | | | |
| Beef Taco | 580 | 48 | 26 |
| Fried Chicken | 470 | 26 | 34 |
| Grilled Chicken | 270 | 10 | 30 |
| *Sides:* | | | |
| **Chili Cheese Fries:** Regular | 800 | 47 | 81 |
| Large | 1190 | 68 | 120 |
| **French Fries:** Regular | 440 | 21 | 60 |
| Large | 640 | 30 | 87 |
| **Parm. Cheese & Herb Fries:** Reg. | 450 | 21 | 60 |
| Large | 650 | 30 | 87 |
| **Onion Rings:** Regular | 440 | 25 | 48 |
| Large | 880 | 50 | 95 |
| *Breakfast:* | | | |
| **Bagels Sandwich:** with Bacon | 450 | 16 | 51 |
| with Sausage | 570 | 29 | 50 |
| **Biscuits:** Bacon, Egg & Cheese | 520 | 35 | 32 |
| Egg & Cheese | 450 | 30 | 31 |
| Sausage & Egg | 600 | 44 | 31 |
| Sausage, Egg & Cheese | 650 | 48 | 31 |
| with Sausage Gravy: Half order | 540 | 37 | 43 |
| Full Order | 1070 | 74 | 86 |
| **Hash Browns:** Shredded | 320 | 26 | 19 |
| Side order, 5 pieces | 260 | 17 | 23 |
| **Skillets:** Country | 1240 | 94 | 63 |
| Portobello & Swiss | 1020 | 83 | 28 |
| *Hand Dipped Milk Shakes: Per Regular* | | | |
| Banana | 690 | 20 | 121 |
| Butterfinger | 840 | 28 | 138 |
| Chocolate | 640 | 20 | 106 |
| Oreo Mint Cookies 'n Cream | 760 | 25 | 124 |

## Subway® (Aug '16)

*6" Sandwich: 6g Fat or Less*

| | C | F | Cb |
|---|---|---|---|

Figures Based on 9 grain wheat bread, lettuce, tomatoes, onions, green peppers and cucumbers. Oil or mayo not included.

| | C | F | Cb |
|---|---|---|---|
| Black Forest Ham | 290 | 4.5 | 46 |
| Oven Roasted Chicken | 320 | 5 | 47 |
| Roast Beef | 320 | 5 | 45 |
| Subway Club | 310 | 4.5 | 46 |
| Sweet Onion Chicken Teriyaki | 370 | 4.5 | 57 |
| Turkey Breast | 280 | 3.5 | 46 |
| Veggie Delite | 230 | 2.5 | 44 |

*6" Sandwiches:* Figures based on 9-grain wheat bread, lettuce, tomatoes, onion, green peppers, cucumbers. Oil or mayo not included.

| | C | F | Cb |
|---|---|---|---|
| Chkn & Bacon Ranch Melt w/ Chse | 610 | 30 | 48 |
| Cold Cut Combo | 360 | 12 | 46 |
| Italian B.M.T. | 410 | 16 | 46 |
| Meatball Marinara | 480 | 18 | 59 |
| Spicy Italian | 480 | 24 | 46 |
| Steak & Cheese | 380 | 10 | 48 |
| Tuna | 480 | 25 | 44 |

*Kids Meal Sandwiches:* Figures based on 9-grain wheat bread, lettuce, tomatoes, onions, green peppers and cucumbers. Oil or mayo not included.

| | C | F | Cb |
|---|---|---|---|
| Black Forest Ham | 180 | 2.5 | 30 |
| Roast Beef | 200 | 3 | 30 |
| Turkey Breast | 180 | 2 | 30 |
| Veggie Delite | 150 | 1.5 | 29 |

*Condiments & Sauces: For 6" Sandwiches*

| | C | F | Cb |
|---|---|---|---|
| Chipotle Southwest, 0.8 oz | 100 | 10 | 1 |
| Honey Mustard, Fat-Free, 0.8 oz | 30 | 0 | 7 |
| **Mayonnaise:** 1 Tbsp, 0.5 oz | 110 | 12 | 0 |
| Light, 1 Tbsp, 0.5 oz | 50 | 5 | 1 |
| Mustard, Yellow or Deli Brown. 2 tsp | 5 | 0 | 1 |
| Olive Oil Blend, 1 tsp | 45 | 5 | 0 |
| Ranch Dressing | 110 | 11 | 1 |
| Sweet Onion, Fat-Free, 0.8 oz | 40 | 0 | 9 |

*Extras: For 6" Sandwiches*

| | C | F | Cb |
|---|---|---|---|
| Bacon Strips (2) | 80 | 5 | 1 |
| **Cheese:** American, 2 triangles, 0.3 oz | 40 | 3.5 | 1 |
| Cheddar, 2 triangles, 0.3 oz | 60 | 5 | 0 |
| Swiss, 2 triangles, 0.3 oz | 50 | 4.5 | 0 |

*Continued Next Page....*

## Subway® cont... (Aug '16)

*Breakfast:*

| | C | F | Cb |
|---|---|---|---|
| **6" Egg White Omelet Sandwiches:** *Includes 9 Grain Wheat Bread* | | | |
| Bacon, Egg White & Cheese | 410 | 13 | 45 |
| Egg White & Cheese | 330 | 8 | 44 |
| Egg White & Cheese with Ham | 360 | 9 | 45 |
| Steak, Egg White & Cheese | 400 | 10 | 46 |
| **6" Regular Egg Omelet Sandwiches:** *Includes 9 Grain Wheat Bread* | | | |
| Bacon, Egg & Cheese | 450 | 18 | 44 |
| Egg & Cheese | 370 | 13 | 44 |
| Egg & Cheese with Ham | 400 | 14 | 45 |
| Steak, Egg & Cheese | 440 | 15 | 46 |
| **8" Pizza:** | | | |
| Cheese | 680 | 22 | 96 |
| Cheese & Veggies | 740 | 25 | 100 |
| Pepperoni | 790 | 32 | 96 |
| Sausage | 820 | 34 | 97 |
| **Flatizza:** *Includes 9 Grain Wheat Bread* | | | |
| Cheese | 400 | 16 | 43 |
| Pepperoni | 500 | 26 | 44 |
| Spicy Italian | 500 | 25 | 44 |
| Veggie | 410 | 17 | 45 |
| **Sides,** Hash Browns, 3.6 oz | 210 | 10 | 28 |

*Salads (6g Fat or Less):* Figures based on lettuce, tomatoes, onions, green peppers, olives & cucumbers. Dressing or croutons not included.

| | C | F | Cb |
|---|---|---|---|
| Black Forest Ham | 110 | 3 | 12 |
| Oven Roasted Chicken | 130 | 2.5 | 10 |
| Roast Beef; Subway Club, av. | 140 | 3.5 | 11 |
| Sweet Onion Chicken Teriyaki, with Sweet Onion dressing | 240 | 3 | 34 |
| Turkey Breast | 110 | 2 | 12 |
| Veggie Delite | 50 | 1 | 9 |

*Salad Dressings:*

| | C | F | Cb |
|---|---|---|---|
| Chipotle Southwest, 1.5 oz | 190 | 20 | 2 |
| Honey Mustard, 1.5 oz | 60 | 1 | 13 |
| Oil & Vinegar, 1.5 oz | 190 | 21 | 0 |
| Ranch, 1.5 oz | 220 | 23 | 2 |

*Soup:* Per 8 oz Bowl

| | C | F | Cb |
|---|---|---|---|
| Clam Chowder | 200 | 11 | 20 |
| Homestyle Chicken Noodle | 110 | 3 | 14 |
| Loaded Baked Potato | 210 | 13 | 15 |
| Poblano Corn Chowder | 150 | 7 | 18 |
| Tomato Basil | 140 | 7 | 15 |

## Subway® cont... (Aug '16)

*Cookies & Desserts:*

| | C | F | Cb |
|---|---|---|---|
| Apple Slices, 1 package, 2.5 oz | 35 | 0 | 9 |
| Chocolate Chip Cookie, 1.5 oz | 200 | 10 | 30 |
| Oatmeal Raisin Cookie, 1.5 oz | 200 | 8 | 30 |
| Raspberry Cheesecake, 1.6 oz | 200 | 9 | 29 |

## Sweet Tomatoes®

**Same Menu & Data as Souplantation ~ See Page 242**

## Swiss Chalet® (Aug '16)

*Starters:*

| | C | F | Cb |
|---|---|---|---|
| Caesar Salad, without Dressing | 90 | 3 | 13 |
| Chalet Chicken Wings (8), with Mild Sauce | 560 | 42 | 4 |
| Cheese Perogies (7) | 420 | 10 | 69 |
| Stuffed Garlic Cheese Loaf, 10.5 oz | 860 | 57 | 63 |
| **BBQ Back Ribs:** *wWth Smoky BBQ Sauce* | | | |
| Half Rack | 460 | 29 | 17 |
| Full Rack | 920 | 58 | 34 |
| **Chicken Pot Pie,** 1 pie | 560 | 32 | 39 |
| **Fish:** 1 piece, 3.1 oz | 230 | 13 | 14 |
| 2 pieces, 6.3 oz | 450 | 27 | 29 |
| Fish & Chips, 2 pieces, with Tartar Sauce & Coleslaw | 1460 | 92 | 122 |
| **Pasta:** Pesto Penne18 oz | 990 | 51 | 113 |
| Spicy Chipotle Linguine, 18.5 oz | 790 | 33 | 103 |
| **Rotisserie Chicken:** *Without Sides* | | | |
| Double Leg, with Skin | 490 | 31 | 0 |
| Half Chicken, with Skin | 530 | 27 | 0 |
| **Quarter Chicken:** | | | |
| Dark meat, without Skin | 160 | 8 | 0 |
| Dark meat, with Skin | 240 | 16 | 0 |
| White meat, without Skin | 220 | 6 | 0 |
| White meat, with Skin | 290 | 11 | 0 |
| **Sandwiches:** *Without Sides* | | | |
| Classic Hot Chicken, white meat | 520 | 11 | 51 |
| Flatbread: Hickory Chicken | 700 | 32 | 70 |
| Southwest Chicken | 710 | 37 | 64 |
| **Stirfry,** Vegetable w/out Rice & Chkn | 590 | 31 | 74 |
| **Wrap,** | | | |
| Rotisserie Chicken Club | 710 | 32 | 57 |
| **Entree Salads:** *Without Dressing* | | | |
| Spinach Chicken Salad | 410 | 16 | 28 |
| Sweet Heat Salad with Chicken | 340 | 9 | 30 |
| West Coast Salad with Chicken | 460 | 21 | 21 |

*Continued Next Page...*

Updated Nutrition Data ~ www.CalorieKing.com
Persons with Diabetes ~ See Disclaimer (Page 22)

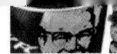
## Swiss Chalet® cont...(Aug '16)

### Dressings/Sauces:

| | C | F | Cb |
|---|---|---|---|
| Caesar Dressing, 1 oz | 180 | 18 | 2 |
| Chalet Dressing, 1 Tbsp, 1 oz | 160 | 14 | 6 |
| Chalet Dipping Sauce, 3.5 oz | 25 | 0.5 | 5 |

### Sides:

| | | | |
|---|---|---|---|
| Creamy Coleslaw | 200 | 14 | 15 |
| Fresh Cut Fries | 530 | 27 | 64 |
| Gravy, 4 oz | 45 | 1.5 | 7 |
| Mashed Potatoes, 5 oz | 150 | 4 | 27 |
| Sauteed Mushrooms, 6 oz | 140 | 1 | 30 |
| Seasoned Rice, 6 oz | 240 | 3.5 | 48 |

### Desserts/Pies:

| | | | |
|---|---|---|---|
| Apple Pie | 440 | 19 | 65 |
| Classic Vanilla Cheesecake | 380 | 25 | 32 |
| Coconut Cream Pie | 540 | 33 | 57 |
| Lemon Meringue Pie | 400 | 11 | 73 |
| Pecan Pie | 590 | 29 | 79 |

## Taco Bell® (Aug '16)

### Burritos:

| | C | F | Cb |
|---|---|---|---|
| ½ lb Cheesy Potato | 490 | 22 | 54 |
| ½ lb Combo | 450 | 18 | 51 |
| 7-Layer | 430 | 16 | 57 |
| Beefy 5-Layer | 500 | 19 | 63 |
| Chili Cheese | 370 | 17 | 40 |
| Shredded Chicken | 400 | 18 | 45 |
| Smothered Beef | 690 | 34 | 69 |
| Smothered Steak | 650 | 28 | 66 |
| XXL Grilled Stuft: Beef | 860 | 41 | 91 |
| Chicken; Steak, av. | 820 | 35 | 88 |

### Fresco Menu:

| | | | |
|---|---|---|---|
| Tacos: Crunchy Beef | 140 | 7 | 13 |
| Soft Tacos: Beef | 160 | 7 | 18 |
| Shrd Chicken; Grilled Steak, av. | 140 | 4 | 16 |

### Fresco Style:

| | | | |
|---|---|---|---|
| Cantina Power Bowls: Chicken | 480 | 20 | 46 |
| Steak | 450 | 21 | 41 |
| Veggie | 430 | 18 | 52 |

### Chalupas:

| | | | |
|---|---|---|---|
| Supreme Beef | 360 | 21 | 31 |
| Supreme Chicken | 340 | 18 | 29 |

### Gorditas:

| | | | |
|---|---|---|---|
| Supreme: Beef | 280 | 12 | 31 |
| Chicken | 260 | 9 | 29 |
| Steak | 260 | 9 | 29 |

## Taco Bell® cont... (Aug '16)

### Fresco Style (Cont.):

| | C | F | Cb |
|---|---|---|---|
| Loaded Potato Griller | 410 | 18 | 50 |
| Soft Tacos: Chicken | 160 | 5 | 16 |
| Spicy Potato | 230 | 12 | 27 |
| Supreme Beef | 210 | 10 | 20 |

### Specialities:

| | | | |
|---|---|---|---|
| Cheese Roll-Up | 180 | 9 | 15 |
| Crunchwrap Supreme | 530 | 21 | 71 |
| MexiMelt | 250 | 13 | 19 |
| Mexican Pizza, 7.5 oz | 550 | 30 | 49 |
| Nachos: BellGrande | 760 | 38 | 84 |
| Supreme | 440 | 23 | 46 |
| Quesadillas: Cheese | 460 | 26 | 37 |
| Steak | 510 | 28 | 38 |

### Tacos:

| | | | |
|---|---|---|---|
| Crunchy: Regular | 170 | 9 | 13 |
| Supreme | 190 | 11 | 15 |
| Double Decker: Regular | 320 | 13 | 36 |
| Supreme | 340 | 15 | 38 |
| Soft: Beef | 180 | 9 | 17 |
| Beef Supreme | 210 | 10 | 20 |
| Chicken | 160 | 5 | 16 |

### Taco Salads:

| | | | |
|---|---|---|---|
| Express Fiesta | 570 | 26 | 63 |
| Fiesta: Beef | 770 | 39 | 77 |
| Chicken | 720 | 33 | 73 |
| Steak | 720 | 34 | 74 |

### Sides: Per Serve

| | | | |
|---|---|---|---|
| Cheesy Fiesta Potato | 230 | 12 | 28 |
| Chips & Guacamole | 320 | 20 | 32 |
| Pintos 'n Cheese, 4.3 oz | 190 | 7 | 22 |

### Condiments:

| | | | |
|---|---|---|---|
| Avocado Ranch Sauce, 0.5 oz | 80 | 8 | 1 |
| Creamy Jalapeno Sauce, 0.5 oz | 70 | 7 | 1 |
| Guacamole, 0.8 oz | 35 | 3 | 2 |
| Salsa Del Sol, 0.5 oz | 5 | 0 | 2 |
| Sour Cream, Reduced Fat, 0.8 oz | 20 | 1.5 | 2 |

### Breakfast:

| | | | |
|---|---|---|---|
| AM Crunchwrap: Bacon | 670 | 42 | 51 |
| Sausage | 700 | 46 | 51 |
| AM Grilled Taco: Bacon | 240 | 14 | 15 |
| Sausage | 230 | 14 | 15 |
| Cheesy Burritos: Tacos: Bacon | 490 | 28 | 37 |
| Fiesta Potato | 520 | 27 | 49 |
| Sausage | 480 | 28 | 36 |
| Steak & Egg | 480 | 25 | 37 |

*Continued Next Page...*

## Taco Bell® cont... (Aug '16)

*Breakfast (Cont):*

| | C | F | Cb |
|---|---|---|---|
| **Grande Scrambler Burrito:** | | | |
| Bacon | 650 | 34 | 64 |
| Sausage | 640 | 34 | 64 |
| **Hashbrown,** 1.9 oz | 160 | 12 | 13 |
| *Sweets:* | | | |
| Caramel Apple Empanada | 280 | 13 | 38 |
| **Cinnabon Delights:** | | | |
| 2 Pack | 160 | 9 | 17 |
| 4 Pack | 310 | 18 | 35 |
| 12 Pack | 930 | 53 | 104 |
| Cinnamon Twists | 170 | 6 | 27 |

*Note: Nutritional data in New York outlets may vary slightly. Please check Taco Bell website*

## Taco Cabana® (Aug '16)

*Cabana Burritos:*
*Includes Flour Burrito & Menu Set Toppings*

| | C | F | Cb |
|---|---|---|---|
| Beef | 980 | 47 | 97 |
| Chicken, Stewed | 900 | 37 | 98 |
| Steak Fajita | 910 | 39 | 96 |
| **Quesadillas:** *Personal, with Guacamole & Sour Cream* | | | |
| Cheese | 710 | 39 | 61 |
| Chicken Breast Fajita; Steak, av. | 765 | 41 | 62 |
| Shrimp Tampico | 820 | 45 | 63 |

**Sizzling Skillets:** *Includes Flour Tortilla, Grilled Onion, Bell Pepper, Rice, Shredded Cheese, Sour Cream, Guacamole, Lettuce & Pico de Gallo*

| | | | |
|---|---|---|---|
| **½ lb, 1 serving:** Brisket | 960 | 46 | 95 |
| Chicken Fajita | 775 | 26 | 95 |
| Mixed Fajita Steak & Chicken | 785 | 28 | 95 |
| Shrimp Tampico; Steak Fajita, av. | 795 | 30 | 97 |
| *Tacos:* | | | |
| Black Bean | 190 | 4 | 34 |
| Carne Guisada | 190 | 6 | 20 |
| **Crispy:** Ground Beef | 200 | 12 | 12 |
| Stewed Chicken | 160 | 7 | 12 |
| **Soft:** | | | |
| Chicken, Stewed | 200 | 7 | 22 |
| Ground Beef | 240 | 12 | 22 |

*Sides & Add-Ons: Per Serving*

| | | | |
|---|---|---|---|
| Black Beans, 4 oz | 80 | 1 | 15 |
| Borracho Beans, 4 oz | 140 | 3 | 20 |
| Guacamole, 3 oz | 110 | 9 | 7 |
| Queso, 3 oz | 110 | 8 | 5 |
| Refried Beans with Cheese, 4 oz | 260 | 14 | 25 |
| Rice, 4 oz | 120 | 0.5 | 25 |
| **Salsa:** Fuego; Roja, 1 oz | 5 | 0 | 1 |
| Verde, 1 oz | 10 | 0 | 1 |
| Sour Cream, 3 oz | 160 | 15 | 3 |

## Taco Del Mar® (Aug '16)

*Baja Bowls:* Per Regular Bowl, with Standard Menu Toppings, without Guacamole, Sour Cream, Jalapenos or Sauce

| | C | F | Cb |
|---|---|---|---|
| **Mondo:** Beef Steak Asada | 500 | 14 | 63 |
| Chicken; Shredded Beef | 520 | 17 | 62 |
| Ground Beef | 570 | 23 | 62 |
| Pork | 500 | 15 | 61 |

*Burritos:* With Standard Menu Toppings, without Guacamole, Sour Cream, Jalapenos or Sauce

| | | | |
|---|---|---|---|
| **Mondito:** | | | |
| Beef Steak Asada | 460 | 12 | 67 |
| Chicken; Shredded Beef, av. | 475 | 14 | 67 |
| Ground Beef | 500 | 17 | 67 |
| Pork | 470 | 13 | 66 |
| **Mondo:** *Per Regular Size* | | | |
| Beef Steak Asada | 810 | 21 | 115 |
| Chicken; Shredded Beef | 840 | 24 | 113 |
| Ground Beef | 880 | 30 | 114 |
| Pork | 830 | 24 | 113 |

*Nachos:* Includes Chips and Standard Menu Toppings without Jalapenos & Sauce

| | | | |
|---|---|---|---|
| Beef Steak Asada; Beef; Chkn, av. | 675 | 31 | 72 |
| Cheese | 620 | 29 | 72 |
| Ground Beef; Fish, average | 700 | 35 | 75 |

*Platters:*

**Enchilada:** *Per 2 Corn Tortillas and Standard Menu Toppings, without Jalapenos or Sauce*

| | | | |
|---|---|---|---|
| Beef Steak Asada (2) | 810 | 27 | 107 |
| Cheese (2) | 810 | 32 | 105 |
| Chicken; Shredded Beef, av., (2) | 845 | 31 | 106 |
| Ground Beef (2) | 890 | 37 | 106 |
| Pork (2) | 830 | 30 | 104 |

**Enchilada/Taco:** *1 Taco, I Enchilada. Includes Corn & Flour Tortillas, Standard Menu Toppings, without Jalapenos or Sauce*

| | | | |
|---|---|---|---|
| Beef Steak Asada | 830 | 28 | 109 |
| Chicken; Shredded Beef, average | 865 | 31 | 107 |
| Fish | 1030 | 48 | 120 |
| Ground Beef | 910 | 38 | 108 |
| Pork | 860 | 31 | 107 |

*Quesadillas:* Includes Flour Tortilla, Standard Menu Toppings, without Sour Cream, Jalapenos and Sauce

| | | | |
|---|---|---|---|
| **Mondito:** Beef Steak Asada | 390 | 17 | 40 |
| Chicken; Shredded Beef, average | 415 | 19 | 39 |
| Ground Beef | 430 | 22 | 40 |
| Pork | 410 | 19 | 39 |

*Continued Next Page...*

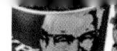 

## Taco Del Mar® cont... (Aug '16)

*Nachos: Includes Chips, Standard Menu Toppings, without Jalapenos and Sauce*

|  | **C** | **F** | **Cb** |
|---|---|---|---|
| **Mondo:** Cheese | 1050 | 62 | 95 |
| Beef Steak Asada | 1150 | 64 | 98 |
| Chicken; Shredded Beef, av. | 1180 | 68 | 97 |
| Ground Beef | 1220 | 74 | 97 |
| Pork | 1170 | 67 | 96 |

*Salads: Includes Shell, Standard Menu Toppings, without Guacamole, Sour Cream or Jalapenos*

|  |  |  |  |
|---|---|---|---|
| **Mondo, Regular:** Chicken | 640 | 32 | 56 |
| Fish | 670 | 34 | 67 |
| Pork | 620 | 31 | 56 |
| Veggie | 720 | 29 | 96 |

*Note: Nutritional Information varies from state to state. Please refer to Taco Del Mar Website*

## Taco John's® (Aug '16)

| **Burritos:** | **C** | **F** | **Cb** |
|---|---|---|---|
| Bean Burrito | 370 | 11 | 53 |
| Beef Grilled Burrito | 590 | 32 | 53 |
| Beefy Burrito | 440 | 21 | 42 |
| Chicken Grilled Burrito | 590 | 30 | 50 |
| Combination Burrito | 410 | 16 | 47 |
| Crunchy Chicken & Potato Burrito | 580 | 27 | 67 |
| Meat & Potato Burrito | 520 | 25 | 57 |
| Super Burrito | 450 | 20 | 50 |
| **Tacos:** | | | |
| Cripsy Taco | 170 | 10 | 11 |
| Soft Shell, Chicken | 190 | 6 | 21 |
| Stuffed Grilled | 540 | 27 | 58 |
| Taco Bravo | 330 | 13 | 38 |
| Taco Burger | 280 | 12 | 29 |
| **Specialties:** | | | |
| Chips & Queso | 430 | 25 | 43 |
| Crunchy Chicken, without sauce | 370 | 18 | 29 |
| **Mexi Rolls:** 2 Pce, w/o Nacho Chse | 280 | 11 | 31 |
| 4 Piece, without Nacho Cheese | 550 | 21 | 61 |
| **Quesadillas:** Beef | 550 | 29 | 46 |
| Cheesy | 450 | 24 | 40 |
| Chicken | 520 | 25 | 45 |
| **Super Nachos:** Small | 420 | 25 | 37 |
| Regular | 790 | 47 | 72 |
| **Super Potato Oles:** | | | |
| Small | 650 | 40 | 59 |
| Regular | 1090 | 67 | 98 |
| **Taco Salads:** Beef, without dressing | 540 | 33 | 40 |
| Chicken, without dressing | 500 | 27 | 39 |
| Crunchy Chicken, without dressing | 630 | 36 | 53 |

## Taco John's® cont... (Aug '16)

| **Wings, Boneless:** | **C** | **F** | **Cb** |
|---|---|---|---|
| Bold Buffalo, 5 oz | 410 | 22 | 30 |
| Honey Habanero, 5 oz | 440 | 18 | 48 |
| Sweet Chipotle, 5 oz | 420 | 18 | 40 |
| **Sides:** | | | |
| Nachos, 5 oz | 380 | 23 | 39 |
| **Potato Oles:** Small | 480 | 27 | 52 |
| Medium | 670 | 38 | 73 |
| Large | 860 | 49 | 94 |
| Refried Beans | 320 | 7 | 46 |
| Side Salad, without Dressing | 40 | 2.5 | 3 |
| **Condiments:** | | | |
| Bacon Ranch, 1.5 oz | 120 | 9 | 10 |
| House Dressing, 1.5 oz | 70 | 7 | 2 |
| Nacho Cheese, 3 oz | 110 | 9 | 5 |
| Salsa, 2 oz | 10 | 0 | 2 |
| Sour Cream, 2 oz | 120 | 10 | 3 |
| **Dessert:** | | | |
| Churro, 2 oz | 200 | 9 | 29 |
| Mexican Donut Bites, 3.2 oz | 290 | 12 | 47 |

## Taco Mayo® (Aug '16)

| **Burritos:** | **C** | **F** | **Cb** |
|---|---|---|---|
| Bean | 450 | 14 | 63 |
| Beef | 515 | 22 | 46 |
| Double, Smothered Double Queso Chicken Platter | 850 | 38 | 84 |
| **Fajita:** Grilled Chicken | 485 | 25 | 43 |
| Grilled Steak | 525 | 28 | 43 |
| **Super:** Beef | 525 | 21 | 56 |
| Chicken | 415 | 18 | 41 |
| **Quesadilla Platter:** | | | |
| Chicken | 675 | 37 | 46 |
| Fajita Chicken | 700 | 39 | 47 |
| Fajita Steak | 725 | 40 | 47 |
| **Tacos:** | | | |
| Crispy Taco, Beef | 160 | 9 | 10 |
| **Soft Taco:** Beef | 230 | 11 | 17 |
| Chicken | 185 | 6 | 16 |
| Taco Burger | 300 | 13 | 28 |
| **Salads:** *As Per Menu Description* | | | |
| Acapulco Chicken | 680 | 50 | 35 |
| **SalsaLita:** Chicken | 280 | 6 | 33 |
| Steak, 12 oz | 305 | 8 | 33 |
| **Taco:** Beef | 705 | 38 | 57 |
| Steak, 11.3 oz | 445 | 25 | 30 |
| **Sides:** | | | |
| Mexicali Rice | 160 | 1 | 36 |
| Refried Beans | 295 | 9 | 43 |
| Potato Locos, Small | 380 | 24 | 36 |

## Taco Time® (Aug '16)

| | C | F | Cb |
|---|---|---|---|
| **Burritos:** | | | |
| Beef, Bean & Cheese | 495 | 17 | 55 |
| Chicken B.L.T. | 695 | 39 | 43 |
| **Big Juan:** Chicken | 575 | 16 | 70 |
| Ground Beef | 635 | 23 | 73 |
| **Casita:** Chicken | 485 | 17 | 42 |
| Ground Beef | 545 | 24 | 46 |
| **Crisp Burrito:** | | | |
| Chicken | 380 | 17 | 33 |
| Ground Beef | 430 | 21 | 36 |
| Pinto Bean | 365 | 14 | 47 |
| **Soft Burrito:** Meat | 425 | 16 | 43 |
| Pinto Bean | 370 | 10 | 54 |
| Veggie | 520 | 17 | 73 |
| **Tacos:** | | | |
| **Crisp Tacos:** | | | |
| Ground Beef, without Sour Cream | 265 | 17 | 12 |
| with Sour Cream | 290 | 19 | 12 |
| **Soft Tacos:** | | | |
| Chicken | 360 | 9 | 40 |
| Ground Beef | 420 | 16 | 43 |
| **Other Favorites:** | | | |
| Cheddar Melt | 250 | 12 | 25 |
| **Chimichanga:** Beef | 645 | 27 | 63 |
| Chicken | 605 | 20 | 63 |
| **Enchilada:** Beef | 290 | 12 | 46 |
| Chicken | 235 | 5 | 51 |
| Nachos Grande | 925 | 43 | 96 |
| **Tostada:** Bean | 230 | 13 | 21 |
| Chicken | 315 | 13 | 22 |
| Ground Beef | 380 | 20 | 25 |
| **Sides:** | | | |
| Chips, Taco, 2 oz | 150 | 3.5 | 27 |
| **Fries:** Cheddar, medium, 7 oz | 500 | 35 | 39 |
| Mexi, medium, 6 oz | 385 | 26 | 38 |
| Stuffed, medium, 7 oz | 465 | 28 | 42 |
| Mexi-Rice, 3.5 oz | 80 | 0.5 | 17 |
| Refritos, with Chips, 6 oz | 230 | 7 | 29 |
| **Salads:** | | | |
| **Regular:** Chicken Taco, 9.5 oz | 310 | 13 | 22 |
| Ground Beef Taco, 9 oz | 370 | 20 | 24 |
| **Tostada Delight:** Chicken, 9 oz | 450 | 19 | 35 |
| Ground Beef, 9 oz | 490 | 26 | 36 |
| **Desserts:** | | | |
| Crustos | 295 | 6 | 58 |
| **Churro:** Plain | 205 | 16 | 17 |
| with Cinnamon & Sugar | 245 | 16 | 27 |

## TCBY® (Aug '16)

| | C | F | Cb |
|---|---|---|---|
| **Soft Serve Frozen Yogurt:** 4 fl.oz | | | |
| Bananas Foster | 100 | 0 | 24 |
| Cake Batter | 120 | 2 | 23 |
| Caramel Supreme | 130 | 1.5 | 27 |
| Cheesecake | 110 | 2 | 23 |
| Chocolate | 110 | 1.5 | 23 |
| Coffee; Golden Vanilla | 120 | 2 | 23 |
| Dutch Chocolate | 100 | 0 | 24 |
| Peanut Butter | 130 | 2 | 26 |
| Silk Almond Nog | 110 | 5 | 31 |
| **No Sugar Added,** Fat Free, | | | |
| average all flavors | 80 | 0 | 22 |
| **Sorbet,** average all flavors, 4 fl.oz | 100 | 0 | 25 |
| **Hand-Scooped Frozen Yogurt:** | | | |
| **Butter Pecan:** Kid's, 4 fl.oz | 120 | 4 | 16 |
| Small, 6.4 fl.oz | 190 | 6.5 | 26 |
| Regular, 12.8 fl.oz | 385 | 13 | 51 |
| **Chunky Choc. Cookie Dough:** | | | |
| Kid's, 4 fl.oz | 160 | 5 | 24 |
| Small, 6.4 fl.oz | 255 | 8 | 38 |
| Regular,12.8 fl.oz | 510 | 16 | 77 |
| **Cookies & Cream:** | | | |
| Kid's,4 fl.oz | 100 | 3.5 | 19 |
| Small, 6.4 fl.oz | 160 | 5 | 30 |
| Regular, 12.8 fl.oz | 320 | 11 | 61 |
| **Peanut Butter Delight:** Kid's, 4 fl.oz | 170 | 8 | 20 |
| Small, 6.4 fl.oz | 270 | 13 | 32 |
| Regular, 12.8 fl.oz | 540 | 26 | 64 |
| **Pralines & Cream:** Kid's 4 fl.oz | 130 | 4 | 19 |
| Small, 6.4 fl.oz | 210 | 6.5 | 30 |
| Regular, 12.8 fl oz | 415 | 13 | 60 |
| **Vanilla Bean:** Kid's,4 fl.oz | 110 | 2.5 | 16 |
| Small, 6.4 fl.oz | 175 | 4 | 26 |
| Regular, 12.8 fl.oz | 350 | 8 | 52 |
| **Cakes:** Per ⅒ Cake | | | |
| Chocolate Lovers Cake | 220 | 6 | 36 |
| Red Velvet Mousse Cake | 190 | 6 | 30 |
| **Pies:** Per ⅒ Pie | | | |
| Cookies & Creme Pie | 320 | 15 | 42 |
| Peanut Buttery Fudge Pie | 340 | 17 | 42 |

## TGI Friday's® (Aug '16)

| Starters: As Served | C | F | Cb |
|---|---|---|---|
| Bacon-Wrapped Stuffed Jalapeno | 480 | 30 | 14 |
| Crispy Green Bean Fries | 900 | 65 | 69 |
| Loaded Potato Skins | 1380 | 98 | 88 |
| Mozzarella Sticks | 820 | 50 | 54 |
| Pan Seared P'stickers | 590 | 25 | 72 |
| Sesame Jack Chicken Strips | 1090 | 35 | 159 |
| Spinach Florentine Flatbread | 540 | 30 | 49 |
| Tuscan Spinach Dip | 870 | 59 | 59 |
| Warm Pretzels w/ Beer-Chse Sce | 1180 | 60 | 125 |
| **Hand-Crafted Burgers:** As Served | | | |
| Cheeseburger | 1250 | 74 | 97 |
| Jack Daniel's Burger | 1510 | 99 | 151 |
| NY Cheddar & Bacon Burger | 1490 | 72 | 108 |
| Sedona Black Bean Burger | 1120 | 55 | 121 |
| Turkey Burger | 960 | 44 | 98 |
| **Sandwiches:** Without Sides | | | |
| California Chicken Club | 640 | 31 | 46 |
| French Dip | 740 | 43 | 49 |
| Jack Daniel's Chicken | 1220 | 62 | 110 |
| **Steaks:** Without Sides | | | |
| Flat Iron | 380 | 26 | 3 |
| NY Strip, 10 oz | 500 | 33 | 4 |
| Ribeye | 560 | 32 | 3 |
| **Chicken & Pasta:** As Served | | | |
| Crispy Chicken Fingers | 1030 | 59 | 87 |
| **Pasta:** | | | |
| Bruschetta Chicken | 950 | 44 | 88 |
| Cajun Shrimp & Chicken | 1110 | 59 | 86 |
| Parmesan-Crusted Chicken | 980 | 57 | 55 |
| **Jack Daniels Grill:** Without Sides | | | |
| Chicken | 530 | 8 | 58 |
| Chicken & Shrimp | 530 | 11 | 67 |
| Flat Iron Steak | 500 | 16 | 57 |
| NY Strip | 620 | 23 | 57 |
| Ribs & Shrimp | 1790 | 78 | 197 |
| **Salads:** Includes Dressing | | | |
| Caesar, with 4 oz Flat Iron Steak | 780 | 62 | 30 |
| Chipotle Yucatan Chicken | 760 | 52 | 35 |
| Pecan-Crusted Chicken | 1080 | 71 | 76 |
| Strawberry Fields Salad | 610 | 47 | 40 |
| **Dressing:** Per 2 oz | | | |
| Balsamic Vinaigrette | 190 | 19 | 4 |
| Bleu Cheese | 200 | 21 | 1 |
| Honey Mustard | 200 | 18 | 8 |
| Ranch | 130 | 14 | 1 |

## TGI Friday's® cont... (Aug '16)

| Signature Sides: | C | F | Cb |
|---|---|---|---|
| Cheddar Mc & Cheese | 470 | 23 | 43 |
| Coleslaw | 90 | 6 | 7 |
| Jasmin Rice Pilaf | 420 | 11 | 72 |
| Mashed Potatoes | 210 | 10 | 21 |
| Seasoned Fries | 320 | 16 | 40 |
| Sweet Potato Fries | 390 | 20 | 50 |
| **Soups:** Per 10 oz Bowl | | | |
| French Onion | 350 | 21 | 25 |
| White Cheddar Broccoli Cheese | 280 | 20 | 18 |
| **Soup Of The Day:** | | | |
| New England Clam Chowder | 500 | 30 | 45 |
| Tomato Basil | 300 | 24 | 20 |
| Tortilla | 210 | 10 | 18 |
| **Desserts:** Per Whole Dish | | | |
| Brownie Obsession | 1200 | 60 | 153 |
| Oreo Madness | 500 | 21 | 76 |
| Vanilla Bean Cheesecake | 920 | 57 | 88 |
| **Signature Slushes:** Per 22 oz Tumbler | | | |
| Blue Raspberry | 280 | 0 | 67 |
| Mango Peach Lemonade | 230 | 0 | 57 |
| Red Bull Passion | 210 | 0 | 54 |
| Ruby Red Bull | 200 | 0 | 51 |

## Thundercloud Subs® (Aug '16)

| Subs: Small, with Standard Toppings | C | F | Cb |
|---|---|---|---|
| **Classic:** BLT | 405 | 17 | 40 |
| Smoked Chicken | 295 | 4 | 40 |
| Turkey | 280 | 4 | 41 |
| **Low Fat:** Hot Pastrami | 430 | 13 | 41 |
| Roast Beef | 315 | 4 | 41 |
| **Signature Subs:** Club | 480 | 19 | 43 |
| California Club | 510 | 23 | 45 |
| NY Italian | 570 | 30 | 42 |
| Office Favorite | 850 | 40 | 81 |
| Texas Tuna | 700 | 45 | 44 |
| Veggie Delite, with Hummus | 360 | 10 | 53 |

## T.J. Cinnamons® (Aug '16)

| Bakery: | C | F | Cb |
|---|---|---|---|
| Cinnamon Roll, Original, 5.3 oz | 505 | 10 | 73 |
| Cinnamon Twist (1), 2.5 oz | 260 | 14 | 33 |
| Sticky Bun Smear with Pecans, 1.3 oz | 180 | 12 | 18 |
| T.J. Cream Cheese Icing, 1 oz | 115 | 5 | 18 |
| **Mocha Chill,** | | | |
| without Whipped Cream, 12 fl.oz | 265 | 4 | 46 |

## Tim Hortons® (Aug '16)

| Breakfast: | C | F | Cb |
|---|---|---|---|
| **Biscuit Sandwich:** | | | |
| Sausage, Egg & Cheese | 530 | 34 | 33 |
| Turkey Sausage, Egg & Cheese | 430 | 23 | 35 |
| **English Muffin Sandwich:** | | | |
| Bacon, Egg & Cheese | 340 | 16 | 30 |
| Steak, Egg White & Cheese | 260 | 7 | 29 |
| **Grilled B'Fast Wraps:** | | | |
| Farmer's Breakfast | 650 | 38 | 54 |
| Steak & Cheddar | 435 | 22 | 40 |
| **Oatmeal,** with Mixed Berries, reg. | 210 | 3 | 44 |
| *Hash Brown,* Regular | 130 | 7 | 16 |
| *Hot Bowls:* Chili, 10 oz | 300 | 16 | 18 |
| Mac & Cheese, 10 oz | 490 | 27 | 48 |
| *Soup:* Chicken Noodle, 10 oz | 120 | 2 | 21 |
| Clam Chowder, 10 oz | 190 | 7 | 23 |
| Potato Bacon Cheddar, 10 oz | 260 | 15 | 23 |
| *Paninis:* Grilled Cheese | 450 | 15 | 57 |
| Grilled Steak & Cheese | 510 | 19 | 58 |
| Grilled Tuscan Chicken | 560 | 20 | 62 |
| **Sandwiches:** | | | |
| **Ham & Swiss** | 380 | 15 | 36 |
| **Turkey Bacon Club** | 510 | 27 | 36 |
| *Wraps,* Chicken/Steak Fajita, av. | 430 | 20 | 40 |
| *Donuts:* Apple Fritter | 290 | 8 | 48 |
| Boston Creme Filled | 220 | 6 | 35 |
| Chocolate, Glazed | 280 | 14 | 37 |
| Chocolate Dip | 190 | 7 | 29 |
| Double Chocolate | 270 | 15 | 32 |
| Football | 230 | 8 | 34 |
| Honey Cruller | 310 | 18 | 37 |
| Old Fashioned, Plain | 210 | 10 | 25 |
| *Timbits:* Chocolate, Glazed | 70 | 3 | 10 |
| Apple Fritter; Honey Dip, average | 50 | 1.5 | 9 |
| Old Fashion, Plain | 50 | 2.5 | 7 |
| *Bagels:* Classic, av., 4 oz | 300 | 3 | 59 |
| Bagel BELT, 9.5 oz | 560 | 24 | 62 |
| *Cream Cheese Spread,* Light, 1.5 oz | 90 | 7 | 3 |
| *Cinnamon Roll,* Frosted | 400 | 14 | 60 |
| *Cookies,* Choc./Oatmeal Raisin, av. | 230 | 10 | 34 |
| *Croissants,* Cheese | 310 | 17 | 30 |
| *Danish,* Maple Pecan | 400 | 19 | 53 |
| *Greek Yogurt,* with Berries, av. | 250 | 5 | 29 |
| *Muffins:* Choc. Chip, 4 oz | 420 | 16 | 66 |
| Blueberry; Fruit; Pecan Ban., av., 4 oz | 350 | 11 | 58 |
| Cran Apple Walnut Bran, 4 oz | 350 | 14 | 54 |
| *Beverages:* Cappuccino, 10 oz | 70 | 0 | 11 |
| Hot Chocolate, 10 oz | 240 | 6 | 45 |
| Latte, 10 oz | 80 | 0 | 12 |
| Mocha Latte, 10 oz | 190 | 6 | 26 |
| Frozen Lemonade, Orig., 12 oz | 140 | 0 | 34 |
| Iced Capp®, w/ Milk, 12 oz | 180 | 2 | 39 |
| Iced Coffee, with Milk, 16 oz | 45 | 0 | 9 |

## Togo's® (Aug '16)

*California Outlet ~ Please check local outlet for menu items and nutritional information*

| *Cold Sandwiches:* Per Regular, with Classic White Bread, without Dressing | C | F | Cb |
|---|---|---|---|
| **Avocado & Cheese** | 630 | 29 | 73 |
| **Black Forest Ham & Cheese** | 560 | 16 | 66 |
| **California Club** | 810 | 46 | 68 |
| **Chicken Salad** | 560 | 21 | 70 |
| **Egg Salad & Cheese** | 640 | 28 | 70 |
| **Hummus** | 650 | 27 | 85 |
| **Roast Beef** | 580 | 9 | 66 |
| **Salami & Cheese** | 945 | 37 | 72 |
| **Turkey & Avocado** | 570 | 20 | 72 |
| **Turkey & Cranberry** | 540 | 7 | 90 |
| *Sandwich Dressings:* | | | |
| Mayo, regular | 150 | 16 | 0 |
| Boom Boom Sauce, regular | 160 | 16 | 3 |
| *Hot Sandwiches:* Regular with White Bread | | | |
| **Chicken** | 500 | 8 | 67 |
| **Meatball** | 870 | 40 | 79 |
| **Pastrami** | 730 | 33 | 69 |
| **Roast Beef** | 580 | 9 | 66 |
| *Signature Sandwiches:* | | | |
| **BBQ Ranch Chicken** | 910 | 39 | 102 |
| **Kickin' Chipotle Roast Beef** | 1100 | 59 | 74 |
| **Pastrami Reuben** | 950 | 52 | 71 |
| **Smokehouse BBQ Pulled Pork** | 800 | 26 | 109 |
| *Toasted Sandwiches:* Regular with White Bread | | | |
| **BBQ Pulled Pork,** with Cheddar | 1090 | 53 | 98 |
| **The Clubhouse** | 850 | 35 | 85 |
| **The Cuban** | 760 | 37 | 62 |
| **The Triple Dip** | 1080 | 50 | 67 |
| **Viva Veggie Wrap** | 600 | 26 | 76 |
| *Salad Wraps:* Includes Spinach Wrap, with Dressing | | | |
| **Asian Chicken** | 590 | 24 | 70 |
| **Chicken Caesar** | 540 | 20 | 65 |
| **Santa Fe Chicken** | 660 | 31 | 70 |
| *Salads:* Per Full Salad, without Dressing | | | |
| **Chicken Caesar** | 210 | 8 | 17 |
| **Farmer's Market** | 160 | 6 | 20 |
| **Santa Fe Chicken** | 410 | 21 | 35 |
| *Salad Dressings:* Caesar, 2.5 oz | 150 | 12 | 8 |
| Buttermilk Ranch, 2.5 oz | 330 | 35 | 3 |
| Italian Vinaigrette, 2.5 oz | 310 | 33 | 2 |
| Thousand Island, 2.5 oz | 310 | 28 | 12 |
| *Soups:* Broccoli Cheddar, 10 oz | 290 | 18 | 24 |
| Garden Veggetable, 10 oz | 90 | 0.5 | 19 |
| New England Clam Chowder, 10 oz | 310 | 20 | 26 |
| Rstd Yukon Baked Potato, 10 oz | 320 | 24 | 18 |
| *Brownie:* Choc. Chunk, 3 oz | 430 | 22 | 54 |
| *Cookies:* Dark Choc. Chunk, 3 oz | 410 | 21 | 53 |
| Oatmeal Raisin, 3 oz | 360 | 13 | 57 |
| Peanut Butter Chip, 3 oz | 410 | 23 | 48 |

**Updated Nutrition Data ~ www.CalorieKing.com**
**Persons with Diabetes ~ See Disclaimer (Page 22)**

## Tropical Smoothie Cafe® (Aug '16)

*Menu & Nutrition May Differ from Outlets to Outlet.
Please Check Instore*

| | C | F | Cb |
|---|---|---|---|
| **Breakfast:** | | | |
| **Wraps:** All American Omelet | 540 | 33 | 37 |
| Peanut Banana Crunch Flatbread | 775 | 39 | 85 |
| Tex Mex Veggie | 485 | 27 | 42 |
| **Toasted Sandwiches:** *Sandwich Only with Set Menu Components* | | | |
| Cranberry Pecan Chicken Salad, on Seedilicious Bread | 495 | 18 | 64 |
| Turkey Bacon Ranch on Ciabatta | 580 | 22 | 53 |
| Ultimate Club on Ciabatta | 645 | 29 | 53 |
| **Toasted Wraps:** *Wrap Only, with Set Menu Components* | | | |
| Hummus Veggie | 675 | 32 | 79 |
| King Caesar Chicken | 635 | 32 | 53 |
| Totally Turkey | 615 | 27 | 54 |
| **Fresh Salads:** *Includes Standard Dressing* | | | |
| Chicken Caesar | 505 | 40 | 10 |
| Loaded Spinach | 575 | 34 | 70 |
| Thai Chicken | 340 | 9 | 38 |
| **Classic Smoothies:** *Per 24 oz with Turbinado* | | | |
| Blimey Limey | 370 | 0 | 99 |
| Blueberry Bliss | 310 | 1 | 78 |
| Jetty Punch | 340 | 0 | 86 |
| Peaches 'N Silk | 315 | 0 | 79 |
| Rockin' Raspberry | 400 | 0 | 100 |
| Sunny Day | 435 | 0 | 108 |
| Sunrise Sunset | 320 | 0 | 81 |
| **Indulgent Smoothies:** *24 oz with Turbinado* | | | |
| Bahama Mama | 475 | 4 | 107 |
| Beach Bum | 520 | 4 | 122 |
| Mocha Madness | 590 | 5 | 126 |
| Peanut Butter Cup | 695 | 20 | 121 |
| **Supercharged:** *Per 24 oz with Turbinado* | | | |
| Health Nut, with Soy | 495 | 5 | 88 |
| Lean Machine | 440 | 0 | 112 |
| Muscle Blaster, with Whey | 440 | 2 | 88 |
| Peanut Paradise, with Whey | 675 | 18 | 101 |

*with Splenda, deduct 200 calories & 50g carbs*

## Tubby's® (Aug '16)

*Subs: Per 8" Regular Wheat Bun, w/out Dressing or Sauce*

| | C | F | Cb |
|---|---|---|---|
| **Deli-Subs:** | | | |
| Ham & Cheese | 500 | 10 | 76 |
| Turkey Breast & Cheese | 530 | 12 | 76 |
| **Grilled Burger Subs:** Big Tub | 630 | 25 | 75 |
| Burger Special | 760 | 33 | 78 |
| Cheeseburger Italiano | 740 | 33 | 76 |
| Pizza Burger | 630 | 25 | 75 |

## Tubby's® cont...(Aug '16)

*Subs (Cont): Per 8" Reg. Wheat Bun, without Dressing or Sauce*

| | C | F | Cb |
|---|---|---|---|
| **Grilled Chicken Subs:** | | | |
| Chicken, Grilled | 440 | 4.5 | 73 |
| Chicken & Broccoli | 520 | 10 | 75 |
| Chicken & Cheddar | 510 | 10 | 73 |
| Chicken Fajita | 520 | 10 | 75 |
| **Grilled Steak Subs:** | | | |
| Portabella Mushroom Steak | 600 | 17 | 80 |
| Pepper Steak & Cheese | 570 | 15 | 76 |
| Steak & Cheese | 560 | 15 | 74 |
| Steak Special | 590 | 16 | 76 |
| **Specialty Subs:** BLT | 580 | 23 | 73 |
| Cold Veggie | 470 | 9 | 79 |
| Italian Sausage | 630 | 26 | 77 |
| Pulled Pork | 660 | 25 | 83 |
| Tuna | 530 | 9 | 74 |

## Uno Pizzeria & Grill® (Aug '16)

| | C | F | Cb |
|---|---|---|---|
| **Appetizers:** *Per Whole Dish* | | | |
| Mozzarella Sticks | 850 | 47 | 80 |
| Muchos Nacos | 1510 | 72 | 174 |
| Onion Rings | 1190 | 56 | 159 |
| **Burgers:** *Without Sides* | | | |
| BBQ Burger, w/ Bacon & Cheddar | 1190 | 70 | 32 |
| Cheddar Bacon Burger | 1170 | 70 | 27 |
| Uno Burger | 910 | 48 | 26 |
| **Entrees:** | | | |
| **Chicken:** *Without Sides Or Breadstick* | | | |
| Baked Stuffed Spinoccoli | 360 | 14 | 10 |
| Chicken Thumb Platter | 480 | 17 | 34 |
| **Deep Dish Pizza:** *Per Pizza* | | | |
| Chicago Classic | 2300 | 164 | 119 |
| Numero Uno | 1850 | 128 | 120 |
| Prima Pepperoni | 1750 | 121 | 114 |
| **Pasta:** *Without Breadstick* | | | |
| Chicken Spinoccoli | 980 | 38 | 107 |
| Deep Dish Mac & Cheese | 1690 | 105 | 120 |
| Shrimp Scampi | 1030 | 53 | 96 |
| **Steak & Seafood:** *Without Sides Or Breadstick* | | | |
| Baked Haddock | 580 | 35 | 12 |
| Brewmasters Grill NY Sirloin | 510 | 14 | 21 |
| Grilled Shrimp & Sirloin | 720 | 33 | 2 |
| **Sides:** | | | |
| Farro Salad, 7.5 oz | 180 | 7 | 31 |
| French Fries, 5.5 oz | 350 | 27 | 25 |
| Red Bliss Mashed Potatoes | 270 | 14 | 34 |
| Roasted Seasonal Veggies, 7.2 oz | 80 | 4.5 | 10 |
| **Dessert:** All American | 650 | 29 | 90 |
| Brownie Bowl | 1160 | 53 | 158 |

## Villa Fresh Italian® (Aug '16)

| *Pizzas:* Per Slice | C | F | Cb |
|---|---|---|---|
| **Neapolitan:** | | | |
| Plain, 7 oz | 440 | 15 | 52 |
| Deluxe, 9 oz | 520 | 21 | 55 |
| Sausage & Pepperoni, 8.5 oz | 570 | 26 | 54 |
| **Stuffed:** Baked Ziti | 920 | 37 | 109 |
| Meat | 910 | 39 | 96 |
| Spinach and Mushroom | 735 | 33 | 80 |
| *Entrees:* | | | |
| Baked Ziti | 860 | 40 | 90 |
| Chicken Marsala | 800 | 25 | 108 |
| Chicken Parmigiana | 870 | 32 | 106 |
| Chicken Scampi | 810 | 29 | 107 |
| Fettuccini Alfredo | 930 | 52 | 87 |
| Mac & Cheese | 1150 | 75 | 86 |
| *Vegetables:* Roasted Potatoes | 210 | 12 | 25 |
| Sauteed, Fresh, 6oz | 80 | 6 | 6 |

## Vocelli Pizza® (Aug '16)

| *Pizzas:* | | | |
|---|---|---|---|
| **Artisan:** *Per ⅛ of Medium Pizza* | C | F | Cb |
| Basil Pesto Primavera | 240 | 10 | 28 |
| Buffalo Chicken | 220 | 9 | 26 |
| Chicken Carbonara | 250 | 10 | 27 |
| Chicken Spinaci | 220 | 8 | 27 |
| Deluxe | 260 | 10 | 29 |
| Hawaiian | 280 | 11 | 30 |
| Meat Magnifico | 280 | 12 | 26 |
| Mexican | 300 | 15 | 28 |
| Philly Steak | 270 | 13 | 25 |
| Quattro Cheese | 270 | 11 | 28 |
| Spring Veggie | 210 | 7 | 28 |
| *Pasta:* Chicken Alfredo, 18 oz | 1080 | 55 | 100 |
| Chicken Parmesan, 20 oz | 1030 | 35 | 132 |
| Chicken Pesto, 18 oz | 1110 | 59 | 99 |
| ***House Baked Subs:*** *On Ciabatta* | | | |
| Buffalo Chicken, 7oz | 310 | 15 | 28 |
| Chicken Parmesan, 7.2 oz | 440 | 18 | 45 |
| Meatball, 7.2 oz | 460 | 23 | 36 |
| ***Salads:*** *Per Regular Size, without Dressing* | | | |
| Antipasta, 16 oz | 270 | 16 | 17 |
| Caesar, 8 oz | 130 | 3 | 5 |
| Mediterranean, 16 oz | 270 | 18 | 17 |
| Tuscan Grilled Chicken, 14 oz | 290 | 13 | 12 |
| ***Wings:*** *Bone In* | | | |
| BBQ, 9 oz | 760 | 53 | 14 |
| Buffalo, 9 oz | 720 | 54 | 2 |
| Garlic, 9 oz | 960 | 81 | 3 |
| Hot Vesuvius, 9 oz | 720 | 54 | 2 |

## Wahoo's Fish Taco® (Aug '16)

| *Bowls:* With White Rice & Black Beans | C | F | Cb |
|---|---|---|---|
| #7 Blackened/Charbroiled Chkn, av. | 860 | 15 | 127 |
| # 8 Charbroiled/Teriyaki Fish, av. | 930 | 22 | 126 |
| #9 Veggie | 760 | 11 | 141 |
| #10 Carnitas/Kahlua Pig, average | 1025 | 25 | 131 |
| *Burritos:* With Brown Rice & White Beans | | | |
| **Banzai:** | | | |
| Blackened or Charbroiled: | | | |
| Chicken | 575 | 16 | 77 |
| Fish, average | 620 | 21 | 77 |
| Mushroom | 490 | 14 | 81 |
| Carne Asada | 565 | 17 | 79 |
| Carnitas | 685 | 23 | 79 |
| Shrimp | 475 | 14 | 77 |
| Vegetarian | 485 | 14 | 82 |
| *Side Kicks,* Corn Tortillas, each | 145 | 2 | 29 |
| *Shredder Sandwiches:* Blackened or Charbroiled | | | |
| Chicken | 360 | 18 | 29 |
| Fish, average | 385 | 20 | 29 |
| Carne Asada | 315 | 18 | 30 |

*For Complete Nutritional Data ~ see CalorieKing.com*

## WAWA® (Aug '16)

| *Breakfast:* | C | F | Cb |
|---|---|---|---|
| **Bagels:** Plain | 260 | 1 | 55 |
| with Reg. Butter | 310 | 7 | 55 |
| Cinnamon Raisin | 290 | 1 | 63 |
| with Regular Cream Cheese | 380 | 10 | 64 |
| Everything | 310 | 6 | 56 |
| **Bowls:** *Without Extras* | | | |
| Creamed Chipped Beef On White | 230 | 6 | 36 |
| French Toasts: without Meat | 340 | 13 | 54 |
| with Bacon | 420 | 19 | 55 |
| with Sausage Crumble | 540 | 32 | 55 |
| with Turkey Sausage Patty | 430 | 20 | 55 |
| Scrambled Egg: with Bacon | 470 | 34 | 10 |
| with Sausage Crumble | 590 | 47 | 10 |
| **Burritos:** *With Scrambled Egg* | | | |
| Bacon | 450 | 23 | 38 |
| Beef Steak & Cheddar Cheese | 480 | 23 | 40 |
| Chicken Steak with Cheddar Chse | 480 | 22 | 40 |
| **Sizzlis:** *Per Sizzli* | | | |
| Bagels: Bacon, Egg & Cheese | 410 | 18 | 43 |
| Pork Roll, Egg & Cheese | 420 | 19 | 43 |
| ***Breaded Chicken Strips:*** | | | |
| 3 piece | 240 | 13 | 16 |
| 5 piece | 400 | 22 | 27 |

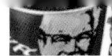

## WAWA® cont... (Aug '16)

*Cold Hoagies:* | **C** | **F** | **Cb**

*On 6" Shorti Roll without Toppings*

| | C | F | Cb |
|---|---|---|---|
| Egg Salad | 650 | 37 | 61 |
| Tuna Salad | 690 | 39 | 63 |
| Turkey | 370 | 5 | 59 |

**Hot Dogs:** *Without Toppings, Mustard or Sauce*

| | C | F | Cb |
|---|---|---|---|
| **All Beef:** ¼ Pound | 420 | 28 | 21 |
| Big Bacon Cheese Dog | 810 | 47 | 57 |

**Hot Hoagies:** *On 6" Shorti Roll without Toppings*

| | C | F | Cb |
|---|---|---|---|
| Beef Steak & Cheddar Cheese | 550 | 19 | 59 |
| Chicken Steak & Cheddar Cheese | 550 | 17 | 59 |
| Meatballs & Cheddar Cheese | 730 | 34 | 75 |

**Soups:** *Per Medium Serving*

| | C | F | Cb |
|---|---|---|---|
| Baked Potato w/ Cheddar & Bacon | 450 | 32 | 28 |
| Chicken Noodle | 190 | 7 | 20 |
| Lobster Bisque | 470 | 38 | 20 |
| Italian Wedding | 210 | 7 | 21 |
| New England Clam Chowder | 330 | 21 | 24 |

**Quesadillas:** *Without Toppings*

| | C | F | Cb |
|---|---|---|---|
| Beef & Cheddar Cheese | 480 | 22 | 39 |
| Cheddar Cheese | 400 | 20 | 38 |
| Chicken & Cheddar Cheese | 480 | 20 | 39 |

**Sides:** *Per Medium Serving*

| | C | F | Cb |
|---|---|---|---|
| Chili | 350 | 16 | 35 |
| Macaroni & Beef | 350 | 11 | 43 |
| Macaroni & Cheese | 500 | 25 | 49 |
| Mashed Potatoes | 470 | 28 | 50 |
| Meatballs in a Cup | 320 | 21 | 17 |
| Seafood Chowder | 210 | 9 | 20 |

**Bakery:**

| | C | F | Cb |
|---|---|---|---|
| **Croissant,** Plain | 280 | 14 | 35 |
| **Muffins:** Banana Walnut | 610 | 33 | 74 |
| Blueberry | 570 | 28 | 72 |
| Chocolate Chip | 680 | 34 | 86 |
| Corn | 640 | 29 | 87 |

**Hot Beverages:** *Per 16 oz, without Extras*

| | C | F | Cb |
|---|---|---|---|
| **Hot Cappuccino,** with 2% milk | 130 | 5 | 13 |
| **Mocha Latte,** with 2% milk | 330 | 7 | 59 |
| **Smoothie,** Strawberry Banana, without whipped cream, 24 oz | 690 | 0 | 180 |

## Wendy's® (Aug '16)

| Breakfast: | C | F | Cb |
|---|---|---|---|
| Artisan Egg Sandwich | 360 | 19 | 29 |
| Honey Butter Chicken Biscuit | 510 | 25 | 52 |
| Morning Melt Panini | 520 | 33 | 33 |
| Sausage & Egg Burrito | 280 | 20 | 14 |
| Seasoned Home-Style Potatoes | 150 | 4 | 26 |

## Wendy's® cont... (Aug '16)

**Cheeseburgers:** *With Standard Toppings*

| | C | F | Cb |
|---|---|---|---|
| Dave's ¼ lb Single | 550 | 34 | 35 |
| Dave's ½ lb Double | 790 | 51 | 35 |
| Dave's ¾ lb Triple | 1070 | 72 | 36 |
| Baconator | 930 | 62 | 33 |
| Double Stack | 390 | 21 | 25 |
| Jr. Bacon Cheeseburger | 380 | 22 | 26 |
| Jr. Cheeseburger | 280 | 13 | 25 |
| Jr. Cheeseburger Deluxe | 330 | 19 | 27 |
| Son of Baconator | 620 | 39 | 33 |

**Sandwiches:** *With Standard Toppings*

| | C | F | Cb |
|---|---|---|---|
| Asiago Ranch Club, with Homestyle Chicken | 650 | 33 | 50 |
| Crispy Chicken | 350 | 17 | 35 |
| Homestyle Chicken | 500 | 21 | 48 |
| Spicy Chicken | 490 | 21 | 46 |
| Ultimate Chicken Grill | 340 | 8 | 34 |
| **Wraps:** Grilled Chicken | 270 | 10 | 24 |
| Spicy Chicken | 370 | 19 | 30 |

**Chicken Nuggets:**

| | C | F | Cb |
|---|---|---|---|
| **Regular:** 6 pieces | 270 | 19 | 15 |
| 10 pieces | 450 | 32 | 26 |
| **Spicy:** 6 pieces | 280 | 17 | 17 |
| 10 piece | 470 | 29 | 29 |

**Dipping Sauce:** *Per 1 oz*

| | C | F | Cb |
|---|---|---|---|
| Barbecue | 45 | 0 | 11 |
| Buttermilk Ranch | 120 | 12 | 2 |
| Honey Mustard | 80 | 6 | 7 |
| Sweet & Sour | 45 | 0 | 12 |

**Garden Sensations Salads:** *Full Size with Dressing*

| | C | F | Cb |
|---|---|---|---|
| Asian Cashew Grilled Chicken | 380 | 14 | 32 |
| BBQ Ranch Grilled Chicken | 600 | 30 | 44 |
| Spicy Chicken Caesar | 790 | 51 | 42 |

**Sides:**

**Baked Potatoes:**

| | C | F | Cb |
|---|---|---|---|
| Bacon & Cheddar | 480 | 17 | 66 |
| Broccoli Cheese | 430 | 11 | 70 |
| Sour Cream & Chives | 310 | 2.5 | 63 |
| **Natural Cut Fries:** Value | 230 | 10 | 30 |
| Small, 4 oz | 320 | 15 | 43 |
| Medium, 5 oz | 420 | 19 | 56 |
| Large, 6.5 oz | 530 | 24 | 70 |
| **Rich Meaty Chili:** Small | 170 | 5 | 16 |
| Large | 250 | 7 | 23 |

**Frosty:**

**Chocolate; Vanilla, average:**

| | C | F | Cb |
|---|---|---|---|
| Small | 340 | 9 | 56 |
| Medium | 460 | 12 | 77 |
| Large | 575 | 15 | 96 |

## Whataburger® (Aug '16)

**Burgers & Sandwiches:**

| | C | F | Cb |
|---|---|---|---|
| A.1. Thick & Hearty Burger | 980 | 54 | 68 |
| Chop House Cheddar Burger | 1100 | 69 | 61 |
| Green Chili Double | 980 | 57 | 61 |
| Honey BBQ Chicken Strip S'wich | 870 | 39 | 90 |
| **Whataburger:** | | | |
| Original | 590 | 25 | 62 |
| Bacon & Cheese | 740 | 36 | 62 |
| Double Meat | 830 | 44 | 62 |
| Jalapeno & Cheese | 680 | 32 | 63 |
| Jr. | 310 | 11 | 37 |
| Triple Meat | 1080 | 63 | 62 |
| **Chicken:** | | | |
| **Grilled:** Chicken Sandwich | 430 | 13 | 49 |
| Chicken Melt | 390 | 12 | 37 |
| **Whatachick'n:** | | | |
| Bites: 6 pieces, without sauce | 380 | 19 | 31 |
| 9 pieces, without sauce | 540 | 27 | 43 |
| Sandwich | 560 | 22 | 69 |
| Strips, 3 pieces, without sauce | 530 | 28 | 42 |
| Taco, Chicken Fajita | 340 | 12 | 29 |
| **French Fries:** Small, 3 oz | 280 | 14 | 35 |
| Medium, 4.5 oz | 420 | 21 | 52 |
| Large, 6 oz | 560 | 28 | 70 |
| **Onion Rings:** | | | |
| Medium, 3.2 oz | 300 | 17 | 32 |
| Large, 4.8 oz | 450 | 25 | 49 |
| **Salad:** *Without Dressing* | | | |
| **Garden:** with Grilled Chicken | 290 | 14 | 11 |
| with Whatachick'n | 430 | 22 | 30 |
| without Chicken | 160 | 10 | 10 |
| **Breakfast:** | | | |
| Cinnamon Roll | 430 | 10 | 79 |
| **Biscuits:** Plain | 290 | 16 | 32 |
| with Gravy | 470 | 29 | 46 |
| Honey Butter Chicken | 560 | 33 | 51 |
| **Biscuit Sandwiches:** | | | |
| with Bacon, 5.8 oz | 480 | 30 | 32 |
| with Sausage | 700 | 52 | 32 |
| **On A Bun:** with Bacon | 350 | 14 | 34 |
| with Sausage | 520 | 31 | 34 |
| **Platters:** | | | |
| with Bacon | 620 | 40 | 36 |
| with Sausage | 790 | 57 | 36 |
| **Taquitos:** | | | |
| with Bacon, Egg & Cheese | 410 | 24 | 28 |
| with Cheese | 360 | 21 | 28 |
| with Potato, Egg & Cheese | 460 | 26 | 38 |

## Whataburger® cont... (Aug '16)

**Desserts:**

| | C | F | Cb |
|---|---|---|---|
| Chocolate Chunk Cookie | 230 | 11 | 31 |
| Hot Apple Pie, 3 oz | 260 | 13 | 34 |
| **Beverages:** | | | |
| **Malts:** Chocolate, 20 oz | 600 | 15 | 107 |
| Vanilla, 20 oz | 550 | 16 | 91 |
| **Shake,** Chocolate, 20 oz | 580 | 15 | 99 |

## White Castle® (Aug '16)

**Note:** *Nutritional Information varies from state to state. Please check instore*

**Sliders:**

| | C | F | Cb |
|---|---|---|---|
| Original | 140 | 6 | 13 |
| Bacon, Cheddar Gr. Chkn | 240 | 12 | 15 |
| Cheese | 160 | 9 | 14 |
| Chicken Breast with Cheese | 390 | 28 | 20 |
| Fish, with Cheese | 340 | 24 | 18 |
| Savory Grilled Chicken | 180 | 7 | 13 |
| Western BBQ Grilled Chicken | 320 | 16 | 28 |
| **Sides:** | | | |
| Cheese Fries, small | 400 | 27 | 35 |
| **Chicken Rings:** | | | |
| 6 rings, 5 oz | 530 | 47 | 12 |
| 9 rings , 7.5 oz | 790 | 71 | 18 |
| **French Fries:** | | | |
| Small, 5.6 oz | 330 | 21 | 32 |
| Medium | 600 | 39 | 57 |
| Sack | 770 | 49 | 76 |
| Fully Loaded Fries, small | 460 | 38 | 20 |
| Mozzarella Cheese Sticks, 3 sticks | 440 | 33 | 22 |
| **Condiments:** *Per Packet* | | | |
| Ketchup | 10 | 0 | 2 |
| Mayonnaise | 60 | 7 | 0 |
| **Sauces:** *Per Packet* | | | |
| BBQ | 10 | 0 | 3 |
| Tartar Sauce | 25 | 1.5 | 1 |
| **Breakfast:** | | | |
| French Toast Sticks, 4 pieces | 460 | 31 | 39 |
| Maple Brown Sugar Oatmeal | 160 | 2 | 32 |
| **Sliders:** Bacon, Egg & Cheese | 210 | 12 | 13 |
| Egg & Cheese | 160 | 7 | 13 |
| Sausage, Egg & Cheese | 310 | 22 | 13 |
| **Toasted Sandwiches:** Egg & Chse | 230 | 9 | 29 |
| Bacon, Egg & Cheese | 340 | 19 | 29 |
| Sausage, Egg & Cheese | 380 | 23 | 29 |
| **Sides:** | | | |
| Hash Round Nibblers: | | | |
| Small | 360 | 28 | 25 |
| Medium | 600 | 46 | 42 |
| Sack | 1440 | 110 | 101 |
| **Dessert:** | | | |
| **On A Stick:** Fudge Dipped Brownie | 250 | 12 | 33 |
| Fudge Dipped Cheesecake | 180 | 10 | 21 |

Updated Nutrition Data ~ www.CalorieKing.com
Persons with Diabetes ~ See Disclaimer (Page 22)

## Wienerschnitzel® (Aug '16)

| *Hot Dogs:* | C | F | Cb |
|---|---|---|---|
| **Original:** *On Standard Bun* | | | |
| Chili | 270 | 12 | 32 |
| Chili Cheese | 320 | 16 | 32 |
| Deluxe; Kraut, Plain, average | 245 | 10 | 31 |
| Pastrami | 350 | 18 | 30 |
| **Original:** *On Pretzel Bun* | | | |
| Chili | 400 | 14 | 55 |
| Kraut; Mustard; Plain; Relish, av. | 370 | 13 | 54 |
| **Angus All Beef:** *On Pretzel Bun* | | | |
| Chicago | 560 | 26 | 61 |
| Chili Cheese | 590 | 32 | 55 |
| Mustard; Relish, av | 515 | 26 | 54 |
| Junkyard Dog, on Seeded Bun | 600 | 36 | 49 |
| *Specialties:* | | | |
| **Corn Dogs:** Regular | 230 | 13 | 31 |
| Mini (6 pack) | 290 | 16 | 28 |
| **Jalapeno Poppers,** (6 pack) | 300 | 16 | 31 |
| *Sides:* | | | |
| **Bacon Ranch Chili Fries:** Original | 1050 | 76 | 76 |
| Large | 1840 | 131 | 133 |
| Chili Cheese Fries | 570 | 32 | 59 |
| **French:** Small | 310 | 16 | 38 |
| Medium | 440 | 23 | 54 |
| Large | 750 | 39 | 92 |
| **Po'taters:** Small | 390 | 27 | 33 |
| Medium | 670 | 47 | 56 |
| Large | 1110 | 78 | 94 |
| **Triple Cheese Dble Bacon Chili Fries:** | | | |
| Original | 1280 | 93 | 72 |
| Large | 1980 | 142 | 125 |
| *Breakfast:* | | | |
| **Biscuits:** Egg, Bacon, Cheese | 450 | 25 | 36 |
| Egg, Sausage, Cheese | 540 | 34 | 40 |
| **Burritos:** Egg, Bacon, Cheese | 370 | 19 | 29 |
| Egg, Sausage, Cheese | 460 | 28 | 33 |
| **French Toast Sticks** | 530 | 28 | 61 |
| Syrup, 1 oz | 120 | 0 | 31 |
| *Desserts:* | | | |
| Banana Split | 820 | 24 | 148 |
| **Cones,** regular: | | | |
| Plain, 5 oz | 250 | 9 | 41 |
| Chocolate Dipped, 5 oz | 450 | 27 | 50 |
| **Freezees:** | | | |
| Chocolate Caramel Crunch | 880 | 39 | 133 |
| Chocolate Covered Strawberry | 980 | 56 | 120 |
| Oreo; M&M | 630 | 25 | 99 |
| Reese's Peanut Butter Cup | 630 | 26 | 97 |
| **Shakes,** average all flavors | 650 | 23 | 110 |
| **Sundaes:** | | | |
| Caramel; Hot Fudge, average | 400 | 15 | 64 |
| Chocolate | 390 | 14 | 64 |
| Strawberry | 370 | 14 | 59 |

## Winchell's® (Aug '16)

| *Donuts:* Per Donut | C | F | Cb |
|---|---|---|---|
| Buttermillk Bars, Choc Iced/Glazed | 420 | 19 | 61 |
| Jelly Filled: | | | |
| Apple with Cinnamon Crumb | 370 | 15 | 53 |
| Raspberry with Glaze | 390 | 13 | 61 |
| Strawberry with Sugar | 380 | 13 | 60 |
| Old Fashioned, Glazed; Maple Iced | 410 | 17 | 60 |
| Raised Ring: Chocolate Iced | 270 | 10 | 41 |
| Sugared | 230 | 9 | 34 |

## WingStreet (Aug '16)

| *Chicken:* | C | F | Cb |
|---|---|---|---|
| **Bone Out Wings:** *Per Wing* | | | |
| Buffalo, Mild | 90 | 4 | 9 |
| Garlic Parmesan | 130 | 9 | 6 |
| Honey BBQ | 110 | 4 | 13 |
| Ranch Rub | 80 | 4 | 6 |
| **Traditional Bone In Wings:** *Per Wing* | | | |
| Buffalo, Medium/Hot | 60 | 3 | 4 |
| Garlic Parmesan | 100 | 8 | 0 |
| Spicy BBQ | 70 | 3 | 6 |
| Sweet Chili | 80 | 3 | 7 |
| *Sides:* Baked Hot Wings, each | 50 | 3.5 | 0.5 |
| Breadstick (1) | 140 | 4.5 | 19 |
| Fried Curly Fries, 1 order | 370 | 20 | 42 |
| Fried Onion Rings, with Ketchup | 860 | 50 | 93 |

## Woody's Bar-B-Q® (Aug '16)

| *Starters:* | C | F | Cb |
|---|---|---|---|
| Breaded Wings (10) | 700 | 47 | 13 |
| Beef Chili Cheese Fries | 805 | 38 | 63 |
| *Dinner Entrees:* without Sides | | | |
| ½ Chicken | 840 | 56 | 0 |
| Baby Back Ribs | 520 | 40 | 2 |
| Pork Sampler | 1010 | 62 | 4 |
| *Sandwiches:* Per Regular, without Sides | | | |
| Beef | 390 | 14 | 28 |
| Pork | 490 | 26 | 29 |
| *Wraps:* Without Sides | | | |
| Beef BBQ | 380 | 13 | 31 |
| Pork | 440 | 21 | 31 |
| *Extras:* BBQ Beans | 170 | 8 | 20 |
| Cobettes | 80 | 1 | 18 |
| French Fries | 185 | 7 | 28 |
| Garlic Toast | 120 | 6 | 14 |
| Green Beans | 50 | 2.5 | 6 |
| Okra | 95 | 1 | 21 |
| Squash | 140 | 1 | 28 |

*For Complete Nutritional Data ~ see CalorieKing.com*

## Yoshinoya® (Aug '16)

*Appetizers:* As Served
*California Outlets May Vary, Check In Store*

| | C | F | Cb |
|---|---|---|---|
| **Asian BBQ Wings:** 4 pieces | 410 | 25 | 21 |
| 6 pieces | 620 | 37 | 32 |
| ***Entrees:*** *As Served* | | | |
| **Angus Steak Bowl:** Regular | 570 | 11 | 97 |
| Large | 850 | 17 | 144 |
| **Beef Bowl:** *With Sauce* | | | |
| Regular | 730 | 27 | 91 |
| Large | 1040 | 38 | 131 |
| With Vegetables: Regular | 650 | 20 | 95 |
| Large | 960 | 29 | 141 |
| **Beef & Teriyaki Chicken Combo:** | | | |
| Large, with skin | 1190 | 36 | 151 |
| Large, without skin | 1150 | 33 | 151 |
| **Teriyaki Chicken Bowl:** | | | |
| Regular, with skin | 790 | 18 | 110 |
| Large, with skin | 1140 | 25 | 165 |
| **Grilled Tilapia:** with Rice & Slaw | 570 | 13 | 91 |
| with Rice & Veggies | 540 | 12 | 88 |
| with Rice, Slaw & Teriyaki Sauce | 620 | 13 | 103 |
| with Rice, Veggies & Teriyaki Sce | 590 | 12 | 100 |
| **Sides,** Clam chowder Soup | 210 | 7 | 34 |
| ***Kid's Meals:*** Beef | 350 | 11 | 48 |
| Teriyaki Chicken with skin | 360 | 7 | 53 |
| Teriyaki Chicken without skin | 340 | 6 | 53 |

*Please note: Relates only to Northern California Menu*

## Z Pizza® (Aug '16)

*Pizzas:* Small, Per Slice

| | C | F | Cb |
|---|---|---|---|
| **Creations:** Berkeley Vegan | 150 | 5 | 21 |
| California | 140 | 4.5 | 18 |
| Casablanca | 180 | 8 | 17 |
| Greek | 140 | 5 | 17 |
| Italian; Mexican, average | 165 | 7 | 17 |
| Provence; Santa Fe | 150 | 6 | 17 |
| Thai; ZBQ, average | 165 | 5 | 19 |
| ***Rusticas:*** *Per Slice* | | | |
| Chicken Sausage | 100 | 3.5 | 12 |
| Curry Chicken & Yam | 130 | 3.5 | 16 |
| Mediterranean; Moroccan, av. | 140 | 8 | 13 |
| Pear & Gorgonzola | 130 | 6 | 14 |
| ***Calzones:*** Meat Calzone | 790 | 36 | 82 |
| Veggie Calzone | 630 | 22 | 86 |
| ***Salads:*** *Small* | | | |
| Arugula, with Balsamic Vinaigrette | 450 | 36 | 24 |
| Caesar Side, with Caesar Dressing | 200 | 16 | 8 |
| California, with Chipotle Ranch | 180 | 13 | 16 |

## Zaxby's® (Aug '16)

*Zappetizers:* With Sauce

| | C | F | Cb |
|---|---|---|---|
| Fried White Cheddar Bites | 780 | 49 | 59 |
| Onion Rings, 5 oz | 830 | 62 | 64 |
| Spicy Fried Mushroom, 5.7 oz | 590 | 46 | 40 |
| Tater Chips, 5.2 oz | 830 | 61 | 62 |
| ***Meal Dealz:*** *Without Drink* | | | |
| Big Zax Snak, with Sauce | 1000 | 56 | 88 |
| Boneless Wings, without sauce | 920 | 57 | 77 |
| Chicken Finger Nibbler, w/ sauce | 1380 | 75 | 143 |
| ***Most Popular:*** *As Served* | | | |
| **Chicken Finger Plate:** Regular | 1300 | 74 | 105 |
| Large | 2050 | 118 | 167 |
| Wings & Things, regular | 1490 | 96 | 91 |
| ***Sandwich Baskets:*** *Includes Fries* | | | |
| Cajun Club | 1100 | 56 | 97 |
| Club | 1300 | 77 | 105 |
| ***Wings & Fingerz:*** *With Sauce* | | | |
| **Buffalo Fingerz:** | | | |
| 5 pieces | 590 | 39 | 15 |
| 10 pieces | 1170 | 78 | 31 |
| **Buffalo Wings:** | | | |
| 5 pieces | 490 | 40 | 3 |
| 10 pieces | 790 | 59 | 3 |
| **Chicken Fingerz:** | | | |
| 5 pieces | 570 | 35 | 19 |
| 10 pieces | 1130 | 70 | 37 |
| ***Zax Kidz:*** *Without Drink* | | | |
| Kiddie Cheese | 840 | 54 | 72 |
| Kiddie Finger | 600 | 37 | 43 |
| Kiddie Nibbler | 580 | 31 | 62 |
| ***Zalads:*** *With Texas Toast, without Dressing* | | | |
| Blue, with Blackened Chicken | 580 | 28 | 36 |
| **Caesar:** | | | |
| with Fried Chicken | 690 | 36 | 39 |
| with Grilled Chicken | 540 | 25 | 31 |
| **Cobb:** Fried Chicken | 835 | 47 | 45 |
| Grilled Chicken | 685 | 35 | 37 |
| ***Salad Dressings:*** | | | |
| Blue Cheese, 1 packet, 1.3 oz | 180 | 19 | 2 |
| Honey French, 1.3 oz | 150 | 12 | 9 |
| Honey Mustard, 1.3 oz | 150 | 13 | 6 |
| Lite Ranch, 1.3 oz | 90 | 8 | 3 |
| Mediterranean, 1.3 oz | 140 | 14 | 4 |
| Ranch, 1.3 oz | 160 | 16 | 2 |
| Thousand Island | 230 | 24 | 3 |
| ***Sides:*** Celery Basket, | | | |
| with 2 cups Ranch Sauce | 420 | 42 | 10 |
| Cole Slaw, 2.2 oz | 140 | 11 | 12 |
| Crinkle Fries, regular, 5 oz | 440 | 22 | 54 |
| Texas Toast, basket, 3 wedges, 4.3 oz | 440 | 20 | 60 |

## Zero Sub's® ~ *see CalorieKing.com*

## Notes on Cholesterol

- **Cholesterol** is a white waxy substance produced mainly by our liver. It is also found in animal food products. Plant foods have no cholesterol.

- **Cholesterol is essential to life.** It is a structural part of every body cell wall and is the building block for vitamin D, sex hormones, and bile acids which help in the digestion of dietary fats. **Cholesterol is also vital for a healthy brain**; and contains some 20% of total body cholesterol.

- **The body makes sufficient cholesterol** for its needs and does not rely on cholesterol in the diet. Dietary fats have a major influence on blood cholesterol levels. (See next page)

- **A high blood cholesterol level increases** the risk of atherosclerosis - the thickening of arteries that can reduce or block blood flow to the heart, brain, eyes, kidneys, sex organs and other body parts.

  **This in turn increases the risk of heart attack,** stroke, blindness, kidney failure, impotence and other blood circulatory problems.

  **Other risk factors which increase the risk of atherosclerosis include high blood pressure, smoking, obesity and uncontrolled diabetes.**

### BLOOD CHOLESTEROL

#### CHECK YOUR RISK!

| Total Cholesterol Level (mg/dl) ▼ | | Risk of Heart Attack ▼ |
|---|---|---|
| 240 and above | ~ | **High Risk** |
| 200 - 239 | ~ | **Borderline/High** |
| Below 200 | ~ | **Desirable** |

❤ **Know your cholesterol level, particularly if there is a family history of heart disease or stroke. If your level is high, see your doctor.**

❤ **All adults should have their cholesterol, HDL and triglycerides tested at least every 5 years.**

### HEART ATTACK WARNING SIGNALS

Many victims die before reaching the hospital by ignoring warning signals and delaying medical help. Symptoms vary and commonly include:

- **Chest pain,** vice-like squeezing or burning sensation in center of the chest or between the shoulder blades, or in the mid-back. Pain may even feel like severe indigestion.
- **Pain** may be felt in the arms, shoulders, neck or jaw.
- **Shortness of breath** often occurs with or before chest discomfort.
- **Other signs,** with or without pain, include a cold sweat, nausea or light-headedness.

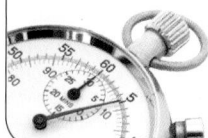

*If you experience any of the above symptoms call IMMEDIATELY for medical help. Every minute counts.*

**Call 9-1-1** *or your emergency number*

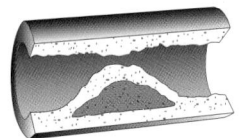

▲ **Atherosclerosis can clog arteries and impede blood flow to the heart or other body organs.**

▼ **A thrombus (blood clot) can form on unstable, festering athero-sclerotic plaque and rapidly block blood flow. A heart attack or stroke can result.**

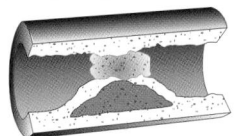

# Fats & Cholesterol Guide

The amount and type of dietary fat has the greatest influence on blood cholesterol levels.

**Fats in food are a mixture of 3 basic types:** saturated, monounsaturated, and polyunsaturated. Animal fats are mainly saturated while plant oils and fish oils are mainly mono- and polyunsaturated.

**Saturated fats** have subgroups known as long-chain, medium-chain, and short-chain fats. Most of the long chain fats raise blood cholesterol, and increase the risk of blood clots and thrombosis leading to artery blockage.

**Long-chain saturated fats** are found mainly in full-cream milk, cheese, butter, cream, fatty meats and sausages, and processed foods.

**Medium-chain fats, as found in virgin coconut oil,** have little effect on LDL-cholesterol but can raise "good" HDL.

**Monounsaturated fats** tend to more selectively lower 'bad' LDL cholesterol and maintain the protective 'good' HDL cholesterol in the bloodstream – but only if they replace saturated fats in the diet. Foods rich in monounsaturates include canola and olive oils, canola margarine, peanuts, and avocados.

**Polyunsaturated fats** consist of two main classes. **Omega-6** polyunsaturates tend to lower blood cholesterol. Rich sources include safflower, sunflower and corn oils.

**Omega-3** polyunsaturated fats can lower blood cholesterol; significantly lower blood triglycerides; and reduce the rise of thrombosis, heart arrythmmia, and artery spasm.

**Best practical omega-3 sources** include canola oil and margarine, soybean oil and fish.

**A balanced intake** of the two omega classes is important for optimal health. For most Americans, slightly increasing omega-3 intake would help attain a more ideal balance.

**Trans fats** from hydrogenated vegetable oils and shortenings should also be avoided. They are common in commercial baked and fried food products such as cakes, muffins, pastries, doughnuts, fried snacks and french fries.

## DIETARY FATS COMPARISON

■ Saturated Fat  ▢ Monounsaturated Fat
Polyunsaturated Fats:
▢ Linoleic (Omega-6)  ■ Alpha-Linolenic (Omega-3)

### OILS — PERCENTAGE CONTENT

| OIL | Saturated | Monounsaturated | Linoleic (Omega-6) | Alpha-Linolenic (Omega-3) |
|---|---|---|---|---|
| CANOLA OIL | 7 | 63 | 20 | 10 |
| LINSEED/FLAX OIL | 9 | 19 | 17 | 55 |
| SAFFLOWER OIL | 9 | 14 | 77 | |
| GRAPESEED OIL | 10 | 22 | 68 | |
| SUNFLOWER OIL | 11 | 23 | 66 | |
| CORN OIL | 14 | 32 | 52 | 2 |
| OLIVE OIL | 14 | 76 | | 10 |
| SOYBEAN OIL | 15 | 23 | 54 | 8 |
| PEANUT OIL | 19 | 45 | 34 | 2 |
| COTTONSEED OIL | 26 | 16 | 58 | |
| PALM OIL | 51 | 39 | | 10 |

### SPREADS & FATS
Saturated Fat includes 'Trans Fats'     ▢ WATER CONTENT

| FAT | Saturated | Monounsaturated | Linoleic | Omega-3 | Water |
|---|---|---|---|---|---|
| LIGHT MARGARINE | 14 | 14 | 21 | | 51 |
| CANOLA MARGARINE | 18 | 45 | 12 | 6 | 19 |
| POLYUNSATURATED MARG | 24 | 20 | 36 | | 20 |
| BUTTER | 57 | | 18 | 2 | 24 |
| LARD | 41 | 47 | | | 12 |
| BEEF FAT | 44 | 37 | 4 | | 15 |

## GOOD SOURCES OF OMEGA-3 FATS

| Plant Sources | Omega-3 Fats (Grams) |
|---|---|
| Canola Oil, 1 Tbsp, ½ fl.oz | **1.5g** |
| Flaxseed Oil, 1 Tbsp | **8g** |
| Soybean Oil, 1 Tbsp | **1.2g** |
| Canola Margarine, 1 Tbsp, ½ oz | **1g** |
| Soybeans, cooked, ½ cup, 4 oz | **0.5g** |
| Walnuts, ½ oz | **0.5g** |

**FISH** - *Per 4 oz Serving*

| | |
|---|---|
| *High Content:* Salmon (Chinook), Tuna, Trout (Lake), Sardines, Herring, Mackerel | **3g** **3g** |
| *Medium Content:* Salmon, (Pink/Red/Coho), 4 oz | **2g** |
| *Fair Content:* Per 4 oz Serving Bass, Catfish, Cod, Grouper, Hake, Halibut, Kingfish, Perch, Pollock, Shark, Trout (Rainbow), Tuna, Crab, Oysters, Blue Mussels, Shrimp, Squid | **0.5-1g** |

### How Much Is Needed?

**As little as 1-2 grams daily of omega-3 fats** may benefit general health. High doses of fish-oil supplements should only be taken as directed by your Healthcare provider.

## Dietary Cholesterol

Cholesterol in food varies in its effect on blood cholesterol level (BCL) from person to person. Much depends on the amount and type of fat and fiber eaten at the same meal.

Any elevating effect of dietary cholesterol on BCL is more likely to occur when the diet is high in saturated fat. Little elevation, if any, generally occurs when dietary fats are balanced in favor of mono- and poly-unsaturated fats (including omega-3 fats).

**Example:** While fish does contain cholesterol, the omega-3 fats can prevent any increase in BCL. Conversely, a meal containing no cholesterol but rich in saturated fat may result in a significant increase in BCL - as well as impairing artery wall functions.

**Consequently, the need to be overly concerned about dietary cholesterol is being de-emphasized in favor of simply limiting total fat, saturated fat, and trans fat in particular – and substituting unsaturated fats (including omega-3 fats).**

**Note:** Persons with familial (genetic) hyper-cholesterolemia should limit cholesterol; and ideally follow a plant based diet.

**The liver usually cuts back its own cholesterol production** in response to cholesterol in the diet. Many people can consume high-cholesterol foods without concern.

However, it is difficult to identify just who is at risk - the so-called 'hyper-responders'. Because over 50% of Americans have a BCL above ideal levels, it may be prudent to limit cholesterol intake to less than 300mg daily, as well as to adopt a heart-healthy diet.

This limitation still allows the inclusion of most foods that are regularly eaten – even the overly maligned egg.

Avocados (like all plant foods) contain no cholesterol. Their fats are mainly monounsaturated and can lower blood cholesterol.

## CHOLESTEROL COUNTER

**Cholesterol is found only in foods of animal origin. Plant foods contain no cholesterol.**

| | Cholesterol mg |
|---|---|
| **Meat** - Average all types: | |
| Lean Meat, cooked, 120g | 100 |
| Fatty Meat, cooked, 120g | 100 |
| Fat, thick strip, 60g | 40 |

*Note: While lean meat and fat have similar amounts of cholesterol, choose lean meat to limit fat intake.*

| | |
|---|---|
| **Chicken/Turkey,** average, 120g | 100 |
| **Organ Meats:** Liver, fried, 4 oz | 500 |
| Brains, beef, pan fried, 3 oz | 1700 |
| **Sausages:** Frankfurter, 40g | 25 |
| Salami, 2 slices, 55g | 40 |
| **Bacon:** 3 slices, cooked, 30g | 20 |
| **Fish:** Fish fillets, average, ckd, 120g | 70 |
| Tuna/Salmon, canned, 100g | 50 |
| Scallops, 9 medium, 3 oz | 30 |
| Prawns, raw, 100g | 110 |
| Oysters, raw, 6 medium, 85g | 45 |
| Crayfish, Crab, cooked, 100g | 70 |
| **Eggs** (Chicken), 1 large | 210 |
| 1 medium | 180 |
| Egg White, *Scramblers* | 0 |
| **Milk/Yoghurt:** Whole, 1 cup, 250ml | 30 |
| Light/low-fat Milk (1%), 1 cup | 10 |
| Skim/Non-fat, 1 cup | 10 |
| **Soy Milk, Tofu, Tempeh** | 0 |
| **Cheese:** Natural/Hard/Cream, 30g | 30 |
| Cottage, low-fat, 2 Tbsp, 40g | 5 |
| Cream Cheese, 30g | 25 |
| **Fats:** Butter, 1 Tbsp, 20g | 45 |
| Margarine, Oils (vegetable) | 0 |
| Mayonnaise, 1 Tbsp | 10 |
| **Cream:** Heavy, whipping, 2 Tbsp, 40g | 40 |
| Light/Sour, 2 Tbsp | 10 |
| **Ice Cream:** Full-fat (10-11%), 100ml/50g | 20 |
| Low-fat (less than 4%), 50g | 5 |
| **Fruit, Vegetables,** Avocados | 0 |
| **Nuts, Seeds, Grains** | 0 |
| **Coffee, Tea, Beer, Wine** | 0 |

*For Comprehensive Food Listings ~ see CalorieKing.com*

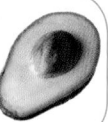

# Blood Cholesterol ~ Diet Hints

## DIETARY HINTS TO LOWER BLOOD CHOLESTEROL

1. **Maintain a healthy weight.**
   If overweight, lose weight with a sensible, low-fat meal plan and daily exercise.

2. **Reduce saturated fat intake by:**
   **(a) eating less dairy fat.** Choose low-fat or fat-reduced varieties of milk, yogurt, soy drinks, cheese, and ice cream.

   **(b) replacing saturated fats** with fats and oils rich in monounsaturated and polyunsaturated fats. Choose vegetable oils such as extra-virgin olive, canola and soybean. Avoid solid frying fats.

   Note: *Promise Active* and *Benecol* spreads contain plant stanol esters which can lower total and LDL cholesterol.

   **(c) eating less fat from meat and poultry**. Choose lean cuts of meat and skinless chicken. Go easy on lunch meats, salami and fatty sausages. Enjoy fish.

   **(d) eating less saturated and trans fats** from baked and fried fast-foods. Avoid deep-fried foods. Avoid donuts, cakes, pastries and cookies unless made with healthier fats and oils.

3. **Increase your soluble fiber intake.**
   Foods rich in soluble fiber include beans, lentils, chickpeas, hummus, nuts, seeds, psyllium-seed husks and psyllium-fiber supplements. Oat bran, rice bran and barley are also good sources, as are fruit, vegetables and avocados.
   (*See Fiber Guide - Page 264-269*).

4. **Eat more soy bean products** such as: soy drinks, tofu, tempeh (cultured soy beans), soy flour, soy vegetarian foods and edamame (fresh green soybeans).

   Soy protein in place of animal protein can significantly decrease high blood cholesterol levels as well as 'bad' LDL cholesterol and blood triglycerides while 'good' HDL cholesterol is maintained. For best results, eat at least 25g of soy protein per day (from 3-4 servings).

5. **Eat more fruit, vegetables, and whole grains** in place of high-fat foods. Aim for 2 fruits and 5 servings of vegetables per day. They also contain valuable antioxidants. The fat of avocados (and most nuts) is mainly unsaturated and can lower blood cholesterol levels.

6. **Limit cholesterol to 300mg per day.**
   (Extra Notes ~ See Previous Page)

7. **Avoid brewed unfiltered coffee** (espresso; plunger-style). Several cups per day may raise blood cholesterol. Filtered coffee is fine.

8. **Spread your food intake over the day.**
   Have 5-6 small meals per day rather than just 2-3 large meals. Nibbling, versus gorging, favors lower blood cholesterol.

## ALCOHOL – WINE

Alcohol is a mixed bag. Moderate amounts of 1-2 drinks daily appear to reduce the risk of heart attack and ischemic stroke in older persons.

However, larger amounts increase the risk of high blood pressure, obesity, heart failure and hemorrhagic stroke, and can aggravate hypertriglyceridemia: as well as many other health hazards. (*See Alcohol Guide – Page 23*)

The speculative benefits of moderate alcohol intake have been overstated in the media. The overriding harmful effects of excess alcohol do not allow its recommendation for any aspects of health promotion.

*Fruit, Vegetables & Tea Also Protect:*
**Red wine and red grapes (more so than white) contain antioxidants which may help protect cholesterol in the blood from becoming oxidized.**

**Many fruits, vegetables, grains, nuts and tea also contain protective antioxidants.**

# How Fats Affect Blood Flow

**Fats in the diet affect more than blood cholesterol levels.** They can also strongly influence blood clot formation and thrombosis, as well as blood flow and ultimate oxygen delivery to body parts and organs.

While advanced atherosclerosis can impede blood flow to the heart and other organs, it is thrombosis (complete blockage by blood clots) or arterial spasm which commonly results in a heart attack or stroke.

**Plant and fish oils rich in omega-3 fats** lessen the risk of blood clots, thrombus formation, and artery spasm by reducing platelet stickiness and adhesion to artery walls. This also reduces inflammation of the artery wall lining. This in turn reduces the risk of atherosclerotic plaque becoming unstable and reactive.

**Omega-3 fats also improve blood flow** by reducing blood viscosity and increasing the flexibility of red blood cells that need to flex and twist on themselves in order to squeeze through tiny narrow capillaries often half their diameter.

**A diet high in saturated fats** (longer chain) has the opposite effect by stiffening red blood cell membranes and increasing blood viscosity, thereby hindering blood flow.

**Stiff red blood cells may also form aggregates that resemble coin stacks.** In narrow blood vessels, this further impedes blood flow and impairs oxygen release through the much-lessened surface area of red blood cell membranes exposed to blood.

**Note:** Smoking, lack of exercise, and stress can have similar adverse effects on thrombosis, red blood cell flexibility, and blood flow.

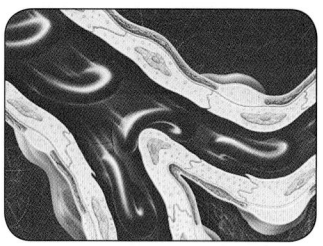

▲ **Picture of Healthy Blood Flow**

*Flexible red blood cells twist and slide through tiny capillaries - often half the diameter of red blood cells.*

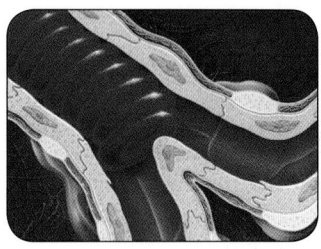

▲ **A Not-So-Healthy Picture!**

*Red blood cells have lost their flexibility and ability to twist and slip through capillaries. They are stacked up, thereby impeding blood flow.*

*A diet high in saturated fats can contribute to this picture - as can smoking, lack of exercise, and stress.*

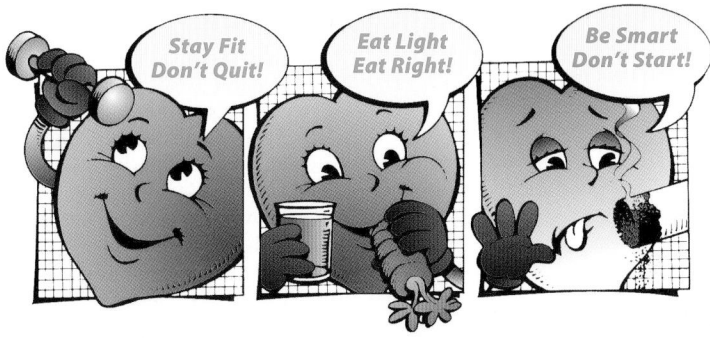

Stay Fit Don't Quit!

Eat Light Eat Right!

Be Smart Don't Start!

# Fiber Guide

## Introduction `Fiber`

Fiber is the general term for those parts of plant food that we cannot digest (although bacteria in the large bowel partly digests fiber through fermentation). It is not found in foods of animal origin (meats, dairy products).

**Fiber promotes intestinal health,** bowel regularity, can benefit diabetes and blood cholesterol levels, and may help prevent colon cancer. High-fiber foods also assist weight control.

**Most Americans don't eat enough fiber – less than 20 grams/day – instead of a healthier 25 to 35 grams/day.**

## Types of Fiber

Plant foods contain a mixture of different fibers in varying proportions. Insoluble and soluble fiber categories are based on their solubility in water. All types of fiber are beneficial to the body.

- ◆ Insoluble fibers (cellulose, hemi-celluloses, lignin) make up the structural parts of plant cell walls.

  **Best food sources** are wheat bran, corn bran, rice bran, wholegrain cereals and breads, beans and peas, nuts, seeds, and the skins of fruits and vegetables.

These fibers absorb many times their own weight in water. They create a soft bulk and hasten the passage of waste products through the intestines.

**They promote bowel regularity,** and aid in the prevention and treatment of uncomplicated forms of **constipation, diverticulosis and hemorrhoids.**

**The risk of colon cancer** may also be reduced by fiber's diluting effect on potentially harmful substances.

- ◆ Soluble fibers **(pectin, gums, mucilages)** are found mainly within plant cells, soy milk (whole bean) and products.

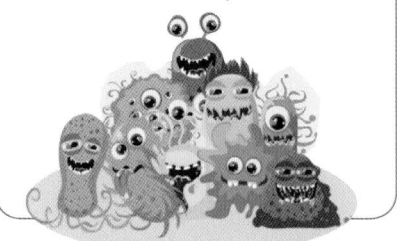

*A fiber-rich diet assists the growth of friendly gut microbes that can benefit our metabolism, weight and blood glucose levels – as well as hunger, mood and our immune system.*

**Best Sources of Soluble Fiber:** Fruits and vegetables, oat bran, barley, beans and peas, prunes, psyllium and flax seed.

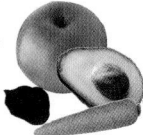

These fibers form a gel which slows both stomach emptying and the absorption of sugars from the intestines. **This helps to control blood sugar levels.**

**Weight control** is also aided by the slower emptying of the stomach and the feeling of **fullness provided by soluble fiber.**

**Soluble fiber can also lower blood cholesterol** by binding bile acids and excreting them. More body cholesterol must then be broken down to supply bile acids for emulsification of dietary fats. **Rice bran, while not high in soluble fiber, can also lower blood cholesterol.**

- ◆ Resistant starch is that part of starchy foods (approx. 10%) which is tightly bound by fiber and resists normal digestion. Friendly bacteria in the large bowel ferment and change the resistant starch into short-chain fatty acids, which are important to bowel health and may protect against colon cancer.

**Starchy foods include** bread, cereals, rice, pasta, potatoes and legumes.

## Fiber & Weight Control

**Fiber can assist weight control** in several ways. Fiber-rich foods such as fresh fruit and vegetables, potatoes and wholegrain bread contain few calories for their large volume (due to their low-fat, high-water content).

**Their bulk fills the stomach** and satisfies the appetite much sooner than fiber-depleted foods. The extra chewing time also contributes to satiety, and gives the stomach time to register a feeling of fullness. Excessive calories are less likely to be consumed.

**Fiber-depleted foods and drinks** are more concentrated in calories; e.g. fats, sugar, candy, soft drinks, fruit juices, alcohol. They require little or no chewing. Large amounts with excessive calories can be consumed before the appetite is satisfied.

**Example:** Whereas one fresh apple might satisfy the appetite, an apple juice drink with the equivalent sugars and calories of 2-3 apples only minimally satisfies the appetite. (See illustration below.)

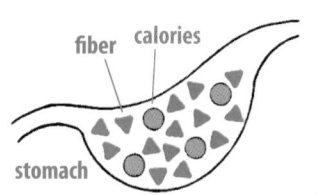

*High-fiber foods fill the stomach. Fewer calories are consumed.*

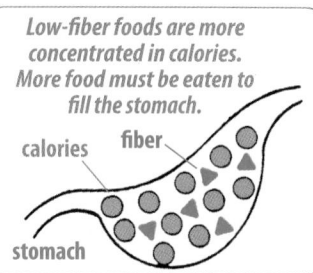

*Low-fiber foods are more concentrated in calories. More food must be eaten to fill the stomach.*

## EFFECTS OF REMOVING FIBER FROM FOOD

*2-3 pieces of fresh fruit produces 1 glass of fruit juice. The removal of fiber concentrates the sugar and calories.*

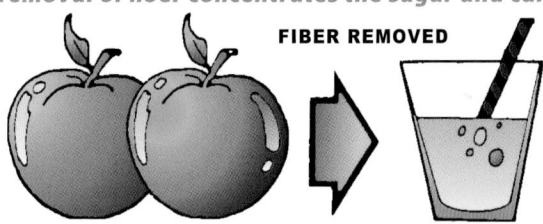

**FIBER REMOVED**

| FRESH FRUIT | (Comparison) | FRUIT JUICE |
|---|---|---|
| High Fiber | ← | Negligible Fiber |
| Low Calorie Density | ← | High Calorie Density |
| Long Eating Time | ← | No Eating Time (Drink) |
| Satisfies Hunger | ← | Does Not Satisfy Hunger |
| Sugar Slowly Absorbed | ← | Sugar More Quickly Absorbed |
| Less Insulin Required | ← | More Insulin Required |
| Supports Gut Microbes | ← | Few Benefits to Microbes |

# Fiber Guide ~ Constipation

## Constipation

**Constipation** can reasonably be defined as a failure to have a bowel movement at least every second day – and just as importantly, without straining or pain.

Typically, constipated stools are too hard, too narrow and too small.

The **main cause** is simply a lack of dietary fiber. Other contributing factors include insufficient fluids, too little exercise, emotional stress, gastrointestinal disease, lack of proper dentition to chew high-fiber foods, and some medications (e.g. some antacids, antidepressants, pain medications).

**Note:** Check with your doctor to rule out any underlying medical problem – especially if you have a change in bowel habits in middle-age or later years.

### DESIRABLE FIBER INTAKE

**Adults:** 25-35gm per day
**Children (under 18):** Age + 5gm
**Example:** 6-year old (6 + 5)= 11gm

### SAMPLE FOOD QUANTITIES
#### For 35 Grams of Fiber/Day

|  | Fiber |
|---|---|
| Breakfast Cereal (higher-fiber) | 5g |
| **plus** 4 slices wholegrain Bread | 6g |
| **plus** 3 servings fresh Fruit | 9g |
| **plus** 1 medium Potato (w. skin) | |
| **or** 1 cup Brown Rice | 4g |
| **or** ½ cup wholegrain Pasta | |
| **plus** 3-4 servings Veggies/Salad | 6g |
| **plus** 1 cup Bean Soup | |
| **or** ¼ cup Baked/Soy Beans | |
| **or** ½ cup Corn/Peas/Lentils | 5g |
| **or** 1¼ oz Almonds (natural) | |
| **or** 3 medium Figs | |

## HINTS TO INCREASE FIBER AND AVOID CONSTIPATION

**1** **Breakfast is an important** contributor to daily fiber intake. Eat high-fiber breakfast cereals (bran-based cereals, oatmeal etc.). Add 1-2 tablespoons of unprocessed bran.

Dried fruits, chopped nuts, soy grits, and seeds are also excellent additions to cereals.

*Note:* A gradual increase in fiber will prevent bloating, gas or pain. People intolerant to bran may benefit from psyllium-based fiber supplements and cereals.

**2** **Drink adequate water daily.** Fiber works by absorbing many times its own weight in water.

**3** **Eat wholegrain breads,** or fiber-enriched breads. They have over double the fiber of regular white bread.

**4** **Enjoy fruit as fresh fruit** with skin rather than as fruit juice. Enjoy wholegrain pasta, barley, brown rice, nuts and seeds.

**5** **Eat more vegetables,** salads and legumes – especially cooked beans, lentils, potatoes with skins, avocado, broccoli, brussels sprouts, cabbage, carrots, celery, and peas.

**6** **Add bran** (barley/rice/wheat) or soy grits to soups, casseroles, yogurt, desserts, cookies, cakes. Also use whole-meal flour or soy flour in place of white flour. Use nuts, seeds, and ground linseed.

**7** **Snack** on fresh or dried fruits, carrot or celery sticks, popcorn, nuts or seeds, wholegrain crackers, high-fiber bars (low-fat). Limit amounts if overweight.

**8** **Exercise regularly** to strengthen abdominal muscles and stimulate the gut. Keep up water intake, especially in warm weather.

**9** **Avoid** indiscriminate and regular use of harsh laxatives. They can overstimulate the intestinal muscles and may make normal bowel activity impossible. It may take several weeks to restore normal bowel function.

## FOODS WITH ZERO FIBER

- **Dairy Products (Milk, Cheese, etc)**
- **Meats, Poultry, Fish, Eggs**
- **Fats/Oils, Sugar/Syrups**
  (Only foods of plant origin contain fiber.)

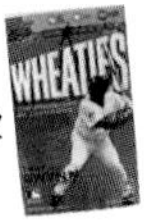

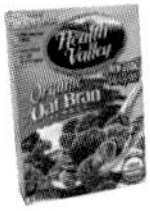

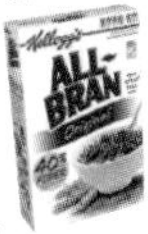

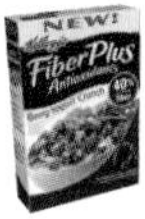

**Fiber** ~ Fiber (grams)

## Breakfast Cereals **Fiber**

### General Mills:

| | |
|---|---|
| Basic 4, 1 cup, 2 oz | 3 |
| Cheerios (Honey Nut; Multigrain), 1 c., 1 oz | 2 |
| Fiber One, ½ cup, 1.1 oz | 14 |
| Multi-Bran Chex, 1 cup, 2 oz | 7 |
| Oatmeal Crisp Almond, 1 cup, 2 oz | 4 |
| Raisin Nut Bran, 1¼ cup, 2 oz | 6 |
| Total, average all types, ¾ cup, 1 oz | 3 |
| Wheat Chex, 1 cup, 2 oz | 6 |
| Wheaties ¾ cup, 1 oz | 3 |

### Health Valley:

| | |
|---|---|
| Amaranth Flakes, ¾ cup, 1 oz | 3 |
| Crunches & Flakes, ¾ cup, 1.9 oz | 4 |
| Fiber 7 Flakes, ¾ cup, 1 oz | 7 |
| Golden Flax, ¾ cup, 1.9 oz | 6 |
| Granola (Low-Fat), ⅔ cup, 2 oz | 6 |
| Healthy Fiber Flakes, ¾ cup, 1.1 oz | 4 |
| Oat Bran Flakes, all types, ¾ cup, 1 oz | 2 |
| Oat Bran O's, ¾ cup, 1 oz | 3 |
| Real Oat Bran, ½ cup, 1.7 oz | 5 |

### Kellogg's:

| | |
|---|---|
| All-Bran, ½ cup, 1.1 oz | 10 |
| All-Bran w. Extra Fiber, ½ cup, 1 oz | 13 |
| All-Bran Bran Buds, ⅓ cup, 1.1 oz | 13 |
| Corn Flakes, Fruit Loops, Smacks 1 cup, 1 oz | 1 |
| Cocoa/Rice Krispies Treats, 1¼ cup, 1 oz | 0 |
| Complete: Wheat Flakes, ¾ c., 1 oz | 5 |
| Oat Bran Flakes, ¾ cup, 1.1 oz | 4 |
| Corn Pops, 1 cup, 1.1 oz | 0 |
| Cracklin' Oat Bran, ¾ cup, 1.7oz | 6 |
| FiberPlus Antioxidants: | |
| Berry Yogurt Crunch, 1 c., 1.9 oz | 10 |
| Cinnamon Oat Crunch ¾ c., 1.1 oz | 9 |
| Frosted Mini Wheats, 24 bisc., 2 oz | 5 |
| Granola w. Raisins, ⅔ cup, 2.1 oz | 3 |
| Raisin Bran, 1 cup, 2.1 oz | 7 |
| Smart Start, Strong Heart, | |
| Cinnamon Raisin, 1 cup, 1.8 oz | 4 |
| Special K, 1 cup, 1.1 oz | 0.5 |

## Breakfast Cereals (Cont) **Fiber**

### Kashi:

| | |
|---|---|
| GoLEAN Cereal, 1 cup, 1.8 oz | 10 |
| GoLEAN Crunch!, 1 cup, 1.9 oz | 8 |
| GoLEAN Bars, avg. (1) | 6 |
| Good Friends: Original, 1 cup, 1.9 oz | 12 |
| Cinna-Raisin Crunch, 1 cup, 1.8 oz | 8 |
| Heart to Heart, ¾ cup, 1.2 oz | 5 |
| 7 Whole Grain Pilaf, ½ cup, cooked, 5 oz | 7 |
| 7 Whole Grain Puffs, 1 cup, 0.7 oz | 1 |

### Quaker:

| | |
|---|---|
| Cap'n Crunch, ¾ cup, 1 oz | 1 |
| 100% Natural Granola, | |
| avg., ½ cup, 1.8 oz | 3 |
| Crunchy Corn Bran, 1 cup, 1 oz | 5 |
| Life Cereal, ¾ cup, 1.1 oz | 2 |
| Oat Bran, ½ cup, 1.4 oz | 6 |
| Oatmeal, average, 1 packet | 3 |

### Post:

| | |
|---|---|
| 100% Bran, ⅓ cup, 1 oz | 9 |
| Alpha Bits, 1 cup, 1 oz | 2 |
| Blueberry Morning, 1 cup, 1.9 oz | 5 |
| Cranberry Almond Crunch, 1 cup, 1.8 oz | 3 |
| Fruit & Bran, 1 cup, 1.9 oz | 6 |
| Grape-Nuts, ½ cup, 2 oz | 7 |
| Great Grains, ⅔ cup, 1.9 oz | 5 |
| Honey Bunches of Oats, ¾ cup, 1.1 oz | 2 |
| Shredded Wheat & Bran, ½ cup, 2 oz | 8 |

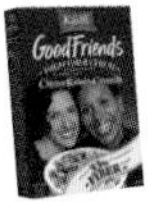

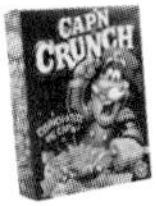

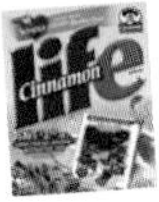

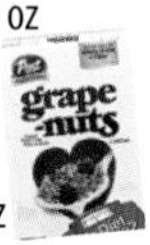

## Brans & Supplements, Metamucil

| | |
|---|---|
| **Oat Bran:** 1 Tbsp (level) | 1 |
| ⅓ cup, (5⅓ Tbsp), 1 oz | 5 |
| **Rice Bran,** raw. ¼ cup, 1 oz | 6 |
| **Wheat Bran,** Unprocessed: | |
| Raw, 1 Tbsp | 1.5 |
| 2 Tbsp (level), ¼ oz | 3 |
| ¼ cup, (4 Tbsp), ½ oz | 6 |
| **Wheat Germ,** Raw, ¼ cup, 1 oz | 4 |
| **Psyllium Seed Husks,** 2 Tbsp | 8 |
| *Fibersure,* 1 heaping tsp | 5 |
| *Metamucil:* Orange, 1 rnd Tbsp, 11g | 3 |
| Fiber Wafers (2) | 6 |

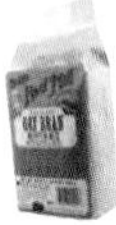

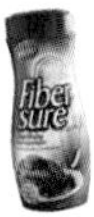

## Hot Cereals, Oatmeal

| | |
|---|---|
| Bulgur (cracked Wheat), ckd, 1 cup | 8 |
| Corn/Hominy Grits, dry, 3 Tbsp, 1 oz | 0.5 |
| Cream of Wheat, cooked, ¾ cup | 1 |
| Oatmeal (uncooked ⅓ cup), ckd, ⅔ cup | 3 |

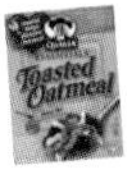

# Fiber Counter

## Breads & Crackers | Fiber

| | |
|---|---|
| **Bread:** White, 1 slice, 1 oz | 0.6 |
| Whole-wheat, 1 slice, 1 oz | 1.5 |
| Wholegrain, 1 slice, 1 oz | 2 |
| Rye, Pumpernickel, 1 oz | 1.5 |
| Bagel/Roll/Bun, 1 medium, 2 oz | 1.5 |
| Pita, whole wheat, 6.5" pocket | 4.5 |
| **Crackers:** Graham, average, 2 | 0.4 |
| Saltine, 4 crackers | 0.4 |
| **Crispbreads,** average, 2 | 4 |
| **Matzo,** 1 board, 1 oz | 1 |
| **Rice Cakes,** average, 1 cake | 0.3 |
| **Tortilla:** Regular, 6" | 0.5 |
| Whole-wheat, 6" | 1.3 |

## Barley, Pasta, Rice & Flours

| | |
|---|---|
| **Barley,** pearled, raw, ¼ cup, 1.7 oz | 8 |
| **Rice:** | |
| White, cooked, 1 cup | 0.6 |
| Brown, cooked, 1 cup | 3.5 |
| *Rice-A-Roni,* average, 1 cup, prepared | 1.5 |
| **Spaghetti/Noodles:** Cooked, 1 cup | 2 |
| Whole-Wheat, cooked, 1 cup | 4 |
| **Flour:** Wheat, All-purpose, 1 cup, 4.5 oz | 3.5 |
| Whole-Wheat, 1 cup, 4.5 oz | 15 |
| Cornmeal, stone ground, 1 cup, 4.5 oz | 13 |
| Carob Flour, 1 cup, 3.5 oz | 41· |
| Rye Flour, 1 cup, 3.5 oz | 15 |
| Soy Flour: Defatted, 1 cup, 3.5 oz | 17 |
| Full-fat, raw, 1 cup, 3 oz | 8 |
| Soy Meal, defatted, 1 cup, 4.5 oz | 14 |

## Frozen Entrees & Dinners

*Average All Brands: Per Serving*

| | |
|---|---|
| Beans/Chili base, average | 6-10 |
| Potato/Pasta base, average | 4-6 |
| Vegetable base, average | 3 |
| Meat/Chicken base, average | 2-3 |
| **Pizzas,** ¼ large, average | 3 |
| **Vegetarian Soy Burgers,** 1 pattie | 4 |

## Soups

| | |
|---|---|
| Chicken Noodle, 1 cup | 0.5 |
| Tomato Soup, average, 1 cup | 0.5 |
| Vegetable Soup, average, 1 cup | 3 |
| *Health Valley:* Per 1 Cup | |
| Black Bean; Minestrone | 8 |
| Tomato | 1 |
| 5 Bean Vegetable; Lentil & Carrots | 10 |
| Mushroom Barley; Vegetable | 4 |
| Split Pea | 8 |
| *Progresso,* High Fiber, all flavors, 1 cup | 7 |

## Fast Foods & Restaurants | Fiber

| | |
|---|---|
| **Hamburgers:** Small, average | 1.5 |
| Large/Whopper, average | 2.5 |
| **Hot Dog,** Regular | 1.5 |
| **French Fries:** Small serving, 2.5 oz | 2.5 |
| Regular/Medium, 3.5 oz | 3.5 |
| **Chicken Nuggets,** 6 pack | 0.5 |
| **Chicken Sandwich,** average | 2 |
| **Taco,** average | 4 |
| **Sundaes,** Shakes, Soft Drinks | 0 |
| *Arby's,* Classic Roast Beef Sandwich | 1 |
| *Denny's:* Grilled Chicken Salad, no bread | 4 |
| Classic Burger, no fries | 4 |
| Club Sandwich, no fries | 2 |
| Grilled Chicken Sandwich, no fries | 4 |
| *Domino's:* 12", Classic/Thin, 1 slice | 1 |
| Deep Dish, 1 slice | 3 |
| Feast Pizza, Classic/Thin, 1 slice | 2 |
| *McDonald's:* Big Mac | 3 |
| Hamburger; Quarter Pounder | 3 |
| Egg McMuffin | 2 |
| Grilled Chicken Caesar Salad | 4 |
| *Pizza Hut: Per 1 Slice, Medium* | |
| Pan Pizza: Cheese, Pepperoni | 1 |
| Supreme | 2 |
| Thin 'n Crispy, Supreme | 2 |
| Hand-Tossed, average all varieties | 2 |
| *Subway:* Sandwich, white roll, av. | 4 |
| With Honey Wheat Roll, average | 3 |
| Salads, average | 4 |

## Cakes, Cookies, Snack Bars

| | |
|---|---|
| **Apple/Fruit Pie,** 1 serving, 4 oz | 2 |
| **Cake:** With plain flour, 1 serving, 3.4 oz | 1.5 |
| With whole-wheat flour, 1 serving | 3 |
| **Carrot Cake,** 4 oz | 4 |
| **Cookies,** oatmeal, (3 small/1 large) | 1 |
| **Donuts,** medium, 1.7 oz | 0.7 |
| **Fruit Cake,** 1 serving, 1.5 oz | 2 |
| **Fig Bars,** 1 cookie, 0.5 oz | 0.7 |
| **Muffins,** Oat Bran (2 small, 1 large), 4 oz | 5 |
| **Granola Bars,** average, 1 bar | 2 |
| *Atkins Advantage Bars,* average | 7 |
| *Clif Bars,* 2.5 oz | 5 |
| *Curves,* Chocolate Peanut Bar, 1 oz | 5 |
| *Fi-Bar Chewy & Nutty,* 1 bar | 1 |
| *Fiber One (Gen. Mills),* 1.4 oz bar | 9 |
| *FiberPlus,* all bars, 1.2 oz | 9 |
| *Health Valley:* Fruit/Granola Bars | 3 |
| Cereal Bars | 1 |
| *Luna Bars,* avg., 1.7 oz | 3 |
| *Special K,* Protein Meal Bar, 1.6 oz | 5 |

## Chocolate, Chips, Popcorn | Fiber

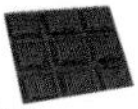

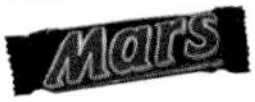

| | |
|---|---|
| **Cheese Balls/Curls/Twists** | 1 |
| **Chocolate,** Hard Candy, 1 oz | 0 |
| **Chocolate with nuts/fruit,** 2 oz bar | 1.5 |
| *Mars Bar,* 1.8 oz | 1 |
| **Potato Chips; corn chips,** 1 oz | 1 |
| **Popcorn,** 3 cups | 3 |
| **Pretzels,** Twists (6) | 1 |

## Nuts, Seeds

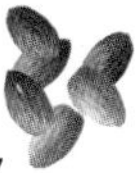

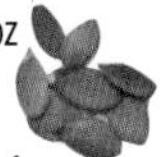

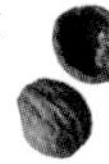

| | |
|---|---|
| **Almonds:** Natural, 25 nuts, 1 oz | 3.5 |
| Blanched (skins removed), 1 oz | 3 |
| **Cashews,** Filberts, Pecans, 1 oz | 1.7 |
| **Peanuts,** Mixed Nuts, Coconut, 1 oz | 2.5 |
| **Peanut Butter,** 2 Tbsp, 1 oz | 2 |
| **Pistachio Nuts,** dried, shelled, 1 oz | 3 |
| **Walnuts,** Black/English, dried, 1 oz | 2 |
| **Seeds:** Amaranth, 2½ Tbsp, 1 oz | 3.5 |
| Flax Seeds, 3 Tbsp, 1 oz | 7 |
| Psyllium Seed Husks, 5 Tbsp, 1 oz | 20 |
| Quinoa Seeds, 3 Tbsp, 1 oz | 1.7 |
| Sesame Seeds, whole, 1 oz | 3.4 |
| Sesame Butter/Tahini, 2 Tbsp, 1.1 oz | 1.4 |
| Sunflower kernels, ¼ cup, 1 oz | 3.8 |
| Teff Seeds, 1 oz | 3.8 |

## Fruit – Fresh

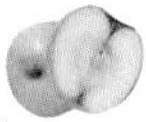

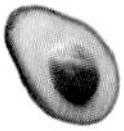

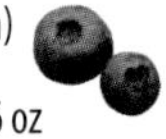

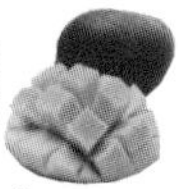

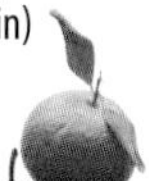

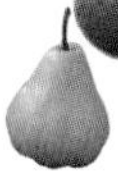

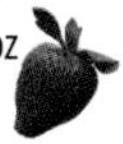

| | |
|---|---|
| **Apples:** 1 medium, 5½ oz (whole) | |
| with skin + core | 3.7 |
| with skin, no core | 3.2 |
| without skin, no core | 1.7 |
| **Apricots,** 2 medium, 4 oz | 1.5 |
| **Avocado,** average, ½ medium | 6 |
| **Banana,** 1 medium, 6 oz (w. skin) | 3 |
| **Blueberries,** ½ cup, 2.5 oz | 1.7 |
| **Cherries,** sweet, raw, 8 fruits, 1.6 oz | 1 |
| **Grapefruit,** average, ½ fruit, 10 oz | 1.4 |
| **Grapes,** 1 medium bunch, seedless, 7 oz | 2 |
| **Kiwifruit,** 1 medium, 2.7 oz | 2.3 |
| **Mango,** 1 medium, 11 oz (whole) | 1.6 |
| **Melons,** Cantaloupe, 4 oz (edible) | 1 |
| **Nectarine,** 1 medium, 4 oz | 1.9 |
| **Olives,** average all types, 7 jumbo, 2 oz | 1.5 |
| **Oranges,** 1 medium (7-8 oz w. skin) | |
| 5½ oz (peeled) | 3.8 |
| **Passionfruit,** 2 medium, 2.5 oz | 5 |
| **Peaches,** 1 large, 6 oz | 2 |
| **Pears,** raw, 1 medium, 6 oz | 4.5 |
| **Pineapple,** 1 slice, 3 oz | 1.2 |
| **Plums,** 2 medium, 6 oz | 1.8 |
| **Strawberries,** 6 medium/3 large, 2 oz | 1 |
| **Watermelon,** 4 oz (edible) | 0.5 |

## Fruit – Dried, Juice | Fiber

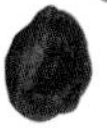

| | |
|---|---|
| **Dried** Fruit: Apricots, 8 halves, 1 oz | 2.2 |
| Dates (3 med); Raisins (2 Tbsp), 1 oz | 1.5 |
| Figs, 3 medium, 1½ oz | 5 |
| Prunes, 3 medium, 1 oz | 2 |
| **Fruit Juice:** Orange/Apple etc, 1 glass | <0.5 |
| Prune Juice, 5 oz | 1.4 |
| Carrot Juice, 8 oz | 1.8 |

## Vegetables

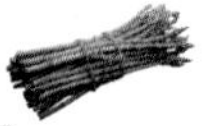

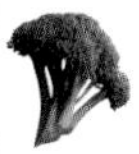

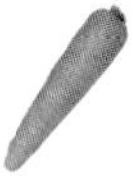

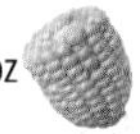

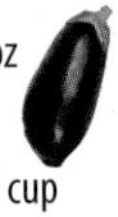

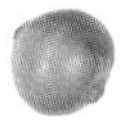

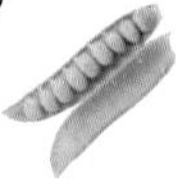

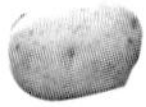

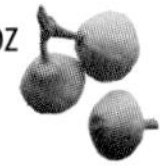

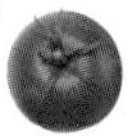

| | |
|---|---|
| **Asparagus,** 4 medium spears | 1.3 |
| **Bean Sprouts,** ½ cup, 2 oz | 1 |
| **Beans:** Snap/Green, ½ cup, 2 oz | 2 |
| Baked Beans in Tom Sce, ½ c, 4.5 oz | 5 |
| Dried Beans, ckd, average, ½ cup | 7 |
| **Beets,** ckd, slices, ½ cup, 3 oz | 1.7 |
| **Broccoli,** cooked, ½ cup, 3 oz | 2.4 |
| **Brussels Sprouts,** ckd, ½ cup, 3 oz | 3.5 |
| **Cabbage:** White, ckd, ½ cup, 2.5 oz | 1 |
| Red, ckd, ½ cup, 2.5 oz | 2 |
| **Carrots,** 1 medium (7½"), ½ cup, 3 oz | 2.5 |
| **Cauliflower,** cooked, 3 flowerets, 2 oz | 1.5 |
| **Celery,** raw, diced, 1 cup, 3.5 oz | 1.6 |
| **Chickpeas (Garbanzos),** ckd, ½ c., 3 oz | 6.5 |
| **Corn:** Kernels, cooked, ½ cup, 2½ oz | 2.5 |
| Corn on the Cob, 1 ear, 5 oz | 4 |
| **Cucumber/Lettuce/Mushrooms,** 2 oz | 0.5 |
| **Eggplant,** raw, sliced, ½ cup , 1.5 oz | 2 |
| **Lentils,** cooked, ½ cup, 3.5 oz | 8 |
| **Mixed Vegetables,** frozen, cooked, ½ cup | 3 |
| **Onions:** Raw, 1 medium, 4 oz | 1.5 |
| Spring Onions, chop., ¼ cup, 1 oz | 0.7 |
| **Peas:** Green, raw, ½ cup, 2.5 oz | 3.7 |
| Cowpeas (Black-eyed), ckd, ½ cup | 10 |
| Split Peas, cooked, ½ cup, 3.5 oz | 8 |
| **Peppers,** sweet, raw, 1 large, 6 oz | 3 |
| **Potatoes:** 1 medium, with skin, 5 oz | 4 |
| 1 medium, without skin | 2.5 |
| ½ cup mashed, 3.5 oz | 1.5 |
| French Fries, small, 2.6 oz | 3 |
| **Spinach,** cooked, ½ cup, 3 oz | 2.2 |
| **Squash:** Summer, cooked, ½ cup, 3 oz | 2.5 |
| Winter, cooked, ½ cup, 3.5 oz | 2.4 |
| **Tomatoes:** 1 medium, 4.5 oz | 1 |
| Tomato Sauce, 1 cup | 0.3 |
| **Soybean Products:** Miso, ½ c., 5 oz | 7.4 |
| Tempeh, cooked, 1 piece, 3 oz | 2 |
| Tofu, ½ cup, 4.4 oz | 0.4 |

## Salads:

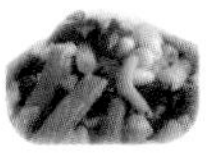

| | |
|---|---|
| **Side Salad,** average | 1 |
| **Bean Salad,** ½ cup | 5 |
| **Coleslaw,** ½ cup | 1 |
| **Potato Salad,** ½ cup | 2 |

# Protein Guide

## General Notes

- **Protein has many important body functions.** It builds and repairs muscle, and is the basis of our body's organs, hormones, enzymes, and antibodies to fight infection.

- **Protein is also an emergency fuel** in the absence of sufficient carbohydrate and fats. For this reason, weight loss should be gradual so as to preserve protein levels in muscle, the heart and other body organs.

- **It is easy to obtain sufficient protein,** even if vegetarian. **Plant proteins are not inferior to animal proteins.** In fact, eating more soy and other plant proteins, and less animal protein, may help to build stronger bones and prevent osteoporosis, and may help to control blood cholesterol levels.

- **When changing to a vegetarian diet,** include soybeans, and other beans, soy milk drinks (calcium-enriched), lentils, tofu, tempeh, nuts and wholegrain breads and cereals. Milk, yogurt, cheese and eggs can enhance nutrient intake.

## Protein & Muscle

- Although muscles are built of protein, protein is not a special fuel for working muscle cells – carbohydrates and fats are.

- In fact, a diet high in protein (and fat) and low in carbohydrate can significantly reduce the performance of endurance sports athletes. **Carbohydrates** are the best fuel for muscles exercised for long periods.

- Any **extra protein** required by athletes and body-builders can easily be obtained from the extra food eaten to satisfy hunger and energy needs.

- Remember, **excessive protein** intake will not build bigger muscles. Any excess is converted and stored as fat. Excess protein can also strain the kidneys, which excrete the waste products of protein metabolism.

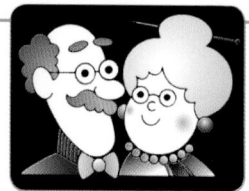

Elderly people (and dieters) must eat sufficient food to ensure adequate protein intake.

Inadequate protein leads to a drop in immune response with greater susceptibility to illness and infections. Muscle strength and muscle mass also drop.

Protein needs are easily met with sensible eating. Athletes who eat enough food for their energy needs can obtain sufficient protein.

## RECOMMENDED DAILY PROTEIN INTAKE
### ~ HEALTHY RANGE ~
(Lower figure is RDA)

| | | PROTEIN |
|---|---|---|
| Children: | 1-3 yrs | 13g-26g |
| | 4-8 yrs | 19g-38g |
| | 9-13 yrs | 34g-64g |
| Males: | 14-18 yrs | 52g-120g |
| | 19+ | 56g-120g |
| Females: | 14+ | 46g-110g |
| Pregnancy: | | 71g-120g |
| Breastfeeding: | | 71g-120g |

**Note:** On lower-calorie diets, aim for higher amounts of protein within the Healthy Range.

## Pro ~ Protein (grams)

| Meat | Pro |
|---|---|
| **Bacon,** 3 medium slices | 6 |
| **Ground Beef Patty,** lean, cooked, 3 oz | 21 |
| **Ham:** Luncheon, 2 slices, 1½ oz | 7 |
| Roasted, 2 pieces, 3 oz | 18 |
| **Lamb chop,** broiled, 3 oz | 22 |
| **Liver,** cooked, 3 oz | 23 |
| **Pastrami,** 2 sl., 1¾ oz | 10 |
| **Pork,** cooked, lean, 3 oz | 24 |
| **Roast Beef,** lean, 2 slices, 3 oz | 24 |
| **Sausages:** Bologna, 2 sl., 2 oz | 7 |
| Braunschweiger, 2 sl., 2 oz | 8 |
| Pork link, thick, 2 oz | 6 |
| Frankfurter, 1⅓ oz | 5 |
| Salami, hard, 3 slices, 1 oz | 7 |
| **Steak:** Average all cuts, lean (no fat) | |
| Small (4 oz raw/3 oz cooked) | 23 |
| Medium (6 oz raw/4¼ oz cooked) | 34 |
| Large (10 oz raw/7¼ oz cooked) | 57 |
| **Veal cutlet,** 1 medium | 23 |
| **Vegetarian,** 1 pattie | 13 |

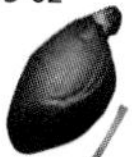

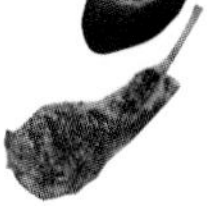

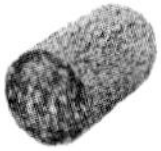

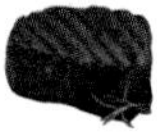

| Chicken/Turkey: *Without Skin* | |
|---|---|
| **Chicken,** cooked: Breast, Roasted, 4 oz | 36 |
| Leg/Thigh,Roasted, 2 oz | 14 |
| ½ Whole Chicken | 60 |
| Drumstick, Rstd, 1 med., 3 oz | 13 |
| **Turkey:** Light meat, cooked, 3 oz | 28 |
| Dark meat, lean, 3 oz | 24 |

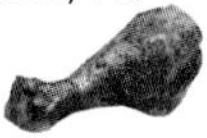

| Fish | |
|---|---|
| **Fresh Fish:** *Per 4 oz, cooked* | |
| Cod, Flounder/Sole, Pollock | 28 |
| Catfish, Haddock, Halibut, M/Mahi | 28 |
| Ocean Perch, Swordf., Orange Roughy | 28 |
| **Canned Fish:** Tuna, Light, 3 oz | 25 |
| White, 3 oz | 23 |
| Salmon, pink, 3 oz | 17 |
| Salmon, red, 3 oz | 17 |
| Sardines, 3 whole (3"), 1¼ oz | 9 |
| Anchovies, 1 can, 1½ oz | 13 |
| **Shellfish:** Crabmeat, 3 oz | 17.5 |
| Clams, raw, 4 large/9 sml, 3 oz | 11 |
| Crayfish, cooked, 3 oz | 20 |
| Lobster, cooked, 3 oz | 17 |
| Oysters, raw, 6 medium, 3 oz | 7 |
| Scallops, 2 lge/5 small, 1 oz | 5 |
| Shrimp, raw, 6 large, 1½ oz | 8.5 |
| **Fish Products:** Fish Sticks, 4 sticks | 10 |
| Fish Portions, in batter, 4 oz | 13 |
| Gefilte Fish, 1 medium ball, 2 oz | 8 |

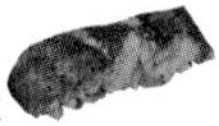

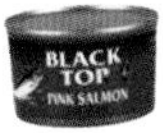

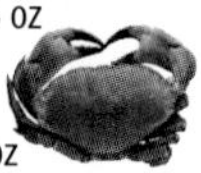

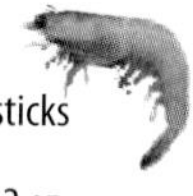

| Eggs | Pro |
|---|---|
| **1 Large Egg,** whole | 6 |
| Egg Yolk | 3 |
| Egg White | 3 |
| **Omelet:** Plain, 2 eggs | 13 |
| Ham & cheese | 17 |
| **Egg Substitutes,** (liquid): | |
| *Egg Beaters,* ¼ cup, 2 oz | 4.5 |
| *Better 'n Eggs/Scramblers,* ¼ cup, 2 oz | 6 |

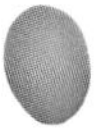

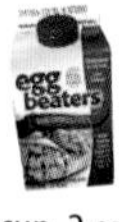

| Milk, Yogurt, Ice Cream | |
|---|---|
| **Milk:** Whole: 2%, 1 cup | 8 |
| Low-Fat (1%); Fat-Free, 1 cup | 8.5 |
| **Chocolate Milk,** 1 cup | 8 |
| **Thick Shake:** Chocolate, 10 oz | 9 |
| Vanilla, 10 oz | 11 |
| **Soymilk,** (fortified), average, 1 cup | 7 |
| *Soy Dream,* Enriched, shelf-stable, 1 cup | 7 |
| **Yogurt,** average all brands: | |
| Plain, 6 oz | 8 |
| Fruit flavors, 6 oz | 7 |
| *Chobani,* Greek, Plain, 6 oz | 14 |
| Soy, fruit flavors, 6 oz | 7 |
| **Ice Cream:** Rich, ½ cup | 2 |
| Regular, Vanilla, ½ cup | 2.5 |
| **Sherbet,** ½ cup | 1 |
| **Custard,** baked, ½ cup | 7 |

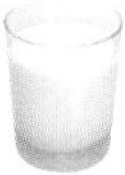

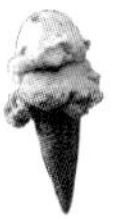

| Cheese | |
|---|---|
| **Hard Cheeses,** average, 1 oz | 7 |
| **Cottage Cheese,** ½ cup | 13 |
| **Cream Cheese,** avg., 1 oz | 2 |
| **Ricotta,** part skim, ½ cup | 14 |

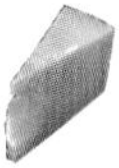

| Bread, Bagels, Biscuits | |
|---|---|
| **Bread:** *With enriched flour* | |
| 1 slice, 1 oz | 2 |
| 4 thin slices, 4 oz | 8 |
| 4 thick slices, 6 oz | 1.2 |
| **Bagel,** plain 2 oz | 6 |
| **Biscuits,** 1 oz | 2 |
| **Pita Bread,** 1 pita, 1½ oz | 4 |
| **Pumpernickel,** 1 slice, 1 oz | 3 |

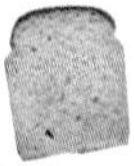

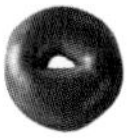

| Infant/Baby Foods | Pro |
|---|---|
| **Infant Formula Milk:** | |
| *Enfamil/Gerber/Similac,* | |
| *Regular/Low Iron* , 5 fl.oz | 2.2 |
| *Isomil/Nursoy/ProSobee,* | 3 |
| **Baby Cereals:** *Average all brands* | |
| Dry, 4 Tbsp, ½ oz | 1 |
| Jars, with fruit, 4½ oz | 1 |

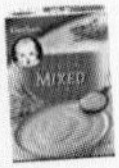

# Protein Counter

## Breakfast Cereals    **Pro**

**Hot Cereals** ~ *Cooked:*

| | |
|---|---|
| **Bulgur,** cooked, 1 cup, 5 oz | 9 |
| **Oatmeal:** Reg., non-fortified, 1 cup | 6 |
|    Instant, fortified, avg., 1 pkt | 4 |
|    *Quaker,* all flavors, ½ cup | 5 |
| **Corn/Hominy Grits:** 1 cup | 3 |
|    *Quaker:* Reg., 3 Tbsp, 1 oz | 2 |
|    Instant White, 1 packet | 2 |
| **Cream of Wheat,** 1 cup | 4 |

**Brands** ~ *Ready-To-Eat*

*General Mills*:

| | |
|---|---|
| Cheerios, Original, 1 cup, 1 oz | 3 |
| Chex, Corn, 1 cup, 1.1 oz | 2 |
| Kix, Original, 1¼ cups, 1 oz | 2 |
| Lucky Charms, Original, ¾ cup, 1 oz | 2 |
| Total, Raisin Bran, 1 cup, 1.8 oz | 3 |
| Wheaties, ¾ cup, 1 oz | 2 |

*Health Valley:*

| | |
|---|---|
| Amaranth Flakes, 1¼ cups, 2 oz | 6 |
| Bran Flakes, with Raisins, 1 cup, 1.8 oz | 5 |
| Corn Crunch-Ems, 1 cup, 1 oz | 2 |
| Oat Bran Flakes, with Raisins, 1 cup, 1.9 oz | 5 |
| Rice Crunch-Ems, 1¼ cups, 1 oz | 2 |

*Kashi:*

| | |
|---|---|
| Good Friends, 1 cup, 1.9 oz | 5 |
| GoLean Crunch!, 1 cup, 1.9 oz | 9 |
| 7 Whole Grain Flakes, 1 cup, 1.75 oz | 6 |

*Kellogg's:*

| | |
|---|---|
| All-Bran, Original, ½ cup, 1 oz | 4 |
| Apple Jacks, 1 cup, 1 oz | 1 |
| Corn Flakes, 1 cup, 1 oz | 2 |
| Low-fat Granola with Raisins ⅔ cup, 2.1 oz | 5 |
| Product 19, 1 cup, 1 oz | 3 |
| Rice Krispies, 1¼ cup, 1.2 oz | 2 |
| Smart-Start Strong Heart, 1 c., 1.75 oz | 4 |
| Special K: All flavors, 1 c., 1.1 oz | 2 |
|    Protein, ¾ cup, 1.1 oz | 10 |

*Post*:

| | |
|---|---|
| Grape Nuts, Original, ½ cup, 2 oz | 8 |
| Raisin Bran, 1 cup, 2 oz | 5 |

*Quaker:*

| | |
|---|---|
| Corn Bran Crunch, ¾ cup, 1 oz | 2 |
| Granola, ½ cup, 1.7 oz | 5 |
| Honey Graham Oh's, ¾ cup, 1 oz | 1 |
| Life, Original, ¾ cup, 1.1 oz | 3 |

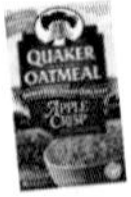

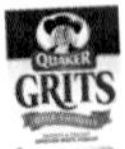

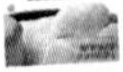

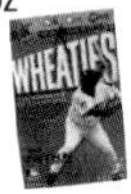

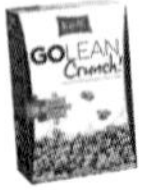

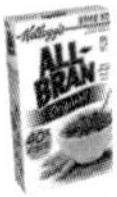

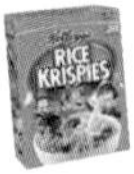

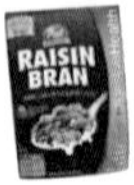

## Brans & Wheatgerm    **Pro**

| | |
|---|---|
| **Oat Bran,** raw, 1 Tbsp | 2 |
| **Rice Bran,** raw, 2 Tbsp | 1 |
| **Wheat Bran,** unprocessed, 2 T. | 1 |
| **Wheat Germ,** 2 Tbsp, ½ oz | 4 |

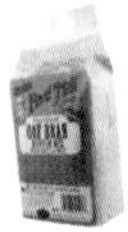

## Grains & Flours, Yeast

| | |
|---|---|
| **Amaranth,** ½ cup, 3.4 oz | 14 |
| **Barley,** ½ cup, 3.2 oz | 12 |
| **Buckwheat Flour,** Whole-groat, 1 cup | 15 |
| **Carob Flour,** 1 cup, 3.6 oz | 5 |
| **Corn Flour,** 1 cup, 4 oz | 11 |
| **Corn Meal,** 1 cup, 4½ oz | 8 |
| **Flour:** White, 1 cup, 5.6 oz | 9 |
|    Wholegrain, 1 cup, 4¼ oz | 16 |
| **Millet,** wholegrain, 1 cup, 3½ oz | 12 |
| **Rye Flour:** Dark, 1 cup, 4½ oz | 18 |
|    Light, 1 cup, 3½ oz | 9 |
| **Soy Flour,** full fat, 1 cup, 3 oz | 29 |
| **Yeast:** Brewers, 2 Tbsp, ½ oz | 8 |
|    Nutritional Yeast Flakes *(Red Star),* 1 heaping Tbsp, ½ oz | 8 |

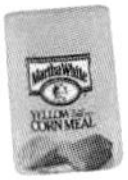

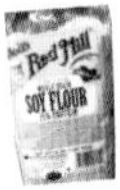

## Rice, Spaghetti, Macaroni

| | |
|---|---|
| **Rice:** Brown/White, average 1 cup cooked, 6½ oz | 5 |
| **Spaghetti/Macaroni/Noodles (enriched):** | |
|    Cooked, 1 cup, 4½ oz | 7 |
|    Canned: in Tomato Sce, ½ cup | 2 |
|      with Meatballs, 1 cup, 8 oz | 10 |
|    Macaroni & Cheese, 1 cup, 9 oz | 8 |

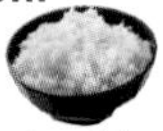

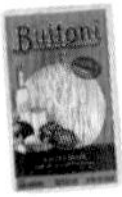

## Soups

| | |
|---|---|
| With Noodles/Vegetables, 1 cup | 3 |
| With Meat/Beans/Peas, 1 cup | 8 |

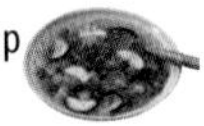

## Fruit

**Fresh/Canned:**

| | |
|---|---|
|    Average, all types, 1 medium/2 small fruit | 1 |
| **Avocado,** ½ medium | 2 |
| **Dried Fruit:** Apricots, 8 halves, 1 oz | 1 |
|    Dates, 6 dates, 2 oz | 1.5 |
|    Figs, 4 medium figs, 2 oz | 2 |
|    Prunes, 5 medium, 1½ oz | 1 |
|    Raisins, 1 oz | 1 |
| **Fruit Juice:** Average, 1 cup | 0.5 |
|    Prune Juice, 6 fl.oz | 1 |
|    Tomato Juice, 1 cup, 8 fl.oz | 1.5 |

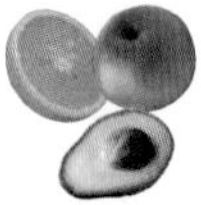

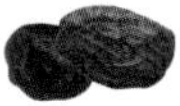

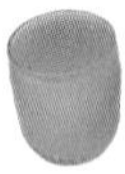

## Vegetables

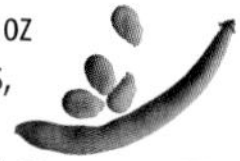

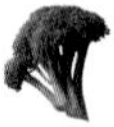

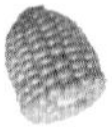

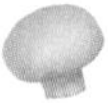

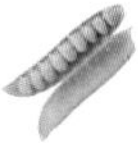

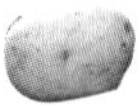

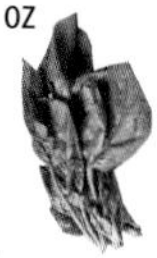

| | Pro |
|---|---|
| **Beans:** Snap/green, ½ cup, 2 oz | 1 |
| Dried: Average all types, cooked, ½ cup | 7 |
| Baked Beans, ½ cup 4½ oz | 5 |
| **Bean Sprouts,** mung, 1 c., 4 oz | 3 |
| **Broccoli,** 3raw, ½ cup, 1½ oz | 1.5 |
| **Cabbage; Cauliflower,** raw, 1 c. 3 oz | 1.5 |
| **Corn:** Raw, ½ cup kernels, 3 oz | 2.5 |
| 1 ear trimmed to 3½" | 2 |
| **Lentils,** cooked, ½ cup, 3½ oz | 9 |
| **Mushrooms,** raw, ½ c., sliced | 1 |
| **Peas:** Green, raw, ½ c., 2½ oz | 4 |
| Split Peas, cooked, 1 cup, 7 oz | 16 |
| **Potatoes:** *Cooked:* | |
| 1 medium, with skin, 5 oz | 3.3 |
| without skin, 4 oz | 2.3 |
| French Fries, small, 2.6 oz | 2 |
| **Potato Salad,** ½ cup, 4 oz | 3.5 |
| **Pumpkin,** ½ cup mashed, 4.3 oz | 1 |
| **Seaweed,** kelp, 1 oz | <1 |
| **Spinach,** cooked, ½ cup, 3 oz | 2.7 |
| **Squash,** ckd, all types, ½ cup | 1 |
| **Tomatoes,** 1 medium, 4½ oz | 1 |
| **Vegetables,** mixed, ckd, 1 cup | 2.5 |
| **Soybeans,** cooked, ½ cup, 3 oz | 14 |

## Tofu, Tempeh, Miso

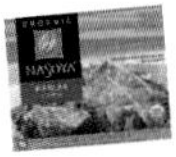

| | |
|---|---|
| Tofu, raw, firm, ½ cup, 4½ oz | 10 |
| Tempeh, ½ cup, 3 oz | 16 |
| Miso, ½ cup, 5 oz | 16 |
| Miso Soup, 1 cup | 3 |
| **Soybean Protein** *(TVP)*, 1 oz | 18 |

## Cakes, Pastries, Pies

(Made with enriched flour)

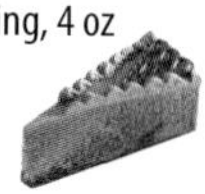

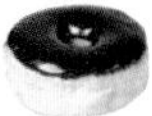

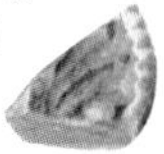

| | |
|---|---|
| Carrot w. cream cheese frosting, 4 oz | 4 |
| Cheesecake, 1 piece, 4 oz | 6 |
| Chocolate, 1 piece, 2 oz | 2 |
| Fruitcake, 1 piece, 3 oz | 4 |
| Plain, 1 piece, 3 oz | 4 |
| **Croissant,** plain, 2 oz | 5 |
| **Danish Pastry,** 1 pastry, 2¼ oz | 4 |
| **Donuts,** average, 2 oz | 4 |
| **Muffins,** average, 1 med., 1½ oz | 3 |
| **Pancakes,** 4" diam., two, 2 oz | 4 |
| **Pies:** Fruit, 1 piece, 5½ oz | 4 |
| Pecan, 1 piece, 5 oz | 7 |
| **Puddings,** average, ½ cup, 4½ oz | 4 |
| **Waffles,** 1 large, 2½ oz | 7 |

## Peanut Butter

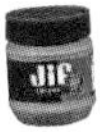

| | Pro |
|---|---|
| **Regular:** 2 Tbsp, 1.1 oz | 8 |
| *Peter Pan Plus,* 2 Tbsp, 1.1 oz | 8 |

## Sugar, Honey, Jam

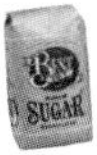

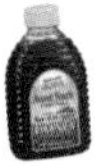

| | |
|---|---|
| **Sugar:** White | 0 |
| Brown, 1 Tbsp | 0 |
| **Molasses:** Light/Med., 1 Tbsp | 0 |
| Blackstrap, 1 Tbsp, ¾ oz | 0 |
| **Corn Syrup,** 1 Tbsp, ¾ oz | 0 |
| **Honey, Jams, Jelly** | 0 |

## Candy, Chocolate, Carob

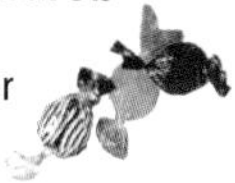

| | |
|---|---|
| **Candy,** sugar-based | 0 |
| **Chocolate:** Plain, 2 oz bar | 4 |
| with nuts, 2 oz bar | 6 |
| **Carob,** plain, 2 oz | 6 |

## Cookies, Crackers, Chips

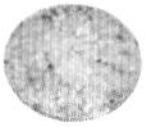

| | |
|---|---|
| **Cookies,** average, 4 cookies | 2 |
| **Crackers,** Graham, 2½" sq., (2) | 1 |
| **Rice Cakes,** average, one | 1 |
| **Corn/Potato Chips,** 1 oz | 2 |

## Nuts:

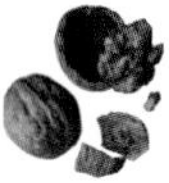

| | |
|---|---|
| Almonds, shelled, 20-25 nuts | 6 |
| Brazil Nuts, 7-8 medium nuts, 1 oz | 4 |
| Cashews, 12-16 nuts, 1 oz | 5 |
| Macadamias, 1 oz | 2 |
| Peanuts, dry rsted, 40 nuts, 1 oz | 6 |
| Pecans, 24 halves, 1 oz | 2 |
| Walnuts, 15 halves, 1 oz | 4 |

## Seeds:

| | |
|---|---|
| Sesame Seeds, dry, 1 Tbsp | 2 |
| Pumpkin Kernels, dry, hulled, 1 oz | 7 |
| Sunflower Seeds, dried, hulled, 1 oz | 6 |
| Tahini, 1 Tbsp, ½ oz | 2.5 |

## Granola & Food/Protein Bars

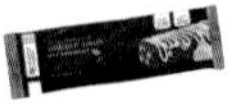

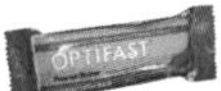

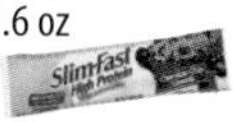

| | |
|---|---|
| **Granola Bars,** average, 1 bar, 2 oz | 2 |
| ***Anytime Health,*** | |
| Meal Repl. Bars, 80g | 20 |
| Snack Bars, 50g | 12 |
| ***Balance*** Bars, Original, average all, 1.76 oz | 14 |
| ***Bariatrix,*** Proti-Bars (1), 1.4 oz | 15 |
| ***Dr Soy,*** Protein Bars, 1.76 oz | 10 |
| ***GeniSoy,*** Protein Bar, 1.6 oz | 15 |
| ***Jenny Craig,*** Bars, av. 1.8 oz | 5 |
| ***Met-Rx,*** "Big 100", av. 3.5 oz | 27 |
| ***Myoplex 30,*** all flavors, 3 oz | 30 |
| ***Optifast 800,*** all flavors, 2 oz | 14 |
| ***PowerBar,*** Energize, 2 oz | 6 |
| ***Slim-Fast,*** Protein Meal Bars, 1.7 oz | 10 |
| ***Special K:*** Protein Meal, 1.6 oz | 10 |
| Protein Snack, 0.9 oz | 4 |

# Protein Counter

## High Protein Drinks **Pro**

| | |
|---|---|
| *Anytime,* Health, | |
| Whey Prot. Isolate, all flav., 1 oz | 25 |
| *Atkins,* Shakes, 11 fl.oz | 18 |
| *Boost,* High Protein, 8 fl.oz bottle | 15 |
| *Carnation,* B'fast Essentials, 11 fl.oz | 10 |
| *Curves,* Protein Drink, 2 scoops, dry | 15 |
| *dotFIT,* First String, | |
| Choc. 2 scps, 2.65 oz | 21 |
| *Ensure,* Plus, 8 fl.oz bottle | 13 |
| *Gatorade,* Protein Recovery Shake, 11 oz | 20 |
| *GeniSoy,* Protein Shake, 1 scoop, 1.2 oz | 14 |
| *Met-Rx,* Meal Replacement, RTD | 40 |
| *Myoplex,* Original Nutrition Shake, 1 pkt | 42 |
| *Optifast 800,* prepared, 8 fl oz | 14 |
| *Slim-Fast Shakes:* Meal, 10 oz can | 10 |
| High Protein Meal, 10 fl.oz bottle | 20 |
| *Special K₂0,* Protein Water, 16 fl.oz | 5 |
| *Weider,* Mass 1000, 4 scoops, 7 oz | 34 |

### Coffee, Tea, Soda

| | |
|---|---|
| Coffee, Coffee Substitutes, 1 cup, 8 fl.oz | 0 |
| Coffee, with 2 oz milk, 1 cup, 8 fl.oz | 2 |
| Caffe latte, large, 16 fl.oz | 12 |
| Cappuccino, large, 16 fl.oz | 8 |
| Frappuccino, average, 16 fl.oz | 6 |
| Hot Chocolate, with milk, 1 cup, 8 fl.oz | 8 |
| Soft Drinks/Soda | 0 |
| Tea, all types | 0 |

### Beer, Wine, Spirits

| | |
|---|---|
| Beer, 12 fl.oz | 1 |
| Wines, red/white, 1 glass | 0 |
| Spirits/Liquor | 0 |

### Fast-Foods/Burgers

| | |
|---|---|
| **Pancakes,** average all outlets, 3 | 8 |
| **Shakes,** Chocolate, 16 fl.oz | 12 |
| **Sundaes,** Average all outlets | 7 |
| *Arby's:* | |
| Chopped Farmhouse Salad, Crispy Chicken | 30 |
| Roast Beef Sandwich: Classic | 23 |
| Max | 45 |
| *Burger King:* Big Fish Sandwich | 18 |
| Double Bacon Cheeseburger | 17 |
| Whopper Sandwich | 22 |

## Fast Foods/Burgers (Cont) **Pro**

| | |
|---|---|
| *Carl's Jr:* | |
| Charbroiled Chicken Club Sandwich | 36 |
| Famous Star Hamburger with Cheese | 28 |
| Super Star Hamburger with Cheese | 48 |
| *Domino's Pizza:* Hand Tossed (12") | |
| Feast, Ultimate Pepperoni, 1 slice | 11 |
| Legend: Buffalo Chicken, 1 slice | 13 |
| Honolulu Hawaiian, 1 slice | 8 |
| *KFC:* Original, Breast | 36 |
| Extra Crispy Tenders, 3 strips | 33 |
| Grilled, Breast | 40 |
| *McDonald's:* Big Mac | 25 |
| Cheeseburger | 15 |
| Chicken McNuggets (6) | 13 |
| Crispy Chicken Classic Sandwich | 24 |
| Filet-O-Fish | 15 |
| Hamburger | 12 |
| Quarter Pounder with Cheese | 30 |
| French Fries: Small, 2.5 oz | 3 |
| Large, 5.4 oz | 6 |
| Salad, with Chicken, average | 26 |
| Shake, McCafe, average, 12 fl.oz | 12 |
| Breakfast: Egg McMuffin | 18 |
| Bacon, Egg & Cheese McGriddles | 19 |
| Sausage Burrito | 12 |
| Sausage McMuffin with Egg | 21 |
| *Pizza Hut:* Per Medium, 1 slice, ⅛ Pizza | |
| Thin 'n Crispy, Supreme | 10 |
| Pan Pizzas, average | 11 |
| Hand Tossed: Pepperoni Lover's | 12 |
| Ultimate Cheese Lover's | 10 |
| *Subway :* 6" Subs with standard toppings, no oil | |
| Applewood Pulled Pork | 25 |
| Meatball Marinara | 21 |
| Spicy Italian | 20 |
| Subway Melt | 23 |
| Turkey Jalapeno Melt | 21 |
| *Taco Bell:* Bean Burrito | 15 |
| Cheesy Gordita Crunch | 20 |
| Chicken Quesadilla | 27 |
| Chicken/Steak Chalupas | 16 |
| Steak Burrito Supreme | 20 |
| Taco Supreme | 9 |
| *Wendy's:* | |
| Asiago Ranch Chicken Club | 38 |
| Dave's ¼ lb Single Burger | 30 |
| Jr Hamburger | 14 |

## High Blood Pressure

**Many American adults** have hypertension (high blood pressure), and are unaware of it. It is generally symptomless, so **have your blood pressure checked annually** – particularly if it runs in the family.

**Untreated hypertension** overworks the heart, damages arteries and promotes atherosclerosis. This in turn greatly increases the risk of heart disease, stroke, blindness, kidney disease and impotence. The earlier hypertension is detected, the sooner it can be brought under control.

### BLOOD PRESSURE CLASSIFICATION

*For Adults Age 18 & Older ~ Not Acutely ill or on Medication (American Heart Association)*

| | DIASTOLIC | | SYSTOLIC |
|---|---|---|---|
| Normal ➤ | Below 80 | and | Below 120 |
| Prehypertension ➤ | 80-89 | or | 120-139 |
| **Hypertension:** | | | |
| Stage 1 ➤ | 90-99 | or | 140-159 |
| Stage 2 ➤ | 100 or more | or | 160 or more |

## Treating Hypertension

**Prehypertension** (in the chart above) means you don't have high blood pressure now but are likely to develop it in the future.

**You can take steps to lessen the risk by adopting healthy lifestyle habits such as:**
- reducing sodium intake
- eating adequate fruit and vegetables
- losing weight if overweight
- limiting alcohol to 2 drinks or less daily
- quitting smoking
- exercising regularly, managing stress.

**Stage 1 hypertension** can often be treated with the above lifestyle changes.

**Stage 2 hypertension** usually requires drug therapy. However, salt restriction, abstaining from alcohol, and the above lifestyle changes will improve the success of drug therapy, and enable smaller drug doses to be prescribed.

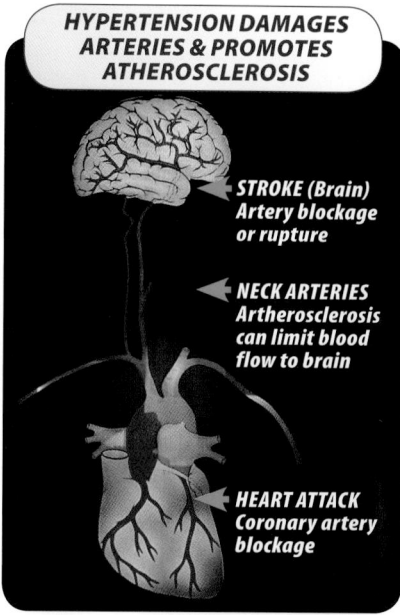

### HYPERTENSION DAMAGES ARTERIES & PROMOTES ATHEROSCLEROSIS

**STROKE (Brain)** Artery blockage or rupture

**NECK ARTERIES** Artherosclerosis can limit blood flow to brain

**HEART ATTACK** Coronary artery blockage

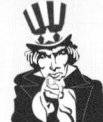

### STROKE
### KNOW THE WARNING SIGNS

**Stroke is a medical emergency! If you notice one or more of these signs, call 9-1-1 or your doctor immediately.**

These signs may be signalling a possible stroke or transient ischemic attack:

- **Sudden weakness** or numbness in your face, arm, or leg on one side of your body.
- **Sudden confusion,** trouble speaking or understanding. Slurred speech.
- **Sudden trouble seeing,** in one or both eyes
- **Sudden trouble walking,** dizziness, loss of balance or coordination.
- **Sudden severe headache** - 'a bolt out of the blue' – with no apparent cause.

*Extra Info: www.stroke.org*

# Salt & Sodium Guide

## Salt & Sodium

- **Sodium is a mineral element** most commonly found in salt (sodium chloride). It also occurs naturally in much smaller amounts in animal and plant foods, and water – normally sufficient for our needs without having to add salt to our diet.

- **Sodium is required** for nerve and muscle function, as well as to balance the amount of fluid in our tissues and blood.
  Sodium acts like a sponge to attract and hold fluids in body tissues.

- **Excess sodium** can cause water retention, and increase the risk of developing hyper-tension. Very high salt intake may also increase the risk of stomach cancer.

- **Too little sodium** may cause low blood pressure (hypotension), and decrease blood flow to the heart, brain and kidneys – especially during exercise. (A certain blood volume is required to sustain the blood pressure needed for adequate blood flow in the capillaries).

## Salt-Sensitive Persons

- **Normally, our kidneys** excrete excess dietary sodium. The thirst we feel after a salty meal is the body calling for water to dilute the sodium, and enable the kidneys to flush out excess sodium.

- **However, 'salt - sensitive'** persons (up to 70% of adults) tend to retain excess sodium (above approximately 3000mg daily) instead of excreting it. Such persons are more likely to develop hypertension and would benefit most from sodium restriction. Assume you are susceptible if there is a family history of hypertension.

- **Although not everyone will benefit, all Americans are being asked to moderate their salt and sodium intake** as a public health measure – particularly because so many do not know whether or not they have hypertension, and also because we do not know just who is salt-sensitive.

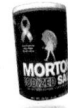

## FINDING HIDDEN SODIUM

On average, **less than one third of our sodium intake comes from the salt shaker.**
The rest is hidden in processed foods that have salt added during manufacture.

Sodium compounds added to food or medicinals can also contribute significant sodium.

**Sodium bicarbonate** in particular is widely used in antacid tablets (such as *Alka Seltzer*) and powders. Sodium bicarbonate contains 27% sodium by weight. Each gram has 270mg of sodium. Large amounts of sodium can be unwittingly consumed – up to 600mg per tablet. (See Antacids ~ Page 280)

**Example:** 2 *Alka-Seltzer* Tablets = 1000mg sodium

**Other sodium compounds** include monosodium glutamate (MSG), sodium ascorbate, sodium nitrite, and sodium citrate.

## POTASSIUM BALANCES SODIUM

Potassium helps to balance sodium by helping the kidneys to excrete excess sodium.
Fruit and vegetables are rich sources of potassium - another reason to ensure you have your 5-7 servings every day.

Nuts also provide potassium as well as magnesium and other heart-healthy nutrients and anti-oxidants. Eat them unsalted.

*Note: This info is only for people with normal kidney function. Also not for persons on potassium-sparing diuretics.*

## ALCOHOL DANGER

*Excessive alcohol intake contributes to hypertension. Susceptible persons should limit alcohol intake to 1-2 drinks per day.*

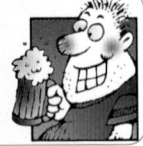

# Salt Sodium Guide

Sodium accounts for only 40% of the weight of salt (sodium chloride). Examples:
1 gram (1000mg) Salt has 400mg Sodium
1 teaspoon (5g) Salt has 2000mg Sodium

## HINTS TO REDUCE SODIUM

- **Cut down use of the salt shaker.** Start with an easy 50% cut in sodium by using Lite Salt (*Morton*) or *Cardia* Salt. Then gradually cut back until you can leave the salt shaker off the table. Sea salt is still high in sodium.

- **Use fresh herbs,** and salt-free seasonings to add flavor to food.

- **Choose low-sodium,** sodium-free, and reduced-sodium products in place of regular, salted products.

- **Check food labels for sodium levels.** FDA Guidelines for sodium descriptors are:
  - **Reduced Sodium:** At least 25% less sodium than the original product
  - **Low Sodium:** 140 mg or less/serving
  - **Very Low Sodium:** 35mg or less/serving
  - **Sodium Free:** Less than 5mg/serving
  - **No Salt Added:** Made without the salt normally added, but still contains the sodium that is a natural part of the food

- **Use reduced-sodium breads,** butter and margarine. Regular varieties are considered high in sodium in view of their significant contribution to our diet.

- **Go easy on salty condiments and sauces** such as ketchup, mustard, soy sauce, spaghetti sauces, and salad dressings. Use low-sodium varieties.

- **Limit pizzas and salty fast-foods.** Check the *CalorieKing.com* food database.

- **Avoid salty snack foods** such as potato chips, corn chips, salted nuts, pretzels and cheesy-flavored snacks. **Choose unsalted** popcorn, nuts or seeds. Eat more fruit.

- **Don't salt children's food** to your taste.

- **Avoid antacids with** sodium bicarbonate (such as *Alka-Seltzer*). They are high in sodium. Look for low-sodium alternatives.

## FOODS HIGH IN SODIUM

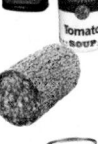

- Bread (4 slices/day), Bagels, Biscuits
- Cheese, Butter, Margarine
- Pickles, Sauerkraut, Olives
- Condiments, Sauces
- Salad Dressings
- Canned vegetables/salads/beans
- Deli Salads (with dressing)
- Frozen/Packaged Meals/Entrees
- Soups: Canned/dry; bouillon cubes
- Meats: Ham, bacon, sausage, luncheon meats, smoked meats
- Canned Fish (in brine/salt)
- Sea Salt, Garlic/Celery Salt
- Snack Foods (potato chips, pretzels)
- Tomato Juice (Canned), V8 Vegetable Juice
- Fast Foods: Pizza, Burgers, Chicken
- *Alka-Seltzer* Antacid

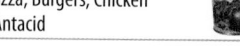

## MODERATE SODIUM

- Meat, Fish, Poultry - Unprocessed
- Milk, Yogurt, Soy Drinks, Eggs
- Peanut Butter
- Breakfast Cereals (less than 200mg/serving)
- Chocolate Candy, Fruit/Nut Bars
- *Reduced Sodium & Low Sodium* Products

## FOODS LOW IN SODIUM

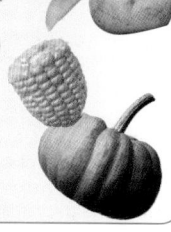

- Products labelled *Very Low Sodium*, or *Sodium Free*
- Bread (No Salt Added)
- Fresh fruits and vegetables
- Canned and Dried Fruits
- Potatoes, Rice, Pasta
- Dried Beans & Lentils, Tofu
- Nuts & Seeds (unsalted)
- Corn & Popcorn (unsalted)
- Pepper, Spices, Herbs
- Jam, Honey, Syrup
- Candy, Gum
- Hard & Jelly Candy
- Coffee, Tea, Alcohol
- Fresh Fruit Juices, Water

# Sodium Counter

**Sodium ~ Sodium (mg)**

## Milk & Dairy Products

| | Sodium |
|---|---|
| **Milk:** Whole/lowfat/skim, average | |
| 1 glass, 8 fl.oz | 120 |
| Whole, low sodium, 1 cup | 5 |
| **Choc Milk,** 1 cup | 130 |
| **Soy Milk,** 8 fl.oz | 30 |
| **Buttermilk,** cultured, 8 fl.oz | 250 |
| **Dry/Powder,** skim, ¼ cup, 1 oz | 110 |
| **Yogurt,** with fruit average, 8 oz | 130 |
| **Cheese:** Bleu, 1 oz | 330 |
| Cottage Cheese, Creamed, ½ cup, 4 oz | 450 |
| *Kraft:* American, 2% milk, 1 sl., 0.7 oz | 230 |
| Philadelphia Cream Cheese Brick, Orig.,1 oz | 105 |
| Parmesan, 1 oz | 425 |
| Process Cheese., average,1 oz | 430 |
| Ricotta Cheese, ½ cup, 4 oz | 110 |
| Swiss, Deli Deluxe, 1 slice | 40 |

## Ice Cream, Frozen Yogurt

| | |
|---|---|
| Icecream, average, ½ cup | 50 |
| Frozen Yogurt, ½ cup | 50 |

## Fats/Oils

| | |
|---|---|
| **Butter/Margarine:** | |
| Regular, 2 Tbsp, 1 oz | 230 |
| Unsalted, reg., 2 Tbsp, 1 oz | 5 |
| **Mayonnaise,** avg., 2 Tbsp, 1 oz | 160 |
| **Oils/Lard/Drippings** | 0 |
| **Cream,** average, 1 Tbsp | 5 |
| *Coffee-Mate:* Powdered, 1 tsp | 2 |
| Liquid, 1 Tbsp | 5 |

## Eggs

| | |
|---|---|
| **Whole,** 1 large | 70 |
| **Omelet: 2 egg,** plain | 220 |
| With 1 oz Cheddar Cheese | 400 |
| *Egg Beaters:* Original, 3 Tbsp | 90 |
| Flavors, average, 3 Tbsp | 140 |

## Meats

| | |
|---|---|
| **Meat,** average all types, cooked | |
| Beef/Lamb/Veal/Pork, 4 oz | 80 |
| **Corned Beef,** cooked, 3 oz | 800 |
| **Bacon,** cooked, 2 slices, 0.5 oz | 270 |
| **Ham,** 3 oz | 1100 |

## Chicken & Turkey

| | |
|---|---|
| **Chicken/Turkey,** cooked, unsalted, 4 oz | 80 |
| **Stuffing Mixes,** average., ½ cup | 500 |

## Sausages & Meats

| | Sodium |
|---|---|
| Bologna, 1 oz | 280 |
| Frankfurter, 2 oz | 640 |
| Ham, chopped, 0.8 oz slice | 290 |
| Liverwurst (Braunschweiger), 1 oz | 320 |
| Pepperoni, 5 slices, 1 oz | 570 |
| Salami: Cooked, 1 oz | 350 |
| dry/hard, 1 oz | 600 |
| Sausage, 1 oz link | 220 |
| Pork, 2 oz patty | 260 |
| *Spam:* Classic, 2 oz | 790 |
| 25% Less Sodium, 2 oz | 580 |
| Turkey Roll, 1 oz | 160 |

## Fish:

| | |
|---|---|
| **Fresh Fish:** average, plain | |
| Cooked, 4 oz, without bone | 60 |
| Broiled w. butter, 4 oz | 150 |
| Breaded & fried, 4 oz | 320 |
| Fish fillets, batter-dipped 3 oz | 350 |
| Fish sticks, 1 oz stick | 160 |
| Gefilte Fish, with broth, 1 pce, 1.5 oz | 220 |
| Herring, pickled, 2 pces, 1 oz | 260 |
| Lobster, meat only, 4 oz | 180 |
| Oysters, fresh, 6 med., 3 oz | 95 |
| **Salmon:** Canned, 3 oz | 460 |
| No Salt Added, 3 oz | 65 |
| **Smoked fish,** average, 3 oz | 650 |
| **Tuna:** Canned, drained, 3 oz | 160 |
| Light, drained, 3 oz | 200 |
| No Added Salt, 3 oz | 40 |
| Spicy Flavored, 5 oz | 260 |

## Entrees & Meals

| | |
|---|---|
| **Frozen Meals,** average | 600-1300 |
| *Lean Cuisine,* average | 700 |
| *Stouffer's,* For One, Beef Pot Roast | 1570 |
| **Dinners,** average | 900-1200 |
| **Side Dishes,** average | 400-600 |
| **Pizza,** frozen, ¼ large, 6 oz | 800-1200 |
| **Microwave,** Cup Meals | 900-1200 |
| **Cup O'Noodles,** average | 1500 |

# Sodium Counter

## Soups

| | Sodium |
|---|---|
| **Condensed:** Average, 1 cup, 8 oz | 800-1000 |
| Low Sodium, average | 70 |
| **Chicken Noodle,** average, 1 cup | 900 |
| **Bouillon Cube,** average | 950 |
| **Ramen Noodle Soup,** av., 3 oz pkg | 1500 |
| **Soup Cups,** average | 850 |
| **Soup Mixes,** average, 1 cup | 900 |

## Condiments, Sauces, Dressings

| | |
|---|---|
| **A-1 Sauce,** 1 Tbsp | 280 |
| **Barbecue Sauce,** 1 Tbsp | 130 |
| **Bragg's Liquid Aminos,** 1 tsp | 220 |
| **Chili Sauce,** 1 Tbsp | 230 |
| **Ketchup:** Tomato, 1 Tbsp | 180 |
| Low Sodium, 1 Tbsp | 20 |
| **Mayonnaise,** 1 Tbsp | 80 |
| **Mustard,** 1 tsp | 70 |
| **Pizza Sauce,** ½ cup | 700 |
| **Salad Dressings,** 2 Tbsp, 1 oz | 160-400 |
| **Spaghetti Sauce,** ½ cup | 500 |
| **Soy Sauce:** 1 Tbsp | 900 |
| Lite, 1 Tbsp | 600 |
| **Sweet & Sour,** ½ cup | 250 |
| **Tabasco,** 1 tsp | 25 |
| **Vinegar,** Lemon Juice | 0 |
| **Worcestershire,** 1 Tbsp | 65 |
| **Tomato:** Sauce, 1 cup | 1200 |
| Paste/Puree (salted), ½ cup | 1000 |
| No Salt Added, ½ cup | 75 |

## Salt & Salt Substitutes

| | |
|---|---|
| **Table Salt:** 1 teaspoon, 6g | 2400 |
| Single Serve package, 1 g | 400 |
| **Cardia Salt,** 1 teaspoon | 1080 |
| **Lite Salt,** 1 teaspoon, 6g | 1200 |
| **Morton,** No Salt Substitute, 1 tsp | 5 |
| **Garlic/Onion/Seasoned Salt,** 1 tsp, 4g | 1350 |
| **Garlic/Seasoned Salt** 1 teaspoon, 4g | 1300 |
| **Sea Salt,** 1 teaspoon, 5g | 2250 |

## Seasonings, Herbs & Spices

| | |
|---|---|
| Baking Powder, 1 tsp, 3g | 340 |
| Baking Soda (Sodium bicarb), 1 tsp, 3g | 810 |
| **Accent,** Flavor Enhancer, 1 tsp | 680 |
| Chili Powder, 1 tsp, 3g | 25 |
| Curry Powder | 0 |
| Lemon Pepper 1 tsp | 340 |
| Meat Tenderizer, 1 tsp, 5g | 1750 |
| MSG (Monosodium Glutamate), 5g | 500 |
| **Mrs Dash,** Blends/Marinades | 0 |
| **Old Bay:** Seasoning, 1 tsp, 2.4 oz | 640 |
| Seasoning, Less Sodium, 1 tsp, 2.4 oz | 380 |
| Pepper, Mustard (dry), 1 tsp | 1 |
| Yeast, Nutritional, 1 Tbsp | 10 |

## Breakfast Cereals

| | Sodium |
|---|---|
| **Kellogg's:** | |
| All-Bran, Original, ½ cup, 1 oz | 80 |
| Special K, Original, 1 cup, 1.1 oz | 210 |
| Corn Flakes, 1 cup, 1 oz | 200 |
| Frosted Mini Wheats, Blueb./Strawb., (25) | 0 |
| Raisin Bran, 1 cup | 210 |
| **Quaker:** | |
| Corn Bran Crunch, ¾ cup, 1 oz | 210 |
| Oh's, ¾ cup, 1 oz | 170 |
| Puffed Rice/Wheat, 2 cups, 1 oz | 1 |
| Simply Granola, average, ½ cup, 1 oz | 30 |
| **General Mills,** Total, ¾ cup, 1 oz | 140 |
| **Oatmeal:** Regular, ¾ cup | 1 |
| **Quaker,** Instant Maple & Brown Sugar (1 pkt) | 260 |

## Breads, Bagels, Crackers

| | |
|---|---|
| **Bread:** Thin Slice, average 1 oz | 140 |
| Thick Slice, 1.5 oz | 210 |
| Low Sodium, 1 oz | 10 |
| **Bagels:** Plain, medium, 2 oz | 200 |
| Large, take-out, average, 4 oz | 550 |
| **Panera Bread,** 3.8 oz | 460 |
| **Biscuits,** average, 1 oz | 180 |
| **Bun/Roll:** 1 medium, 1.5 oz | 200 |
| Large, 4 oz | 560 |
| **Crackers:** Saltine, 2 crackers | 70 |
| Low Salt, 2 | 25 |
| Graham, 2 regular | 50 |
| **Croissant,** Plain, average, 2 oz | 280 |
| **Rice Cakes,** average | 25 |
| **Ritz Crackers,** Hint of Salt, 1 oz | 60 |
| **Ry-Krisp,** Crispbread, Sesame, 0.7 oz | 70 |

## Cookies, Cakes, Desserts

| | |
|---|---|
| **Cookies:** Average, 2-3 cookies, 1 oz | 100 |
| Average, 1 cookie, 2.5 oz | 180 |
| **Baked Custard,** ½ cup | 100 |
| **Brownie,** 1.5 oz | 130 |
| **Carrot Cake,** 8 oz | 650 |
| **Cheesecake,** 7 oz | 350 |
| **Cinnamon Sweet Roll,** 2 oz | 250 |
| **Danish,** Apple/Fruit | 250 |
| **Donut,** average | 150 |
| **Muffins:** 1 medium, 2 oz | 150 |
| 1 extra large, 4 oz | 300 |
| **Pancakes,** (4"), x 3 | 360 |
| **Fruit Pies,** average, 7 oz | 600 |
| **Pudding:** Average, ½ cup | 160 |
| Jell-O Instant Pudding Mix, ¼ pkg | 360 |
| **Waffles:** Home-made, 7", 2.5 oz | 350 |
| Frozen: Average, 1.2 oz | 260 |
| **Aunt Jemima,** Homestyle, av., 2.5 oz | 480 |

# Sodium Counter

## Fruit & Juices

| | Sodium |
|---|---|
| **Fresh Fruit,** average all types, 1 serving | 1 |
| **Dried/Canned Fruit,** ½ cup | 1 |
| **Fruit Juice:** Fresh, sqz'd, 6 fl.oz | 1 |
| Commercial, aver., 6 fl.oz | 20 |
| **Tomato Juice** (Campbell's), 8 fl.oz | 680 |
| Low Sodium (No Salt Added), 8 fl.oz | 140 |
| **V8 Vegetable** (Campbell's): | |
| 11.5 fl.oz bottle | 880 |
| Low Sodium, 5.5 fl.oz can | 80 |

## Vegetables

**Fresh/Frozen (No Salt Added):** Per ½ Cup

| | Sodium |
|---|---|
| Asparagus, Bean Sprouts, Corn | 3 |
| Beets, Carrots, Celery, ½ cup | 40 |
| Broccoli, Cabbage, Cauliflower | 10 |
| Cucumber, Green Beans, Mushroom, Okra | 3 |
| Onions, Peas, Potato, Pumpkin, Squash | 3 |
| Peppers, Hot Chili, raw, each | 3 |
| Spinach, Turnips, ½ cup, cooked | 40 |
| Tomato, 1 medium, 5 oz | 10 |
| **Canned:** Asparagus, 4 spears | 300 |
| Beans, baked in tomato sauce | 450 |
| Beets, ½ cup, 3 oz | 240 |
| Corn Kernels, ½ cup, 3 oz | 190 |
| Creamed, ½ cup, 4.5 oz | 330 |
| Mushrooms w. butter sce, 2oz | 550 |
| Peas, ½ cup, 3 oz | 250 |
| Sauerkraut, ½ cup, 4 oz | 750 |

## Pickles, Olives

| | Sodium |
|---|---|
| **Olives:** pickled: Green, 1 large | 90 |
| Ripe/black, 1 large | 40 |
| **Pickles:** Bread & Butter, 4 slices, 1 oz | 200 |
| Dill, 1 pickle, 2.5oz | 900 |
| Sweet, 1 gherkin, 0.5 oz | 130 |

## Soybean Products

| | Sodium |
|---|---|
| **Miso (Soy Paste),** ¼ c., 2.5 oz | 2500 |
| **Soybean Protein Isolate,** 1 oz | 280 |
| **Tempeh,** Natural, ½ cup, 3 oz | 5 |
| **Tofu,** average, ½ cup, 4 oz | 5 |

## Jam, Honey, Syrups

| | Sodium |
|---|---|
| **Jam/Jelly,** 1 Tbsp | 2 |
| **Honey/Maple Syrup,** 1 Tbsp | 1 |
| **Log Cabin,** Syrup, 1 fl.oz | 35 |
| Lite, 1 fl.oz | 90 |

## Peanut Butter

| | Sodium |
|---|---|
| **Peanut Butter:** Regular, 2 Tbsp, 0.5 oz | 190 |
| *Jif,* Low Sodium, 2 Tbsp | 65 |
| *Trader Joe's,* Unsalted, 2 Tbsp | 5 |

## Snacks, Nuts

| | Sodium |
|---|---|
| **Cheese Balls/Curls,** 1 oz | 280 |
| **Cheetos,** 1 oz | 290 |
| **Corn/Tortilla Chips:** average, 1 oz | 220 |
| *Fritos,* Lightly Salted, 1 oz | 80 |
| **Granola bars,** average, 1 bar | 80 |
| **Nuts:** Plain, unsalted, 1 oz | 1 |
| Lightly salted, 1 oz | 80 |
| Salted or Honey Roasted, 1 oz | 160 |
| **Popcorn:** Plain (unsalted), 1 cup | 1 |
| Flavored, average, 1 cup | 60 |
| Salt added, 1 cup | 180 |
| **Potato Chips:** Plain, 1 oz | 160 |
| *Lay's,* Lightly Salted, 1 oz | 85 |
| Flavored, average, 1 oz | 200 |
| **Pretzels:** Regular, 3, 1 oz | 450 |
| Soft, salted, large | 1000 |

## Candy, Chocolate

| | Sodium |
|---|---|
| **Chocolate,** milk, 1 oz | 30 |
| **Fudge,** chocolate, 1 oz | 55 |
| **Candy Bars,** average, 1.5 oz | 60 |
| **Hard Candy,** 1 oz | 10 |
| **Licorice,** 1 oz | 30 |

## Beverages, Alcohol

| | Sodium |
|---|---|
| **Coffee or Tea,** 1 cup | 1 |
| **Cocoa: Dry,** plain, 1 Tbsp | 0 |
| Mix, average, 1 envelope | 120 |
| **Quik,** 2 tsp | 35 |
| **Soft Drinks,** average, 8 fl.oz | 20 |
| **Mineral Water:** Perrier, 8 fl.oz | 5 |
| *Gatorade,* Thirst Quencher, 8 fl.oz | 110 |
| *Red Bull:* 8.4 fl.oz can | 105 |
| Sugar Free, 8.4 fl.oz | 200 |
| **Water,** Average, 1 cup, 8 fl.oz | 5 |
| **Alcohol:** Beer, average, 12 fl.oz | 15 |
| Wines, average, 4 fl.oz | 10 |
| Spirits (distilled), 1.5 fl.oz | 1 |

## Antacids ~ Alka-Seltzer

| | Sodium |
|---|---|
| Alka-Seltzer: *Per Tablet* | |
| Original; Heartburn | 570 |
| Extra Strength | 590 |
| Lemon Lime | 500 |
| Gold | 310 |
| *Alka-Mints,* chewable | 0 |
| *Bromo Seltzer,* ¾ capful | 760 |
| *Picot,* 1 packet, 5g | 670 |
| *Rolaids,* All types | 0 |
| *Tums,* Regular/Extra Strength | 0 |

## Cold & Flu ~ Alka-Seltzer Plus

| | Sodium |
|---|---|
| Effervescents, average, 1 tablet | 480 |
| Fast Crystal Packs; Liquid Gels | 0 |

## Fast-Foods & Restaurants — Sodium

**Burger King:**

| | Sodium |
|---|---|
| **Burgers:** Cheeseburger | 540 |
| **Double Bacon Cheeseburger** | 800 |
| **Hamburger** | 460 |
| **Whoppers:** Original | 910 |
| With Cheese | 1260 |
| Whopper Jr. with Cheese | 640 |
| **Chicken Sandwich,** Original | 1170 |
| **Sides:** French Fries, medium, salted | 570 |
| Onion Rings, medium | 1080 |
| **Breakfast,** Ham, Egg & Cheese Croissan'wich | 1080 |

**Denny's:**

| | Sodium |
|---|---|
| **Burgers:** Bacon Avocado Cheeseburger | 1490 |
| Spicy Sriracha | 2100 |
| **Sandwiches:** Club | 2180 |
| Prime Rib Philly Melt | 2340 |
| **Dinner:** Brooklyn Spaghetti & Meatballs | 2480 |
| Sirloin Steak | 1260 |
| Sides: Broccoli | 20 |
| French Fries, salted, 6 oz | 110 |
| Red-Skinned Potatoes | 590 |
| **Soup:** Chicken Noodle, 12 oz bowl | 1130 |
| Clam Chowder, 12 oz bowl | 1870 |
| **Breakfast:** Buttermilk Pancakes (2), w/ Marg. | 1210 |
| Moons Over My Hammy Omelette, w/ Hash | 2560 |
| Hearty Breakfast Skillet | 2050 |
| Sides: Hash Browns, 1 serving | 410 |
| Hearty Breakfast Sausage | 840 |
| **Dessert,** Apple Pie, 1 slice, 14 oz | 750 |

**Jack In The Box:**

| | Sodium |
|---|---|
| **Burgers:** Bacon Untimate Cheeseburger | 2190 |
| Hamburger | 680 |
| Jumbo Jack with Cheese | 1310 |
| Sandwiches: H'style Ranch Chicken Club | 1910 |
| Sourdough Grilled Chiken Club | 1490 |

**KFC:**

| | Sodium |
|---|---|
| **Chicken Breast:** Original | 1140 |
| Extra Crispy | 1140 |
| Grilled | 730 |
| **Popcorn Nuggets,** | |
| Family Tray | 4670 |
| **Sandwich,** Crispy Twister | 1300 |
| **Tenders,** Extra Crispy Tenders, Family Tray | 310 |
| **Wings,** HBBQ Hot (1) | 270 |
| **Sides:** Macaroni & Cheese | 830 |
| Mashed Potatoes with Gravy | 530 |
| Potato Wedges | 810 |

## Fast-Foods & Restaurants — Sodium

**McDonalds:**

| | Sodium |
|---|---|
| **Burgers:** Big Mac | 970 |
| Cheeseburger | 680 |
| Double | 1050 |
| Hamburger | 490 |
| Quarter Pounder with Cheese | 1110 |
| **Chicken McNuggets:** 6 pieces | 540 |
| Spicy Buffalo Sauce, 1 package, 0.8 oz | 540 |
| **Sandwich,** Buttermilk Crispy Chicken | 900 |
| **French Fries:** Small, 2.6 oz | 130 |
| Medium, 3.9 oz | 190 |
| Large, 5.9 oz | 290 |
| Ketchup, 1 package, 10g | 90 |
| **Breakfast:** Egg McMuffin | 750 |
| Big Breakfast, reg. size Biscuit | 1560 |
| Hash Browns, 2 oz | 310 |
| Hotcakes, with Syrup & Whipped Margarine | 590 |
| Sausage McGriddle | 1030 |
| Southern Style Chicken Biscuit, regular bisc. | 1180 |
| **Desserts/Shakes:** Hot Fudge Sundae | 170 |
| Strawberry McCafe Shake, 12 fl.oz | 160 |

**Pizza Hut:**

| | Sodium |
|---|---|
| **Pan Pizza:** *Per ½ Medium Pizza, 4 Slices* | |
| Meat Lovers | 2960 |
| Cheese; Cock A Doodle Bacon | 2000 |
| Pepperoni Lover's | 3080 |
| Pepperoni; Buffalo State of Mind, av. | 2420 |

**Subway:**

| | Sodium |
|---|---|
| **6" Lowfat Sandwich:** *W/ Set Menu Board Toppings, no oil* | |
| Chicken, oven roasted | 610 |
| Roast Beef | 660 |
| Subway Club | 800 |
| Sweet Onion Chicken Teriyaki | 770 |
| **6" Sandwiches:** *W/ Set Menu Board Toppings, no oil* | |
| Chicken Bacon Ranch Melt with Cheese | 1050 |
| Meatball Marinara | 920 |
| Spicy Italian | 1490 |
| **12" Footlong** ~ Double the above figures | |

**Taco Bell:**

| | Sodium |
|---|---|
| **Burritos:** Combo, 8.2 oz | 1380 |
| Supreme, Chicken; Steak | 1090 |
| **Chalupa Supreme**, Chicken; Steak | 530 |
| **Gordita Supreme**, Steak | 530 |
| **Nachos:** BellGrande | 1310 |
| Supreme | 860 |
| **Specialties,** Cheese Quesadillas | 980 |
| **Tacos:** Chicken, Soft | 480 |
| Crunchy Supreme | 340 |

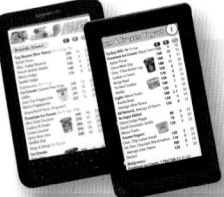

## e-BOOK EDITIONS
### NOW AVAILABLE FOR
### KINDLE • 0 iPAD • iPHONE
**Fully Searchable & Enhanced**

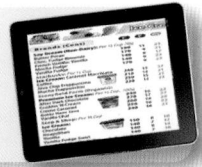

# Index E - J

**FAST-FOODS INDEX**
**~ PAGE 175 ~**

**FAST-FOODS INDEX ~ PAGE 175 ~**

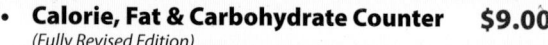
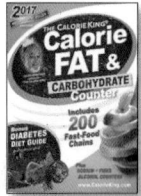
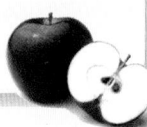
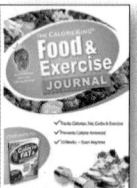
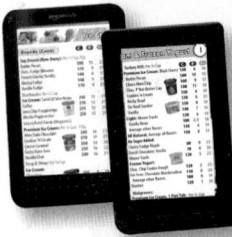
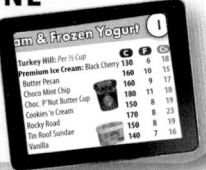
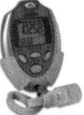  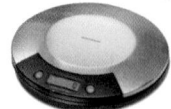 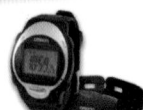
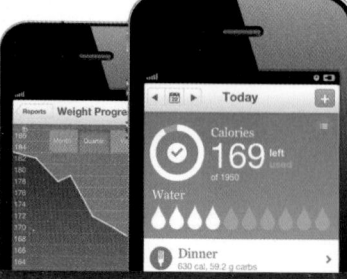
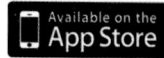